What Others Have Said

... about Circumcision: The Painful Dilemma

Circumcision: The Painful Dilemma will stand as a moving social document of our times. It will serve as a beacon of light to all who seek truth and understanding, and greatly broaden our appreciation of what it means to be human. Your book, with its wonderful sense of balance, provides the total spectrum of information that any lay or professional reader would need in order to form a rational opinion on the subject of circumcision. Your emphasis on the unique individuality of every newborn child with certain rights no less genuine than those of any adult, deserves the highest commendation. In spite of the element of tragedy indicated by the suffering and complications of an unnecessary surgical procedure on newborns, the book comes through in a warm and positive way, and one is left with a sense of enlightenment as well as commitment that our future newborn sons may establish themselves in this world intact, and "at peace."

T.D. Swafford, M.D.
Group Health Medical Center, Seattle, WA

Rosemary Romberg has given us the definitive book on circumcision ... American physicians should study the book carefully, especially the authoritative chapter on "Complications of Circumcision." I enthusiastically join Rosemary Romberg in her well-documented, comprehensive condemnation of modern hospital circumcision.

Robert S. Mendelsohn, M.D.
Evanston, IL
Author of *Confessions of a Medical Heretic.*

Thank you very much for the opportunity to review the manuscript for your book on circumcision. I was very impressed by the extensive research which you have conducted and your attention to detail. A most important aspect of the manuscript which is not covered by other authors is the letters from parents describing in personal terms their experiences with circumcision and non-circumcision ...

William W. Pope, M.D., M.P.H.
Deputy State Health Officer,
Garrett County Health Department, Oakland, MD

Fascinating lore-both of history and the religions! A veritable encyclopedia! ... the mothers' letters on routine neonatal circumcision are priceless!

It has material I shall want to quote when I raise issues of why today it is so important for us to examine our routine practices and our cultural attitudes to see if they still work for us and fit the needs of individuals today striving to live consciously and at the highest possible level of harmony with each other and this small planet of ours.

Men and women will thank you for giving the tools and knowledge with which to make conscious decisions about what are issues of real import to our hearts and psyches.

Suzanne Arms
Author of *A Season to be Born; Immaculate Deception: A New Look at Women and Childbirth; Five Women, Five Births* (video); *Adoption: A Handful of Hope; Best-feeding: Getting Breastfeeding Right for You* (co-authors Mary Renfrow & Chloe Fisher); *Seasons of Change: Growing Through Pregnancy & Birth; Imma-culate Deception II: Myth, Magic & Birth; Giving Birth: Challenges & Choices* (video).

Circumcision; The Painful Dilemma looks to be *the classic* on circumcision. One day 20th Century archivists will choose your book to give the most comprehensive history on an ancient and almost forgotten barbaric ritual. May it rest in peace. Your book is a tremendous contribution towards that end (of circumcision).

Jeannine Parvati Baker
Author of *Prenatal Yoga and Natural Birth; Hygieia: A Woman's Herbal*, and *Conscious Conception: Elemental Journey Through the Labyrinth of Sexuality.*

I strongly endorse your thesis opposing circumcision, as do a goodly number of physicians and sexologists. I consider that you have written a fair-minded and tho-rough review of all the pros and cons. Your book will be extremely useful as a reference source as well as a policy statement.

John Money, Ph.D.
Professor of Medical Psychology and
Associate Professor of Pediatrics
The Johns Hopkins University School of Medicine Baltimore, MD

I am excited by your manuscript. I feel it's an extremely important piece of work ... Your manuscript is forcing me to re-examine some of my thinking. Thank you for the challenge.

John C. Glaspey, M.D.
Clinical Director of Nurseries,
Milwaukee County Medical Complex Perinatal Center
Medical College of Wisconsin, Milwaukee, WI

Rosemary Romberg has not missed a dimension in her approach to circumcision, or more accurately, her denunciation of it ... This book will educate prospective parents enormously, and this is where purely textbook treatises have fallen short.

Richard J. Eliason, M.D.
General and Pediatric Urology
Salt Lake City, UT

This is a good book ... your parent and doctor interviews are (the) strongest and most interesting sections. You asked good questions and got good response.

Tonya Brooks
President – Association for Childbirth at Home, International,
Los Angeles, CA.

I am so pleased that you sought out the available Information on circumcision and have given us a book. I am glad to endorse it ... The Information Is needed so very much. Misconceptions abound about what circumcision Is, why it is done, how it is done, the effects from doing It, parents' right to informed consent, and the PAIN ... Parents, even with family centered care are likely to be unaware of what happens to their babies ... The structure for circumcision surgery is there. It is difficult to stop this routine surgery and interesting that the American Academy of Pediatrics does not support It.

Constance Bean
Author of *Methods of Childbirth; Labor & Delivery; An Observer's Diary.*

Thank you for your incredible focus on male circumcision. It is a needed book and will, I am sure, have a strong effect on the people of this nation. Your work represents so much time and thought on the issue. I appreciate you and your work ... I salute you for your dedication to a most worthy topic ...

Your stories from mothers are wonderful. I have always appreciated testimony, and I was very appreciative of yours. Your personal story brought tears to my eyes.

You have done a monumental job and I commend you on it. I have great hopes for your material and will encourage many to read your book.

Raven Lang
Author of *The Birth Book.*

What a piece of work! You deserve a Ph.D. for reviewing and detailing all these aspects of circumcision.

Gail Sforza Brewer
Author of *What Every Pregnant Woman Should Know: The Truth About Diets and Drugs in Pregnancy; The Pregnancy After 30 Workbook; Right From The Start.*

Whatever is done to stop the practice of circumcision will be of immense importance. There is no rational, medical reason to support it. And no one is aware of the deep implications and life-lasting effect. The work you are doing is of *immense* value.

Dr. Frederick Leboyer
Author of *Birth Without Violence.*

CIRCUMCISION
The Painful Dilemma

Second, Revised Edition

Rosemary Romberg

edited by Ulf Dunkel

Copyright © 1985-2020 Rosemary Romberg †, 2021 Ulf Dunkel
All rights reserved.

First published in 1985 by Bergin & Garvey Publishers, Inc.

This Second Edition of the book was edited and revised on the basis of the revised online version of the book by the author herself until shortly before her death and then by a group of intactivists led by John Adkison and Ulf Dunkel.

The editor has no responsibility for the persistence or accuracy of URLs for external or third-party Internet websites referred to in this publication and does not guarantee that any content on such websites is, or will remain, accurate or appropriate.

No part of this publication may be used or reproduced in any manner whatsoever without written permission from the editor except in the case of brief quotations embodied in critical articles and reviews.

Editor:
Ulf Dunkel
Bergkamm 2
DE-49624 Löningen
Germany

With the consent of Rosemary Romberg's widower, Steve Wiener, all proceeds from the sale of the second edition of this book will go to the financing of the author's blog, Peaceful Beginnings, and the IntactiWiki information website of the editor.

Designations used by companies to distinguish their products are often claimed as trademarks. All brand names and product names used in this book are trade names, service marks, trademarks and registered trademarks of their respective owners. The publisher and the book are not associated with any product or vendor mentioned in this book. None of the companies referenced within the book have endorsed the book.

ISBN 13: 979-8683021252
Second, Revised Edition (rev. state: 2021-09-05)

Printed by *kindle | direct publishing*, an Amazon division.

Table of Contents

What Others Have Said 1
Dedications By Her Family 14
Thanks To 16
In Memoriam 18
From Dr. Leboyer 19
A Thankful Book Review 20
Foreword I 21
Foreword II 23
Editor's Remarks 25
The Author's Own Story 26
Dedication 37

1 The History of Circumcision 38
   1.1 The Reasons for Circumcision 41
      1.1.1 Hygiene 42
      1.1.2 Cosmetic Value 43
      1.1.3 Tribal Identity or Mark of Adulthood 44
      1.1.4 A Means of Diminishing Sexual Desires 45
      1.1.5 Enhancement of Sexuality 45
      1.1.6 Fertility 46
      1.1.7 A Mark of Subjugation for Conquered Enemies and Slaves 48
      1.1.8 A Mark of Purity 48
      1.1.9 A Test of Endurance 49
      1.1.10 Symbolic Castration 50
      1.1.11 Menstrual Envy 51
      1.1.12 Sacrifice 51
   1.2 Conclusion 53
   1.3 Informational Resources 53

2 Female Circumcision 55
   2.1 Reasons for Female Circumcision 58
      2.1.1 Cleanliness 58
      2.1.2 Congenital Hypertrophy 58
      2.1.3 Preservation of Virginity 58
      2.1.4 "To Raise the Value of the Woman" 59
      2.1.5 A Means of Lessening Sexual Desire 59
      2.1.6 Shifting the Center of Sexual Sensation 59
   2.2 Why Has Female Circumcision Not Been Practiced to the Extent of Male
      Circumcision? 60
   2.3 Complications of Female Circumcision 61
   2.4 Female Circumcision in the United States During the 20th Century 62

  2.4.1 Episiotomy 64
 2.5 Conclusion 66
 2.6 The Question No One Would Answer 66
 2.7 Female Circumcision: Indications and A New Technique 70
  2.7.1 Instrument for Female Circumcision 71
  2.7.2 Technique of Circumcision 72
  2.7.3 Clamp for Procedure 73
 2.8 In Regards to Male Genital Mutilation vs. Female Genital Mutilation ... 74
 2.9 Informational Resources 75

3 Circumcision and Judaism 79
 3.1 Blood Taboos 81
 3.2 The Significance of Cutting 84
 3.3 Sacrifice 84
 3.4 Fertility 85
 3.5 Identity as a People 86
 3.6 Why Did the Jews Choose to Circumcise Infants? 86
 3.7 Why the Eighth Day? 88
 3.8 The Jewish Circumcision Ceremony 90
  3.8.1 The Shalom Zachor 90
  3.8.2 The Night Before the Bris 90
  3.8.3 The People Involved in the Bris 90
  3.8.4 The Chair of Elijah 91
  3.8.5 Prayers and Procedures that Begin the Bris 91
  3.8.6 Miloh – The Cutting of the Foreskin 92
  3.8.7 Periah – The Tearing of the Inner Membrane 93
  3.8.8 Mezizah – The Suctioning of the Blood 95
  3.8.9 Procedures Immediately After the Operation 95
  3.8.10 Treatment of the Amputated Foreskin 96
  3.8.11 The Festive Meal Following the Bris 97
  3.8.12 Feelings at the Time of the Bris 97
 3.9 Circumcision and Anti-Semitism 98
 3.10 Conflicts Within Judaism Concerning Circumcision 101
  3.10.1 Mohelim vs. Doctors 102
  3.10.2 Use of Clamps 104
  3.10.3 Mezizah 105
  3.10.4 Attempts by the Jewish Reform Movement to Abolish Circumcision 107
  3.10.5 Mutilation of the Body 108
  3.10.6 Attitudes about Circumcision by Jews Today 109
  3.10.7 The Jewish Ideal of Kindness 110
  3.10.8 Considerations of Today's Jewish Parents 112
 3.11 Interview with Rabbi F.S. Gartner 115
 3.12 Interview with Elizabeth & Marsh Pickard-Ginsberg 123

   3.13 A Letter From a Jewish Mother 134
   3.14 Informational Resources 134

4 Circumcision and Christianity 139
   4.1 Circumcision and the History of Christianity 139
   4.2 Jesus' Circumcision 142
   4.3 An Ancient Holy Relic – The Prepuce of Christ 144
   4.4 The Meaning of Circumcision for Today's Christian 145
   4.5 Informational Resources 149

5 Infant Male Circumcision As a Medical Practice In 20th/21st Century USA 151
   5.1 The Recent History of Infant Circumcision 151
   5.2 Are the Jews to Blame? 159
   5.3 The Medical Profession as a "Pseudo-Religion" 161
   5.4 The Perspective of Medical Professionals 163
   5.5 Is Profit an Important Motive? 166
   5.6 The Factor of Insurance Coverage 168
   5.7 Delivery Room Circumcision 170
   5.8 Coercion and Unauthorized Circumcision 173
   5.9 The Perspective of Expectant and New Parents 175
   5.10 Circumcision Techniques: Gomco and Plastibell 183
       5.10.1 The Gomco technique 183
       5.10.2 The Plastibell technique 185
   5.11 Conclusion 187
   5.12 Interview with Dr. Howard Marchbanks, M.D. 192
   5.13 Interview with Paula Coleman, R.N., Camarillo, CA 194
   5.14 Interview with Nancy & Frank Ring (young parents) 201
   5.15 Letters from Parents of Circumcised Sons 208
   5.16 Informational Resources 219

6 Circumcision and Sexuality 220
   6.1 The Question of Homosexuality 226
   6.2 Author's Addendum 229
   6.3 Informational Resources 229

7 Circumcision and the Military Service 234

8 The Circumcision of a Three-year Old 240

9 The Circumcision of an Adult 245

10 Foreskin Restoration 248
   10.1 Informational Resources 251

11 Complications of Circumcision 256
- 11.1 Meatal Ulceration 257
- 11.2 Meatal Stricture 262
- 11.3 Hemorrhage 264
- 11.4 Infection 266
- 11.5 Retention of Plastic Bell Ring 269
- 11.6 Concealed Penis 270
- 11.7 Urethral Fistula 273
- 11.8 Phimosis of Remaining Foreskin 275
- 11.9 Urinary Retention 277
- 11.10 Glans Necrosis 278
- 11.11 Injury and Loss of Glans 279
- 11.12 Excessive Skin Loss 280
- 11.13 Skin Bridge 282
- 11.14 Vomiting, Apneic Spells 283
- 11.15 Sewing of Penile Skin to the Glans 284
- 11.16 Laceration of Penile or Scrotal Skin 284
- 11.17 Undetected Hypospadias 285
- 11.18 Preputial Cysts 285
- 11.19 Complications of Anesthesia 285
- 11.20 Tuberculosis and other Diseases from Mezizah 286
- 11.21 Strangulation of the Glans by Hair 286
- 11.22 Recurrence of Pneumothorax 288
- 11.23 Pulmonary Embolism 288
- 11.24 Keloid Formation 290
- 11.25 Lymphedema or Elephantiasis of Skin 290
- 11.26 Reaction of Older Sibling 290
- 11.27 Cosmetic Problems 291
- 11.28 Loss of Penis 291
- 11.29 Informational Resources 295

12 Urinary Tract Infections and Infant Circumcision 301
- 12.1 Observations Reported by Others 303
  - 12.1.1 Non-Surgical Preventability 304
  - 12.1.2 Comparative Pain and Trauma 307
  - 12.1.3 Medical "Just In Case-ism" 309
  - 12.1.4 The Purpose of Surgery 309
  - 12.1.5 "Knives Versus Washcloths" – Medical Dictatorship Versus Wholeness of the Body and Personal Autonomy 310
- 12.2 Conclusion 310
- 12.3 Informational Resources 311

13 Penile Cancer 314

- 13.1 What is Cancer of the Penis? How Does it Develop? What are its Causes and Related Factors? 315
- 13.2 Laboratory Experiments That Have Tested the Alleged Carcinogenic Properties of Smegma 318
- 13.3 Socioeconomic Factors Related to the Incidence of Penile Cancer 319
- 13.4 Worldwide Distribution of Penile Cancer 321
- 13.5 Methods of Treatment of Cancer of the Penis 323
- 13.6 Conclusions 326
- 13.7 Informational Resources 329

14 Sexually Transmitted Infection **331**
- 14.1 Yeast Infections 333
- 14.2 Benign Transient Lymphagiectasis 333
- 14.3 Conclusion 334
- 14.4 Informational Resources 335

15 Circumcision and HIV/AIDS **343**
- 15.1 Research to Find a Reason for Circumcision 343
- 15.2 Refuting Biased Research 348
- 15.3 CDC's Misleading Headlines 369
- 15.4 Conclusion 372
- 15.5 Informational Resources 373

16 Prostate Cancer **374**
- 16.1 Informational Resources 377

17 Cervical Cancer **378**
- 17.1 Factors Related to Cancer of the Cervix 379
  - 17.1.1 Ethnicity 379
  - 17.1.2 Socioeconomic Status 380
  - 17.1.3 Personal Hygiene 380
  - 17.1.4 Age of First Coitus 381
  - 17.1.5 Marriage 382
  - 17.1.6 Childbearing 383
  - 17.1.7 Use of Contraceptives 384
  - 17.1.8 Sperm Contact 385
  - 17.1.9 Diet 385
  - 17.1.10 Coal Tar Douches 386
  - 17.1.11 Nidah – Jewish Ritual Abstinence Following Menstruation 386
  - 17.1.12 Menstrual Disorders 387
  - 17.1.13 Sexually Transmitted Disease 387
  - 17.1.14 Chronic Cervicitis and Lacerations to the Tissues 388
  - 17.1.15 Vaginal Discharge 388

17.1.16 Hormones 389
17.1.17 Number of Sexual Partners 389
17.1.18 Circumcision Status of Sexual Partner 390
17.2 Controlled Experiments with Smegma 393
17.3 Conclusions 395

18 Is Circumcision Traumatic For a Newborn Baby? 397
18.1 Scientific Investigations in Regard to the Infant's Reaction to Circumcision 404
18.2 The Awareness and Consciousness of the Newborn 407
18.3 Is There a Relationship Between Circumcision and Sudden infant Death Syndrome? 415
18.4 A Possible Link Between Infant Circumcision and Autism 421
18.5 Primal Pain – Interview With The Primal Institute 423
18.6 Reports About Circumcisions 435
    18.6.1 Shawn's Circumcision 435
    18.6.2 One Man's Story 436
18.7 Interview With a Pediatrician About Pain 438
18.8 Interview With the Founder of the Association for Childbirth At Home 440
18.9 Conclusions 444
18.10 Informational Resources 445

19 The Intact Penis 452
19.1 The Care of the intact Penis 452
19.2 What About the Problems that the Intact Male May Encounter? 455
    19.2.1 Phimosis 456
    19.2.2 Infection of the Foreskin 463
19.3 The Intactivism Movement 466
    19.3.1 Intactivism Goals 474
19.4 Interviews and Letters 474
    19.4.1 Dr. Paul M. Fleiss, M.D., Los Angeles, CA. (Pediatrician) 474
    19.4.2 Interviews with Mothers 476
    19.4.3 Letters from Parents of Intact Sons 480
19.5 MALE Circumcision REMOVES 16+ Functions. Do you know what they are? 503
    19.5.1 Frenar Band, or Ridged Band 503
    19.5.2 Mechanical Gliding Action 503
    19.5.3 Meissner's Corpuscles 503
    19.5.4 Frenulum 503
    19.5.5 Dartos Fascia 504
    19.5.6 Immunological System 504
    19.5.7 Lymphatic Vessels 504
    19.5.8 Estrogen Receptors 504
    19.5.9 Apocrine Glands 504
    19.5.10 Sebaceous Glands 505

- 19.5.11 Natural Glans Coloration 505
- 19.5.12 Length and Circumference 505
- 19.5.13 Blood Vessels 505
- 19.5.14 Sensation of the Prepuce 506
- 19.5.15 Sensation of the Corpora Cavernosa 506
- 19.5.16 Sensation of the Glans 506
- 19.6 Other Losses 506
- 19.7 Informational Resources 507

20 Timeline 513

21 Use of Infant Foreskins in Cosmetics, Skin Grafts and Other Industries 524
- 21.1 As Concerned Consumers What Can We Do? 538
- 21.2 Informational Resources 540

22 Humane Alternatives in Infant Circumcision? 544
- 22.1 Informational Resources 550

Appendix A: Glossary 552

Appendix B: Bibliography 561

Appendix C: Books About 574
- Appendix C.1: Male Genital Mutilation / Intactivism 574
- Appendix C.2: Female Genital Mutilation 575
- Appendix C.3: Pregnancy, Birth, Infancy & Child Raising 576

Appendix D: Resources Online 579
- Appendix D.1: Facebook Sites & Groups 579
- Appendix D.2: Websites 580

Dedications By Her Family

**In loving memory of Rosemary Romberg,
Author, Wife, Mother, Grandmother, and Champion of Infant Rights.**

The passing of a loved one can be a profoundly sad and grief filled experience. And yet, it can also be a time to celebrate. Celebrate a life well lived. Celebrate the creation of a successful and loving family. And perhaps most of all, celebrate that loved one's contributions to the betterment of the voiceless and helpless all across our Mother Earth. It has been my honor and privilege to have shared my life with Rosemary Romberg for more than 50 years. And although my contributions to *Circumcision: The Painful Dilemma* have always been in the realm of providing support to Rosemary and our family, without this support her seminal book could not have been written. She passed peacefully surrounded by her entire loving family on February 7th, 2020. Since then I have collected and provided her updated materials to the volunteer editors who have completed and published this newly revised Second Edition of her book. My profound appreciation is extended to all those who supported and continue to support her work.

I first met Rosemary in 1967. We married in 1970 and it was her greatest desire to begin a family. The result was six beautiful babies that grew into amazing adults. She developed a lifetime interest and great empathy for all children which led her to begin writing *Circumcision: The Painful Dilemma* after the birth of her third son. The cause for infant rights became a lifelong passion for Rosemary and she was active in the movement right up until her final days. Rosemary's religious beliefs profoundly influenced her sense of empathy and her desire to help others. So let us remember and celebrate how much her life's work improved the lives of so many others. It is my sincere hope that this second edition of Rosemary's book will continue to keep her spirit alive in the minds, hearts and souls of everyone she touched in her life, and will continue to support her life's passion far into the future.

Stephen Paul Wiener
February 2021

The ability to see clearly – through the fog of biases foisted upon us by whatever culture we're born into – is a rare skill. My mom had that to such an extraordinary degree that I could almost see it as a superpower. My mom was a loving mother, a fierce activist for all the world's babies, and – in my eyes – still a superhero. I miss her, and I admire her.

Jason Stephen Wiener
February 2021

From my earliest memories, I grew up infused and entwined with my mom's passion and commitment to helping others, as I helped her staple pamphlets, stuff envelopes, and prepare mailings for hundreds of people searching for answers and information. Through a child's eyes, this was all part of normal life, but now that I am grown with two children of my own, I find myself continuously reminded and inspired by what an extraordinary individual she was, tirelessly helping out infants around the world while taking the time to raise her kids and make each one of us feel valued and cherished. It would have been her greatest wish that her words continue to reach people and her legacy be continued.

Lisa (Wiener) Humphrey
February 2021

A mother's love is a singularly powerful force. I am humbled to think that the love I cherished while growing up has been shared to thousands of infants around the world. It takes a truly compassionate, kind soul to care and advocate so much for the rights of those who she had never met. But that was my mother. The kindest, most nurturing soul one could ever hope to meet. It gladdens my heart to know that her legacy will continue to live on in this book, in the work she accomplished, and of course in the loving family that she helped to raise. And so let us strive to hold on to some of that love and to share it with those in our lives; to our friends and family, and to strangers alike.

Kevin Robert Von Wien
February 2021

Thanks To

I wish to express gratitude to the following people:

To the wonderful people who publish **Mothering Magazine**. Shortly after I began this research I wrote a letter which appeared in the Winter 1978 issue of their magazine. In that letter I requested that people write to me about their experiences concerning circumcision. An incredible amount of communication filled with valuable information and encouragement reached me as a result of that letter. Their publication of my article (which I now title "Circumcision: My Own Story") which was published in their Winter 1981 issue brought me even more wonderful contacts and support.

To **Constance Bean** for writing the chapter "The Circ Room" in her book *Labor and Delivery, An Observer's Guide*. This chapter upset me terribly, but contributed to my decision to write this book.

To **Dr. Frederick Leboyer**, for awakening people to the fact that newborn babies are sensitive, feeling individuals. Why were we unable to realize this before *Birth Without Violence* opened our eyes?

To **the late George Soule** who helped me immensely with my research and gave me continued moral support. We all miss you so much since you left us in 1990.

To **Jeffrey R. Wood**, for giving me encouragement and moral support, and for founding INTACT Educational Foundation.

To **Dave Beauvais** for his help in preparing the original manuscript for publication.

To the late **Jeannine Parvati Baker** who has been an inspiration to me. You left this earth much too soon and I miss you every day.

To **Suzanne Arms** whose wonderful photographic skills have provided many of the pictures I have used. The fire and energy that went into your world changing book *Immaculate Deception* has inspired me and so many others to speak out as well against medical absurdities.

To **Marilyn Milos**, RN whose maternal regret and heartbreak mirrors my own. Your undying energy, strength and determination have carried intactivism so much further than I ever could have done on my own.

To **Richard Angell** for urging me to update this book and make it available to others on line.

To **Duane Voskuil** for all of your help with the computer scanning.

To **John A. Erickson** whose clear, concise writings and "in your face" style of presenting information has packed a far greater "wallop" than even I have dared to try. Thank you for encouraging me and admonishing me through all these years. You also left this earth much too soon and we all continue to miss your dedication and support.

To **U-Alabio** who carried my website and book on Wikipedia at one time.

To **Janet Boyd** for your tireless generosity, help and computer skills in continuing to carry my website and book and your endless patience with me as we've trudged through every glitch, typo and re-write along the way.

To **Brother K and all of the "Bloodstained Men"**. Your pure energy and guts that go into every demonstration has cranked all of intactivism up into an entirely new dimension.

To **the many other people**, too numerous to list, who have shared their knowledge, experiences, feelings, and concern that in so many ways have contributed to this book.

To **my husband Steve**, and **my three sons Eric, Jason, and Ryan**, all of whom have been "victims of the system," but are beautiful people nonetheless. Without them this book never would have been written.

To my daughter **Lisa**, who was conceived, carried, and born while this project was underway. May you grow up to live in a happier, saner world.

To my mother, **Mary Jo Romberg**, who left this world in 1999 after 88 years of life. Your immense intelligence, sensitivity towards people, and compassion for children gave me the foundation for my own career as a mother, researcher, writer, activist, and creative craftsperson.

To my father, **Harland G. Romberg**, who left this world in 2003 at age 93. You never could understand me or acknowledge my work, but I'm sure I've inherited much of your brilliant mind and solid Germanic stubbornness nonetheless.

To my youngest two children, **Kevin and Melissa**, born in 1985 and 1989, after this book was first written. **Kevin**, you were just an embryo inside of me when my garage was filled with copies of my book's first edition. The first male in our family, after countless generations, to grow up with all parts of your body. To you it seems like no big deal. But your emphatic announcement at age seven, upon having circumcision explained to you, – "NO!! That is **NEVER** going to happen to **ME!!**" – has been our most powerful statement yet. Wouldn't every baby say the same, if only they too could speak?

Melissa, born at home, in our bathtub, – the simplest birth of all. At age 42, 6th baby, 3 prior miscarriages, – others tried to tell me I didn't have the right to the kind of birth I wanted. Little girl, priceless treasure, filled the hole left by other births gone wrong, other daughters gone from this world too soon. You were our little "tomboy", living in a world filled with softball games and puppy dogs. Now you are all grown up (too soon for Mommy!) May your life be filled with rewards. May the world allow you to be whatever you want to be.

Finally, to my precious grandchildren – **Sonya, Marina, Julia and my perfect grandson Logan**. You have all brought me so much joy and the most honorable title of "Grandma." May you face a world filled with positiveness, love and fulfilled promises, free from unspoken assaults on any children of the future.

In Memoriam

The following people were all dear to my heart and immensely helpful to me and to intactivism as a whole. These people have now left this earth but will remain in our hearts forever.

- Jim Bigelow, Ph.D.
- Gary Burlingame
- Jonathon Conte
- Robert Darby
- John A. Erickson
- Paul M. Fleiss, M.D.
- Lorna Kellogg
- Van Lewis
- Paul Mason
- D.C. McKnight, D.C.
- Dr. Robert Mendelsohn
- Ashley Montague
- Elizabeth Noble
- Jeannine Parvati Baker
- James Peron
- Thomas J. Ritter, M.D.
- My dear brother, The Rev. Theodore E. (Ted) Romberg
- My parents Harland G. and Mary Jo Romberg
- Daniel Seely
- George Soule
- Thomas D. Swafford, M.D.

From Dr. Leboyer

Dear Rosemary Romberg.

Yes, whatever is done to stop the terrible practice of circumcision will be of tremendous importance.

There is no rational, medical reason to support it.

It is done just as a habit with no one being aware of why it is done.

And, much worse, no one being aware of the deep implications and life-lasting effect. Once we remember that all that takes place during the first days of life on the emotional level, shapes the pattern of all future reactions, we cannot but wonder why such a torture has been inflicted on the child. How could a being who has been aggressed in this way, while totally helpless, develop into a relaxed, loving, trusting person? Indeed, he will never be able to trust anyone in life, he will always be on the defensive, unable to open up to others and to life.[1]

There has been, recently, a large, international survey conducted by the World Health Organization regarding what takes place, in Africa, with young women at the stage of puberty. The public opinion was stunned and revolted finding out the tortures and mutilations (removal of clitoris and so on) inflicted.

The practice of circumcision is of exactly the same nature and level. And we call ourselves "rational and developed" !

At least these young women are conscious and they are told that it is a sort of test, an act of courage. Although, in fact, it is meant to make them submissive to men and insure that they will never challenge man's power.

But there is no such consciousness in the newborn.

The torture is experienced in a state of total helplessness which makes it even more frightening and unbearable.

Yes, it is high time that such a barbaric practice comes to an end.

And the work you are doing is of immense value.

With best wishes,

Dr. Frederick Leboyer

author of *Birth Without Violence,*
NY, Alfred A. Knopf, 1976

---

[1] I am not able to fully agree with such a fatalistic statement. However, I still believe that Dr. Leboyer's concerns about the circumcision trauma are of great value and must be shared. – *Rosemary Romberg.*

A Thankful Book Review

When my daughters were born six and three years ago I was relieved not to have to face the circumcision decision. Although I had reservations about the procedure, I was not sure enough to withstand the pressures to have a son circumcised. It was with great interest then that I received Rosemary Romberg's book while pregnant with my third child.

Rosemary Romberg is a childbirth educator who, after having her own three sons circumcised, decided to research the subject and write a book presenting the facts about circumcision. What she found was overwhelming evidence that circumcision is an unnecessary practice which became advocated as a medical procedure late in the 1800's because it was thought to cure or prevent masturbation. Routine circumcision of infants became increasingly common in the early 1900's as more births were occurring in hospitals. For too many years the procedure has been accepted as a routine by uninformed parents. One by one the author debunks the arguments surrounding the "benefits" of circumcision and "dangers" of non-circumcision. She has thoroughly investigated her subject and presents the reader with much, if not all, of the research which has been done on the subject. While not all readers will want to read through them, the studies are painstakingly summarized for those who are interested. If Ms. Romberg's book has one fault it is that its length may seem too imposing to some readers. However, the book is organized in such a way that it is easy to pick and choose the chapters that one wants to read in depth and skim through the others.

The fact of the matter is that most of us, particularly women, know very little about the anatomy of the penis and how circumcision is done. For years mothers automatically signed consent forms thinking that circumcision was a natural and necessary procedure which was not painful to the newborn. Even though the American Academy of Pediatrics stated as early as 1971 that routine circumcision of all boys was not medically warranted, parents have continued to have the procedure done so that their sons will not be "different."

Ms. Romberg has included many illustrations and photographs in her book. We see the medical instruments used in circumcision, babies undergoing the procedure, and intact boys. There is a chapter on the care of the intact penis – which is actually very simple. In fact, it is pointed out that many of the health problems which have been associated with non-circumcision are the result of parents being instructed to force the foreskin back in order to wash under it. By the time a boy is about three years old, the foreskin will have separated naturally from the glans so that retraction need not be forced. *(Sometimes normal separation of the foreskin from the glans can take longer than this, even into adolescence for some. – R.R.)* In addition to all of the information the author has compiled she has included personal accounts both from parents who had their sons circumcised and those who did not.

When I finished reading *Circumcision: The Painful Dilemma*, I felt that there was no way to justify circumcising my unborn baby should it turn out to be a son. Obviously one can argue that the book is biased – in fact even the title makes it clear where the author stands. However, I believe Ms. Romberg when she states that she did not undertake her exhaustive work with conclusions drawn beforehand. In the absence of any clear medical benefit from circumcision, it is hard to dispute the author's powerful statement that, "Immediate circumcision is unquestioningly totally disregarding of the infants feeling in his introduction into this world. It constitutes the absolute antithesis on non-violent birth. However, welcoming the baby into the world with non-violent birthing techniques, only to subject him to circumcision a few days later is nothing but hypocritical!" For too long those of us who have espoused natural, gentle childbirth have failed to see this contradiction.

William was born on August 7, 1985. Hours later we brought our son home – intact. Thank you, Rosemary Romberg.

Carole Kavanagh
Boston Association for Childbirth Education Newsletter, April-June 1985

Foreword I

After reading Rosemary Romberg's carefully researched book, *Circumcision, The Painful Dilemma*, one wonders why there still exists such a diversity of opinion on the subject. Routine neonatal circumcision obviously is unnecessary and serves no sensible purpose. But in arriving at this seemingly logical conclusion, one discounts the all pervasive sexual opinions and emotions that reside in each one of us.

Males in particular, because of their convex genital makeup, visually confront, and probably assess, their penises many times. Each day the male awakens with an erection. The penis must be touched when washing, dressing, and directing the urinary stream. A man usually regards his penis as an extremely valued possession, and in its frequent perusal, cannot fail to associate with it emotions, reminiscences, and possible fantasies. These factors then enter into any evaluation of neonatal circumcision by physicians and laymen alike. To different people the act of circumcising carries varying weight and significance. To some it is a removal of a piece of skin of no relevance. To others it represents a covenant with God, or a rite of passage. To still others it is an irrational, cruel, desensitizing mutilation.

Coldly appraised, circumcision is clearly a surgical procedure involving a subtraction. The sensitive foreskin is lost. The delicate glans is forever exposed to toughening abrasive trauma. The mobility of the loose penile skin sheath, a function that greatly facilitates sexual dalliance, is destroyed. Logically, how does one legitimize a "routine" operation upon a normal structure? Normalcy in itself interdicts any interference. Consider the paradox of absurdities associated with neonatal circumcision. The patient does not give his consent. Anesthesia is rarely used. There are no legitimate surgical indications for the procedure. And the operation entails many risks and possible complications: death, psychic trauma, hemorrhage, infection, urethral damage, excessive skin removal, etc.

A poet-philosopher once wrote: "One sees what one knows." This aptly applies to today's prevailing sexual milieu in the United States regarding the prepuce. Most American women have never seen a foreskin, least of all a foreskin on an erect adult penis. They have no concept of its function or merit. Most American physicians are circumcised males, and of necessity expound their views on the merits of circumcision from a base of incomplete penile sensitivity.

How does one find fault with the beauty and perfection of the normal infant's body? What quirk in our psyche causes us to focus upon the male prepuce as a mistake of creation, to be removed by our flawed judgment, believing that now the penis is improved and more acceptable?

Rosemary Romberg's book is exceedingly timely. Each year in the United States, 1.3 million male infants are circumcised. Since the 1940s, when hospital deliveries became commonplace and circumcision became almost routine, well over fifty million males have been subjected to this worthless operative procedure.

Ms. Romberg is a dedicated childbirth educator who has been mesmerized by the beauty of birth. The infant is to be brought into this life with gentleness, and accepted with love. But into Ms. Romberg's rational humane perusal of birth, a most serious incongruous event has appeared that offends her sensibilities – circumcision of the male infant, an act that brings pain. In her humanity and concern, Ms. Romberg has set about studying why this painful procedure is inflicted upon male infants. She has delved thoroughly and extensively into this subject of infant circumcision and has moved from a position of neutrality to one of dogged condemnation.

The author presents her material in a mildly judgmental way and arrives at an obvious conclusion: circumcision of infants is unnecessary. It is difficult to refute Ms. Romberg's reasoned presentation. Any unbiased reader must agree with her.

This book should be read by all prospective parents, but especially by all physicians. Ms. Romberg's advice and counsel would bring greater love and gentleness to all mothers and infants.

Clear heads, gentle hearts, and common sense eventually shall prevail. Rosemary Romberg's scholarly treatise hopefully shall lead to the discontinuance of circumcision of newborn males.

Thomas J. Ritter, M.D., F.A.C.S.

Foreword II

> *"Theirs not to make reply,*
> *Theirs not to reason why,*
> *Theirs but to do and die."*
> — Alfred Lord Tennyson

Mankind is presumably the highest species inhabiting the earth and is generally thought to consist of a few leaders and many followers. In ages past, a premium was placed on conformity. Natural law declares survival for the fittest. The establishment has traditionally suggested a dangerous lack of fitness must be done away with before it can spread. Those who successfully struggled their way to the top know best. Through enforced ignorance the masses were kept rigidly in line to ensure survival of civilization and its ruling hierarchies. Then, in a relative instant, a vast knowledge explosion occurred as the age of science and reason dawned. The ensuing revolution in human thinking made leaders accountable for their actions and allowed followers to fearlessly ask just where they were being led and for what reason. Today we are in the midst of great behavioral sciences experiments while before us lies a perilous but promising future.

In the present age, humanity's main concern is rightfully the prevention of a nuclear holocaust. The question of routine circumcision may seem a comparatively minor issue, worthy of barely more than a casual mention – hardly subject matter for an entire book. Yet circumcision is a time-honored institution that interacts directly with powerful sex drives, therefore demanding intense study of what the various attitudes concerning it reveal about our inner selves. In truth, does not the indiscriminate lopping off of any normal body structure, quite apart from whatever arbitrarily designated religious values it may imply, represent an expression of utter contempt for nature? Shouldn't it be plain that for genuine satisfaction in life to be realized, man and nature must work harmoniously together, and in fact can do so at any level of technological development? What is ultimately to be gained by seeking escape from reality?

Symbolically speaking, circumcision is an issue to which we can all relate in some way. In my own case, I had experienced a difficult childhood. It seemed that everyone, parents, teachers and friends alike, had let me down, with nowhere to turn except toward my uncertain perception of God. In Sunday school I had been taught that the best way to discover the Almighty was by reading the Bible, so at the age of twelve I began at the beginning with the Book of Genesis. Needless to say, I didn't get very far before encountering strange new words about which I was afraid to ask. But I knew how to use the dictionary and shortly was able to figure out why all boys were not alike. With scarcely more than a vestige of childlike innocence remaining,

I somehow discovered within myself the instinctive conviction that a truly loving, infinitely intelligent heavenly Father could never be so inconsistent as to create man one way and then want him another. Much later in life, I learned that the popular religious argument in favor of circumcision states that God did not make man exactly as he wanted him because it is man's duty to perfect himself through the fulfillment of a divine command. Fortunately by this time I had outgrown my anthropomorphic concept of a Deity and was able to see the physical perfection of man in his unaltered form as an inspiration for the striving to manifest spiritual perfection through thinking and doing good instead of evil.

The American public, so overwhelmed by materialistic values and motives, is in the process of being informed that routine circumcision is medically unnecessary and even harmful. The media has done a cautious but good job of covering a subject which until recently was avoided like the plague. Independent volumes published within the past few years have presented in a well documented and extremely convincing manner the facts about circumcision upon which this book serves to reinforce and expand. But if it takes a woman to view this most masculine topic in a thoroughly objective manner, then for this reason alone we should be grateful that Rosemary Romberg has written her treatise. The sincere reader will, however, have many more reasons to develop a profound sense of gratitude. In her capacity as an experienced mother, the author presents her subject as only one in her position can, for that wonderfully feminine quality known as motherly love motivates an intimate concern for the feelings and security of the helpless newborn. And yet her viewpoint is broad enough to see the controversy for what it really is, essentially not a medical debate at all, but rather a question of whether or not individual freedom of choice should be preserved in an age where the acknowledgement of infants' rights is increasingly regarded as a practical prerequisite to becoming a parent. Ms. Romberg is further blessed with sufficient modesty to realize that her book is by no means the last word on circumcision. Research into the operation's hidden psychological consequences is just starting to gain a measure of priority, so Romberg's primary purpose is to provide a much needed impetus for further scientific investigation.

At the beginning I wrote of leaders and followers. If we are going to use labels at all, then the number of categories must be made adequate. It appears now that another distinct variety of human beings is emerging who are intent on neither leading nor following the mainstream, and demonstrably capable of conscientious self government. People of this exciting new breed ask simply for the privilege of being themselves without interference. It is primarily in recognition of people such as this, including those yet unborn, that this book has been written.

Jeffrey R. Wood
Wilbraham, MA,
Founder of *INTACT Educational Foundation*

Editor's Remarks

I know Rosemary Romberg since I got into the topic of circumcision in 2012. After translating some books on the subject, I asked Rosemary in 2018 for permission to translate her famous book into German and distribute it. She gladly agreed, but asked me to wait until she had revised and expanded the book, which was then available in a partly updated online version only.

I offered to help revise her book. Other intactivists also offered their help. Unfortunately, Rosemary's health deteriorated more and more, so that she had to pause working on the book more and more often. I promised her to continue her work if necessary. She passed away in February 2020.

Thanks to the generous help of her husband, Steve Wiener, I was able to maintain additional data and bring it up to date. Other intactivists also helped and contributed to the now completely revised Second Edition of the book.

Rosemary added sections named "Informational Resources" to various chapters of the online version of her book. I have reviewed and resorted them alphabetically, added titles and clickable links for the ebook version of the Second Edition. Where the URLs originally chosen by the author are no longer available online, I have used new URLs for the same content. Where content could no longer be found on active websites, the replacement URLs refer to the Internet Archive or to content saved in the IntactiWiki pool.

For the printed version, all listed URLs are available on the author's website at circumcisionthepainfuldilemma.wordpress.com.

All references are now formatted in the concise AMA notation. The journals cited are abbreviated according to ISO 4. You can find all information about the journals in the IntactiWiki article "Journal" at en.intactiwiki.org/wiki/Journal.

I would like to thank the following persons for their help:

John Adkison, Gerald E. Boor, Ken Brierley, Robert Clover Johnson, George Hill, Brother K, James Loewen, Jason Metters, Marilyn Milos, Reed Nelson, Philip David Smith, Daniel Strandjord, and last, but not least, Steve Wiener for his trust and frankness.

Ulf Dunkel, April 2021

The Author's Own Story

I am an American middle class woman. I have a college degree and consider myself intelligent. I am a person who actively seeks to inform and educate myself about all matters that will concern my children and myself.

However, like many Americans, I grew up uninformed about one important matter. All my life I believed that penises were supposed to look a certain way with the rounded "head" exposed at the end. I assumed that all males were born with penises like that. I had no awareness that they should look any different or that anything had been cut off.

I had heard of the term "circumcision." I knew that the Bible mentioned it and that it had something to do with the penis. I knew that people thought of circumcision as a good thing and that it somehow had something to do with cleanliness. I had no understanding of what circumcision involved or why it was done. People seldom discussed the subject. I rarely thought about it.

I am married to a Jewish man. We do not actively practice the Jewish faith. However, I knew that circumcision of infant males was important to Jewish people.

The following is my own personal account of the birth and circumcisions of my own three sons. It is a story of sincerity, seeking, pain and growth, which led to my decision to write this book:

It is 1972. Steve and I are excitedly expecting our first child. I want to do everything possible to make things right, perfect, and beautiful for this child that we already love so much. We attend Lamaze classes together. Steve will be by my side in the delivery room. I plan to give birth without medication. I also am looking forward to nursing my baby.

I discuss birth with a friend of mine. She has two little sons. Eagerly we share our ideas about birth and breastfeeding. Then she says, "Another thing that we decided was not to have our boys circumcised. It seems to me that if that skin was not meant to be there, they would have been born without it."

To me her idea seems strange. "Oh, that doesn't appeal to me. Circumcision seems cleaner," I reply. "Also, I've read that a newborn baby does not have a highly developed pain response and that circumcision doesn't hurt them the way it would if it were done at a later age. Besides, Steve is Jewish and his family would object if we did not have our son circumcised."

Later, at my obstetrician's office the doctor asks me, "Now, do you want the baby circumcised?"

I giggle, "Yes, but only if it's a boy."The author' son Eric in the delivery room.

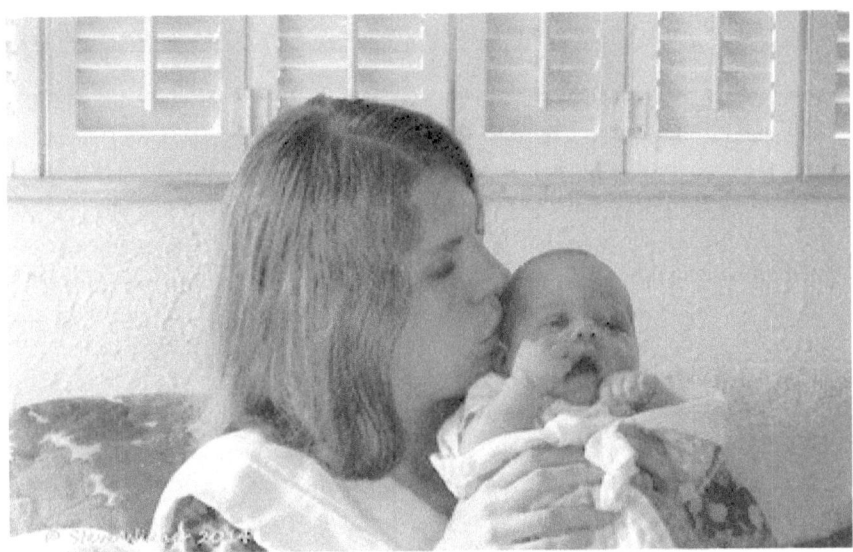

Rosemary and baby Eric as a newborn

May 27, 1972, after hours of challenging, exhausting labor, I push our child into the world. I am on the delivery table, on my back, with my legs up in stirrups. Steve is by my side. I have had no medication and am fully conscious. In the mirror I watch the baby's head emerge, and then the body. "That's the baby!! That's the baby!!"

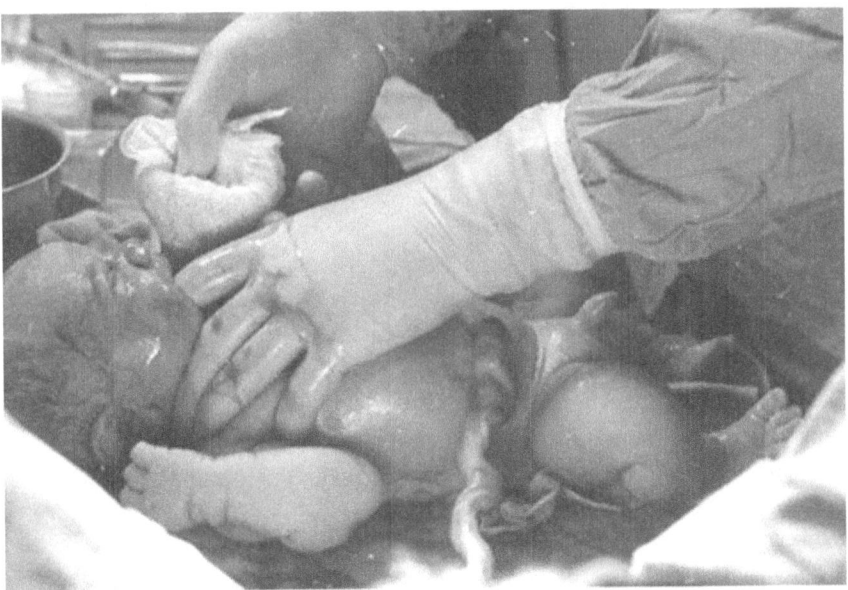

The author's son Eric in the delivery room.

Steve exclaims excitedly. Now the baby is down on a table in front of me. I can hear him crying but I cannot see. The doctor informs us, "You have a boy."

"Honey, we have a little boy! I can't believe it!"

Our son Eric is held up in front of us, wailing and screaming, and then handed to the nurse who carries him down the hall to the central nursery. We are unbelievably excited over the birth of our first child! But now the three of us are sent our separate ways. Eric is in the nursery. I am taken to the recovery room. Steve must go home.

Before he leaves Steve talks to our doctor and then tells me: "He says you did a great job with natural childbirth! He's going to circumcise the baby for us in the morning."

It is now the 9 a.m. feeding. Finally I hold Eric for the first time, twelve hours after his birth. He does not nurse. His body is wrapped in blankets with only his head visible. Mothers are not allowed to unwrap their babies. Soon the nurse takes him away. Eric is brought to me again for feedings at 1 p.m. and at 5 p.m. but still he does not nurse. I am wondering if there is something wrong with me. I ask the doctor if we can go home the following day. Maybe once we are home I'll be able to get him to nurse.

It is the 9 p.m. feeding. Eric is 24 hours old and finally nurses. I am beginning to feel like this baby is mine.

It is the afternoon of the second day. Eric and I are ready to go home. Steve has brought some diapers and baby clothes. A nurse changes and dresses Eric while we watch. This is the first time I get to see my baby's body. The end of his little penis is bright red from his circumcision. Eric was circumcised some time the previous day, before he had ever even nursed. Possibly it was done before I had even held him. The nurse gives me a small tube of petroleum jelly and instructs me, "Put this on his circumcision each time you change his diaper until it heals. Also, apply alcohol to his umbilical stump until it dries up and falls off."

Now Eric and I are home. I am still exhausted from the hours of agonizing labor. I am in great pain from my episiotomy. My uterus cramps with after-labor contractions. My nipples are sore and blistered from my first attempts to nurse. Soon my breasts become painfully engorged. That subsides and then I develop a breast infection. My entire body feels like a raw mass of blood and pain, as if I've been put through a meat grinder!! But it will be okay if it means bringing a beautiful, healthy baby into the world to hold and love. Eric is a good sweet baby and is nursing well. His only problem is that he screams frantically during every diaper change. A friend suggests, "Maybe it's because of his circumcision." I agree, "Yeah, maybe so."

Soon Eric and I both heal and become bonded to each other. Despite our poor start in the hospital and our painful postpartum adjustment, we are now a happy, loving mother-child couple.

Months later I show a friend the pictures we took of Eric in the delivery room. She comments, "That's what they look like before they're circumcised."

I ask her, "You had your two boys circumcised, didn't you?"

"Yeah, but my sister's two kids aren't," she replies. "Their father didn't want to have it done. Their little penises look so funny!"

1974. I am pregnant with our second child. I have become a Lamaze instructor. I now know much more about pregnancy, birth and babies than I did the first time. This time we want to hold, love, and be with our baby from the beginning. We consider giving birth at home so that we will not be separated from our baby.

I find a hospital with a "family centered" maternity department. My doctor is supportive and enthusiastic about our desires. With this birth I will nurse the baby on the delivery table and have immediate rooming in.

October 31, 1974. Again I am pushing on the delivery table. Steve is by my side. This time the stirrups are lowered and my back is raised. We watch our child emerge into the world. "It's another BOY!!" we all shout at once "Waah!!" Jason cries softly while the doctor suctions him and "milks" and clamps the cord. The baby is placed on my abdomen on top of the drapes while I gaze at him lovingly. Then he is wrapped up and given to me to nurse. It is beautiful to gaze into his eyes and get to know Jason. The doctor sews up my episiotomy. Soon the nurse takes Jason away to the nursery to weigh him and clean him up. I shower and eat lunch. Then the baby is brought to my room and we stay together from then on.

The following morning the doctor comes back to examine us and to circumcise Jason. He wheels the baby across the hall in his plastic bassinet. I feel anxious, expecting to hear a lot of screaming. In about 15 minutes the doctor brings Jason back. "He didn't really cry about being circumcised. He fussed and spit up a little bit afterwards," the doctor informs us. I feel relieved. We go on to talk about breastfeeding and other things. With rooming in I change the baby's diapers. I know to apply petroleum jelly to his circumcision wound, as I had with Eric.

Shortly afterwards I walk down the hall. The nurse's aide is cleaning some instruments and shows me the device that was used to circumcise the baby. It is a metal gadget that fits over him with a hole where the baby's penis comes through and another part that comes down and clamps the foreskin. I find it interesting. I had imagined that the doctor trimmed off the foreskin freehand fashion. Then she says, "Maybe I shouldn't show this to you. This could get a mother upset."

"No, that's okay."

I give Jason's circumcision no further concern. The baby and I stay together for the rest of the day and night and go home the following day. We go on to form a new, happy, mother-child nursing relationship.

1977. I am now pregnant with our third child. We are going to have this baby at home with a midwife. I have Dr. Leboyer's book *Birth Without Violence*. We will use some of his ideas for this baby's birth. Eric and Jason had both screamed frantically

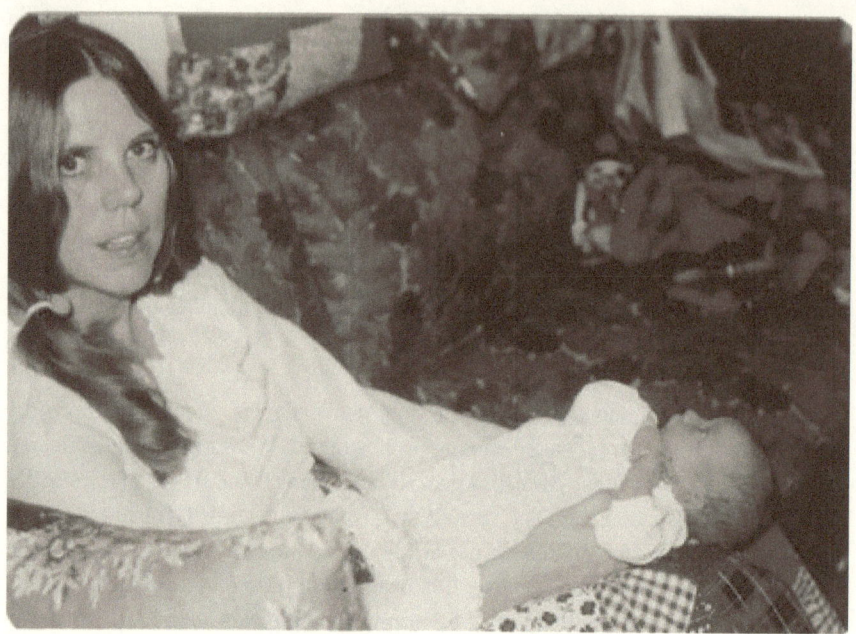
The author and son Jason as a newborn.

at birth, the way we had, at the time, expected all babies to behave. The lights had

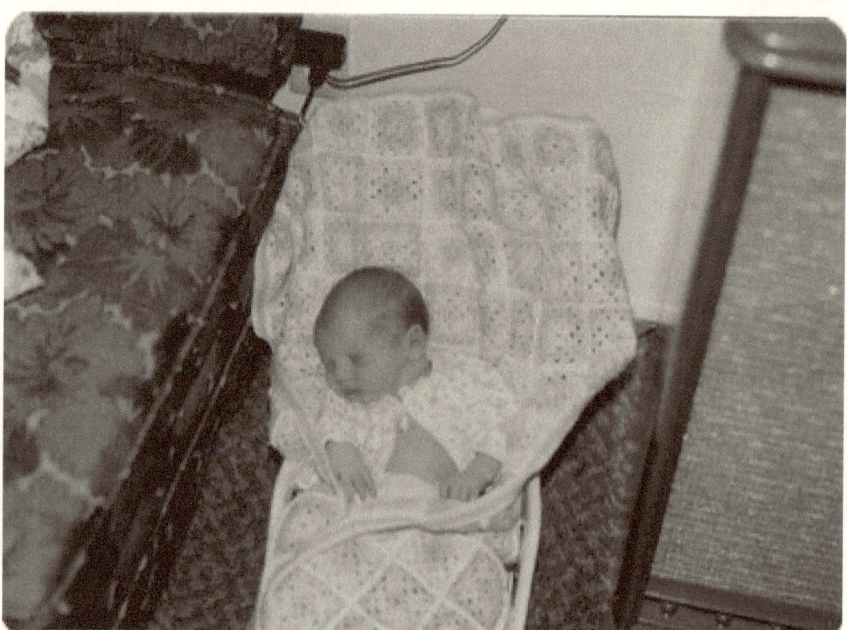
Rosemary's son Jason as a newborn.

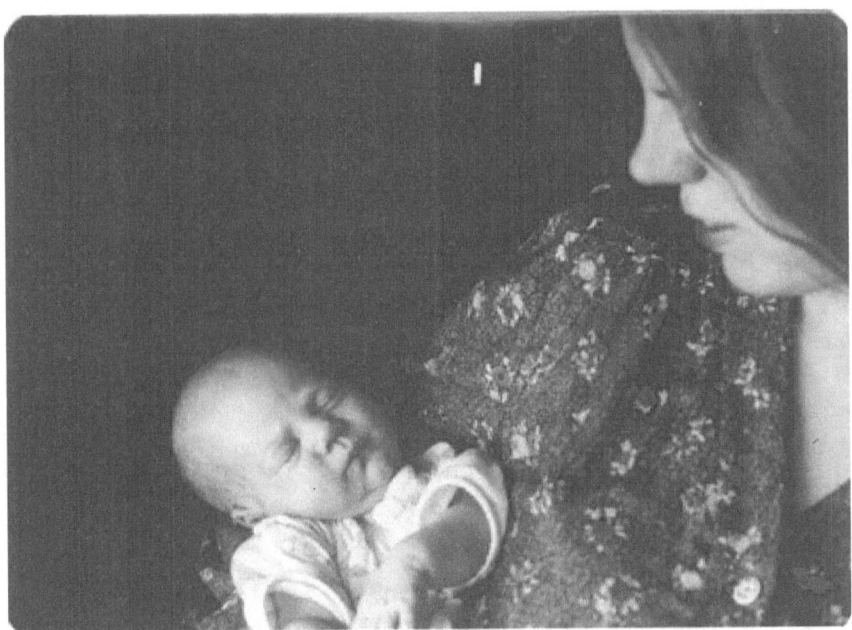

The author and son Ryan as a newborn.

been bright, people had been noisy, and their cords had been cut right away. Leboyer presents some radically different ways to treat a newborn baby.

Our new baby will be welcomed into the world at home, into loving arms, peace, and contentment. We will use dim lighting in our birth room. We will speak softly to the child. We will massage and caress the infant. We will wait a while before cutting the cord. We will not use silver nitrate in the baby's eyes. This child is very special, and his or her birth will be beautiful, pure, and perfect.

I am taking additional training in childbirth education, to teach home birth oriented classes. I am studying obstetric textbooks, attending seminars, and learning much more about pregnancy, birth, and babies.

One day an idea occurs to me. I tell Steve: "You know what I've been thinking? If this baby is a boy, I'd like to not have him circumcised."

"Oh, no." He replies, "They can get terrible infections if they're not circumcised."

"Well, I suppose with your being Jewish, you wouldn't want a son not to be circumcised."

"No, being Jewish isn't the reason. I just think it's necessary for their health."

"It just seems with all of the other neat things that we are going to be doing for this baby's birth, not circumcising would be another 'natural' thing to do."

My mind is full of questions. I have seen other baby boys who were not circumcised. The longer, straight penis has a "strange" appearance to my American middle class eyes. I do not know whether it is better for a baby to be that way or to be circumcised. But I guess our third son would not like being different from his two brothers or his Daddy. Being neither male, nor Jewish, maybe it is not my place to suggest not circumcising.

Early in the morning, April 25, 1977, our third child silently emerges into the world on the bed in our dimly lit room. Steve and our midwife catch the baby together. "It's a boy." our midwife says softly. Ryan's little body is placed on my tummy and I massage and caress him. He coughs, sputters, and starts to breathe quietly. His body is relaxed and there is no crying. The skin-to-skin contact is a warm, beautiful experience that I never had with my other two babies. Eric and Jason are standing by the bed, awestruck by the birth of their tiny new brother.

After about ten minutes the cord stops pulsating and we cut it. I put Ryan to the breast. He nuzzles but does not nurse. Steve takes off his shirt and snuggles Ryan against his bare chest. I work at expelling the placenta. Ryan is again placed in my arms and now begins nursing. In the dim light his little eyes open and he looks at me.

In a little while the midwife examines Ryan's perfect little body. "Are you going to have him circumcised?" she asks. She tends to favor it. Her own son is circumcised. "Yes." I reply absently. I am not thinking about it right now.

It's about 4:30 a.m. The midwife and my other friend leave. Steve sleeps on the couch. The kids go back to their beds. Ryan and I are alone in the birth room together. He is so tiny, 7 lbs. 3 oz., the littlest of my three babies. He has a perfect little round head and is fair and blond. His face is tiny and sweet and bespeaks a

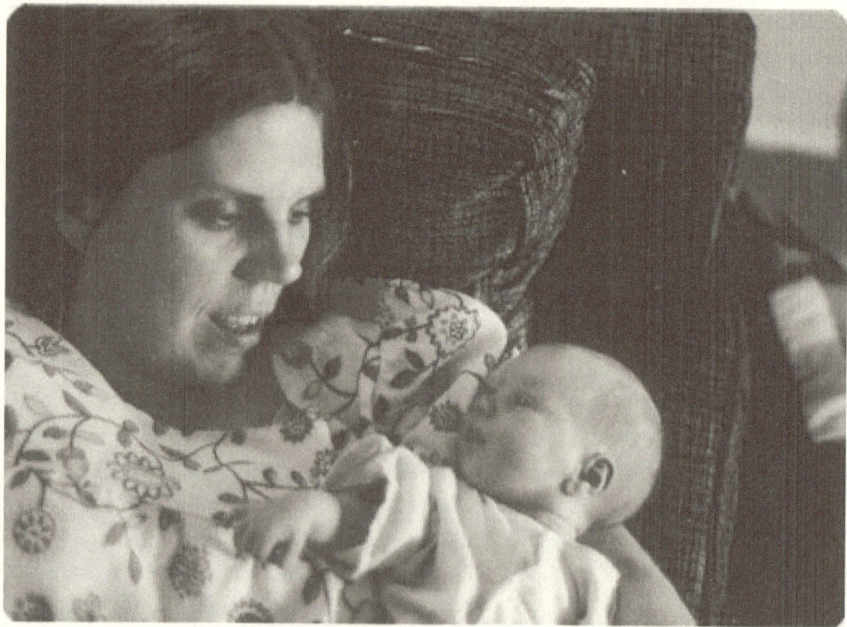

Rosemary and newborn son Ryan.

calmness brought about by his most peaceful birth. It's hard to believe that anything so little and fragile could be real.

In the days that follow, Ryan sleeps and nurses peacefully and never leaves my side. I had always thought that newborn babies were squalling little bundles of appetite and nerves that did not become cute or enjoyable until they were about two to three months old. But this little baby evokes an ethereal tranquility that I have never seen before. He drifts between sleep and wakefulness and makes little smiles just like the pictures in Dr. Leboyer's book totally happy and trusting of this world.

"Why is Ryan's penis different from mine?" asks Eric who is almost five.

"Ryan hasn't been circumcised yet," I explain.

"What is 'circumcised'?"

I explain to Eric that baby boys are born with this skin on the end of their penises but most parents have it cut off. "We will take Ryan to a doctor and have him cut the skin off of the end of his penis."

"Why?"

"Oh, it's supposed to be easier to keep clean."

Ryan's appointment with the pediatrician is on Monday morning. He will be eight days old. The doctor wants us to take the baby to the hospital for a vitamin K shot and PKU test first. We stop by his office to get a prescription for this. I sit in the car and feel like crying. I had my baby at home so I could avoid all of these traumatizing medical procedures. I made so many plans to have his birth be beautiful and perfect. Right now I feel helpless. "Please, can't we just not have any of this stuff done!"

Monday morning arrives. My mother comes over to watch the older boys. "Too bad he has to be hurt," she says sympathetically, as I leave the house with little Ryan. I sigh, resignedly, and say to him, "But we have to make you match your Daddy and your brothers."

Steve meets me at the doctor's office. We go into an examining room. Ryan is sleeping peacefully and trustingly in my arms. My stomach feels like a lump of lead. Nothing has ever felt so wrong! Silently I communicate to him, "I would rather die than let anything hurt your precious little being. And yet this has to be."

The nurse tells me to undress the baby. I say to the doctor, "They showed me the clamp device that they use when our last baby was born in the hospital. Is that what you use?"

"Yeah," he mumbles. He acts as if that is something that parents should not know about. Then suddenly he ushers Steve and me out of the room. I had assumed that I would stay with him!! He tells us to leave the building and suggests a nearby hamburger stand where we could go and eat. This baby has never been separated from me from the moment he was born!! How could you expect me to eat at a time like this??!!

"We use a topical anesthesia on the baby's skin, but it will be painful," he says honestly.

We leave the building and sit on a bench. My baby is inside there! I have no idea what is going on! My maternal, protective instincts are totally violated! It is as if we were helpless children. Steve reminds me of the joke about a "Jim Dandy" being a guy who was circumcised with a pinking shears. Finally enough time has passed that I say, "Let's go back in."

The baby's screams fill the entire building! The nurse leads us back into the room. Ryan is lying on the table. A diaper is half around him. The end of his penis is bright red!! There is blood on the diaper!! He is crying pitifully, a high-pitched wail that I have never heard out of him before. I pick him up and embrace his tiny body close to mine. "Oh, no! Don't hold him like that!" the doctor warns me. I shouldn't put pressure on his wound. So I cradle him in my arms as the doctor leads us into another room. As soon as we sit down I start to nurse Ryan.

"Right now you are doing the very best thing you can for him," the doctor assures me. "Sucking will really help ease the pain."

He gives us advice about various aspects of baby care. Between attempts to nurse Ryan continues to wail frantically! I hear very little of what the doctor says.

Steve leaves and I sit in the waiting room, continuing my attempts to nurse and comfort Ryan. Vaguely his tense, anguished little body reminds me of the way Eric and Jason had been as newborns. A nurse comes by and says, "Hey, it will be all right."

"I know, this is my third baby."

"You just look so upset."

I take Ryan out to the car. He no longer wants to nurse. Mercifully he drifts off to sleep and I drive home. I feel like I am taking home a different baby. He wails in pain again as I carry him back into the house. My mother adds her sympathy to his traumatized condition. I place him on his side in his buggy where he falls asleep again. About three hours later he awakens with another painful wail. I change his diaper and put petroleum jelly on his circumcision. He nurses again and from then on no longer cries about it.

That evening we go out to the "class reunion" of my midwife's childbirth classes. Ryan seems content and peaceful again. I keep him in my arms most of the evening. "I'll never let anything hurt you like that again, I promise."

Weeks later, Ryan was to start cooing and smiling like all normal, healthy babies. But I was never to see those beautiful, mystic, Leboyer newborn-baby smiles again. Ryan was past his pain, But my own heart was to ache about this for a long time. Again and again I was to ask myself, "Why?"

Why did I have the courage and resolve to go outside the medical system and have a home birth, but was unable to question this?!

Why was it so important to me to have his birth be totally peaceful in so many ways, with dim lights, soft voices, and no silver nitrate, and then turn around and do this?!

Why, when I had been a childbirth educator for several years, when I have gone out of my way to educate and inform myself about so many things concerning birth and babies, when I am probably more knowledgeable about most of these matters than 99% of all parents, did I still know virtually *nothing* about circumcision?!

Five months after this experience I awakened out of my feelings of torment, guilt, and horror, to my decision to write this book. It is my profession, as a childbirth educator, to educate expectant parents about all matters that concern their babies. Why aren't people being educated about circumcision?

I did not know where to begin. The many books in my personal childbirth education library said little or nothing about the subject. A visit to my local library yielded little more. Even books on surgery gave only a sentence or two to circumcision. I approached many of my friends about their experiences with the operation, and conducted many of the interviews that appear in this book.

However, despite Ryan's heartrending experience, I *did not start my research being anti-circumcision*. I was even undecided over whether or not I would choose circumcision again should I ever have another son. I fully intended to write a book that was *neutral* on the subject. I had planned that this book would present the pros and cons of both choices, guiding parents to either direction as best suits their lifestyles.

♦

I began this research with the American middle class belief that male circumcision surely conferred many benefits. Therefore I did not skew the results of my research nor the personal accounts herein to conform to a pre-conceived anti-circumcision bias. Instead, it has been the personal accounts and facts that have educated *me*.

The personal accounts in this book tell many stories. Some are from parents of circumcised sons, all expressing remorse over their decision. Some are from parents of intact sons, all expressing peace and satisfaction with their choice. *I have not received any letters from parents of circumcised sons who were happy about their decision, nor any letters from parents of intact sons who were unhappy about it.*

These personal accounts, along with the *facts* I have uncovered, have led me to a strong stand against routine infant circumcision. If the *facts* supported cutting off the foreskins of infant males as a beneficial, justifiable operation, I would have presented that in this book. Instead, I have learned that none of the medical arguments for circumcision are justified, and while I believe that people's religious beliefs require a certain degree of careful consideration and sensitivity, have found that the other so-called "social" reasons have little solid basis.

Three significant concerns surround the issue of infant circumcision:

First, the operation is painful to the newborn infant. Feelings of tenderness and protection surround most of our attitudes about tiny babies. *Why* then have we considered it okay to strap the baby down and proceed to pinch and smash his foreskin, tear it away from his glans, and then clamp and cut it off? Usually this is done without anesthesia. Circumcision was often deliberately intended to be a means of torture of slaves and in primitive initiation rites. Today, if an older child or adult is to undergo circumcision, anesthesia is used. *Why* do we believe that infants either feel no pain or that their feelings are unimportant?

Secondly, is the foreskin a useless piece of tissue an "anomaly" in need of surgical correction? Is the human male body made wrong the way it normally comes into the world? Or does the foreskin serve a purpose? Can we improve on the body by cutting part of it off?

Thirdly, *do we have the right*, in the absence of true medical need, to alter another person's body *without his permission? Does* a person have the right to keep all parts of his body? Isn't each person's foreskin rightfully his? If so, aren't parents who consent to circumcision and doctors who perform the operation taking something away from that child?

These concerns and many more will be examined in the following chapters.

Dedication

This book is dedicated to:

All of the baby boys who have yet to be born into this world ... with the sincere hope that the beginnings of your lives may be peaceful and joyous, and that you may live in this world whole and complete as you were intended to be.

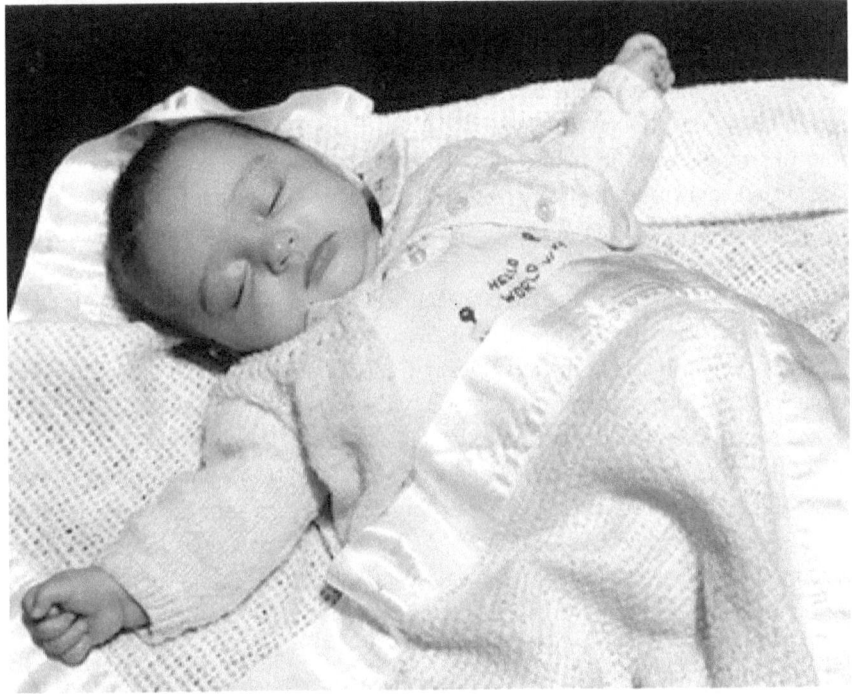

Newborn Welcome to the World. © Suzanne Arms

1   The History of Circumcision

A curious behavior has existed among people from the early beginnings of human existence. Many people have felt a desire to draw blood from, cause severe pain to, and alter the appearance of various parts of the human body – frequently the bodies of their children – in particular the male genital organ.

The penis is normally formed with skin extending over and protecting the more delicate glans. This skin is commonly known as the "foreskin." The procedure of amputating this skin is known as "circumcision." The word is derived from Latin terms which literally mean "cutting in a circle" because a circular piece of foreskin is most commonly cut off.

Who were the first people to practice circumcision? When were the first foreskins cut off? How was it done originally? What was the age and status of the individuals who first relinquished their foreskins? And, most importantly ... why? No definite answers are known. Most history that covers a practice as ancient as this is based on conjecture and speculation. It is almost certain, however, that foreskin amputation is one of the oldest types of surgery.

The first written account of circumcision according to today's knowledge appears in the Bible, with the Hebrew patriarch Abraham's "covenant" with God.[1] The Biblical account is part of the late Priestly Code which was written during the fifth century B.C. (More about this in Chapter 3 "Circumcision and Judaism".)

Other artifacts predate the Old Testament account by many centuries. Drawings on walls of ancient Egyptian tombs and temples date back to approximately 2400 to 2600 B.C.[2] Other historians have given these same relics estimated ages ranging from 3503 to 3335 and 1300 to 1280 B.C.[3] Egyptian mummies estimated as old as 6,000 years also have shown evidence of circumcision.[4]

Some historians have speculated that circumcision has been practiced for more than 5,000 years among the native tribes of the West Coast of Africa.[4]

Very likely, circumcision dates back as far as the stone age. According to one writer

> "... from the stone knives used for the operation ... (circumcision is) a custom reaching back into 'hoary antiquity.' "[5]

---

1   Genesis 17: 10-12
2   Wrana P. Circumcision. *Historical Review.* 385.
3   Schneider T. History of Medicine, "Circumcision and 'Uncircumcision' ". *SAMJ.* 1976-03-27; 556.
4   Remondino PC. *History of Circumcision.* NY: Ams Press Inc.; 1974: 22-23 (original edition, F.A. Davis Co., 1891).
5   James T. A Causerie on Circumcision, Congenital and Acquired. *SAMJ.* 1971-02-06; 45: 151.

1 – The History of Circumcision

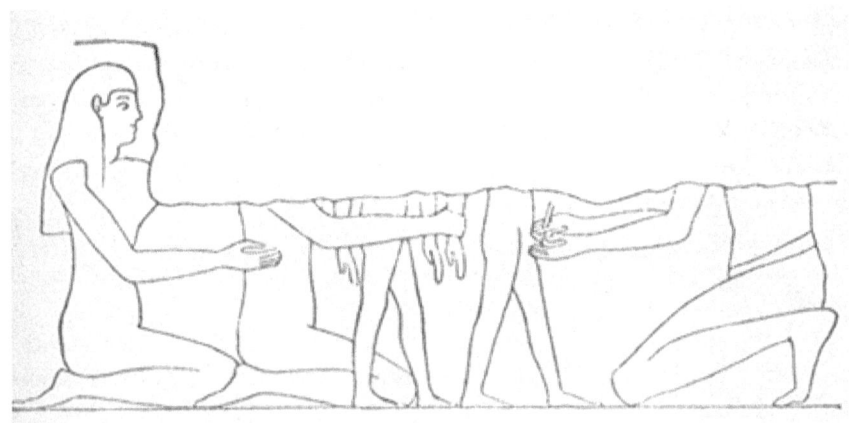

ANCIENT EGYPTIAN RELIEF SHOWING CIRCUMCISION *(after Chabas)*
From Bryk F. *Sex & Circumcision: A Study of Phallic Worship and Mutilation in Men and Women.* North Hollywood, CA: Brandon House; 1967:307.

Speculation also abounds as to which people originated the practice. It is known that circumcision has been practiced among peoples of Semitic origins – specifically the ancient Egyptians, Hebrews, Babylonians, Assyrians, and Moslems, as well as many tribes in Africa, Australia, the South Sea Islands, and sporadically among the Indian tribes of North and South America.

Groups who have practiced circumcision are a *minority* both throughout history and today. Circumcision is presently practiced by approximately one-seventh of the world's population. Most people leave the penis intact. However, attention is usually given to what a culture *does* rather than *does not* do.

It is impossible to determine with which group the practice originated. A plausible speculation is that circumcision originated with the common stock from which the Semitic peoples have sprung.[6]

It is not known whether the practice originated with one group of people and was later copied by others, or if it developed independently among a number of different groups. The fact that different types of phallic mutilation were practiced among different peoples, and that different groups have offered widely divergent reasons for the practice suggests that it very likely had more than one origin.

Very rarely has circumcision been performed on adults. Almost never has it been the *personal* choice of the individual. Adult circumcision was largely confined to converts to religions such as Islam or Judaism, and to slaves and conquered warr-

---

6   Loeb EM. The Blood Sacrifice Complex. *AAA, Memoirs.* 30: 15.

iors.[7] Most peoples performed circumcisions on their sons, most commonly during adolescence between the ages of 11 and 17. Usually this was a part of an adolescent initiation rite in which young boys "became men." Many tribes, especially in Africa, have observed what anthropologists call "bush time" in which the young boys are taken away from their homes and village for a number of months and undergo rigorous training to be hunters and warriors.

Only a very few groups have performed circumcision on younger children.[8, 9] With the exception of Judaism, and the medical profession in 20th century America, infant circumcision has been rare.[10, 11]

Many other types of mutilation of the penis, other than amputation of the prepuce, have been practiced. Historians have often included these under the broader definition of "circumcision."

The simplest ritual was a gashing of the prepuce, without removing any skin. This type of "circumcision" has been attributed to the peoples of the South Sea islands and to a few native tribes in Mexico and South America. This variation may have stemmed from an earlier practice of amputation of the prepuce. It is also possible that foreskin amputation itself was derived from an earlier ritual of gashing the foreskin.[12]

Among the Massai and the Kikuyu in Africa, the males are "half circumcised – the lower part of the foreskin not being cut away at all, but hanging atrophied for the rest of the owner's life." [13]

The more bizarre practice of subincision, the slitting of the entire underside of the penis through to the urethra, was performed by Australian and New Guinea aborigine tribes. This took place during an initiation rite, usually preceded by a "conventional" circumcision a few weeks before.[14, 15, 16]

The Hottentot tribe of Africa did not practice circumcision, but practiced partial castration, removing one testicle of their infant males. Speculations as to the motivation for this practice range from "making the young men better runners" [17] to "preventing the birth of twins" [18] in a tribe which routinely killed the smaller of twins.[18]

---

7 Bryk F. *Sex & Circumcision: A Study of Phallic Worship and Mutilation in Men and Women*. North Hollywood, CA: Brandon House; 1967: 80.
8 Ibid., pp. 80, 59, 73, 74, 155.
9 Wrana, pp. 388-9.
10 Bryk, pp. 91, 263.
11 Remondino, pp. 46-7.
12 Bryk, p. 264.
13 Ibid., p. 65.
14 Ibid., pp. 90, 128.
15 Remondino, p. 56.
16 Bettelheim B. Symbolic Wounds. In: Lessa WA, Vogt EZ, ed. *Reader in Comparative Religion*. 2nd ed. NY: Harper & Row; 1965: 237-8.
17 Remondino, p. 60.
18 Bryk, pp. 123-4.

A few groups practiced perforation of the glans, following foreskin amputation. A metal rod with a small ball at each end was worn in the glans, some believing this to be a sexual stimulant.[19] Other groups inserted a similar device such as a wooden peg which infibulated the foreskin over the glans, as a male chastity device.[20]

The most extreme practice of all involved stripping of the skin from the navel to the anus, including the skin of the penis and scrotum of a young bridegroom. This occurred among the Yesidis in Vilajat Assir in Yemen.

> "The one being circumcised may not cry out nor wail or he would be despised and forsaken by his bride, who witnesses the procedure. Hot oil is put on the wound. People often die of the consequences, many leave the tribe." [21]

A few peoples have practiced a "mock circumcision ceremony." The Nive, of a South Pacific island, perform a ceremony in which the operator performs a mimic operation on his own finger. When a Hindoo joins a sect of Paira of Mahadev Mohammedans in Mysore, a betal leaf is substituted for the foreskin and cut off.[22] A ritual such as this suggests that at one time actual circumcision was performed by the people, which was later abandoned with the ritual remaining.

One historian comments:

> "Circumcision by amputation of the prepuce appears, with comparatively few exceptions, to be confined to the Semitic races and to those who have come under their influence." [23]

1.1 The Reasons for Circumcision

Many explanations have been offered for foreskin amputation and other types of phallic mutilation. Varying peoples appear to have had different reasons for practicing circumcision. Groups who practice it often do not know the true reason. When asked they will frequently offer another reason considerably changed from the original motivation. Some explanations are interrelated. Therefore, scholars are challenged to find the original motivations for the practice. However, some are more plausible than others. Twelve of the most commonly given reasons are:

---

19 Ibid., pp. 134, 211-2.
20 Ibid., pp. 227-8.
21 Ibid., p. 137.
22 Wrana, p. 390.
23 Ibid., p. 389.

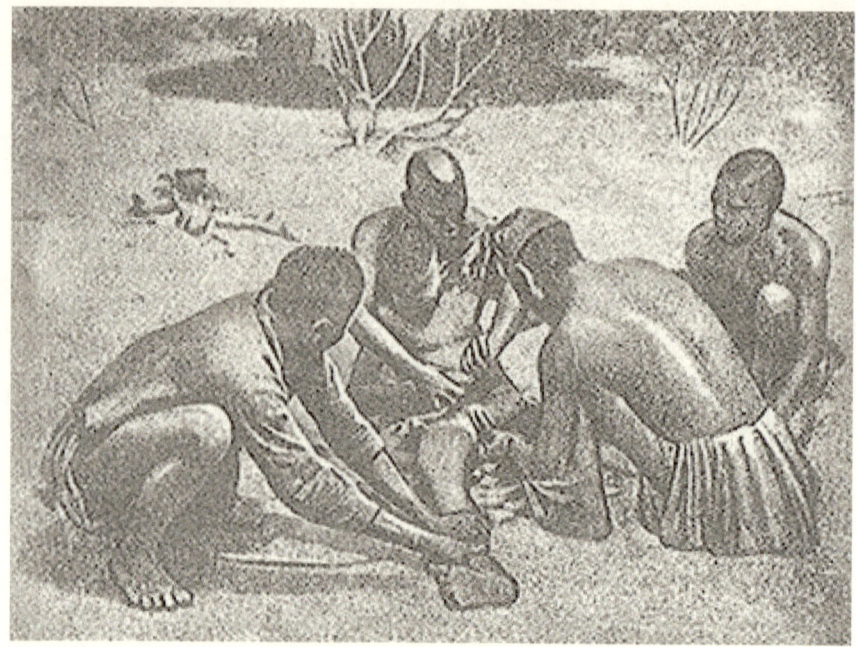

From Bryk F. *Sex & Circumcision: A Study of Phallic Worship and Mutilation in Men and Women*. North Hollywood, CA: Brandon House; 1967: 70.

1.1.1 Hygiene

When American people think about the supposed reasons for circumcision, this explanation usually first comes to mind. Frequently the casual observation has been made that most peoples who have practiced foreskin amputation have lived in lands with hot climates, in either tropical or desert environments. Some historians have offered the speculation that circumcision was therefore desired for cleanliness. Some groups who have practiced the rite believe it is necessary for hygienic purposes.

However, most scholars refute the idea that cleanliness was ever the original motivation for the practice. According to Felix Bryk:

> "... One must have a pretty poor knowledge of the mentality of primitive man, to think seriously for one moment that hygienic motives moved him to introduce and make obligatory a general preventive measure ... it contradicts primitive psychology." [24]

---

24 Bryk, p. 100.

"An uncommonly large number of peoples that practice circumcision show, on the contrary very little passion for cleanliness, and it is hardly to be assumed that they make an exception of the masculine organ in particular. There must be another psychic motive that induced them to undertake the operation." [25]

The fact that many groups practiced simple gashing of rather than amputation of the foreskin, and that foreskin amputation may have been preceded by an earlier practice of foreskin bleeding supports the idea that cleanliness had nothing to do with its origins. The other variations of phallic mutilations described can in no way be indicated to offer any hygienic value. Additionally, many groups which practiced foreskin amputation also practiced female genital mutilation, which is certainly not necessary as a hygienic measure, although some also believe that female circumcision confers cleanliness to women.

There is no evidence that people living in lands with *colder* climates had *more* opportunities to bathe. Historical accounts of people in snowy climates often cite the common practice of wearing the same outfit of clothing throughout the entire winter, never undressing or bathing until spring. Frequently running water was scarce, heating supplies limited, and regular bathing was an unobtainable luxury in colder climates. Perhaps one may perspire less in a colder environment. On the other hand, people in warmer lands often could more readily bathe in nearby bodies of water, which could not be so easily accomplished in freezing temperatures.

However, most primitive peoples in warmer climates usually wore little or no clothing. Therefore, the penis was more readily on view. Perhaps this is why people in warmer lands were more likely to cut or amputate the foreskin. People in colder climates, out of necessity wore more clothing, and the penis was always out of view. This may be the reason that such people did not practice phallic mutilation.

Foreskin amputation "for cleanliness purposes" is clearly a superficial, "after the fact" explanation, made by people who are unaware of its more complex origins.

1.1.2   Cosmetic Value

Was phallic mutilation a practice similar to ear piercing, body tattooing, scarification, or plates in the lips? Were foreskins originally amputated because people believed that penises looked better that way?

Curiously, in the historical literature, little mention has been made of circumcision being a "cosmetic" measure. Like cleanliness, this too appears to be a superficial, secondary explanation of the practice, rather than a primary motivation.

One author writes:

---
25   Ibid., p. 140.

> "While (other deformations) serve the purpose of imparting to the organ in question a specific ornamentation by means of lip plug, earring, etc. that is to enrich the organ artificially, this point of view of the esthetic in the treatment of the masculine sexual organ is, with few exceptions, absolutely unfounded. It is not a question of embellishment, but of injury, that is applied to it." [26]

The fact that foreskin gashing rather than amputation was practiced among many peoples also refutes the idea of cosmetic value. Also, female circumcision was practiced among many of the same peoples and most versions of the female counterpart have little obvious effect on the outward appearance of the female genitals. It appears that the blood and pain caused by the operation was more important to its meaning than the change in appearance of the organ.

1.1.3 Tribal Identity or Mark of Adulthood

Was the circumcised penis a "membership badge" signifying "belonging" to one's group? Since circumcision was commonly a part of adolescent initiation rites, the circumcised penis did become a "mark of adulthood" – obviously since only children had penises with foreskins.

Considerable social value has surrounded the perpetuation of foreskin amputation. Since the procedure was obviously quite painful, societal pressure was necessary to motivate the young boys to cooperate with the ritual. Refusal to have it done became indicative of cowardice. The social ostracism would have been a greater trauma and punishment than the initial pain of the operation.

According to one author, describing an African tribe:

> "Whoever does not have himself circumcised is considered a boy all his life, and not only by the men, but also by the women, who despise and ridicule him as one. He is regarded as civilly dead, ... incurs the loss of all honors, may not witness any assemblage, and no one takes his advice ... and finally, one who is uncircumcised may not marry." [27]

Frequently, circumcision did become a means of tribal identification among many peoples. Speculation has been made that it served to identify one's own during battle, perhaps originating from the barbaric custom of amputating the genitals of slain or even living enemies conquered in battle as victory "trophies". The circumcised penis being a means of identifying the victim as an enemy or of one's own tribe. However,

---

26 Ibid., p. 170.
27 Ibid., p. 84.

when tribes living in close geographical proximity all practiced foreskin amputation, the circumcised penis' value in "tribal identity" was weakened.

It appears that tribal identity was not the primary motivation for circumcision in many cases, although it did serve that purpose in some instances.

1.1.4 A Means of Diminishing Sexual Desires

Some have believed that amputation of the foreskin was intended to weaken the sexual organ and counteract excessive lust.

Philo, an ancient writer, saw in circumcision:

> "... the excision of the passions which bind the mind. For since among all passions, that of intercourse between man and woman is greatest, the lawgivers have commanded that the instrument, which serves this intercourse, be mutilated, pointing out, that these powerful passions must be bridled, and thinking that not only this, but all passions would be controlled through this one ..." [28]

Other writers have accused the foreskin of causing masturbation, bed-wetting, involuntary erection, "psycho-/pathological reactions" and "wicked moral crimes!" [29]

Evidence does exist that intact men do have greater sexual sensation due to the greater sensitivity of the protected glans, and that the foreskin is an erogenous zone in itself. Whether enhanced sexuality is considered beneficial or evil, and dulled sexuality undesirable or "morally beneficial" depends on prevalent cultural attitudes which constantly change. Our society is in the painful process of growing away from the Victorian prudishness of the previous centuries, towards general acceptance and enjoyment of sexuality. (More will be covered in future chapters about how circumcision as a modern medical fad finds its roots in the masturbation phobia of the Victorian era.) Hopefully our current trend towards greater acceptance of sexuality will accompany the trend of leaving our infant sons intact.

1.1.5 Enhancement of Sexuality

In direct contradiction to the above, many groups connected foreskin gashing or amputation with phallic worship, believing that the procedure enhanced sexuality. Some believed that coitus was impossible with the prepuce intact. Circumcision as part of an adolescent initiation rite conferred not only adult status, but was meant to be an introduction into sexual life.

---
28 Ibid., p. 94.
29 Ibid., pp. 102-3.

When the penis has its foreskin, the only time that the glans is normally exposed is during erection. One theory is that men originally retracted the foreskin as an erotic measure, to give the penis a look of being erect, and later, for the same reason, decided to cut off the foreskin, to give the penis a "permanently erect look." [30]

Sometimes the young intact male may have a tight frenulum, the band of skin between the inner lining of the prepuce and the glans, which has been called a "sign of virginity". Occasionally this can be a hindrance to coitus, at least during his first attempts. This may have been the basis for the belief that coitus without circumcision was impossible or dangerous, and thus may have been a motivation for foreskin amputation. Similarly, girls occasionally have tight hymens, in rare cases necessitating surgical intervention to clip the hymen before she can have intercourse. Some people have practiced *routine* hymenotomy for reasons similar to those given for circumcision.

1.1.6 Fertility

The concept of circumcision enhancing sexuality or as a necessary prerequisite to adulthood and sexual life links directly with the idea that circumcision increased or was necessary for fertility. The procedure was frequently part of primitive fertility rites.

Even with today's scientific knowledge, the process of conception and childbearing is awe-inspiring. It is little wonder that desire for many offspring and elements of magic and sacrifice centered around fertility rituals played a predominant role in the lives of primitive peoples.

In this perspective, circumcision served as a method of "dedicating the genital organ to the gods." The prepuce was, in effect, sacrificed to the gods to insure numerous offspring. The foreskin is the only part of the male organ which can easily be cut off, yet allow the individual to procreate. In some instances the amputated prepuce took on magical elements, becoming a charm that the individual carried with him at all times to ensure fertility.[31] Among one African tribe the same knife that was used for circumcision was subsequently used for severing the umbilical cords of the man's children.[32]

Some believed that the foreskin was, if not a hindrance to copulation, an obstacle to procreation. Failing to understand the nature of the foreskin which becomes drawn

---

[30] Ibid., p. 198.
[31] Ibid., p. 143.
[32] Ibid., p. 43.

1 – The History of Circumcision

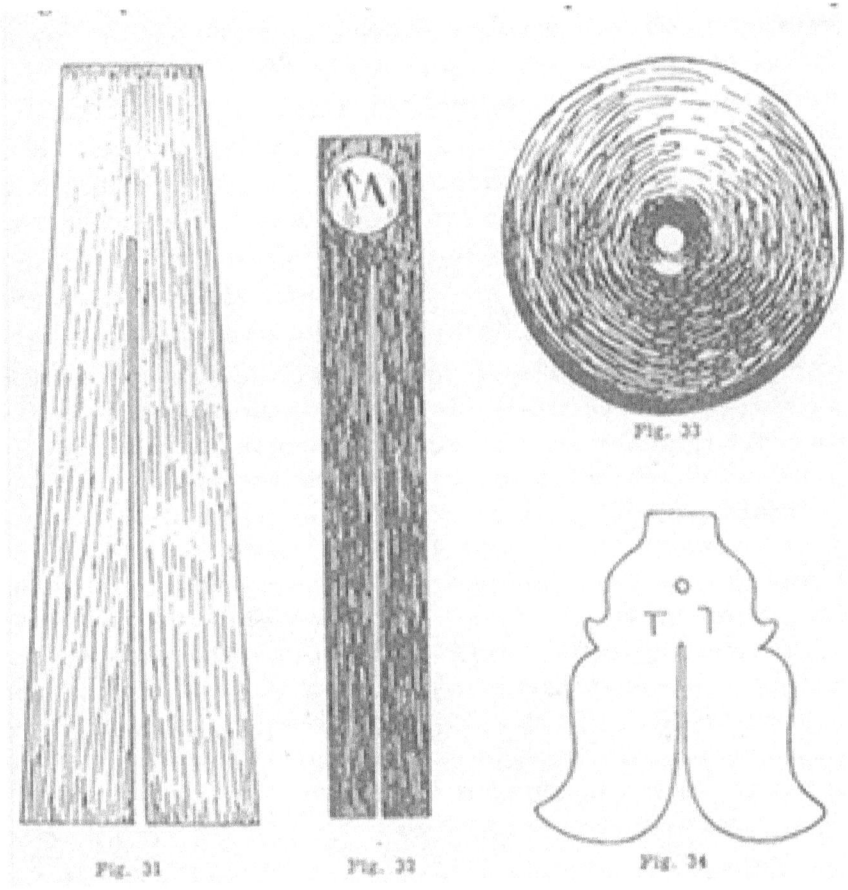

CIRCUMCISION INSTRUMENTS OF THE TURKS AND JEWS
Fig. 31. Split Slab of Wood. Fig. 32. Split Reed. Fig. 33. Perforated Plate Through Which the Foreskin Is Drawn. Fig. 34. Barzel of the Jews: the Foreskin Is Drawn Through the Slit.
From Bryk F. *Sex & Circumcision: A Study of Phallic Worship and Mutilation in Men and Women.* North Hollywood, CA: Brandon House; 1967: 244.

back, fully exposing the glans during erection and copulation, some believed that the semen "became lost in the folds of the foreskin." [33, 34]

Of course if circumcision truly did grant fertility and if the foreskin truly was a hindrance to conception, the human race would have long ago ceased to be. Humans existed for eons prior to the innovation of foreskin amputation. It can be easily noted

---
33 Ibid., p. 93.
34 Ibid., p. 104.

that entire populations throughout the world, including most parts of Asia and Europe reproduce regularly although circumcision is not practiced. If the prepuce were indeed a hindrance to fertility, it would be a convenient birth control device today, but this certainly is not the case.

1.1.7 A Mark of Subjugation for Conquered Enemies and Slaves

It is doubtful that this was ever an original motive for circumcision, but some foreskins have been cut off for the above reason.

Some have suggested that circumcision was a means of identification of slaves.[35] Possibly it replaced earlier, more dangerous practices of amputating an extremity of or castrating of slaves. Or perhaps, since slaves were a marketable commodity, circumcision was performed supposedly to increase their fertility. Some have speculated that the Jews, who were at one time slaves of the Egyptians, adopted circumcision for this reason.[36]

The suggestion has been offered that circumcision was a mark of subjugation inflicted upon conquered warriors by their victors, in lieu of punishment by death. There are some true accounts of this. In other cases, however, there may be some confusion in terminology as to exactly what was being cut off of conquered warriors. Among many tribes the phalluses of conquered warriors were amputated and brought home as "trophies." Old Testament accounts describe warriors collecting the foreskins of their conquered enemies. Others speculate that it was amputated phalluses, not foreskins that were actually collected. (In recent centuries Puritanistic attitudes have changed the meaning of some words when the Bible has been translated.)

1.1.8 A Mark of Purity

In direct contrast to circumcision being a mark of subjugation and humiliation, some considered foreskin amputation to be a holy act, and a means of purification. In ancient Egypt circumcision was at one time limited to the priesthood and was done in addition to the shaving of all body hair. Not only foreskins, but hair was considered unclean.[37]

Philo suggested that circumcision was "purifying" in that it likened the glans of the penis to the heart in appearance. This is hardly plausible, for the concept of a "Valentine" heart shape is a modern concept, not anything like a real, physiological heart. Also the concept of "love" or "purity" originating in the organ which circulates

---

[35] Remondino, pp. 29-30.
[36] Burger R, Guthrie T. Why Circumcision? *Pediatrics*. 1974-09; 54: 362.
[37] Remondino, preface.

1 – The History of Circumcision

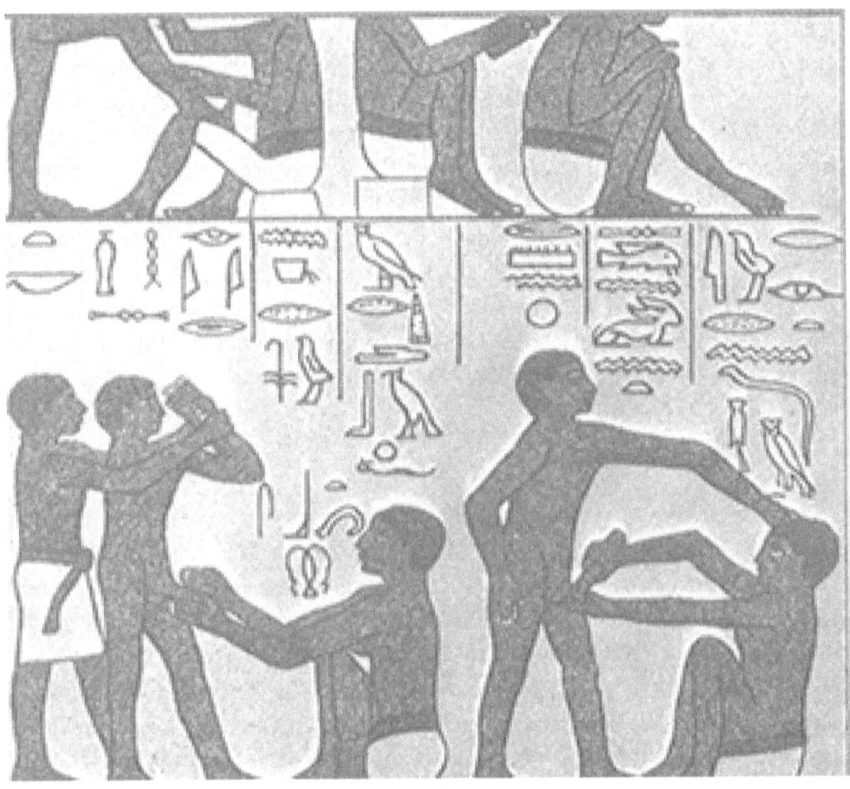

EGYPTIAN CIRCUMCISION *(ancient relief)*
From Bryk F. *Sex & Circumcision: A Study of Phallic Worship and Mutilation in Men and Women.* North Hollywood, CA: Brandon House; 1967: 238.

blood, does not appear to be prevalent among primitive peoples. This is a peculiarly Western idea.

Another writer comments: "It was not the heart that was to be imitated, ... but rather the phallus [erect penis]." [38]

1.1.9 A Test of Endurance

In primitive societies circumcision was frequently a part of adolescent initiation rites. Perhaps it was simply one more of a number of types of torture which the young boys had to endure in their initiations. Excruciation, torture, and subjection were part

---

38 Bryk, p. 104.

of their declaration of manhood.[39] Frequently this accompanied practices such as cutting other areas of the skin, knocking out teeth, piercing of the ear or nose.[40]

The question is raised: was the pain inflicted the original motivation for circumcision? Or was the prepuce being bled or amputated for other reasons, but since it also happened to be painful became consequently connected with the element of torture?

Circumcision of infants and young children appears to be a later adaptation of earlier practiced adolescent circumcision. Did the peoples involved have the desire to torture infants and small children? Did they amputate the prepuces of infants and young children because they were less able to resist? Or did they operate on the premise that infants and young children do not feel pain?

1.1.10 Symbolic Castration

The circumcision of adolescent boys, and other torments that accompanied initiation ceremonies have been explained as punitive, hostile acts on the part of fathers towards their young sons. Symbolic castration motives have been suggested, circumcision being a means of squelching potential incestuous desires of the young men by the fathers who were hostile towards their sons' developing sexuality.[41]

This theory has plausibility in tribes in which older men married young girls and marriage for men was delayed until quite late in life. It was not their own mothers that the young boys desired, but the young wives of the older men.

Some have suggested that circumcision derived from earlier practices of actual castration. Castration can result in profuse bleeding, has had a high mortality rate. Also it obviously prevents continuation of the lineage, making it generally impractical. Hence circumcision, being less dangerous and damaging, was substituted.

Documented studies have linked castration anxieties and motivations to circumcision. One Turkish doctor studied a number of Turkish children undergoing ritual circumcision who manifested definite castration anxieties.[42]

In another study, maternal-infant sleeping arrangements of various primitive societies were analyzed in conjunction with whether or not the young boys were circumcised in adolescence. The rates of circumcision were considerably higher in groups in which the mother and baby slept together and the father slept separately (64%), than in groups where the mother, father, and baby slept together (20%), or the mother and father slept together, but baby slept separately (22%).[43] (The presumption

---

39 Ibid., p. 98.
40 Ibid., pp. 141-2.
41 Ibid., p. 151.
42 Ozturk OM. Ritual Circumcision and Castration Anxiety. *Psychiatry.* 1973-02; 36: 49-60.

here is that circumcision of the infant was motivated by the father feeling jealous or "replaced" by the child if he must sleep separately from his wife.)

1.1.11   Menstrual Envy

One of the most curious and fascinating theories is that subincision and possibly circumcision developed because men are envious of the female and her sexual organs. Females have a natural process of bleeding from their genitals which begins during adolescence, marks the end of childhood and initiation into womanhood, and is directly linked with fertility. In some cases men have ritually bled their penises in an attempt to simulate menstruation. The subincision operation of splitting the urethra was apparently an attempt to make the penis look like a vulva.[44]

Peoples who have practiced subincision rite, primarily tribes in New Guinea and Australia, use parallel names for menstrual bleeding and the bleeding from the subincision wound. When the penis is periodically incised, the term for the operation translates as "men's menstruation."[45]

Myths tell of such things as an ancient totemic bird that threw a boomerang which circumcised the male tribal ancestor and cut the vulva of his wives so that they bled, causing their monthly menstrual periods. Among some tribes, menstruation was considered a punishment for women for inventing circumcision.[45]

Relatively few groups have formal initiation rites for young women. Perhaps this is because nature bestows "initiation" on them through menstruation and childbearing. Male envy of the female reproductive process applies to birth as well as to menstruation. Giving birth is definitely a "test of endurance" that introduces the woman into womanhood and motherhood. Some societies practice "couvade," a ritual in which the father goes through a mimic labor and delivery while the mother actually gives birth. Frequently the men imagine birth to be much more difficult than it is in reality. In similar fashion, possibly out of the same motives of envy, in today's society, birth has been taken out of the control of women and is dominated by the male oriented medical profession. (Thankfully today women doctors and competent midwives are doing much to place birth back into women's domain.)

1.1.12   Sacrifice

The elements of sacrifice and magic were definitely involved in the ancient practice of circumcision. This relates to what has been previously discussed concerning cir-

---

43 Kitihara M. A Cross-cultural Test of the Freudian Theory of Circumcision. *Int J Psychoanal Psychother.* 1976; 5: 541.
44 Bettelheim, p. 231.
45 Ibid., p. 238.

cumcision supposedly increasing fertility and the rite being connected with phallic worship.

Throughout history circumcision has always been connected with religious ritual. Giving up one's foreskin has been presented as giving up a part of one's body to the gods. Circumcision appears to be a milder form of more drastic types of sacrifice.

E.M. Loeb presents an in-depth study tracing the ancient origins of circumcision and relating it to other primitive sacrificial customs of *finger sacrifice, cannibalism, human sacrifice,* and *bleeding of the body.*[46]

Cannibalism was not normally based on need for food. Instead it had sacrificial, magical, or revenge motivations. Human sacrifice interconnects with cannibalism in that sacrifices of humans were intended to be food offerings to gods. Frequently sacrifice was made of conquered enemies and slaves, but child sacrifice also took place.[47]

The blood involved in all types of sacrifice has always been an extremely important facet of the ritual. Blood confers life, therefore numerous religious rituals, both primitive and modern, are centered around blood or the concept of blood. (For example Communion or Mass [Eucharist] among Christians, and Koshering of meats by Jews.) In primitive rituals, sometimes the priests smeared themselves with blood, or temple doors and statues were smeared with blood. Sometimes wounds were made all over the bodies of children amidst great solemnities perhaps to insure a bountiful harvest or consecrate the child to the gods.[48, 49]

Elaborate rituals surrounding the treatment of the amputated foreskin, such as burying it, burning it, preserving and keeping it, or hiding it in a totem tree, support the magical, sacrificial nature of the act.[50, 51, 52]

The previously discussed "mock" circumcision ceremony carried out by some groups, suggests the religious and sacrificial nature of the procedure. Similarly, the fact that the Jews proceed with the circumcision ceremony and draw blood from the penile skin of a baby born without a foreskin, illustrates the religious significance of the ritual in and of itself.

Some have suggested that the Jewish practice of infant circumcision was preceded by earlier rites of infant sacrifice.[50] However, this theory does not appear plausible because most historians agree that circumcision of infants was a relatively late acquisition of all peoples, preceded by earlier adolescent circumcision.[51]

---

46 Loeb, p. 3.
47 Ibid., p. 6, 9.
48 Bryk, p. 114.
49 Ibid., p. 140.
50 Ibid., p. 112.
51 Ibid., p. 119.
52 Loeb, p. 23.

Loeb concludes that neither was human sacrifice the cause of circumcision nor circumcision the cause of human sacrifice, but both related to each other and stemmed from cannibalism. In his opinion, circumcision developed when victims could not be found for sacrifice, so a part of the body was offered instead. Some peoples chopped off fingers, or bled parts of the body, while others amputated the foreskin.[52]

1.2 Conclusion

It is doubtful that purposes of hygiene or cosmetic value were original motivations for amputating the prepuce. The practice may have arisen out of ancient sacrificial rituals which relate directly to fertility, which in turn relate to its being part of an adolescent initiation rite which prepared the boy for adulthood and sexual functioning. The operation, being painful, was viewed as a test of endurance, although it is questionable that this was its primary purpose. Some connect this with a ritual torture which relates to castration wishes on the part of fathers toward their sons. This in turn suggests circumcision to be a procedure which diminishes the sexuality of adolescent boys. Some groups circumcised slaves and captured warriors, perhaps as a substitute for castration. Among other groups it was a mark of the ruling or priestly class and was considered an act of purity. Individual groups have bled and mutilated the phallus out of a wish to copy female menstruation. Circumcision also imparted a mark of tribal identity on the group although it is doubtful that this was the primary motivation for the procedure. Circumcision consists of amputating the prepuce, but the term also extends to other variations of phallic mutilation such as subincision and gashing of the foreskin. Circumcision began as an adolescent initiation rite and much later was changed in some groups to a procedure that was done to babies and small children.

1.3 Informational Resources

- 5 Insane Ways Fear of Masturbation Shaped the Modern World:
    cracked.com/article_19520_5-insane-ways-fear-masturbation-shaped-modern-world.html
- Abraham, Moses and circumcision, the conundrum of the three Covenants: (Gn. 15, Gn. 17 & Ex. 20):
    academia.edu/2095572
- Ancient Origins of Jewish Ritual Circumcision In Modern Society:
    web.archive.org/web/20150717231348/http://www.gnosticliberationfront.com/ancient_origins_of_jewish_ritual_circumcision.htm
- Circumcision: Then and Now: cirp.org/library/history/peron2
- Dogon Circumcision Cave Painting:
    miscellaneous-pics.blogspot.com/2011/08/dogon-circumcision-cave-painting.html

- Don't Blame Your Grandparents: Circumcision became routine without parents' permission: circumstitions.com/1941.html
- History of Circumcision: cirp.org/library/history
- Kilimanjaro and Its People: A History of Wachagga, their Laws, Customs and Legends, ...: amazon.com/dp/1138010898
- Religious Traditions and Circumcision *(ancient origins and tales, good pictures / Larue)*: come-and-hear.com/editor/br-circum-history/index.html
- The history of circumcision *(Dunsmuir / good pictures)*: cirp.org/library/history/dunsmuir1
- The riddle of the sands: Circumcision, history and myth: academia.edu/9899840
- The troubled history of the foreskin: arstechnica.com/science/2015/02/the-troubled-history-of-the-foreskin
- To Mutilate in the Name of Jehovah or Allah: Legitimization of Male and Female Circumcision: pubmed.ncbi.nlm.nih.gov/7731348

2   Female Circumcision

Women and girls have also had a variety of tortures, blood rites, and mutilations performed on their genitals. Many people in Western society are unaware that females can be "circumcised". Some think the idea is a joke. When made aware of the reality of the practice, most in the Western world find it repugnant. Yet the origins of female genital mutilation and the justifications for its practice are very much similar to those of the male counterpart.

Like male circumcision, the origins of the female counterpart are vague and difficult to trace. Many speculations exist as to its beginnings.

Most historians agree that female circumcision was developed by many of the same people who practiced male circumcision, but probably originated much later. It appears to have had a number of different origins, and at one time was practiced by many people who have since abandoned it.

According to Hathout:

> "The origins of female circumcision is [sic] rooted too distantly in human history to be fruitfully traced. The ritual has always been so widespread that it cannot have arisen from a single origin. Although always entangled in beliefs and superstitions with a mystical or religious background, the various peoples practicing it do not conform to a common racial, social or religious pattern. As a matter of fact no continent in the world has been exempt ..." [1]

Like male circumcision, the female operation has been widely practiced by Semitic peoples. Many Moslem peoples and Egyptians still practice this rite. It is believed that the Israelites at one time also circumcised their female children.[2] This is significant, for our current (United States) medical fad of infant male circumcision has come about partially as a result of Jewish influence. If the Jews still circumcised their female infants, perhaps Non Jewish Americans too would also be circumcising their baby girls!

The practice of female genital mutilation has been widespread throughout many parts of the world, although it has not been practiced nearly to the extent of that of its male counterpart.

In Africa, the ancient Egyptians, Mohammedans, Gallas, Abyssinians, the Bantu tribes of Kenya and many other African tribes ... In Asia the ancient and modern Arabs and the Malays of the East Indian Archipelago ... In Australia by many

---

[1]   Hathout HM. Some Aspects of Female Circumcision. *Obstet Gynecol.* 1963-06; 70: 505.
[2]   Bryk F. *Sex and Circumcision: A Study of Phallic Worship and Mutilation in Men and Women.* Hollywood, CA: Brandon House; 1967: 270-1.

tribes ... Some Indian tribes in eastern Mexico, Peru, and Western Brazil ... and the Skopizy of Russia[3] are listed among the people who have, and in some cases still do practice the female procedure.

Circumcision of female infants has been rare. Abyssinian infant girls are circumcised on the 8th day after birth. In Arabia it is sometimes done a few weeks after birth.[4] The Ikito and the Kashbo of Africa also circumcise their infant girls during the first few weeks of life.[5]

Many other peoples have circumcised little girls ranging in ages from 3 to around 10. These include the Somalis, Sudanese, Coptics, and Egyptians. Sometimes the operation involves two steps, circumcision of the clitoris which is done at an earlier age, and infibulation, the artificial closing together of the vaginal lips, which is done a few years later.[4]

Among most other groups, the procedure is performed in early adolescence as some form of initiation rite signifying her entrance into womanhood and marriageability. This has been the practice in Peru, Australia, ancient Egypt, and the Bantu tribes.[4, 6]

Among the Masai in Africa the operation is performed shortly after marriage. Among the Swahili and Guinea people the procedure is performed after childbirth.[4]

A number of different types of mutilations have been included under the broader category of female "circumcision."

Some groups have practiced a deliberate elongation of the clitoris and labia minora – from artificial, mechanical manipulation, reaching lengths as long as 10 cm. The Hottentot tribe of Africa practiced this and the protuberance has been referred to as the "Hottentot Apron." Possibly it was considered sensual or beautiful. Some claimed that it made intercourse easier, or perhaps was connected with Lesbianism.[7] Bettelheim proposes that it developed out of women's envy of males and desire to have a penis-like organ.[8]

A few groups practiced artificial defloration, the rupturing of young girls' hymens prior to the first intercourse. Perhaps this was for magical or social reasons, or to spare the bridegroom the disagreeableness of the blood. The Totonacs of ancient Mexico cut the hymens of month-old infant girls.[9] Artificial enlargement of the vagina was practiced among tribes that practiced subincision of males.[10]

3   Schaefer G. Female Circumcision. *Obstet Gynecol.* 1955-08; 6(2): 235-6.
4   Worsley A. Infibulation and Female Circumcision; A Study of a Little-Known Custom. *J Obstet Gynaecol Br Emp.* 1938; 45: 690.
5   Bryk, pp. 273-4.
6   Ibid., pp. 272-3.
7   Ibid., pp. 276-8.
8   Bettelheim B. Symbolic Wounds. In: Lessa WA, Vogt EZ, ed. *Reader in Comparative Religion.* 2nd ed. NY: Harper & Row; 1965: 239-240.
9   Bryk, p. 281.
10 Ibid., p. 280.

Infibulation involves the artificial closing up of the vagina, usually accompanied by the excision of the clitoris and labia minora. These two practices together have been the most commonly practiced type of female genital mutilation.

Among the Sudanese:

> "... The major part of one labium and the whole clitoris are removed by the first sweep of the razor, followed by excision of the corresponding part of the other labium ... the two cut edges of skin [are clamped] between the two limbs of a split cane tied together at the end. More modern users make use of thread and needle ... This operation aims at fusion between the right and left sides, leaving an orifice that often barely admits a fingertip, and through which urine and the menstrual flow find an outlet." [1]

Usually this is done by a woman whose trade is to circumcise girls, but is not medically trained. No anesthesia is used and usually the girl is screaming and struggling frantically. Therefore the ultimate outcome of the operation is often haphazard. The operation prevents the loss of virginity, or in cases where it has been lost, makes it appear that she is still a virgin. Intercourse is impossible, therefore shortly before marriage another operation is performed to enlarge the opening. Additional surgery is needed at the time of childbirth. The scar in the labia is cut away during delivery to make the vagina large enough for the child to pass. Usually the wound is then artificially tightened and "freshened up" again for her husband's benefit.[11]

Clitorectomy refers to the excision of the clitoris. Usually this involves the amputation of the clitoris, as well as the prepuce ("hood" of the clitoris), labia minora and part of the entrance of the vagina. This is practiced in many Moslem countries, and in parts of Africa and South America.[12] This mutilation appears to be a modification of the more damaging practice of infibulation, as a compromise among people who cannot be persuaded to do away with the operation entirely. Even today, this custom is too deeply ingrained among these people to be abandoned, so a less radical operation is replacing infibulation.[13]

The Omagua of North Peru excised the tip of the glans clitoris. The Kalihari perforated the clitoris.[14] These are rare variations of female genital mutilation.

The amputation of the female prepuce alone, the fold of skin that normally covers the clitoris, is most closely analogous to typical male circumcision. This has been relatively rare throughout history, but like male foreskin amputation, has also been a

---
11 Ibid., pp. 281-3.
12 Ibid., pp. 284-5.
13 Mustafa AZ. Female Circumcision and Infibulation in the Sudan. *J Obstet Gynaecol Br Commonw.* 1966-04; 73: 303.
14 Bryk, p. 287.

medical fad in the United States within recent decades. While female genital mutilation parallels its male counterpart in its practice and development, although to a lesser extent, the motivation was clearly not to remove the prepuce and expose the clitoris.

2.1 Reasons for Female Circumcision

2.1.1 Cleanliness

Some people have believed that circumcision of females is desirable for cleanliness. "That thereafter the women may be able the more conveniently to wash themselves ..." [15] or "... to keep the women from stinking." [16]

One writer explains:

> "Cleanliness and freedom from offensive secretions in the hot weather is another excuse. These are all fabricated arguments to justify a barbaric custom that probably started as a tradition alone, [which] however, [are] responsible for its survival today in spite of the efforts made to eradicate it." [3]

2.1.2 Congenital Hypertrophy

Some peoples who have practiced female circumcision apparently have a congenital enlargement of the clitoris and elongated labia minora that was considered ugly and undesirable, and thus a hindrance to marriage.[14]

2.1.3 Preservation of Virginity

Infibulation results in a tiny vaginal opening which makes intercourse impossible. Bryk comments on the Egyptian practice:

> "... In Egypt they must deprive the women of their natural rights and convert them into insensible machines for the greater security of the husband." [17]

He also cites the practice of artificially tightening the vaginas of prostitutes to put them on the market as "fresh girls." [17]

---

[15] Ibid., p. 289.
[16] Ibid., p. 294.
[17] Ibid., pp. 283-4.

2.1.4 "To Raise the Value of the Woman"

In countries where female circumcision was a long-cherished tradition, the operation became a necessary part of the woman's social status, or "... both a commandment of necessity for sexual intercourse and a simple duty of decency." [15]

Female circumcision was universal in Islam and no Arab would marry a girl "unpurified" by it. "Son of an uncircumcised mother" is a sore insult. [18]

Recent laws attempting to protect young girls from the mutilation have often gone unheeded because it has been impossible to find husbands for uncircumcised girls, and it is considered a disgrace for a woman not to marry. [3]

Additionally, a bride who lacks virginity can be rejected by her husband, or put to death on her wedding night. Therefore clitorectomy with infibulation, "a chastity belt forged of her own flesh," was a matter of her own protection. [19]

Certain Islamic families have had an inherited tradition of their women being female circumcisers, thus giving them a position of prestige in the community. These people have had a social and economic motive for perpetuating the custom. [19]

2.1.5 A Means of Lessening Sexual Desire

Excision of the clitoris is frequently explained as for the purpose of lessening sexual desire – protecting the morals of women and girls, making them passive, or preventing masturbation or nymphomania ... during a time when it was believed that masturbation led to idiocy or insanity. [13, 15]

2.1.6 Shifting the Center of Sexual Sensation

There is a Freudian theory, now largely refuted, that women experience two types of orgasms, clitoral orgasm being "immature" and vaginal orgasm being "mature." The possibility is offered that the clitoris is excised to "remove the erogenic zone from the front of the vagina by the extirpation of the organ most sensitive for the sexual libido ..." [18]

However, it is dubious that any primitive tribes or ancient civilizations had any Freudian concepts of clitoral and vaginal orgasms. It has now been proven that all female orgasms are physiologically identical, the clitoral orgasm during masturbation seeming more intense because there is nothing in the vagina. However it has been noted that in victims of clitorectomy, orgasm is sometimes still possible with the

---

18 Bryk, p. 290.
19 Morgan R, Steinem G. The International Crime of Genital Mutilation. *Ms.* 1980-03; 67+98.

clitoris removed, with the sensation evidently becoming centered in the surrounding tissue.

Other miscellaneous reasons for the procedure include fertility,[14] the clitoris being believed to cause the death of a woman's children,[15] to make women more easily accessible to men,[16] legal status – a woman cannot inherit property without having been circumcised,[4] a required introduction into womanhood,[3] or a "second birth." [20]

A highly educated, modern-day Egyptian woman relates her reasons for desiring circumcision for her daughter in terms uncomfortably similar to our own society's popular platitudes for circumcision of infant males:

"... A young Egyptian woman physician ... was expecting a baby and was asked by a Danish scholar, Henny Harald Hansen, about the reasons for these mutilations. She informed him that 'if the child she was expecting should be a girl she would circumcise her herself.' The young woman gave several reasons. The first was religious: she was a Muslim. The second was cosmetic: she wanted 'to remove something disfiguring, ugly and repulsive.' Thirdly, the girl should be protected from sexual stimulation through the clitoris. The fourth reason was tradition. 'The young doctor argued in support of her intention to respect tradition that the majority of husbands preferred their wives to be circumcised.' " [21]

2.2 Why Has Female Circumcision Not Been Practiced to the Extent of Male Circumcision?

Little has been discussed in the historical literature about this. The following are possible explanations:
– Among many peoples women may have simply not been *important* enough to warrant a special ritual such as circumcision. For example, among the ancient Hebrews the male infant was considered in need of and deserving of the special purification, consecration, and dedication supposedly afforded by the *Brith* ceremony. The Hebrews were an extremely patriarchal social order and females were of lower social status. Jewish female infants may not have been considered important enough to need a similar rite.
(See Chapter 3 "Circumcision and Judaism".)
– If menstrual envy, as discussed in the previous chapter, was a motivation for male circumcision and other male genital mutilations, then women had a natural

---
20 Ibid., p. 295.
21 Daly M. African Genital Mutilation: The Unspeakable Atrocities Gyn Ecology. Ch. 5 in: *The Metaethics of Radical Feminism*. Boston, MA: Beacon Press; 1978: 165. Her reference: Henny Harald Hansen, "Clitoridectomy: Female Circumcision in Egypt Folk", 1972/73; 14-15: 18.

process of blood extruding from their genitals as proof of fertility and signifying entrance into adult status.
- The male prepuce is readily visible, and usually it can be casually noted whether or not the individual has undergone circumcision. The female genitalia are not readily visible, and only closer scrutiny would indicate whether or not she has been circumcised. Therefore such motivations as "tribal identity," "cosmetic value" and "changing the outward appearance of the organ" have not tended to operate as strongly to perpetuate the female operation as they have with male circumcision.
- The highly vascular nature of the tissue of the female genitalia, as compared with the male foreskin, has very likely made female circumcision more dangerous. Rates of hemorrhage, infection, and death have been higher for female circumcision than for its male counterpart. This may very possibly be the reason that many people have abandoned the female operation.
- Male circumcision has been almost exclusively under the control of men and the female operation has been controlled by women. Apparently the whole idea of genital mutilation was *originally* a *male* practice, as it appears that female circumcision developed more recently. Perhaps females had more *common sense* and therefore less desire to cut up their own or their daughters' genitals. Or perhaps maternal protective urges intervened to prevent harm from befalling their daughters, while they had no such control over the circumcision of their sons. (Certainly men are equally *capable* of being caring and protective of their children, but such traits have frequently not been allowed to develop in males in many cultures.)

2.3 Complications of Female Circumcision

Numerous complications resulting from female circumcision have been reported. Shock can result from the initial trauma as the operation is usually done without anesthesia, or it may follow hemorrhage.[22]

Hemorrhage is a frequent complication which has resulted in anemia, lowered resistance to infection, and death.[22] Apparently death from female circumcision was fairly common in ancient times.[3]

Injuries to the urethra, bladder, vagina, perineum, anal canal, and Bartholin's glands have resulted – especially since the operation is frequently done by an untrained person with a struggling, unanesthetized girl.[23]

---

22 Mustafa, p. 304.
23 Worsley, p. 687.

Infections have been common, including tetanus, septicemia, abscesses, infections of the urethra and bladder, chronic pelvic infection, inflammation of the connective tissue, and pockets of pus. Infections from this operation have been fatal.[22, 23]

Retention of urine, due to damage of the urethra, or as a response to the immediate trauma have been reported.[22]

Epidermoid cysts – pockets within the tissue filled with puslike material, have been common. These are usually caused by outer skin being incorporated into the wound as it heals.[22, 24, 25]

Other complications include infertility due to chronic pelvic infections or obstruction preventing intercourse, excessive menstrual bleeding, painful menstruation, retention of menstrual blood, keloid scar formation, vaginal calculi ("stones" of smegma), and painful intercourse.[22, 23]

Repeated pregnancies can be an indirect result if intercourse is painful, causing women to seek pregnancy as temporary relief from sexual demands.[26]

Difficulties in pregnancy and delivery caused by obstruction of the vulva and necessitating surgical intervention to insure safe delivery have also been reported.[27]

2.4 Female Circumcision in the United States During the 20th Century

The amputation of the female prepuce and subsequent exposure of the glans clitoris has been performed on women and little girls by the modern medical profession, particularly in the 1950s – for many of the same reasons as are offered for male circumcision.

One doctor, in an article that was published in a medical journal in 1958, advocated circumcision of female children for the following reasons:

> "... The infant clitoris is hidden. The prepuce covers it at birth. The midline raphe is invariably intact. ... It may remain intact into late multiparous life. ... When the raphe does not open, smegma accumulation can cause trouble. If the raphe opens only a pinpoint, bacteria can enter to cause contamination of the debris. Then come the symptoms of irritation, scratching, irritability, masturbation, frequency, and urgency. In adults ... dyspareunia (painful intercourse) and frigidity ... The same reasons that apply for the circumcision of males are generally valid when considered for the female." [28]

---

24 Hathout, pp. 506-7.
25 Onuigbo W. Vulval Epidermoid Cysts in the Igbos of Nigeria. *Arch Dermatol.* 1976-10; 112: 1405-6.
26 Morgan & Steinem, p. 67.
27 Dewhurst CJ, Michelson A. Infibulation Complicating Pregnancy. *BMJ.* 1964-12-05: 1442.
28 McDonald CF. Circumcision of the Female. *GP.* 1958-09; 17(3): 98-9.

During the 1950s it was popular to circumcise women who were non-orgasmic or climaxed only with difficulty. One doctor who performed the operations wrote:

> "Women can have a redundancy (excessive amount of tissue) and phimosis (inability to retract) of the prepuce" and advocates the operation: "1.) If the patient is adipose ... this operation may help cure her adiposity (fat) by relieving psychosomatic factors, 2.) If the husband is unusually awkward or difficult to educate, one should at times make the clitoris easier to find. [!] 3). If the clitoris is quite small and difficult to contact." [29]

In response to the fad of circumcising women to cure frigidity, Dr. Money says:

> "Some people would tell you they've had better sex after a nose-job operation." He insists that while some women do report improved orgasm capacity after circumcision, the effect is psychological.[30]

The operation is described:

> "After an injection of novocaine the doctor uses a 4-inch forceps to pull back the prepuce, makes a small ½-inch slit in it, and removes the elliptical piece of skin ... however, ... the inner lips serve as a protective shield for the clitoris and if too much is removed it could leave the clitoris dangerously exposed." [30]

It is curious that doctors like this are concerned about exposing and traumatizing the very sensitive glans clitoris, but appear to lack concern or awareness that the glans of the intact male is similarly sensitive and equally exposed to trauma if the prepuce is cut off.

Interestingly enough, female circumcision was, during recent decades, purported to decrease a woman's sexuality. In 1936, in an article written in a medical publication by a doctor, it was seriously suggested that women more passionate than their husbands be circumcised to *reduce* their sex drive.[30]

It appears doubtful that circumcision of the female confers any sexual benefits. Circumcision of females is *not* necessary for personal hygiene, *if* they can be taught necessary washing procedures. The following are instructions for female hygiene which appear in a recently published book:

---

29 Rathmann WG. Female Circumcision, Indications and a New Technique. *GP.* 1959-09; 20(3): 115-120.
30 Schultz T. Female Circumcision: Operation Orgasm. *Viva.* 1975; 2(6): 53-4, 104-6.

"All that is required for adequate hygiene is to keep the outside labia and clitoral area clean, using soap and water. Inadequate hygiene can produce unpleasant odors and interfere with lovemaking, but frequent washing of the external genitalia will be sufficient to prevent any unpleasant odors. It may be necessary to retract the foreskin of the clitoris, and using a cotton swab or piece of gauze, remove any accumulation of smegma. Male genitals also need frequent washing, as females are no more 'dirty' than males." [31]

2.4.1 Episiotomy

I added these comments of mine in honor of the late Sheila Kitzinger, a leading pioneer in the beginning natural child birth movement of the 1970's and earlier. She boldly labeled episiotomy as the "Western version of female genital mutilation." – R.R.

There is another form of female genital mutilation that is *extremely* common in Western society today. It is performed regularly among today's medical profession. Episiotomy involves the cutting of the perineum, the skin between the vagina and the anus, to enlarge the vaginal opening at the time of birth. After delivery, the severed skin and internal muscle tissue are stitched back together. This is normally done under local anesthesia, unless a stronger type of medication was used for the birth. Initial healing often causes severe pain, burning upon urination, and difficulty with defecation. Subsequent intercourse may be difficult for months. For many women, the pain caused by the healing of the episiotomy is much greater than any pain experienced with labor or delivery. This pain can definitely disrupt bonding with the baby and adjustment to motherhood.

Expectant mothers in America have been led to believe that they cannot give birth vaginally without episiotomies. They have been told that they will either tear badly or be left with a "gaping hole" for a vagina, if episiotomy is not done. Some people believe that the baby will not come out at all unless this cut is made. The rate of episiotomies for vaginal births in American hospitals has been nearly 100%. Some doctors cut the mother's skin before the baby's head is even in the birth canal. Doctors have even been known to perform episiotomies after the baby's head has emerged spontaneously – so convinced are they that this surgery must be done.

Most midwives and some progressive doctors gently massage the perineum, applying oil or hot compresses to ease the tissues around the baby's head.

Why has the genital mutilation of episiotomy taken over the American birthing scene?

---

31   Kline-Graber G, Graber B. Woman's Orgasm. *Popular Library.* 1975; 9: 99.

The traditional position in which a woman is placed on the delivery table, flat on her back with legs spread-eagled up in the air in stirrups gives her less control over her body and hampers her ability to give birth naturally. When birth takes place in a bed or mat on the floor – which is the choice for most women giving birth at home or in birth centers – she is free to assume whatever position she desires. Less stress is placed on the perineum, particularly if she assumes a side lying or hands and knees position.

Doctors are trained to do episiotomies, and tend to assume that this is a necessary procedure. Some do not know how to deliver a baby without doing this. Perhaps for a male doctor, massaging a woman's perineum seems too personal and time-consuming. Doing a quick surgical cut and repairing it is a more impersonal "medical" procedure, which more readily fits into his or her way of thinking.

Normal vaginal birth is a simple, natural process. Doctors have been accused of turning birth into surgery in order to make their role in birth indispensable and give themselves something to do of a medical nature.

Most importantly, many male doctors readily admit to doing episiotomies "for the husband" on the idea that stitching up the vagina tightly will make future sex relations more stimulating for him. Other countries' practices of infibulation and subsequent "freshening" and tightening of this area following childbirth, ring far too familiar a bell for today's mother who has experienced a typical delivery in an American hospital. Women have been led to believe that they will no longer be sexually desirable after childbirth unless this operation is done. However, the first attempts at intercourse following a still-healing episiotomy, even if it offers a degree of "tightness" for her husband or partner, usually involve considerable pain and tension for her and consequently will bring about less pleasure for either partner.[32]

The discomfort that a man feels when recovering from adult circumcision appears to be similar to the pain and soreness that a woman experiences following an episiotomy. Interestingly, many male doctors advocate infant circumcision on the grounds that it is "so painful for a grown man to be circumcised," yet regularly give women episiotomies with little or no concern for *their* discomfort. One medical doctor who has been a popular proponent of natural childbirth advises expectant parents that "Newborn babies pay little attention" to being circumcised, and tells husbands "... do not let your wife build up a mighty issue over these simple little cuts" (episiotomies),[33] but that "... swelling and pain is terrific ..." [34] when grown men have circumcisions. Apparently the thinking of our male-dominated medical profession

---

32 Haire D (Co-President International Childbirth Education Association). The Cultural Warping of Childbirth. *ICEA News. 1972;* special issue: 24.
33 Bradley RA. Ch. 8: Does My Wife Have To Be Cut? In: *Husband-Coached Childbirth – If We Have a Boy, Should He Be Circumcised?* NY: Harper & Row; 1965: 142.
34 Ibid., p. 159.

has been that only grown men have feelings – and that women and infants do not have feelings worthy of consideration!

Like many other medical interventions in birth, episiotomy is justified in a small percentage of cases, perhaps 5-10% of all vaginal births. A breech birth or a sudden drop in fetal heart tones indicates the need to deliver the baby as quickly as possible and an episiotomy will speed up this process. A large baby and a tight, unrelaxed perineum or a frantic, uncooperative mother may also indicate need for episiotomy. Most midwives want to be trained and equipped to do episiotomies if necessary, but wish to reserve its use to cases of true need rather than making it a routine procedure.

2.5   Conclusion

As a woman, and mother of two daughters, I find the descriptions of female genital mutilation horrifying and can only approach them with gratitude that for many people these practices have fallen into antiquity. However, with my primary concern being circumcision of infant males in this country, I am also acutely aware of the discrepancy over the fact that tremendous protest and public outrage has been expressed over the practice of female genital mutilation in other countries, while we are still struggling to develop similar awareness and outrage over the male genital mutilation that is rampant in our own country!

I have no interest in having myself or my daughters circumcised. I believe that they and I are capable of keeping ourselves clean and can function normally in our natural states. I never realized that female hygiene was so "complicated." Women are rarely given specific instructions for cleaning themselves or for caring for the genitals of their infant daughters. In actuality, female hygiene is *more complicated* than male hygiene since women and girls frequently do not wipe themselves correctly and can contaminate their vaginas with feces.

Perhaps modern-day female circumcision can be of benefit to a few select females. Similarly, perhaps male circumcision can be of benefit to some males. However, if circumcision of either males or females were being done only to people who personally desired it or had true medical need for the operation, both practices would be extremely rare.

2.6   The Question No One Would Answer

A courageous Egyptian feminist tells the truth of her own genital mutilation – and the beginning of a life devoted to saving other women.

"I was six years old that night when I lay in my bed, warm and peaceful in that pleasurable state which lies halfway between wakefulness and sleep. I felt something move under the blankets, something like a huge hand, cold and rough, fumbling over my body, as though looking for something. Almost simultaneously another hand, as cold and as rough and as big as the first one, was clapped over my mouth, to prevent me from screaming.

They carried me to the bathroom. I do not know how many of them there were, nor do I remember their faces, or whether they were women or men. The world seemed enveloped in a dark fog. Perhaps they put some kind of a cover over my eyes. All I remember is that I was frightened and that there were many of them, and that something like an iron grasp caught hold of my hand, and my arms, and my thighs, so that I became unable to resist or even to move. I also remember the icy touch of the bathroom tiles under my naked body and unknown voices and humming sounds interrupted now and then by a rasping metallic sound which reminded me of the butcher when he used to sharpen his knife before slaughtering a sheep for the 'Eid' [festival].

My blood was frozen in my veins. I thought thieves had broken into my room and kidnapped me from my bed. I was afraid they were getting ready to cut my throat, which was what always happened with disobedient girls in the stories my old rural grandmother told.

I strained my ears trying to catch the metallic, rasping sound. The moment it ceased, I felt as though my heart had stopped beating, too. I was unable to see, and somehow my breathing seemed to have stopped. Yet I imagined the rasping sound coming closer and closer to me. Somehow it was not approaching my neck as I had expected, but another part of my body, somewhere below my belly, as though seeking something buried between my thighs. At that very moment, I realized that my thighs had been pulled wide apart, and that each of my legs was being held as far away from the other as possible, as though gripped by steel fingers that never relinquished their pressure. Then suddenly the sharp metallic edge dropped between my thighs and cut off a piece of flesh from my body. I screamed with pain despite the tight hand held over my mouth. The pain was like a searing flare that went through my whole body. After a few moments, I saw a red pool of blood around my hips.

I did not know what they had cut off, and I did not try to find out. I just wept, and called out to my mother for help. But the worst shock of all was when I looked around and found her standing by my side. Yes, it was she. In flesh and blood, right in the midst of these strangers, she was talking to them, and smiling at them, as though they had not just participated in slaughtering her daughter.

They carried me to my bed. Then I saw them catch my four-year-old sister in exactly the same way they had caught me. I cried out with all my might. No! No! I could see my sister's face held between the big rough hands. It had a deathly pallor. Her wide black eyes met mine for a split second, a glance of terror that I can never forget. A moment later, she was gone, behind the door of the bathroom where I had just been. The look we exchanged seemed to say: 'Now we know what it is. Now we know where our tragedy lies. We were born of a special sex, the female sex. We are destined in advance to taste of misery, and to have a part of our body torn away by cold, unfeeling hands.'

My family was not an uneducated Egyptian family. On the contrary, both my parents had been fortunate enough to have a very good education, by the standards of those days. My father was a university graduate and that year had been appointed General Controller of Education for Menoufa, then a province of the Delta region north of Cairo. My mother had been sent to French schools by her father who was director general of army recruitment. Nevertheless, this custom of clitoridectomy for girls was very prevalent then, and no girl could escape having her clitoris excised, regardless of her social class or whether her family lived in a rural or an urban area. When I recovered from the operation and returned to school, I asked my friends about what had happened to me, only to discover that all of them, without exception, had been through the same experience.

For years, the memory of my clitoridectomy continued to track me down like a nightmare. I had a feeling of insecurity, fear of the unknown, waiting for me at every step I took into the future. I did not know if there were other such surprises being stored up for me by my mother and father, or my grandmother, or the people around me. Since that day, society had made me feel that I was a girl, and I saw that the word 'Bint' [girl] when pronounced by anyone was almost always accompanied by a frown.

Time and again I asked myself why girls were made to undergo this barbaric procedure. But I could never get an answer to this question, just as I was never able to get an answer to the questions that had raced around in my mind the day that both my sister and I were clitoridectomized.

Somehow this question seemed to be linked to other things that puzzled me. Why did they favor my brother when it came to food? Why did he have freedom to go out of the house? Why could he laugh at the top of his voice; run and play as much as he wished, when I was not even supposed to look into people's eyes directly? My duties were primarily to help in cleaning house and cooking, in addition to studying. My brother, however, was not expected to do anything but study.

My father was a broad-minded man who tried as best he could to treat his children equally. I used to feel sorry for my young girl relatives when they were forced out of school in order to get married to an old man just because he owned some land, or when their younger brothers could humiliate and beat them because boys could act superior to their sisters. My own brother tried to dominate me, though my mother used to say that a girl is equal to a boy. I used to rebel, sometimes violently, and ask why my brother was accorded privileges not given to me, despite the fact that I was doing better than he was at school. Neither my mother nor my father ever had any answer except: 'It is so.' I would retort: 'Why should it be so?' and back would come the answer, unchanged: 'Because it is so.'

Even after I grew up and graduated as a doctor in 1955, I could not forget the painful incident that made me lose my childhood, that deprived me during my youth and for years of married life from enjoying the fullness of my sexuality and the completeness of life that can only come from psychological equilibrium. Nightmares followed me throughout the years, especially during the period when I was working as a medical doctor in rural areas where I often had to treat young girls who had come to the outpatients' clinic bleeding profusely after this mutilation. Many died as a result of the primitive way in which clitoridectomies were performed. Others were afflicted with acute or chronic infections from which they sometimes suffered for the rest of their lives. And most, if not all, became the victims of sexual or mental distortions later on as a result of this savage experience.

My profession also led me to examine patients from other Arab countries where excision of all external genitals and even infibulation are practiced, and where I found even worse stories than those I had experienced and seen at home. In Egypt, the removal of the clitoris is often not complete. Sometimes only the tip is cut – a modification of the operation practiced by educated parents who understand the sexual and psychological dangers of total excision, but who feel prevented by tradition from not doing the operation at all.

Although the practice is declining rapidly in Egyptian cities, clitoridectomy is still done regularly in the villages.[35] Clitoridectomy is only one of the measures by which the patriarchy reinforces the values of monogamy. Up until recently in some parts of Egypt, a woman could be killed if she was not a virgin on her wedding night and a wife could be killed if she was unfaithful to her husband. Because the woman has a powerful sexuality, the male-class society must enforce

---

35 The Cairo Family Planning Association held a seminar, "Bodily Mutilation of Young Females," [in 1979] and concluded that "female circumcision" is medically and psychologically harmful. The meeting called for a national campaign to educate and involve parents, medical staff, women's associations, and religious scholars, and to formulate legislation.

monogamy with powerful measures – physically, psychologically, morally, and legally.

Since the day of my terror, I have realized that I had to find my own answer to the question that no one would answer. From that day extends a long path that has led to these words."

Nawal el Saadawi

Nawal el Saadawi is an Egyptian physician and writer who is well known throughout the Arab world for her books on the status, psychology, and sexuality of women, and her novels and short stories.

Before 1972, these works were published in Egypt where Dr. Saadawi worked, first in rural areas, then in Cairo hospitals, and finally as director of education in the Ministry of Health; she was also the editor of Health *magazine. The publication of her book,* Women and Sex, *led to her dismissal as both director and editor, and her work was no longer accepted for publication in her own country. Now published in Lebanon, her books remain best-sellers in most Arab countries, but are forbidden in Saudi Arabia and Libya. Only one of her books is available in English.*

At 48, Dr. Saadawi continues to write and to organize. She was a founder of the African Women's Association for Research and Development in 1977 and is now director of the African Training and Research Center for Women (United Nations Economic Commission for Africa) in Addis Ababa, Ethiopia.

Reprinted, with permission, from *Ms.* Magazine, March 1980, p. 68-69.

2.7 Female Circumcision: Indications and A New Technique

This Chapter 2.7 is quoted from Rathmann WG. GP. 1959-09: 20(3): 115-20:

"Redundancy or phimosis of the female prepuce can prevent proper enjoyment of sexual relations; yet some modern physicians overlook indications for circumcision. Indications for, and relative contraindications against, use of this procedure are presented, and a new technique is described. Properly carried out, circumcision should bring improvement to 85 to 90 per cent of cases – with resulting cure of psychosomatic illness and prevention of divorces."

2 – Female Circumcision

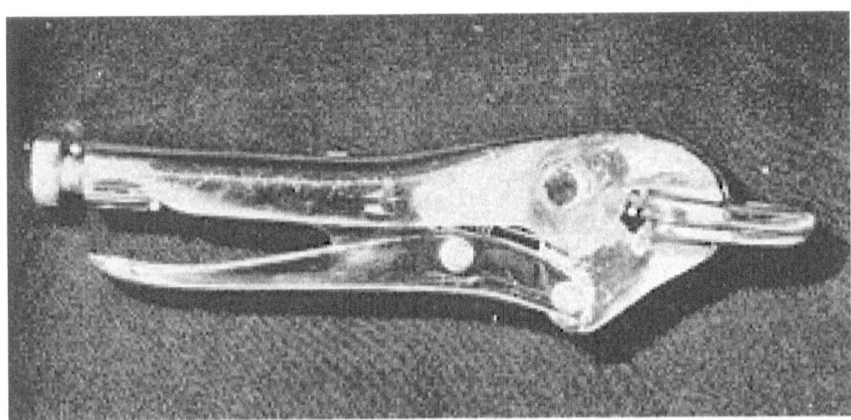

Fig. 1: Jaws closed.

2.7.1 Instrument for Female Circumcision

"Note the adjustment screw on tip of handle to adjust the pressure applied by the jaws. After the surgeon clamps the instrument, it remains in place without effort. The instrument is seven inches long."

For comparison of medical instruments used for male foreskin amputation, see noharmm.org/instruments.htm on the web.

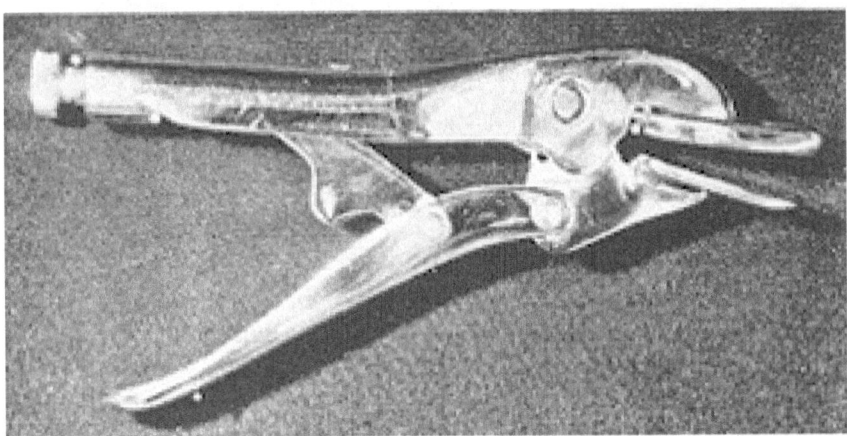

Fig. 2: Jaws open.

Circumcision – The Painful Dilemma

2.7.2 Technique of Circumcision

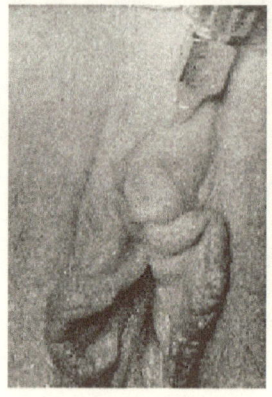
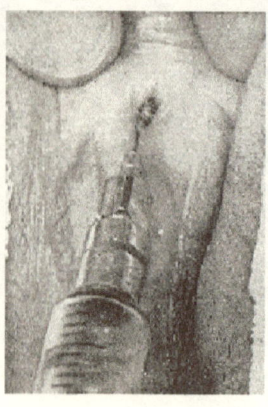
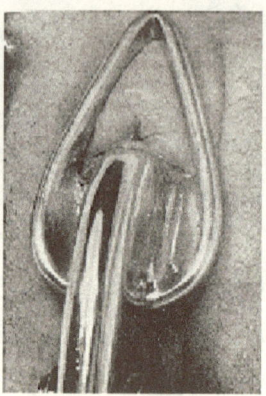

Fig. 3: Site of entry for the first four injections

Fig. 4: Injecting close to each side of clitoris. Site of clitoris marked with dye

Fig. 5: Phimosis freed, redundant prepuce clamped four or five minutes

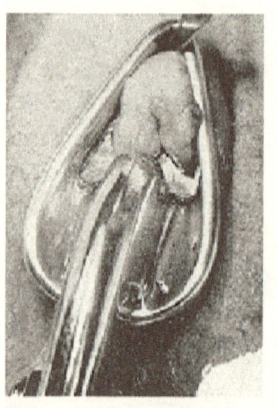
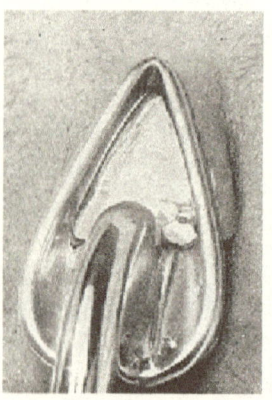
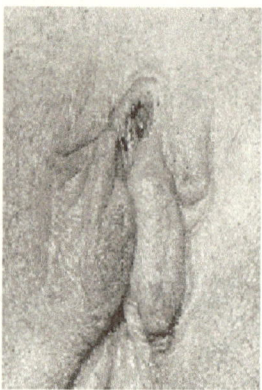

Fig. 6: Excision, prepuce within clamp

Fig. 7: Appearance before removing clamp

Fig. 8: Clamp removed. Compare with Figure 5

"It seems that such a relatively minor procedure should not require much detailed description. However, the fear of scar tissue formation, bleeding and the lack of a descriptive technique in the usual surgery texts, might prevent some physicians from attempting it. A few lines will be devoted to my previous technique, then a more simplified technique will be described.

Allow two weeks before the next menstrual period. Give ¾ gr. seconal one-half hour prior to surgery. Trilene inhalation makes the injection of 2 per cent Xylocaine or Nesacaine less painful. Most of the injection for adequate anesthesia can be made from one point, starting at the mid-line, about one inch anterior to the edge of the prepuce. The first injection is made three-eighths inch deep, to each side of the clitoris (Figure 3). Without removing the needle from the skin, the anesthetic is then injected subcutaneously to the base of the lateral attachment of the prepuce. The needle is then removed and injections are directed cephalad, as close as possible to the sides of the clitoris (Figure 4). This latter injection reduces the discomfort of separating the phimosis. The clitoris itself is not injected.

The prepuce is then freed with a blunt probe. More Trilene is occasionally needed at this time, but the rest of the surgery should be painless. The operative area is resterilized.

In the past, two long mosquito forceps were used to help perform the circumcision. They maintained the proper relationship of the internal and external skin layers and controlled the bleeding prior to suturing. Because the procedure was technically difficult and time consuming, I developed a clamp to be used for the procedure (Figures 1 and 2)."

2.7.3   Clamp for Procedure

"This instrument is seen with jaws open in Figure 2 and closed in Figure 1. It is simply a 'vise-grip' pliers with strong, specially designed jaws for this procedure. After opening, the lower triangular plate or jaw (which is not perforated), is placed under the prepuce and the jaws are partially closed. A tooth thumb forceps is then used to reach through the hole in the upper jaw and pull the desired amount of prepuce into the clamp (Figure 5). The adjusting screw on the handle of the pliers can be turned to adjust for the various thicknesses of prepuce before the pliers are clamped. The cam action not only exerts adequate pressure to compress the tissues at the narrow lower edge of the upper jaw, but also sets itself so that no more force is needed by the operator.

After a lapse of five minutes, the surgeon uses a scalpel to excise the prepuce within the upper jaw, being careful to stay close to the inner wall of the clamp (Figure 6). After the triangular piece of excised prepuce is removed, only the lower blade can be seen (Figure 7). The jaws are then opened and the clamp removed. On a thin prepuce, sutures are not necessary (Figure 8). When there is a doubt whether they are needed, however, the edge is reinforced with a few 5-0 plain catgut sutures on an atraumatic needle. This technique is extremely simple, accurate and bloodless. It has given excellent results because of the reduced healing time and absence of scar tissue."

Author's Addendum:

2.8 In Regards to Male Genital Mutilation vs. Female Genital Mutilation

In recent years there has been a considerable and well justified outcry over the many forms of cutting of female genitalia.

Immigrants to the U.S., primarily from Moslem countries, have wished to continue their centuries old custom. During the 1990's the American Academy of Pediatrics attempted to approve of a ritual nick of the genitalia of young girls, not out of medical need but of social custom for these people. Vast public opposition to this caused the AAP to withdraw their approval and in 1997 a law was passed making all forms of female genital mutilation illegal in the U.S. Sadly the custom still persists in the Moslem world and among some African tribes. In the U.S. some still do it illegally, sometimes sending their daughters outside of the country to undergo circumcision. (Sadly in 2018 a judge declared the U.S. law against female genital mutilation "unconstitutional" and acquitted the doctor who had been charged with performing this act.)

Countless feminists have joined the chorus of opponents of female genital mutilation. Sadly, when those of us who also oppose male genital mutilation have tried to chime in, too often we've been met with scorn and denial. Our only answer has to be "pure cultural blindness." Female genital mutilation, however accepted and embraced it may be in cultures other than our own, is universally repugnant and abhorrent to American eyes. There is no question but to forbid it. The male counterpart has been deeply culturally ingrained in the U.S. as the unquestioned norm. I once received a phone call from a man asking "Why would anybody be opposed to circumcision?" The concept has blinded our sensibilities. The challenge to crawl out of our fog of apathy and confusion, to question how we treat our children, to respect the human body in its original form, and to accept our sexuality in its fullness, has been a decades long struggle.

Some feminist voices have been angry when male rights against genital mutilation have been introduced. Hence there are feminist mothers who parade and protest for female freedom from genital mutilation, yet have passively accepted society's urges when their own sons were born and unquestionably circumcised. The following is my answer:

We are all one humanity. Society has many unfair situations which must be questioned and changed. Some inequities favor males, others favor females. But we are all together in this universe. We all exist from equal input from a father and a mother. We all begin, in our embryonic state, with equal equipment eventually morphing into ovaries, vaginas and uteri, or penises and testes. The majority of us form hetero–sexual unions. Regardless of our sexual orientation, we all form friendships with people of both genders. Every fertile woman is capable of conceiving and birthing a child of either gender. I doubt that there is an opponent of male genital mutilation (aka circumcision) that does not also oppose the female counterpart. One gender pitted against the other will get us nowhere. Intactivism comprises an equal amount of male and female voices.

2.9 Informational Resources

- 18 U.S. Code § 116. Female genital mutilation: law.cornell.edu/uscode/text/18/116
- 3 Survivors Reveal the Brutal Reality of Female Genital Mutilation:
    cosmopolitan.com/lifestyle/advice/a6504/female-genital-mutilation-survivor-stories
- 50 years on, Canada lawyer yet to get over her circumcision trauma: timesofindia.indiatimes.com/city/
    mumbai/50-years-on-canada-lawyer-yet-to-get-over-her-circumcision-trauma/articleshow/50884200.cms
- "A Tiny Cut": Female Circumcision in South East Asia:
    theislamicmonthly.com/a-tiny-cut-female-circumcision-in-south-east-asia
- Alternative to Genital Mutilation Emerges For Kenya's Maasai Girls:
    hooded2016.wordpress.com/2016/03/29/alternative-to-genital-mutilation-emerges-for-kenyas-maasai-girls
- America's Forgotten History of Female Circumcision: sites.google.com/site/completebaby/female
- Anatomy: Development of the Male and Female Foreskin:
    hooded2016.wordpress.com/2016/03/28/anatomy-development-of-the-male-and-female-foreskin
- Between moral relativism and moral hypocrisy: reframing the debate on "FGM": academia.edu/10197867
- Boys and girls alike: aeon.co/essays/are-male-and-female-circumcision-morally-equivalent
- British girls undergo horror of genital mutilation despite tough laws:
    theguardian.com/society/2010/jul/25/female-circumcision-children-british-law
- Circumcision in the Female: Its Necessity and How to Perform It: noharmm.org/CircintheFemale.htm
- Circumcision Is Male Genital Mutilation: returntonow.net/2016/05/10/circumcision-male-genital-mutilation
- Circumcision of Males / Females:
    canadiancrc.com/Circumcision_Genital_Mutilation_Male-Female_Children.aspx
- Circumcision of the Female: noharmm.org/circumfemale.htm
- Debates about FGM in Africa, the Middle East & Far East: religioustolerance.org/fem_cirm.htm
- Doctor Testifies Surgeon Secretly Circumcised Woman: cirp.org/news/1996.10.30_Turner
- Double Standard: dropbox.com/s/gcwd6dof26x9gyc/1380094_598713180178190_1272291232_n.jpg
- Female Circumcision and Clitoridectomy in the United States: A History of a Medical Treatment:

amazon.com/dp/158046498X
- Female Circumcision as Sexual Therapy: The Past and Future of Plastic Surgery?:
  hooded2016.wordpress.com/2016/04/07/female-circumcision-as-sexual-therapy-the-past-and-future-of-plastic-surgery
- Female Circumcision: Indications and a New Technique: noharmm.org/femcirctech.htm
- Female genital mutilation: forwarduk.org.uk/violence-against-women-and-girls/female-genital-mutilation
- Female Genital Mutilation – Professional Neglect; Legitimate Moral Panic:
  hilaryburrage.com/2012/05/05/fgm-professional-neglect-legitimate-moral-panic
- Female Genital Mutilation (FGM): plan-international.org/sexual-health/fgm-female-genital-mutilation
- Female genital mutilation (FGM) and male circumcision: should there be a separate ethical discourse?:
  blog.practicalethics.ox.ac.uk/2014/02/female-genital-mutilation-and-male-circumcision-time-to-confront-the-double-standard
- Female genital mutilation (FGM) frequently asked questions:
  unfpa.org/resources/female-genital-mutilation-fgm-frequently-asked-questions
- Female Genital Mutilation (FGM): What You Need To Know: globalgiving.org/fgm
- Female Genital Mutilation *(Google: huge assortment of images)*:
  google.com/search?q=female+genital+mutilations&source=lnms&tbm=isch
- Female genital mutilation *(WHO)*: who.int/en/news-room/fact-sheets/detail/female-genital-mutilation
- Female genital mutilation *(Wikipedia)*: en.wikipedia.org/wiki/Female_genital_mutilation
- Female Genital Mutilation and Male Circumcision – Don't Compare Them?: hooded2016.wordpress.com/2016/04/22/female-genital-mutilation-and-male-circumcision-dont-compare-them
- Female Genital Mutilation In Britain: Professional Culpability, Public Responsibility, Private Peril:
  hilaryburrage.com/2012/04/29/fgm-in-britain-professional-culpability-public-responsibility-private-peril
- Female Genital Mutilation Is Child Abuse Too; So Why NO Enquiries About Ignoring It?: hilaryburrage.com/2012/10/25/female-genital-mutilation-is-child-abuse-too-so-why-no-enquiries-about-ignoring-it
- Female Genital Mutilation on the Rise in the U.S.: newsweek.com/fgm-rates-have-doubled-us-2004-304773
- Female genital mutilation on the rise in the United States: news.trust.org/item/20130311121900-e7lda
- Female genital mutilation or cutting: womenshealth.gov/a-z-topics/female-genital-cutting
- Female Genital Mutilation: The Difficult Debates:
  hilaryburrage.com/2012/05/11/fgm-the-difficult-debates-female-international
- Female Genital Mutilation: The Reason Of My Sleepless Nights. No Girl Should Ever Face What I Faced!:
  hooded2016.wordpress.com/2016/03/27/female-genital-mutilation-the-reason-of-my-sleepless-nights-no-girl-should-ever-face-what-i-faced
- Female Genital Mutilation: What It Does To A Woman:
  npr.org/sections/goatsandsoda/2017/05/06/526766230/female-genital-mutilation-what-it-does-to-a-woman
- Female Genital Mutilation: Why Does This 'Holiday' Horror Endure?:
hilaryburrage.com/2012/09/10/female-genital-mutilation-why-does-this-holiday-horror-endure
- Female genital mutilation: Why Egyptian girls fear the summer:
  edition.cnn.com/2015/06/25/middleeast/egypt-female-genital-mutilation

- Female Genital Mutilation/Cutting: A Global Concern:
  unicef.org/media/files/FGMC_2016_brochure_final_UNICEF_SPREAD.pdf
- Feminine and masculine sexual mutilation, the greatest crime against humanity: academia.edu/2095540
- Feminism, sexism and sexual mutilation: academia.edu/1006015
- FGM defended on the same grounds as MGM: circumstitions.com/FGM-defended.html
- FGM: 'My daughter will never be cut. It stops with me':
  theguardian.com/society/2014/dec/13/fgm-my-daughter-will-never-be-cut-it-stops-with-me#show-all
- FGM/MGM: Similar Attitudes & Misconceptions:
  www.drmomma.org/2010/06/fgmmgm-similar-attitudes-misconceptions.html
- Forced infant circumcision harms transsexual women too:
  hooded2016.wordpress.com/2016/03/27/forced-infant-circumcision-harms-transexual-women-too
- History of Female Circumcision in the United States:
  www.drmomma.org/2009/09/history-of-female-circumcision-in.html
- "I think male circumcision is worse than an incision of the girl.":
  thelibertarianrepublic.com/think-male-circumcision-worse-incision-girl-aayan-hirsi-ali
- Is Female Genital Mutilation an Islamic Problem?:
  meforum.org/1629/is-female-genital-mutilation-an-islamic-problem
- Kenya: 20 girls forcefully circumcised in FGM saga:
  thisisafrica.me/politics-and-society/20-girls-14-forcefully-circumcised-kenya
- Legislation on Female Genital Mutilation in the United States:
  reproductiverights.org/sites/default/files/documents/pub_bp_fgmlawsusa.pdf
- Male and Female Circumcision: www.drmomma.org/2011/04/male-and-female-circumcision.html
- MGM/FGM A Visual Comparison: www.drmomma.org/2008/01/mgmfgm-visual-comparison.html
- My Submission To The UK Home Affairs Parliamentary Select Committee Inquiry On Female Genital Mutilation: hilaryburrage.com/2014/02/12/my-submission-to-the-uk-home-affairs-parliamentary-select-committee-inquiry-on-female-genital-mutilation
- Nigeria's female genital mutilation ban is important precedent, say campaigners: theguardian.com/society/2015/may/29/outlawing-fgm-nigeria-hugely-important-precedent-say-campaigners
- #NoFGM: A Listing For Action & References On Female Genital Mutilation:
  hilaryburrage.com/2012/06/25/nofgm-a-listing-for-uk-action-references-on-female-genital-mutilation
- Obama calls for end to female genital mutilation in Africa while US has highest rates of male circumcision:
  nhregister.com/columns/article/Forum-Obama-calls-for-end-to-female-genital-11341360.php
- Politically Correct Research: When Science, Morals and Political Agendas Collide:
  joseph4gi.com/2013/02/politically-correct-research-when.html
- Posttraumatic Stress Disorder and Memory Problems After Female Genital Mutilation:
  taskforcefgm.de/wp-content/uploads/2010/03/FGM__Trauma.pdf
- Schools Must Safeguard Girls From FGM; But How?:
  hilaryburrage.com/2014/07/26/schools-must-safeguard-girls-from-fgm-but-how
- Support for female circumcision stirs controversy in US: smh.com.au/lifestyle/health-and-wellness/support-

- for-female-circumcision-stirs-controversy-in-us-20100521-w1uz.html
- The Childhood Origins of Terrorism:
  psychohistory.com/books/the-emotional-life-of-nations/chapter-3-the-childhood-origins-of-terrorism
- The day I saw 248 girls suffering genital mutilation:
  theguardian.com/society/2012/nov/18/female-genital-mutilation-circumcision-indonesia
- The Gambia bans female genital mutilation:
  theguardian.com/society/2015/nov/24/the-gambia-bans-female-genital-mutilation
- The Number of Victims of Female Genital Mutilation is Much Higher Than We Thought:
  friendlyatheist.patheos.com/2016/02/11/the-number-of-victims-of-female-genital-mutilation-is-much-higher-than-we-thought
- The Other FGM Debate: Is Male Circumcision (MGM) Also Child Abuse?:
  hilaryburrage.com/2012/06/03/the-other-fgm-debate-is-male-circumcision-also-child-abuse
- The Other Side Of The Circumcision Debate: huffpost.com/entry/895132
- The role of men in abandonment of female genital mutilation:
  bmcpublichealth.biomedcentral.com/articles/10.1186/s12889-015-2373-2
- To Mutilate in the Name of Jehovah or Allah: Legitimization of Male and Female Circumcision:
  pubmed.ncbi.nlm.nih.gov/7731348
- Under Debate: Female Circumcision: scienceline.org/2010/07/under-debate-female-circumcision
- What is female genital mutilation and where does it happen?:
  theguardian.com/society/2014/feb/06/what-is-female-genital-mutilation-where-happen
- What Is Female Genital Mutilation? An Introduction To The Issues, And Suggested Reading: hilaryburrage.com/2016/04/01/female-genital-mutilation-an-introduction-to-the-issues-and-suggested-reading
- What is FGM?: endfgm.eu/female-genital-mutilation/what-is-fgm
- What is FGM? Everything you need to know about female genital mutilation:
  independent.co.uk/life-style/health-and-families/health-news/what-fgm-everything-you-need-know-about-female-genital-mutilation-9580935.html
- Why circumcision is the same as FGM *(Peter Lloyd, The Suffragent)*:
  hooded2016.wordpress.com/2016/03/31/peter-lloydthe-suffragent-why-circumcision-is-the-same-as-fgm
- Women were circumcised to stop harassing men for 'vigorous action in bed' – Migori Doctor:
  hooded2016.wordpress.com/2016/04/07/women-were-circumcised-to-stop-harassing-men-for-vigorous-action-in-bed-migori-doctor
- Would you circumcise your daughter?:
  womanuncensored.blogspot.com/2009/12/would-you-circumcise-your-daughter.html

Videos:

- "Circumcision is OK" say women and men: youtu.be/wcJNAtn-c6I
- FGM (Female Genital Mutilation): youtu.be/nBvqW9Jde7A

3 Circumcision and Judaism

GENESIS: CH. 17:
7 AND I WILL ESTABLISH MY COVENANT BETWEEN ME AND THEE AND THY SEED AFTER THEE.
8 AND I WILL GIVE UNTO THEE, AND TO THY SEED AFTER THEE, THE LAND WHEREIN THOU ART A STRANGER, ALL THE LAND OF CANAAN, FOR AN EVERLASTING POSSESSION; AND I WILL BE THEIR GOD.
9 AND GOD SAID UNTO ABRAHAM THOU SHALT KEEP MY COVENANT THEREFORE, THOU AND THY SEED AFTER THEE IN THEIR GENERATIONS.
10 THIS IS MY COVENANT WHICH YE SHALL KEEP, BETWEEN ME AND YOU AND THY SEED AFTER THEE: EVERY MAN CHILD AMONG YOU SHALL BE CIRCUMCISED.
11 AND YE SHALL CIRCUMCISE THE FLESH OF YOUR FORESKIN, AND IT SHALL BE A TOKEN OF THE COVENANT BETWIXT ME AND YOU.
12 AND HE THAT IS EIGHT DAYS OLD SHALL BE CIRCUMCISED AMONG YOU, EVERY MAN CHILD IN YOUR GENERATIONS, HE THAT IS BORN IN THE HOUSE, OR BOUGHT WITH MONEY OF ANY STRANGER, WHICH IS NOT OF THY SEED.
13 HE THAT IS BORN IN THY HOUSE, AND HE THAT IS BOUGHT WITH THY MONEY, MUST NEEDS BE CIRCUMCISED: AND MY COVENANT SHALL BE IN YOUR FLESH FOR AN EVERLASTING COVENANT.
14 AND THE UNCIRCUMCISED MAN CHILD WHOSE FLESH OF HIS FORESKIN IS NOT CIRCUMCISED, THAT SOUL SHALL BE CUT OFF FROM HIS PEOPLE; HE HATH BROKEN MY COVENANT [...]
23 AND ABRAHAM TOOK ISHMAEL HIS SON, AND ALL THAT WERE BORN IN HIS HOUSE AND CIRCUMCISED THE FLESH OF THEIR FORESKIN IN THE SELFSAME DAY AS GOD HAD SAID UNTO HIM.
24 AND ABRAHAM WAS NINETY YEARS OLD AND NINE WHEN HE WAS CIRCUMCISED IN THE FLESH OF HIS FORESKIN.
25 AND ISHMAEL HIS SON WAS THIRTEEN YEARS OLD, WHEN HE WAS CIRCUMCISED IN THE FLESH OF HIS FORESKIN.
26 IN THE SELFSAME DAY WAS ABRAHAM CIRCUMCISED, AND ISHMAEL HIS SON.
27 AND ALL THE MEN OF HIS HOUSE, BORN IN THE HOUSE, AND BOUGHT WITH MONEY OF THE STRANGER, WERE CIRCUMCISED WITH HIM.[1]

The origin of circumcision is lost in prehistory, but it predates the Biblical account by at least thousands of years. Biblical scholars, estimating when Abraham

---
1 Genesis: Ch. 17: 7-14, 23-27.

Circumcision – The Painful Dilemma

must have lived, based on the proclaimed lifespans of subsequent patriarchs, at some point decided that if such a covenant actually occurred, it must have happened around 1713 B.C.[2] The Biblical account, however, is part of the late Priestly Code which was written during the fifth century B.C.[3] Therefore, the story of the Abrahamic covenant was repeated orally through countless generations before it was written down in the account that we know of as Genesis.

Although faithful Jews accept this agreement between Abraham and God as a literal event, some more skeptical scholars believe Jewish leaders at some point may have decided that circumcision of Jewish males would ensure that Jewish identity would never be compromised by the contrary beliefs of other surrounding societies.

Moses, who was raised by the Egyptians who did not circumcise infants, apparently was never circumcised. A mysterious account appears in Exodus, in which God becomes angry about Moses' lack of circumcision, and Moses' wife, Zipporah remedies the situation:

EXODUS: CH. 4:

24 AND IT CAME TO PASS BY THE WAY OF THE INN, THAT THE LORD MET HIM AND SOUGHT TO KILL HIM [MOSES].

25 THEN ZIPPORAH TOOK A SHARP STONE AND CUT OFF THE FORESKIN OF HER SON, AND CAST IT AT HIS FEET, AND SAID "SURELY A BLOODY HUSBAND THOU ART TO ME." SO HE LET HIM GO; THEN SHE SAID, "A BLOODY HUSBAND THOU ART, BECAUSE OF THE CIRCUMCISION." [4]

It appears that despite the covenant with Abraham, circumcision was practiced only sporadically by the Hebrews during ancient times. Under Joshua, several generations later, circumcision took on a new meaning. Joshua was instrumental in making the ritual obligatory for all Israelites. Evidently all the Hebrew males that came out of Egypt were circumcised, but those born in the wilderness during the forty year aftermath were not circumcised. Therefore God called upon Joshua to enforce circumcision upon all the people. From thereon, circumcision became universal among the Hebrews.[5]

There is also a Biblical account of an outrageous misuse of circumcision. A number of soldiers were conquered in a battle and subsequently circumcised. Then, three days later, when the men were too sore to fight, Simeon and Levi, Dinah's brethren, "took each man his sword, and came upon the city and slew all the males." [6]

---

2 Waszak SJ. The Historic Significance of Circumcision. *Obstet Gynecol.* 1978-04; 51(4): 500.
3 *Interpreter's Dictionary of the Bible*, Vol. I., p. 629.
4 Exodus: Ch. 4: 24-6.
5 Joshua: Ch. 5: 2-9.
6 Genesis: Ch. 35: 24-5.

Further on in the Old Testament, mention is made of the metaphorical "circumcision of the heart." In other words, mere cutting of the flesh is not enough without inner fervor and commitment to the religion's ideals. Jeremiah especially preached this message:

JEREMIAH: CH. 4:
4 CIRCUMCISE YOURSELVES TO THE LORD, AND TAKE AWAY THE FORESKINS OF YOUR HEART, YE MEN OF JUDAH AND INHABITANTS OF JERUSALEM.[7]

The unsolved riddle is *why* ...? Why does a religion with the dignity of Judaism, one of the major religions of the world with widespread influence in Western thought, place central importance upon cutting off part of the penis?

3.1 Blood Taboos

Fears and superstitions about blood have prevailed among many primitive peoples. Fear of blood pollution is mentioned repeatedly in the Old Testament.
One writer explains:

> "The sight of blood brought consternation into the mind of primitive man. He was unable to account for its mysterious power. In one moment he saw a person flushed with life and strength; in another moment he saw this same person inert, motionless, helpless and dead, only because the blood had oozed from his body. He was dead beyond all efforts to revive or resuscitate ...
>
> Primitive man was awed by the puzzling element of life that was in that blood. He began to fear it. Thus was born the superstitious belief that blood had power within itself to wreak vengeance or bring injury upon another. For fear of being contaminated by the mysterious power inherent in blood, primitive man could conceive of no other way to avoid contamination than by making taboo those capable of polluting others; and if contaminated, then some form of blood expiation was necessary for purification ... primitive belief of blood contamination brought into existence elaborate and myriad forms of blood expiation, from that of uttering a prayer upon the killing of an animal to the cutting off of the foreskin of a male child, on the eighth day (after) its birth." [8]

In particular, concern about blood contamination and impurities was directed toward any woman with an "issue of blood" such as during menstruation and following

---

7   Jeremiah: Ch. 4: 4.
8   Lewis J. *In The Name of Humanity!* NY: Eugenics Publishing; 1956: xii-xiii (preface).

childbirth. In Leviticus, laws that concerned blood taboos surrounding menstruation and postpartum bleeding are clearly written out. Anything that is touched by a woman who is menstruating, recently delivered, or otherwise bleeding vaginally is considered unclean. Anything that she lies on or sits on is contaminated. Anyone who touches her bed or anything that she has sat on must wash his clothes and bathe himself. If a man has sex with her during this time he is considered unclean for seven days. After the woman has finished bleeding she is still unclean for seven days. "Nidah" is the name given to this traditional Jewish practice (today largely abandoned) by which women abstain from sexual relations during menstruation and for seven days thereafter. The period of abstinence is followed by a ritual, "purifying" bath called "mikvah" before she and her husband can resume marital relations.[9]

These fears and taboos surrounding women's vaginal bleeding were obviously a manifestation of an extremely patriarchal society which considered women inferior beings. In regards to the postpartum period, the law states:

LEVITICUS: CH. 12:

2 SPEAK UNTO THE CHILDREN OF ISRAEL SAYING, IF A WOMAN HAVE CONCEIVED SEED, AND BORNE A MAN CHILD, THEN SHE SHALL BE UNCLEAN SEVEN DAYS: ACCORDING TO THE DAYS OF THE SEPARATION FOR HER INFIRMITY SHALL SHE BE UNCLEAN.

3 AND IN THE EIGHTH DAY THE FLESH OF HIS FORESKIN SHALL BE CIRCUMCISED.

4 AND SHE SHALL THEN CONTINUE IN THE BLOOD OF HER PURIFYING THREE AND THIRTY DAYS: SHE SHALL TOUCH NO HALLOWED THING, NOR COME INTO THE SANCTUARY, UNTIL THE DAYS OF HER PURIFYING BE FULFILLED.[10]

The infant boy, of necessity, had to be in contact with his mother following birth. Some authors have interpreted the above passage in Leviticus to mean that the newborn infant boy was considered "unclean" due to contact with his mother who was bleeding, and the blood of his circumcision was an "atonement" for this impurity ... a protection against evil forces.

It must be noted that today, with modern plumbing, disposable sanitary pads and tampons, menstruation and postpartum bleeding can be dealt with easily. In a primitive land without flushing toilets, showers, or modern sanitary products, the same process was certainly much more disagreeable. Additionally, women can die from excessive postpartum bleeding. Today such hemorrhages can be treated readily with medications and procedures which were not available to primitive peoples. Occasio-

---

9   Leviticus: Ch. 15: 19-28.
10 Leviticus: Ch. 12: 2-4.

nal encounters with death from hemorrhage following childbirth also certainly contributed to primitive peoples' fear of this bleeding.

Yet another consideration – among peoples who practiced early marriage, repeated pregnancies, large families, and prolonged breastfeeding, most women did not experience regular menstrual cycles. Usually only the barren woman, who was in a position of shame and sorrow, experienced regular monthly periods. Therefore menstruation was a less familiar occurrence to such people and when it did occur it was often connected with the stigma of being unable to conceive.

But is the "impurity" of the mother's postpartum bleeding the true, original reason for the circumcision of Jewish infant males? At best it appears to be only a partial explanation.

Most historians believe that circumcision of male infants by the Jews was preceded by the practice of adolescent circumcision. Therefore it cannot have *begun* as a postpartum blood taboo. Also, when the Abrahamic covenant was established and Abraham circumcised himself and his son Ishmael, there was no menstruating or recently delivered woman around to necessitate a "blood atonement."

If baby boys were considered in a state of danger and impurity from the mother's postpartum blood, and therefore in need of circumcision, why wasn't a similar rite necessary for equally "contaminated" baby girls? Were female children not "important" enough to warrant such "consideration?" Were infant girls at one time circumcised, but the practice proved too dangerous for females? Were mothers able to protect their girl children from this painful procedure, but lacked similar control over the fate of their male children?

Women also had to care for their children during menstruation, but children were not made to go through a similar "purifying" rite every time their mother menstruated. Women frequently had to care for their older children during the postpartum period, but these children were not put through any blood purification rite as a result.

However, the blood shed by the infant during circumcision definitely is an important part of the ritual. The occasional baby born without a foreskin must still have the ceremony with a small amount of blood drawn from his penis or another part of his body. Among Orthodox Jews, modern clamp devices cannot be used for circumcision because they do not allow for enough bleeding.

There are references in Jewish literature which associate the blood shed by the infant during circumcision with the blood of the sacrificial Passover lamb, and also with the blood of the Jewish martyrs.[11, 12]

---

11 Shechet J. *The Layman's Guide to the Covenant of Circumcision.* 1973: 3.
12 Isaac E. The Enigma of Circumcision. *Commentary.* 1967-01; 55.

3.2 The Significance of Cutting

Erich Isaac comments on the act of cutting in itself being an important aspect of the Jewish circumcision ritual:

> "... the ancient custom of using cutting or dismembering rites in connection with treaty and covenant obligations ... Jeremiah mentions a dismembering rite similar to Abraham's first covenant ceremony. The nobility of Judah pledge themselves to set their slaves free by dividing a calf and walking through the parts ... The whole notion of cutting as a covenant sign seems strange to us, for we associate covenants and treaties with binding together. Yet it was the *cutting* of the Gordian knot by Alexander the Great which was to bind Asia and Europe together, and even today we cut silk ribbons when inaugurating bridges and highways. We thereby symbolize the joining together of places that were previously separate. In terms of ancient ritual too, the act of severing was not symbolic of separation, but rather of a prior and subsequent state of wholeness." [13]

3.3 Sacrifice

Blood taboos and atonement interconnect with the concept of sacrifice as related to circumcision. There has been considerable speculation that circumcision either shared a common origin with or developed as a more humane replacement of human sacrifice.

Jewish historical sources often state this clearly:

> "A man who brings his son to be circumcised is to be compared to a High Priest bringing a meal offering and libation to the Temple altar." [14]

> "... By fulfilling the Commandment of Circumcision every person has an opportunity to bring a sacrifice to the Almighty." [15]

Sacrifice of animals in the form of burnt offerings placed upon the altar of the Temple was a frequent practice of the ancient Hebrews. Such a sacrifice was required of a woman following the birth of a child ... further evidence that she was considered to be in a state of "impurity" and in need of "atonement." [16]

---

13 Ibid., p. 54.
14 Hertzberg A. *Judaism*. Washington Square Press. 1961: 75.
15 Schechet, p. 17 (Menoras Haraor).
16 Leviticus: Ch. 12: 6-8

Belief in evil spirits prevailed among the ancient Hebrews. The mother and child were considered in danger during the first eight days prior to circumcision – the operation somehow "warding off" evil spirits.

Carter explains:

"All diseases were manifestations of the wrath of God for transgressions or due to the attack of demons or to the breach of a taboo or to the Evil Eye. The whole world was filled with demons; every phase and every form of life was ruled by them and they had to be cajoled, appeased, bribed and rewarded. ALL people believed in demons, among whom Lilit was a favorite. In the Talmud she is the wife of Adam before Eve was created and became the mother of demons – those creatures whose haunts were 'uncultivated wilds and deserts and bleak summits of mountains.' Lilit was a nocturnal specter bent on mischief. She caused men to waste their seed (semen) and weakened boy babies during the first eight days. (One of the attempts to explain circumcision after the origin had been forgotten may have been inspired by the legend of Lilit.)" [17]

3.4　Fertility

Circumcision was connected with a promise of fertility on the part of God to the Hebrew people. In Genesis it is clearly stated along with the Abrahamic covenant:

"... FOR A FATHER OF MANY NATIONS HAVE I MADE THEE. AND I WILL MAKE THEE EXCEEDINGLY FRUITFUL, AND I WILL MAKE NATIONS OF THEE, AND KINGS SHALL COME OUT OF THEE ..." [18]

Other evidence of the relationship between circumcision and fertility is illustrated in the use of the term "circumcision" in reference to fruit trees and fields to be harvested. In Leviticus mention is made of "uncircumcised" trees, the fruit of such trees being "taboo" during the first three years of production.[19]

Reference is also made to

"... the feast of circumcision of the field ... It is the marriage feast of the field as an introduction to its actual time of fertility." [20]

17　Carter N. *Routine Circumcision: The Tragic Myth.* London, England: Londinium Press. 1979: 26.
18　Genesis: Ch. 17: 5-6.
19　Leviticus: Ch. 19: 23-4.
20　Weiss C. Ritual Circumcision; Comments on Current Practices in American Hospitals. *CLP.* 1962-10; 1(1): 223.

(While "circumcised fields" and "uncircumcised trees" sounds ludicrous to us, undoubtedly much of the meaning is lost in translation!)

All of this indicates the concept that fertility, through circumcision, is not merely a matter of removing a supposed physical handicap of the foreskin as a hindrance to conception, but that the act, or sacrament of circumcision, as a ritual, is being offered in return for the gift of fertility from the deity.

3.5 Identity as a People

Possession of a penis that lacks its foreskin has often served to signify membership within the group for many peoples, including the Jews. This appears to be a result of the practice rather than the original motivation.

The Jews were without a homeland for centuries, until Israel was re-established in the 1940s. Therefore, Jews have been a unique cultural group throughout the world's history. They have frequently been misunderstood, shunned and persecuted for many reasons including their practice of circumcision. Frequently other peoples have forbidden Jews from practicing the rite. Due to both their lack of a homeland throughout the ages and the persecutions that they have suffered for practicing circumcision, the circumcised penis has become a symbol of common identity for Jews. Reverse psychology came into effect, with the attempts of others to put an end to Jewish circumcision making the Jews more determined than ever to perpetuate the rite – while other practices such as sacrificing animals or observance of Nidah have been largely abandoned by Jews today.

Another consideration is the fact that circumcision is an event that occurs only once in an individual's lifetime and is an "all or nothing" condition. Therefore the Jew who is not strongly observant in some aspects of his religion may, for example, eat only Kosher foods during Passover and other special Jewish observances, but eats pork and other non-Kosher foods on ordinary days. But one either has a circumcised penis or he has a penis with its foreskin.

3.6 Why Did the Jews Choose to Circumcise Infants?

The vast majority of circumcisions throughout ancient history were performed on older individuals, usually adolescents during initiation rites, or captured slaves and enemies. Circumcision of infants and small children has been a relatively recent innovation.

Bryk mentions that the Hebrew terminology "hatan" meaning "bridegroom" apparently also means "newly circumcised" and "hoten" – father in law – means the same as "circumciser." [21]

The Biblical account in which Zipporah, to appease the Lord's wrath, circumcises their son, throws the severed foreskin at Moses' feet and calls him a "bloody husband," has been interpreted as meaning "You are now that to me, what you should have been as a bridegroom, that is one consecrated for marriage through such a shedding of blood." [22]

These instances suggest that at one time among the ancient Hebrews, or their predecessors, circumcision was an initiation rite through which the youth became marriageable." [21]

If the rite did begin as a procedure done to adolescents why was it changed to infancy? Young Jewish men observe an "adolescent initiation ritual" – a Bar Mitzvah ceremony when they reach the age of 13. This is preceded by years of study of the Torah and Jewish history. Bar Mitzvah is the official Jewish introduction into "manhood." Did the precursor of this rite include circumcision at age 13 as well? If Jewish boys today were being circumcised at the time of their Bar Mitzvah instead of as infants, would the operation have remained as popular as has infant circumcision? Would our present-day medical profession have been as eager to follow suit and advocate routine circumcision of teen-aged non-Jewish boys?

Bryk comments:

"It is no wonder that the marriageable youth, considering the fear circumcision must have exercised, resisted the establishment of the new custom. It can be determined almost exactly, even among the Jews, how long it took for the custom of circumcision to become firmly established. The young people generally offered opposition to it and had to be coerced by means of whippings, threats of death, and torture." [23]

Therefore it appears that somewhere in prehistory the ancient Hebrews switched to circumcising infants because it was easier. The infant could not put up any resistance, nor express his needs or feelings except by crying. Of course, in ancient times people had no effective anesthesia, suturing, or antiseptic procedures for surgery. Therefore circumcision of older individuals was much more painful and risky than it is today. Perhaps during previous ages the amputation of the foreskin of an infant who healed rapidly and grew up with no conscious memory of the event, did appear more

---

21 Bryk F. *Sex & Circumcision: A Study of Phallic Worship and Mutilation in Men and Women.* North Hollywood, CA: Brandon House; 1967: 36.
22 Ibid., p. 37.
23 Ibid., p. 217.

humane than performing the same procedure on an older child or an adult. However, today with effective modern anesthesia, suturing and sterile techniques, the argument that "circumcision is less painful for babies" is hardly balanced!

The platitude that newborn babies have little or no feelings is not a *new* concept. In the 13th century the Jewish scholar Moses Maimonides comments:

> "This law can only be kept and perpetuated in its perfection, if circumcision is performed when the child is very young, and this for three good reasons. First, if the operation were postponed until the boy had grown up, he would perhaps not submit to it. Secondly, the young child has not much pain, because the skin is tender, and the imagination weak. For grown-up persons are in dread and fear of things which they imagine as coming, some time before these actually occur. Thirdly, when a child is very young, the parents do not think much of him because the image of the child, that leads the parents to love him, has not yet taken a firm root in their minds. That image becomes stronger by the continual sight. It grows with the development of the child, and later on the image begins again to decrease and to vanish. The parents' love for a newborn child is not so great as it is when the child is one year old, and when one year old, it is less loved by them than when six years old. The feeling and love of the father for the child would have led him to neglect the law if he were allowed to wait two or three years, whilst shortly after birth the image is very weak in the mind of the parent, especially of the father who is responsible for the execution of this commandment." [24]

3.7 Why the Eighth Day?

Why has the eighth day of life been the particular day chosen for Jewish circumcision?

In the Bible certain numbers often have had significance. The earlier discussion of circumcision being a blood atonement from the contamination of the mother's postpartum blood mentioned that the baby and mother were considered to be in a state of danger from evil spirits for the first seven days and were then redeemed and purified on the eighth day by circumcision.

Most new mothers are stronger and more recovered from childbirth after the first week. If a newborn baby is not going to survive, he is most likely to succumb during the first few days after birth.

One Jewish scholar quotes:

---

24 Maimonides M. *The Guide for the* Perplexed. NY: Dover Publications; 1956: 378-9.

"... What is the reason that a child is circumcised on the eighth day? Because the Almighty had mercy on the baby and required waiting until the baby gathers his strength ..." [25]

Maimonides comments:

"The circumcision must take place on the eighth day ... because all living beings are after birth, within the first seven days, very weak and exceedingly tender, as if they were still in the womb of their mother. Not until the eighth day can they be counted among those that enjoy the light of the world." [26]

Today it is a known medical fact that newborn babies are deficient in vitamin K, a blood clotting factor, during the first few days of life. Normally vitamin K is produced by intestinal bacteria. For a newborn baby the digestive process is just beginning. Not until after the first week are his intestines fully functioning with vitamin K stores at normal levels. Today artificial vitamin K injections are available for newborn babies and are almost always given as a precautionary measure to all infant boys who are to undergo circumcision.[27]

In previous times, when artificial vitamin K injections did not exist, perhaps circumcision was safer, with the baby running less risk of hemorrhaging, if circumcision was delayed until after the first week. One wonders if the practice of postponing circumcision until the 8th day came about as a result of tragic instances of trial and error. (Of course if the baby is ill or premature, Jewish law provides that the circumcision rite is to be delayed until he is healthy enough to withstand the operation.)

Another reason that Jewish ritual circumcision is delayed until the eighth day is that in Jewish tradition there is a celebration held for the newborn infant on the first Friday night, which is the beginning of the Jewish Sabbath (Jewish Sabbath is observed from sundown on Friday to sundown on Saturday) after his birth and before the Bris. This observance is called the "Sholom Zochor." Eight days must elapse before the circumcision ceremony to insure that a Sabbath will occur before the Bris.[28]

---

25 Shechet, p. 6 (Devorim Rabon 6).
26 Maimonides, p. 379 (quoting Leviticus 12: 27).
27 Korones SB. *High-Risk Newborn Infants*. St. Louis: The C.V. Mosby Co.; 1976: 188.
28 Shechet, p. 5.

3.8 The Jewish Circumcision Ceremony

3.8.1 The Shalom Zachor

The Hebraic word "shalom" means completeness and peace. "Zachor" means male. The celebration for the infant male on the Sabbath preceding the Bris is a feast which has been described as filled with a sense of Jewish spirit of happiness, good feeling, and love called "nachas" (parental bliss).[29]

3.8.2 The Night Before the Bris

"Van Nacht" is the term for the night before the day of "entering into the covenant of Abraham." The custom is to be awake and guard the newborn from forces that seek to disrupt the observance of this important "Mitzvoh" (Divine Commandment). Traditionally candles are burned. This relates directly to the belief in evil spirits which supposedly endanger the mother and infant prior to the Bris. Food and drink are served and prayers and Psalms are recited.[25]

3.8.3 The People Involved in the Bris

It is considered a great honor to participate in a Bris. Many people are involved in the actual circumcision ceremony.

A "Godmother" and "Godfather" are selected (usually a husband and wife, but sometimes a father and daughter or mother and son).

> "The mother hands her child to the Godmother and by this act signifies her consent to entrust the child to God's care. The Godfather takes the child and hands him to a designated individual whose honor is to place the infant on a cushion on the 'Kidei Shel Eliyohu' (chair of Elijah)." [25]

The Godfather, called "Sandek" is described as "he who holds the child during the 'Miloh' " (cutting). He sits on a table or in an elevated chair to facilitate the "Mohel's" maneuvering during the course of the "Bris." He is usually the rabbi of the community or its most illustrious figure. It is the most important honor bestowed at the "Bris." [21]

Other people involved in the Bris include "Amido Livrocho – He who holds the child during the recitation of prayers and name giving" and "Brochos" – He who recites the prayers, usually the 'Mohel' himself, and then gives the name.[29]

---

29 Ibid., pp. 13-4.

Whenever possible it is preferable to have a "minyan" – ten men over the age of 13, including the father and the mohel, present at the Bris.

Sometimes the Bris ceremony is performed in the synagogue. In modern times the ceremony more commonly takes place in the parents' home. Some hospitals, especially in communities with large Jewish populations, have special rooms available for this purpose.

3.8.4 The Chair of Elijah

The prophet Elijah is invited to all Jewish Bris ceremonies and a special chair is set aside for him, placed to the right of the Sandek. The Mohel recites certain prayers and then the father lifts the child (out of the chair of Elijah) and places him in the lap of the "Sandek." [29]

One author explains the significance:

> "Elijah championed the covenant when the Children of Israel had forsaken it, and thus had a special role in the ceremony. It is suggested by some in discussing the symbolism of the rite that the story of Elijah's resuscitation of the widow's son may mean that the symbolic presence of the prophet refers to the possible need for the first aid should there be any complication at the operation, threatening the life of the child." [30]

3.8.5 Prayers and Procedures that Begin the Bris

> "At the loud call of one of those present, boys bring the instruments necessary for the ceremony, a flaming torch, the knife, powder to spread on the wound, a bandage to tie up the wound, a goblet of wine, and basin of oil and another of sand, and take their places near the circumcisor. At the door of the synagogue the Godfather receives the child from the hands of the Godmother, brings it to the gathering, and the mohel cries 'Blessed be the newborn!' The whole gathering repeats these words. Then the Godfather lays the child on his lap ..." [31]

According to Remondino, the Mohel recites the following as the operation commences:

> "Blessed be Thou, O Lord our God, King of the Universe, Creator of the fruit of the vine! Blessed art Thou, O Lord our God! Who hath sanctified His beloved

---

30 Conard R. Side Lights on the History of Circumcision. *Ohio State Med J.* 1954-08; 50(8): 771.
31 Bryk, p. 50.

from the womb, and ordained an ordinance for His kindred, and sealed His descendants with the mark of His holy covenant; therefore, for the merits of this, 0 living God! Our rock and inheritance, command the deliverance of the beloved of our kindred from the pit, for the sake of the covenant which He hath put in our flesh. Blessed art Thou, 0 Lord, the Maker of the Covenant! Our God and the God of our fathers! Preserve this child to his father and mother, and his name shall be called in Israel, A, the son of B. Let the father rejoice in those that go forth from his loins, and let his mother be glad in the fruit of her womb, as it is written: 'Thy father and mother shall rejoice, and they that begat thee shall be glad.' The father of the child then says the following grace: 'Blessed art Thou, 0 Lord our God, King of the Universe! Who hath sanctified us with His commandments, and commanded us to enter into the covenant of our holy father, Abraham.' The congregation answers: 'As he hath entered into the law, the (nuptial) canopy, and the good and virtuous deeds." [32]

Bryk relates another most curious variation of the mohel's prayer:

"After the mohel has spoken on the institution of circumcision, as it is known from the Bible, and implored the blessing of God, he thanks God that the child has not been born a woman or slave [!]. As a sign of the seal of God, he implores: that the circumcision might keep the child from sexual acts with animals, be it mammal or bird, with a non-Jewess, with an unmarried woman, with the bride in the house of his father-in-law, against intercourse 'in the manner of beasts,' against intercourse during menstruation, and against masturbation. He is never to change his religion, neither of his own free will nor by force. The concluding words are: 'and receive my service in this mitzvah (duty), as if I had brought a sacrifice to thine altar, even as the sacrifice of Isaac.'

After the blessing of the mohel and then of the father, the congregation present pronounces the following words: 'As he has here been initiated into the covenant, so may he enter into the Torah, into matrimony, and into all good deeds.' " [33]

3.8.6 Miloh – The Cutting of the Foreskin

"The securely wrapped child is placed so that the penis is easily accessible, and ... the mohel pronounces a Hebrew prayer and then makes the cut (chituch). He takes the member by the thumb and forefinger of his left hand and then rubs it

---

[32] Remondino PC. *History of Circumcision from the Earliest Times to the Present.* NY: Ams Press. 1974: 149 (1st ed.: F. A. Davis. 1891).
[33] Bryk, p. 57.

several times gently to evoke an erection; he then takes hold of the outer and inner lamellae of the foreskin on both sides and draws them down over the glans, pressing them smooth, by lifting his hand upward at the same time and thus giving the member a vertical position. The mohel now takes a pair of small pincers in the thumb and forefinger of his right hand and inserts the foreskin into the crack in such a manner that the glans comes to be behind it and the foreskin that is to be cut away in front of it. Then he takes hold of the knife ... With one vertical motion downwards he cuts off close to the plate the part of the foreskin that is before it ... If this has been done according to prescription, then, after the cut has been completed, the outer lamella of the foreskin is drawn back over the crown of the glans, the glans itself is clipped at the tip, resulting in an opening about the size of a pea." [34]

Furthering the description:

"As he takes hold of the knife, he says in a loud voice, 'Praised be Thou, O Lord, our God, King of the earth, who hast consecrated us and hast commanded circumcision unto us.' At the last word he cuts away the foreskin and throws it into the pot of sand. To stanch the blood somewhat, he takes a sip of wine, besprinkles the wound with it, and, if the child becomes weak, its face also ..." [35]

3.8.7 Periah – The Tearing of the Inner Membrane

Originally only the first step, the cutting off of the prepuce, was done. Jews, wishing not to be identified as such, soon learned to pull down the remaining foreskin over the glans, stretching it to make it appear as if they had never been circumcised. Therefore the act of Periah, the uncovering of the glans following the amputation of the foreskin, by which the remaining foreskin mucosa is torn back, usually with the Mohel's sharp fingernails, is done to prevent this from happening.

"Directly after the cut has been made the mohel puts the tip of his thumb nail (which, as a rule, has been cut long, lancet-shaped), or, as is generally customary now, a lancet-shaped pair of scissors into the opening of the inner lamelia of the foreskin, grasps the foreskin by it with the help of both index fingers, splits it on the back of the glans by means of slitting up to the crown of the latter, and shoves the slit foreskin up over the glans. Finally the mohel tears the whole foreskin off

---

34 Ibid., p. 47.
35 Ibid., p. 51.

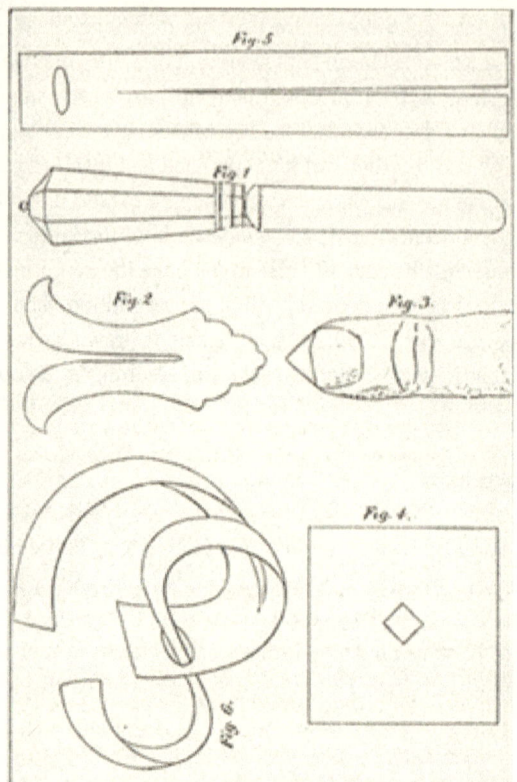

CIRCUMCISION INSTRUMENTS OF THE JEWS *(after Collins)*
Fig. 1. Circumcision knife. Fig. 2. Barzel. Fig. 3. Pointed fingernail. Fig. 4. Square cut linen cloth. Figs. 5 and 6. Bandage (longuette).
From Bryk F. *Sex & Circumcision: A Study of Phallic Worship and Mutilation in Men and Women.* North Hollywood, CA: Brandon House; 1967: 48.

> all around the corona of the glans by taking hold, with his thumb and forefinger, of the flaps of the foreskin ..." [34]

According to Jewish law, in the Joreh Deah no. 246,

> "The tender covering under the skin is to be rent with the nails. Circumcision without tearing is equivalent to no circumcision at all." [36]

---

36 Ibid., p. 54

Today most Reform and Conservative mohelim have abandoned the older techniques, believing the modern clamp devices for circumcision to be safer and more humane. If a bell and clamp device such as the Gomco clamp is used, by which the small metal bell is first inserted beneath the foreskin and over the glans, then the clamp applied and the foreskin sliced off, the act of Periah is unnecessary because the bell automatically forces the glans away from the inner lining and membranes. Orthodox Jews do not believe in the use of clamp devices (because not enough blood is shed) and therefore continue to practice Periah. Some practitioners insist that the use of instruments is safer for this procedure because fingernails are not sanitary. Others insist that

> "... circumcisors can feel much more sensitively and surely with their thumbnails, knowing just when to stop tearing, than they could with a knife or pair of scissors ..." [37]

Probably both techniques are equally painful for the baby.

3.8.8 Mezizah – The Suctioning of the Blood

The third step of the Jewish circumcision procedure is for the Mohel to apply his mouth directly to the newly circumcised penis and suction the first drops of blood.

> "Now follows the exsuction of the wound in such a manner that the mohel takes the circumcised member into his mouth and with two or three draughts sucks the blood out of the wounded part. He then takes a mouthful of wine from a goblet and spurts it, in two or three intervals, on the wound." [34]

This apparently was intended as a technique to stop the bleeding. Mezizah has been largely abandoned in the 20th century. The few who still practice it today usually use a small glass tube for the suction instead of direct application of the mouth. Many complications have resulted from Mezizah and the practice is surrounded by considerable controversy which will be discussed shortly.

3.8.9 Procedures Immediately After the Operation

> "... Then [the mohel] bandages the child with linen, wraps it up again, and washes his mouth and hands. Once again the Godfather faces him with the child

---
37 Ibid., p. 53.

and the circumcisor concludes the procedure with a prayer, that God keep the child alive and that he afford his parents much joy." [35]

"Many hold the child over sand or water, that the holy blood may flow into it. In fact those standing about have to wash their faces with the mixture of blood and water. The water has usually been boiled beforehand with aromatic and narcotic ingredients. Or the mohel pours the blood mixed with wine behind the cabinet in which scrolls of the law are kept." [33]

3.8.10   Treatment of the Amputated Foreskin

Commonly the amputated foreskin is buried in a small bowl of sand that is provided, a custom which apparently originated with the Israelites' desert ancestry. Some Jewish groups burned the foreskin instead, in the manner of a sacrificial offering. Yet another practice is described as follows:

"The days preceding the circumcision, the foreskin of a child previously circumcised is put into the mouth of the infant who is about to undergo the operation [...]!

It is a wonderful charm; the night before circumcision, measures were taken to ward off attacks by demon Lilit. After circumcision, the bloody foreskin is placed in a bowl containing water and spices, and each member of the congregation as he leaves the Synagogue, would bathe his hands and face." [38]

According to another writer:

"... On the death of the Mohel, or Circumciser, the foreskins of the children he had circumcised were sometimes buried with him to drive away the demons and destroyers who would seek to do him harm after death. It is also commonly believed by the Orthodox that some form of magic prevails over those who have circumcised a certain number of children. This is supposed to prevent putrefaction of their mouths, as well as to prevent their mouths from becoming food for worms after their deaths!" [39]

---

38   D'Alba A. *Circumcision, the savagery of the cradle.* Galen Medical Publications; 1979: 26.
39   Lewis, p. 63 (quoting Jewish Encyclopedia, Vol. 4, p. 95).

3.8.11 The Festive Meal Following the Bris

This is called the "Seudo Shel Mitzvo": (The Meal in Honor of the Commandment of Circumcision) which is considered a religious feast.

> "Throughout the millennia a regular meal was served with fish, meat and 'Shabbos Chalas' but in our American society where everyone is in a hurry to get to his office and job, a hasty meal is served, usually bagels, lox, and coffee with liquors and cakes." [40]

3.8.12 Feelings at the Time of the Bris

A wide range of feelings on the part of the adult participants in the circumcision ritual has been related by different authors:

> "... All celebrate the reception of a new member, with brandy and honey cakes, hearty 'mazeltovs' and innumerable toasts ... God is increasing the number of His Chosen. His people are fulfilling their part of the pact, the promise of the future is one step nearer to fulfillment, and in the present a living source of joy and honor to the family has been added for all to admire ..." [41]

In contrast, another writer condemns the ritual:

> "The rite is retaliation for parricidal wishes ... In primitive rites, this affect is reinserted in action – the boys are beaten mercilessly, and made to run the gauntlet. In the Jewish ceremony, too, an effort is made to bring the appropriate sadistic affect into conjunction with the act – and this is done by the recitation of a formula ... the congregation recites 'If this act is performed timidly, or with a soft heart, it is null and void.' At the same time, the sadistic affect is projected and bound in the strict institutionalization of the ritual ... This is the celebration: the relief at the lifting of the father's guilt and removal of the anxiety by the accepted mutilation of himself in the person of his son." [42]

A modern day Rabbi describes the occasion in terms of specialness and holiness:"It is a milestone in the lives of both the parents and the youngster." [25]

---

40 Shechet, p. 15.
41 Zborowski M, Herzog E. *Life is With People*, NY: Schocken Books; 1952: 318-9.
42 Malev M. The Jewish Orthodox Circumcision Ceremony – Its Meaning from Direct Study of the Rite. *J Am Psychoanal Assoc.* 1966: 14: 513.

"Rabbi Shimon ben Yoichoi said: 'Come and observe! There is nothing more beloved to a person than his son, yet he circumcises him; why is this so? Rabbi Nachman bar Shmuel said: 'In order to fulfill the will of the Creator. A person sees blood spilling from the circumcision of his son and accepts it with joy.' Rabbi Hanino said: 'Not only is that so, but the person also pays the expenses incurred and celebrates the day as a Holiday ...' " (Midrash Tanhumo-Tazrea).[43]

3.9 Circumcision and Anti-Semitism

Throughout history, Jews have been hated and persecuted by other groups of people. Frequently their practice of circumcision has been a target of such persecution.

In some instances people who left the penis intact ridiculed the Jews and other groups who practiced circumcision, considering the penis with an exposed glans to be ugly, ridiculous, or obscene in appearance. In ancient Greece:

"The Greeks in everyday life did not wander around in the nude. However, for the Greeks nudity was an inherent part of the aesthetics of athletic competition ... The Greeks had clearly defined ideas about masculine beauty and fine distinctions were made about forms of nudity. While most peoples of the Mediterranean were circumcised, the Greeks and Romans were vehemently opposed to circumcision. It's thought that the Greeks preserved the foreskin believing that this would maintain the sensitivity of the glans ... [A story is told about a] ... team of circumcised non-Greeks who turned up at the Olympic Games in Roman times and became the laughing stock of the assembled Greek athletes – so much so that the next day, the foreigners returned with false foreskins! The foreskin was essential to Greek modesty. The bared glans was considered indecent and even obscene – probably because normally it was on view only when the penis was erect, which was, except in the case of satyrs, never in public." [44]

If circumcision is one of the oldest forms of surgery, "uncircumcision" – an operation to make the penis appear that it still has its foreskin, is one of the second oldest types of surgery.

The following is a description of the practice of the Jews who came under Greek influence and wished to appear as if they had not been circumcised: "The Hellenizers pulled this fragment [of foreskin] forward manually, stretched it, and even applied blistering agents thereto, in order to make it cover the glans." [45]

---

43 Shechet, p. 10.
44 Conrad A. What's Behind the Sports Myths About Sex? *Sex Med Today*, 27.
45 Tushnet L. Uncircumcision. *Med Times*. 1965-06; 93(6): 588.

(It was because of this that the second step, "Periah," was added to the Jewish circumcision ritual, to prevent the individual from becoming "uncircumcised.")

Under some rulers the Jews were forbidden to practice circumcision. The motivation for this was not simply a matter of not liking the looks of circumcised penises, nor of merely picking on Jews by forbidding them from practicing one of their religious rites. Circumcision was believed to grant fertility. Therefore, theoretically, circumcision meant more Jewish people, a situation not desired if one hated Jews.

The decree of Antiochus, 167 B.C., consigned every Hebrew mother to death who dared to circumcise her offspring.[46]

Adrian, A.D. 130, inflicted the death penalty. Antoninus, A.D. 140, for a time permitted it, but in A.D. 160 it was again forbidden. When Christianity became the official state religion under Constantine, A.D. 315, Jews were permitted to circumcise their own children, but not non-Jews. A liberal view was taken by Charlemagne, then for about three centuries the whim of various ruling princes governed the matter. From about A.D. 700 and approximately seven centuries thereafter, while Spain was the cultural center of Jewry and was under the rule of the Moors, persecution was cruel.[47]

Sometimes in times of persecution the Jews performed circumcisions secretly on their dead, "that the spirit of the law of their fathers might be carried out." [48]

The Jewish circumcision rite has persisted throughout history, in part as a result of the Jews' lack of a homeland and repeated persecution by others. Remondino comments:

"No custom, habit, or rite has survived so many ages and so many persecutions. Other customs have died a natural death with time or want of persecution, but circumcision, either in peace or in war, has held its own, from the misty epochs of the stone age to the present." [49]

During times when Jews were hunted down by their enemies, possession of a circumcised penis oftentimes became a disadvantage, serving as a mark of identity by which he could be singled out as a Jew. During Hitler's regime this was especially so:

"Escape from the Ghettos set up by the Germans in Poland was difficult but possible. On the 'Aryan side', life for the Jew remained dangerous. No matter how

---

46 Remondino, p. 63.
47 Conard, p. 773.
48 Remondino, p. 67.
49 Ibid., p. 68.

'good' the visage nor how well-forged the Kennkarte (identification documents), the male Jew carried with him incontrovertible proof of his origin.

The blackmailers and extortionists known as schmaltzovniks (from the Polish szmalec' meaning 'fat') used circumcision as the criterion of Jewishness ...

These scum would approach their victims with the words, 'Hand over your fat.' They were a terrible plague upon the Jews who lived on the Aryan side. In addition to the Gestapo, SS men, and others who hunted them relentlessly, the Jews lived in constant danger from these dregs of Polish morality, who make a business of Jewish lives. Hundreds were engaged in this hateful occupation – searching out the unfortunates who now lived on Aryan documents or who hid under the protection of Gentiles ... Jews who had nothing and were not profitable were handed over to the Nazis. Others had to pay monthly blackmail. When they finally had nothing left for the blood tax, they were handed over to their fate ... They operated in gangs ... They would pull their victim into a doorway or an alley and rip open his trousers, looking for the fateful sign ..." [50]

During the Nazi holocaust, various methods of "uncircumcision" were attempted as a life-preserving measure to enable the Jewish male to hide his identity. The operation basically consisted of freeing the inner shaft of the penis from the surrounding skin, pulling the skin forward, drawing the scrotal skin onto the shaft of the penis and making a new "foreskin" out of the penile skin in front. Attempts were also made to construct a foreskin, made of skin grafted from another part of the person's body. Additionally, many Jewish male infants were left with prepuces intact, in the hopes that they would escape torture and extermination under Hitler.[51]

Many writers have commented on the psychology of anti-Semitism as it relates to circumcision. Included in Freud's theory about the "castration complex" is his idea that: "Society despises the woman and the Jew ... the woman because she is missing a penis and the Jew because he is missing part of his penis." [52]

One author explains:

"... [Circumcision] is a partial actual castration and promotes anti-Semitism by making Jews despised as women; that the circumcised state is used to work out bisexual fantasies with the removed foreskin representing the female part; ... in the service of anti-Semitism, it may cause the Jew to be regarded as castrated and effeminate, or conversely as a sacrifice of a portion of the phallus to ensure preservation of the male portion ..." [53]

---

50 Tushnet, pp. 590-1.
51 Ibid., pp. 592-3.
52 Glenn J. Circumcision and Anti-Semitism. *Psychoanal Q.* 1960; 29: 397-8.
53 Malev, p. 510.

Another writer comments:

> "The circumcised Jew is often represented as a mutilated person and this fantasy is repeatedly stated in the literature. An uncanny feeling is said to exist in some to whom a Jew is a reminder that one can be castrated. The unconscious fantasy develops that a mutilated people desire revenge and want to circumcise (castrate) the non-Jew." [52]

In the United States today, where most non-Jewish males have also been circumcised, the above situation does not exist. Although routine neonatal circumcision as a medical procedure has not come about as a result of any conscious Jewish plot to deprive the rest of America of their foreskins, the American Jew is at an "advantage" in that he is hardly unique by having a circumcised penis. Many Jews have felt reassured by our medical system's endorsement of circumcision as a supposed "health" measure.

Now that the medical advisability of circumcision has been found lacking, and concern grows for the feelings of infants and the rights of individuals, the trend is increasing for American parents to leave their sons intact. In the future, Jews may again be the only people to cut off infant foreskins. It is hoped that the rest of us will develop attitudes of tolerance and understanding for other peoples' religious beliefs and anti-Semitic attitudes will not result. Certainly the anti-Semitism that prevailed in the past over circumcision was not out of concern for the feelings of tiny babies!

Author's note: Please note here – for anyone who has read the original 1985 version of my book and may have wondered why there was a large gap between the paragraphs on p. 50 – there had been a paragraph here that Bergin & Garvey decided to delete [and then didn't bother to correct the paste up!] The essence of what I said was as follows:

While most ethnic stereotypes are rarely valid and should never be used to demean or belittle any group, I cannot help but wonder in empathy with the commonly held image of the Jewish mother. She has been typified as unusually protective, controlling and continually worried about her children, especially her sons. This behavior may have true justification in that the Jewish mother was forced to witness the torture of her newborn infant when she was powerless to protect him.

3.10   Conflicts Within Judaism Concerning Circumcision

There are three major branches of Judaism. Reform Judaism is the most liberal, Conservative is in-between, and Orthodox adheres the most strictly to the old traditions and laws. Within these groups are different factions and a vast range of conflicting beliefs about a large number of Jewish observances, including circumcision.

3.10.1 Mohelim vs. Doctors

Should Jewish ritual circumcision be a medical procedure performed in a hospital, or does this detract from its religious significance? Should the operation be done by a mohel or a doctor? Who is better skilled and qualified to perform the operation?
For the Orthodox, Jewish circumcision is not valid unless a mohel performs the operation. A modern-day mohel writes:

> "Thus it follows that a 'Bris-Miloh' should be performed only by a competent, Torah observant Jew, who understands the significance of 'Miloh' and its proper application. It does not make sense for a Jew who is having this noble 'Mitzvah' performed, not to avail himself of the opportunity to have the circumcision performed in the correct and prescribed way. A competent 'Mohel,' trained in the age-old method used by the Jewish people in accordance with 'Halacha' (Jewish Religious Law), and trained to take advantage of the most current medical knowledge is the most appropriate person to perform a 'Bris.' " [54]

Other branches of Judaism feel differently, for frequently the Bris is performed with a doctor doing the operation and a rabbi officiating the ceremony with prayers and recitations. Preferably the doctor should be Jewish, but sometimes non-Jewish doctors are called upon to perform the circumcision for a Jewish Bris. While most mohelim are rabbis, some Jewish doctors are licensed as mohelim.

A newer variation, practiced by some Reform Jews is the "Baby Naming" ceremony. Several years ago my husband and I attended such a celebration. The parents had chosen to have their son circumcised shortly after birth in the hospital, because their insurance would cover the cost, rather than pay the substantial sum of money required for a mohel to perform the same operation at a Bris. Their baby was about two months old when they had his "Baby Naming" ceremony, complete with a large feast, many friends and relatives present, and a rabbi who performed a ceremony for the baby, saying prayers, naming him, and dedicating him to a life within Judaism. (Some have combined the ceremony with the *Pidyon ha-ben*, a redemption ceremony which takes place on the thirty-first day after the birth of a first-born son.) Some factions of Judaism would consider this a sacrilege.

The argument over whether a mohel or a doctor is better qualified to circumcise babies is similar to the controversy over obstetricians versus midwives. The medical

---
54 Shechet, p. 4.

profession claims that mohelim, simply by virtue of not being medical professionals, are automatically less competent. In the past much of this criticism was based on the mohelim's lack of medical equipment and the less than sanitary practices of tearing the prepuce with the thumbnail and the sucking of the wound. Proponents of mohelim claim that the following of a "4,000 year old technique" is safer than that of "an average surgeon whose technique and instruments seem to change with every decade." [55] This is questionable however, for most mohelim today *do* use modern medical techniques for the procedure. Four thousand years ago circumcision was usually done with a flint knife.

Much of the concern over safety is based less on which type of operator is more competent than over the fact that the Orthodox Jews do not believe in using modern clamp devices for circumcision. Therefore, the baby circumcised by the older techniques runs a greater risk of hemorrhaging.

There is concern that a doctor would lack the religious "spirit" of the Bris, his presence making it seem merely a surgical procedure. One Rabbi comments:

> "Brith [Bris] Milah is a most sacred religious ceremony. Its whole purpose is not medical and there is a vast difference between the normal medical approach and the requirements of Brith Milah. Thus, Jewish religious requirements are not met by mere surgical circumcision." [56]

Circumcision is the *only* operation that a mohel is usually trained to do. The Jewish Bris ceremony takes place in a highly religious atmosphere with many people present. These factors would tend to cause the mohel to be more conscientious about his technical skill. No doctor specializes in doing circumcisions. He either delivers or cares for babies, and does circumcisions as a sideline – the operation being only one of his many medical skills. To most doctors, infant circumcision seems trivial compared to the more serious operations that they must do. Routine circumcisions of newborns are usually performed hastily in a hospital nursery with only a nurse or two present. Frequently a doctor may circumcise three or four babies after he "makes his rounds" of patients, and before he goes to his office. The setting hardly has the same "aura" that surrounds the Jewish Bris. Therefore the doctor may not be as likely to be as conscientious about performing circumcisions.

There are probably more differences between the skills of *individual* operators, than there are between doctors and mohelim *per se.*

---

55   Mendelsohn RA. Circumcision View Solicited. *People's Doctor* (newspaper column). Hayward, CA. 1978.
56   Wood, JR. "The Circumcision Controversy", Information sheet for INTACT Educational Foundation, quoting Rabbi Morris Shoulson, author of *Circumcision in Jewish Law and Modern Medical Practice.*

Where the Bris should take place is also widely debated. As with birth, the hospital is better equipped to handle emergencies. Blood is available for transfusion. Doctors are readily available to handle complications. On the other hand, the home lends a more personal atmosphere to the occasion. Also, the chances of infection tend to be greater in a hospital with its resistant strains of germs. A Bris performed in a synagogue would certainly emphasize the religious nature of the ceremony, although today it is not common to perform a Bris in that setting.

If mohelim are to perform circumcisions, they should seek to avail themselves of as much skill, knowledge, modern techniques and equipment as possible. These are certainly not the exclusive property of doctors.

3.10.2   Use of Clamps

In ancient times circumcision was performed with knives, often with a precursor of the clamp device called a *barzel*, which kept the foreskin up over the glans while the knife severed it. Earlier techniques employed flint knives or pieces of stone.

Today nearly all doctors, and most mohelim use modern clamp-type devices for infant circumcision. The precursor to the Gomco clamp was invented by a Jewish physician, Hiram Yellen, in the late 1800s. The present Gomco clamp, with its metal bell and circular clamp, was developed in 1934 by Aaron Goldstein.[57] "Gomco", the medical company that supplies this device, is an abbreviation of "Go(ldstein) M(edical) Co(mpany)." [58]

This device, and others based on the same concept such as the Plastibell (See Chapter 5.10.2 "The Plastibell technique") usually produce an even, symmetrical cut. The sealing of the edges by the clamp minimizes the amount of bleeding and accompanying dangers.

A Rabbi explains the Orthodox' opposition to the use of clamps:

"This 'Midrash' [interpretation of the Scriptures in reference to the Blood of the Passover Sacrificial Lamb and the blood of circumcision] teaches us the great importance of blood flowing during circumcision and that a 'clamp' or 'clamping instrument' which prevents bleeding in a 'Bris-Miloh' may not be used. Rabbinical authorities in Jerusalem and throughout the world have asserted that the usage of 'clamps' or 'clamping instruments' that prevent bleeding during circumcision is not in accordance with 'Halachia' [Jewish Religious Law]." [11]

---

57 Carter, p. 69.
58 Yellen HS. Discussions of Bloodless Circumcision. *Brochure for Gomco Surgical Manufacturing Corp.* Buffalo, NY (from *AJOG.* 1935-07).

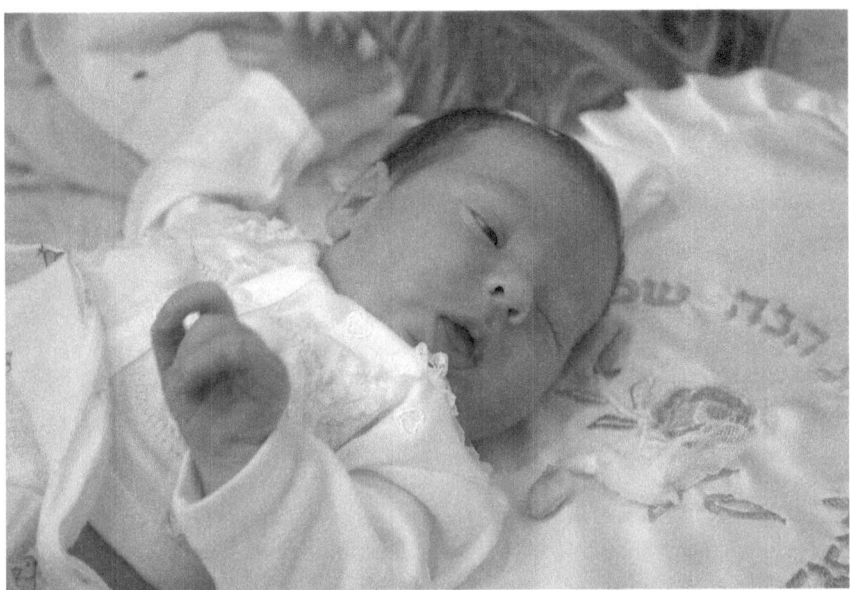

Infant after brit. Source: Wikipedia

Other Rabbis, among the Conservative and Reform branches, recognize the dangers of excessive bleeding in a tiny baby and believe that the drops of blood that are shed with the initial dorsal slit are sufficient to fulfill this part of the scriptural requirements.

3.10.3 Mezizah

The third step of the circumcision ritual, in which the Mohel applies his mouth to the baby's freshly circumcised penis, has been surrounded with an extreme amount of controversy and consternation.

> "The 'mohel' took some wine in his mouth, and applying his lips to the mutilated organ, sucked the wound, expelling the mixture of blood and wine into a receptacle especially provided for the purpose. This suction was repeated several times, after which the operation was completed by apposing the skin and mucosa back of the glans and applying a retentive dressing of linen ..." [59]

In the old tradition this act was considered "the greatest honor of all." [60]

---
59 Kiser EF. Ceremonial Circumcision. *N Engl J Med.* 1930-10-23; 203(17): 836.
60 Zborowski & Herzog, p. 319.

At one time there was a stipulation:

"If ... mezizah has not been performed upon it, it is at least to be considered circumcised (as opposed to if periah is omitted) but such a mohel shall hereafter be denied the practice of the berith (Bris) because he has omitted a hygienic (!) measure." [61]

One author speculates about a number of possible motivations for mezizah:

"It may represent the most infantile concept of the mode of implementation of castration ... It may reflect the blood- – brotherhood of males ... an analogy to that portion of the primitive rites in which blood from the incised penis is permitted to drip into the water, which is then drunk by the elders of the tribe. It may be an affectionate reaction by the grandfather for the mutilation inflicted.

Following removal of the prepuce, the mohel recites this sentence: 'O, Living God, command to preserve our beloved flesh from destruction' ... suggest-[ing] another meaning for the sucking at the penis – which is plainly a passive homosexual act. It may be the reflection of another ... defense against castration, universally present in repression, and frequently rising to overtness, namely homosexuality ..." [62]

Others deny that Mezizah had any overt homosexual or sadistic motivations, but believe it was merely the only means known at the time for stopping the bleeding.

"... Persons wounding their fingers will instinctively carry them to their mouth, and it may be that the suction practiced by the Hebrews had its origin in this natural hemostatic suggestion. Wine as a hemostatic aid and as an emblem of thanksgiving and an acceptable offering naturally came in as an accessory." [63]

Tragic results have occurred due to Mezizah:

"Cases of disease and even death have repeatedly occurred as a result of this unhygienic measure including, children being infected with syphilis or tuberculosis, or conversely circumcisors receiving inherited maladies from their patients. During the years 1805-1866, eight syphilis epidemics have been known from London to Krakow, caused by syphilitic circumcisors. In Krakow over 100 cases

---

[61] Bryk, p. 56.
[62] Malev, pp. 514-5.
[63] Remondino, pp. 151-2.

were listed (1833). Even in the year 1923 ... two four month old children were infected by one and the same circumcisor with skin tuberculosis in the penis." [36]

Because of the dangers, Mezizah has been almost abandoned by many factions of Judaism, in recent years. Among some extremists who could not be persuaded to abandon the practice, direct application of the mouth has been replaced with the use of a small glass tube.

3.10.4 Attempts by the Jewish Reform Movement to Abolish Circumcision

During the 1800s the Jewish Reform movement exerted considerable effort to abolish the ritual of circumcision. In 1892, the requirement of circumcision for adult converts to Judaism was abolished (except for the Orthodox) "... on the grounds that it is 'a measure of extreme cruelty when performed upon adults.' " [64]

Attempts were made to abolish circumcision altogether. Baltz proposed that not children, but adults, be circumcised when they came into the full possession of their faculties, and then only the tip of the foreskin. [65]

Others attacked it due to the "low standard of the art of ritual circumcision from the sanitary point of view." Few regulations existed, and many children were greatly endangered and exposed to disease.

Others spelled out:

"A.) Circumcision could be derived from no moral law but from an Abrahamitic. Consequently circumcision did not by any means make one an Israelite.
B.) The commandment of circumcision did not appear among the laws in the Pentateuch.
C.) Moses did not have his sons circumcised.
D.) According to Joshua all those born in the desert during the forty-year period were not circumcised.
E.) From the fact that the daughters of Israel enter Judaism without any rite at all, it may be concluded that according to the principles of the Mosaic belief it is birth that makes one a Jew, and one born of Jewish parents belongs to the Jewish religious community so long as he does not forsake his belief." [65]

Felix Adler also opposed Jewish ritual circumcision:

---

64 Lewis, p. 153.
65 Bryk, pp. 234-6.

"To Adler, at that time a professor of philosophy at Columbia University and soon thereafter founder of the Ethical Culture movement, this ritual appeared as 'simply barbarous in itself and utterly barbarous and contemptible in its origin.' Coming from a former rabbinical student and son of the leading Reform rabbi, Samuel Adler, this declaration called forth sharp condemnation even from Isaac Mayer Wise, one of the recognized leaders of the Reform movement ... The issue was debated time and again in both Germany and America. Yet circumcision has remained the accepted form of admission to the Covenant of Abraham among the overwhelming majority of Reform Jews.

On the other hand few reformers entertained the same scruples about other provisions of Talmudic law, especially those relating to the Sabbath commandment or to ritually permissible food ..." [66]

3.10.5 Mutilation of the Body

LEVITICUS: CH. 19:
28 YE SHALL NOT MAKE ANY CUTTINGS IN YOUR FLESH FOR THE DEAD, NOR PRINT ANY MARKS UPON YOU: I AM THE LORD.[67]

Many critics of Jewish circumcision find that the practice conflicts with the basic Jewish laws against most pagan practices of cutting of the flesh or mutilation of the body. Isaac comments on this paradox:

"Circumcision is a surprising rite to find prescribed in the Bible. It was, of course, widely practiced among Israel's pagan neighbors: ... the whole tenor of the Bible is against the pagans and their practices. Moreover, it is, in general, strongly opposed to any form of bodily mutilation or deformation, ritual or otherwise. Thus tattooing and scarification, for example, are forbidden for the explicit reason that the Israelites are the children of God." [56]

Yet another puzzle in Old Testament writings is the concept that "God created man in his own image." (Genesis: 1: 26) Did God really make a mistake when he created the male body? If he had wanted men to be without foreskins, why did he not simply create them that way?

D'Alba comments:

---

66 Schwarz LW (ed). *Great Ages and Ideas of the Jewish People*. NY: The Modern Library; 1956: 366.
67 Leviticus: Ch. 19: 28.

"Amazing inconsistency! What motivates this attitude of having God in special rendezvous with Abraham in order to tell him that he must cut off his prepuce? Who created this prepuce anyway? God, of course. Who was not aware of His mistake for attaching to the organ of procreation and life itself such filthy imperfection ...? In the first place, why didn't Jehovah notice this imperfection after creating Adam, and revise His masterpiece afterwards?" [68]

3.10.6 Attitudes about Circumcision by Jews Today

Not all Jews are content with or accepting of circumcision. Many do question it. Some Jewish parents have chosen to leave their sons intact. Others agonize over the decision. Some Jewish parents choose circumcision with no feelings of religious observance, but merely out of conformity to the American middle class, or belief that they have ascribed to a medically preventive measure.

A modern day Rabbi, seeking to preserve the significance of ritual circumcision for Jews, finds the act glorified and beautiful:

"The Almighty praised-be-He wanted to permanently affix a symbol on the bodies of the people He chose to be called in His name. The purpose of this symbol is to physically differentiate the Chosen People from others, just as they are distinct spiritually and differ in their actions.[69] The 'Golden Circle'[70] [circumcision] was perpetuated as the symbol because this is the source from which the perpetuation of the species emanates. Circumcision completes and perfects the physical appearance of the body. The Almighty desires the character and traits of the Chosen People to be perfected and He wants this perfection to be accomplished through human action. The reason the Almighty does not create the human being complete in the mother's womb, is to indicate to us that just as the physical aspects of the body can be made better by human deeds, so it is within human power to perfect the soul by correcting one's actions." [71]

In contrast, a personal letter from a friend tells of feelings of outright hatred that some Jews have for circumcision:

---

68 Isaac, pp. 51-2.
69 Yet many other groups, including the American middle class, also practice circumcision, therefore the Jews certainly are not unique in their practice. – R.R.
70 It is most interesting to note that the crippled, deformed feet of women in ancient China, which resulted from tightly binding the feet of little girls, have been referred to as "Golden Lotuses." (Daly M. Ch. 4: Chinese Footbinding: On Footnoting the Three-Inch 'Lotus Hooks'. In: *Gyn Ecology*. Boston, MA: Beacon Press; 1978) What is there in human mentality that wants to attribute "goldenness" to body mutilation? – R.R.
71 Shechet, p. 16.

"... Some of the most adamant and powerful arguments AGAINST the practice have come from Jews! I once had some very close Jewish friends. The mother was such a great person. They were from Germany. We had many very long talks about circumcision, and she was so much against the practice you wouldn't believe it! She told me ... 'In America you don't see it like you would if you were in Germany. You see, NO boys are circumcised except the Jews ... In this way it is very easy indeed to see clearly the definite negative effects it has upon Jewish boys and men! ... That's our religion and my own son is circumcised too ... but I think it is time the Jewish people gave up this horrible ancient practice in accordance with every day modern living.' She was so disgusted that so many Jewish doctors actually forced young mothers into having their baby circumcised ... with very harsh words for Jewish doctors, as she felt they were the ones REALLY responsible for routine circumcision in our hospitals. Once I knew the son of a rabbi who told me 'It is quite impossible for me to put into words the deep-seated hate ... pure HATE ... I have for circumcision. I mean ALL circumcision. It is ugly, disfiguring and most unaesthetic!' So the general public's opinion that ALL Jewish people are all for circumcision is not true either. Many of the leaders feel the same way ... 'It has worn out its time,' etc. I recall well one Jewish Boy Scout who told me ... 'Why should I have to go all through my life with my penis all exposed and skinned back ... just to belong to some Congregation? No matter WHAT my father says, I think it's a hell of a lousy deal ...' " [72]

3.10.7   The Jewish Ideal of Kindness

Few people, especially parents, doctors, or mohelim *want* to believe that the infant feels any significant pain as his foreskin is smashed, slit, torn back from his glans, clamped and sliced off. No one who performs circumcisions on babies does so out of any *deliberate* intent to torture infants. It is with great difficulty that people are coming to accept the fact that the newborn is indeed a sensitive, feeling human being who is just as capable of feeling pain as any other person. If it is true that the infant experiences a severe amount of pain while undergoing circumcision, then the practice conflicts with the basic Jewish ideals of kindness, compassion to other living beings, and commandments not to assault another or cause pain to any living creature.

---

[72]   Pablo de la Rosa (personal correspondence).

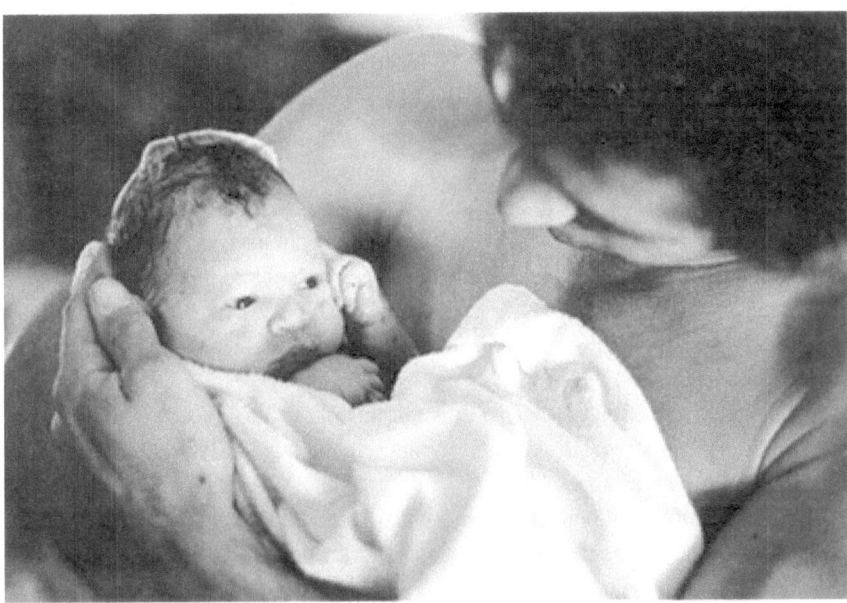

Dad and baby. © Suzanne Arms

" 'If a man shows no mercy,' says an ancient source, 'what difference is there between him and a beast which can callously stand by and not feel the anguish of its fellow creature?' " [73]

"The Torah prohibits the torture or causing of pain to any living creature. One is duty bound to save every living creature from pain or distress …" [74]

"It is forbidden to assault another. One who physically assaults another violates Torah commandment …" [75]

"The first words of any introduction to the Jewish daily way of life must speak of kindness, because we believe that Jewish religious faith and ritual observance aim, above all, to achieve a perfection of the human relationship and to create a better society … When the Talmud speaks of the characteristics of Israel, it does not do so in terms of the unique ritual observances and disciplines. Rather it adopts humane criteria: 'Three characteristics does this people possess: they are merciful, modest, and perform deeds of kindness' (Yevamot 79a)." [76]

---

[73] Donin HH. *To Be A Jew.* NY: Basic Books; 1972: 45.
[74] Ibid., p. 54.
[75] Ibid., p. 57.
[76] Ibid., p. 41.

3.10.8 Considerations of Today's Jewish Parents

All people's religious beliefs and practices must be respected. My own major concern, and the primary focus of the anti-circumcision movement has been directed against circumcision as an American medical fad that has come about within the past few decades, not the Jewish ritual that has existed for thousands of years.

If only Jews were circumcising their babies, I may not have written this book, yet a book about circumcision would not be complete without consideration of the Jewish practice. This is not meant to be construed that I have no concern for Jewish babies. As a non-Jew I may have considered the Jewish ritual simply out of my area to question.

Religious tolerance is important, although this places the anti-circumcision activist in a "can't win for losing" situation. What stand to take in regard to Jewish ritual circumcision has been the stickiest aspect of the entire dilemma. For the underlying tenet of religious and individual tolerance is "one should be free to do whatever one wishes as long as it does not hurt anyone." But neonatal circumcision DOES hurt someone – the helpless infant involved!

If we take a stand against Jewish ritual circumcision we run the risk of being labeled anti-Semitic. Yet if we take a stand of tolerance for the Jewish ritual, others accuse us of not caring about the pain inflicted on Jewish babies. For certainly the Jewish baby feels just as much pain and torment when his foreskin is cut off as does any other baby. He knows nothing about the ancient Jewish laws and traditions. All he knows is that his body is being assaulted. And the Jewish male is just as deprived of his foreskin as any other circumcised male.

However, those of us who oppose infant circumcision should look to the examples throughout history of other groups who have wished to put an end to Jewish ritual circumcision. Whatever their motivations, their efforts have been futile. Pressures upon the Jews to stop circumcising, coming from outsiders, have only left the Jews more determined than ever to perpetuate the rite. The lesson is: *Only the Jews themselves can decide whether or not to continue circumcising their babies.* If Jewish ritual circumcision is to come to an end (and there are many Jews today who would like the practice to stop!) that effort will have to come from *within* Judaism. If this is to happen, it will have to begin with many individual Jewish parents personally deciding to leave their sons intact, before Judaism as a whole makes a united effort against it.

Jewish parents of baby boys should not *automatically* choose circumcision. They are challenged to do a great deal of thinking about how much the Abrahamic covenant truly means to them. For many Jews today, circumcision has little meaning as a religious observance, yet they still choose it according to the same platitudes that the rest of us have heard – the supposed medical arguments, beliefs that "it is cleaner" or "looks better," or for mere conformity. I have heard, Jews describe circumcision as a "tradition" among their people, but have little awareness of the religious meaning ascribed to the Bris ceremony.

If the Abrahamic covenant has little or no meaning for Jewish parents, then they should question circumcision along with everyone else. Certainly Jewish parents who leave their sons intact (and there are many today!) will encounter questioning and criticism from their relatives, but many non-Jewish American parents with intact sons encounter the same from their families. Practices in all aspects of child rearing have changed so drastically within the past several years that almost all new parents encounter some criticism over many things such as natural birth, prolonged breast-feeding, "on demand" feeding (instead of schedules), delayed starting of solid foods, dolls for boys … the list could go on endlessly. Conflicts between family members can be heartrending, but should not stop us from doing what we believe is best for our children.

Conformity and acceptance by the group is an important consideration, and some Jewish parents have made the decision that having an intact penis within a culture where the circumcised penis is the norm would be more "traumatic" than the initial pain of the operation and the lifelong deprivation of one's foreskin. However, non-Jewish American parents are faced with the same pressures of "conformity." This concern will only remain as long as everyone "follows the herd," but will soon change as more and more parents choose to leave their sons intact.

Jewish parents who decide that their infant sons must be circumcised can take a number of considerations to help ease the baby's trauma:

1. Perhaps a local injection, a dorsal nerve block, can be used to help ease the baby's initial pain. Because this is medication, a doctor would probably have to administer it, even if a mohel were to do the operation. Opinions will vary about the use of this, for some believe that the ritual is "null and void" unless the infant feels a great deal of pain. Please refer to Chapter 22 "Humane Alternatives in Infant Circumcision?" for further discussion of this technique.
2. *Do* have genuine concern for your baby's feelings as he is being cut, and during the following days as he heals. Give him a lot of love and physical contact by holding him close. A child fares better from any injury if he can sense his parents' genuine concern.
3. Remember that the baby born in the past had all the benefits of the "old fashioned" concepts of baby care that today's new parents are struggling to relearn. The baby born in previous ages was always born at home or in a home-like setting and immediately after birth was placed in his mother's arms. He was always breast-

fed, usually for the first couple of years of his life. Too many of today's babies experience the first days of life away from their mothers in a sterile hospital nursery, and know only lifeless bottles instead of their mother's breasts for nourishment. So if your baby must undergo circumcision, do all the other positive, beneficial things that you can for him. Give birth to your baby in a loving, non-traumatic environment. Nurse him at the breast the way God intended all babies to be fed. Have him grow up in a loving and caring environment. All these things are important to his well-being, whether or not he keeps his foreskin.

Jewish parents who wish to leave their infant sons intact, yet wish to do something in observance of the Abrahamic covenant can consider a number of other alternatives.

Recently a midwife wrote about the following observance:

"Last year a baby boy was born to Jewish parents.. The parents wanted to give the child a *brith* without inflicting the pain of circumcision. On the eighth day friends were invited to their home. A friend who is a rabbinical student read the appropriate scriptures, blessed the child with a Jewish name and at the time of circumcision a large organic carrot was produced and the tip severed. It was a joyous moment for all involved.

You will all have your own personal reaction to this ceremony. For those who want to keep with the tradition, but do not feel it is necessary to cause your newborn unnecessary pain, try cutting a carrot! Do it with sincerity, respect and love. We can only pray for God's Blessings and offer our actions unto him. Perhaps this is the alternative some of you have been looking for." [77]

As another option, I have been told that in Russia, Jews follow a ritual for the newborn, but do not amputate the foreskin, but instead only draw one drop of blood from the prepuce in observance of the ceremony. In some countries, where the rest of the population has intact penises, Jews also have wished to keep their foreskins. This may be less contradictory to the ancient covenant than it appears, for there is considerable speculation that during ancient times the prepuce was merely gashed and bled rather than cut off.

As was previously discussed, some Reform Jews have a "Baby Naming Ceremony," a Jewish ritual for the male infant, without circumcision (circumcision having been previously done in the hospital). Perhaps some progressive rabbis would be willing to perform a similar ceremony for a baby who was not circumcised, because the parents wished to spare him the trauma. One Jewish couple who wished to leave their infant son intact reported the following:

---

[77] Burns NR. Alternative Circumcision? *Mothering.* 1979; 13: 85.

"We went to a Reform temple and had Joshua 'named' at a Sabbath service. We now have a certificate with his Jewish name and the family is happy because now he's 'Jewish.' The rabbi never asked and we never volunteered the information that Joshua wasn't circumcised." [78]

Regardless of the various personal choices that will be made by individuals, it must be strongly emphasized that this book, and the growing movement opposing infant circumcision, have absolutely no intention of being anti-Jewish. For Jews too are becoming increasingly concerned about circumcision. Some are choosing against it for their own sons. Many are concerned that a large number of Jewish parents chose it only as a supposed medical consideration, similar to routine immunization, rather than as a religious rite. (For the devout Jew, medical circumcision is not considered "true" circumcision.) Many Jews advocate circumcision *only* as a religious observance, and urge non-Jewish parents not to follow suit.

Rabbi Moses Maimonides summed it up in the 13th century: "No one ... should circumcise himself or his son for any other reason but pure faith ..." [79]

Today, even that faith is being questioned by some.

You may want to check out these "Jewish Movement Resources" on my *Peaceful Beginnings* website.

3.11 Interview with Rabbi F.S. Gartner

(Bellingham, Washington)

The following interview with Rabbi Gartner is the only one in this book that is in favor of circumcision. I of course disagree with much of what he has to say. However, I do consider his views worth sharing.

He was an older man who was born in Europe and lost several relatives during the Nazi regime. This interview took place in 1979. Rabbi Gartner died in 1984 at the age of 86.

Prior to this interview I showed him a copy of the proposed outline for this book. Included in the outline was mention of the Chapter 18 "Is Circumcision Traumatic For a Newborn Baby?" Because he saw this, he was quite defensive about this point, insisting that the operation could not possibly be painful for a baby.

I include this interview with little comment. I made no attempt to argue any of the points on which he and I disagreed. I only ask that this interview be read in context with the rest of the book. – R.R.

---

78 Steinberg, Linda (personal correspondence).
79 Maimonides, p. 378.

Rabbi Gartner: Circumcision is not an exclusively Jewish rite. It was, and still is practiced among peoples all over the world. Today many European and American Christians practice circumcision for reasons of health. According to some physicians, circumcision is beneficial in avoiding cancer.

Rosemary: I have articles that present both sides of that question. Many would disagree with that.

G: It is estimated that one-seventh of the world's population are practicing circumcision at present. In ancient times the Egyptians and the Phoenicians, just as the Jews, practiced circumcision. The Philistines, Syrians, and Canaanites were not circumcised. The Arabs circumcised their sons at the age of 13 years. This is based on Genesis: 17: 25: "And Ishmael was the son. His son was 13 years old when he was circumcised in the flesh of his foreskin." Since the Mohammedans base their beliefs to a certain degree on the Bible and the Pentateuch, they still usually practice circumcision at the age of 13. It's not a very comfortable procedure, as you can well imagine.

R: I'm sure it isn't at any age.

G: In the past they didn't use anesthesia. It was painful and the boys had to really be "heroes." The Jews circumcise on the eighth day, which is, according to every authority I know, the ideal day for circumcision. Sensitivity is still at a low and the coagulation which goes back to 30% in the earlier days is restored normally at the eighth day. That's the ideal day as far as sensitivity, pain and feelings.

R: You believe that they're less sensitive to pain on that day than any other day?

G: Yes, definitely. I've performed quite a few hundred circumcisions and very often I didn't even hear a peep out of the baby. The baby is held comfortably and sucks on a piece of sugar. We put the sugar on a piece of gauze and the baby doesn't even react. It reacts when you spread the legs. The baby doesn't want to be tied down. That has to be done for reasons of security.

R: Do you use the circumcision board where the baby is strapped down?

G: I usually use it. Sometimes a nurse would hold the legs. I usually do it in the hospital or at home. The Jewish hospitals in large Jewish cities have special rooms set aside for the festivities that take place. Everything is done in the hygienic way. That's my main concern.

In Hebrew, *Brith* is the right pronunciation. This means covenant. We used to pronounce it *Briss* because of the old fashioned way of pronunciation of Hebrew. The Israeli pronunciation has taken over more recently.

It's a sign of the covenant of Abraham. Circumcision assumed a deep spiritual meaning. It is still the outward mark of belonging to the Jewish community. The hostility of other groups has only intensified the determination of Jews to continue circumcising. Circumcision has been performed in secret and very often turned the Jews into martyrs. Jews were ready to and did die for their belief. They call this "Al-Kiddush-Hachem," "for the sanctification of God's name." The circumcision ceremony has become a religious ceremony of great significance. Attached to it are benedictions, joy, and feasting. Oil lamps were burned and the operation is done by a specially appointed skilled man known as Mohel.

In the Middle Ages, the ceremony was transferred from the home to the synagogue and the "Chair of Elijah" was added. Also the Sandek, which means "Godfather," the assistant to the mohel was added to the circumcision ritual.

In modern times the Reform Jews in Western Europe discarded circumcision together with other rituals, but later restored it. Often it was performed during modern times by a physician if there was no qualified mohel available. The mohel has to have special training which he gets in hospitals.

During the 19th century the ceremony again was reverted to the home instead of the synagogue. Circumcision has to be performed even on the Sabbath. Also it is done on Yom Kippur, the day of atonement, which is the holiest day in the Jewish calendar. At the circumcision ceremony, the baby is given the Hebrew name.[80]

R: Do they do any kind of ceremony for baby girls?
G: There are some people who circumcise women too. I think it was practiced in Abyssinia. The clitoris was cut. There is no circumcision for a girl in the Jewish religion. The girl is named in the synagogue, usually within a week.
R: What is the cultural significance of circumcision for Jewish people?
G: It's not cultural significance. You consider civilization or culture a form of development of a people, then circumcision became a part of the Jewish civilization, the culture. But it is strictly a religious ceremony.
R: Is it important as a cleanliness measure?
G: Cleanliness is practiced, especially in modern times. In ancient times I don't know what they did. There must have been some by not knowing about germs. I use disinfectants and I scrub my hands and use surgical gloves. I don't think it's necessary though, because babies have a wonderful capacity. They're healthy and young.[81]
R: They heal very rapidly. What method do you use when you circumcise?
G: We used to use a knife. Now we use a clamp. I use the Gomco because the religious requirements of shedding some blood: "Thou shalt deliver some blood ..."

---

80 Some modern Jewish parents give their children, both sons and daughters, a name in Hebrew in addition to a conventional "American" name. Frequently the conventional name (by which the child will be known) and the Hebrew name are chosen to start with the same letter sounds. – R.R.
81 I was trying to ask him, "Do Jewish people consider circumcision an important measure of personal body cleanliness?" He misunderstood the question and thought I was asking him about cleanliness measures taken during the operation. – R.R.

the blood is enough from cutting with a clamp. I cut it, and I leave the clamp on, so I draw a little bit of blood. The eighth day is very important, but for reasons of health we postpone circumcision. Also if a woman lost two children to circumcision, her third boy is not to be circumcised. This applies to her sister's sons too. It means that this [an inherited tendency to have bleeding problems] is in the family. If there's a danger to life, it takes precedence over any ritual or commandment.

R: I have heard of a theory that circumcision of newborn males originated as a "blood sacrifice" in order to purify the infant from the "contaminated" blood of his mother from giving birth. What are your comments on this?

G: This is *theory*. You can let your imagination go haywire! But we have other sources besides theory! I am sick and tired of theories! I am not the person to agree with this! It's a sign of the covenant between God and Abraham and his successors that this has to be practiced.

R: I have also heard of a theory that circumcision of newborn males began as a "token sacrifice" replacing the earlier practice of sacrificing the baby. This would have been far back in ancient times.

G: The Jewish religion is completely against that! The practices of the ancient Babylonians had the sacrifice of children to the God Moloch and burned the children alive. This was an abomination to the Jewish people. The greatest part of the Jewish religion deals with commandments not to follow those practices and never to be cruel! The Jewish tradition teaches us to be kind to animals too, and not to cause any pain. The laws of killing animals were made for this reason. People were too cruel and the Jews were always considered to cause the least pain. So this is completely out of line for the Jews. We never sacrificed. We were warned in the scripture never to fall back on this abomination.

R: Why has the ritual of circumcision persisted among Jewish people, even when they no longer choose to observe other practices such as dietary laws?

G: Perhaps it is because Jews are not a nation. Therefore it's a mark of civilization that Jews have developed. *[sic: Israel officially became a nation in 1948. – R.R.]*

R: Even among some Jewish people who have dropped following the Kosher diet and so forth?

G: Yes, and are not observant, but they still want to be classified as Jews.

R: Of course in the United States most males are circumcised, so being circumcised does not set one apart as being Jewish.

G: Yes, the Christians do it for health reasons. I know there are some opinions saying that this is not true, but I have spoken to doctors. They say that when a person is not circumcised, in old age he suffers with cleanliness problems. Then the circumcision has to be performed in old age, and it's not a very pleasant procedure. From a hygienic point of view, physically, circumcision is of tremendous value.

R: I have read descriptions of the three basic steps to the Jewish ritual. They are described as the "milah" which is the cutting off of the foreskin, the "periah" which is the pushing back and tearing of the inner membrane with the thumbnail, and "mezizah" in which the blood is sucked from the baby's penis. Is the ritual still done in this manner?

G: The milah is the cutting off of the foreskin, but this is done in modern times not by tearing the foreskin. It is done with scissors. Then the glans comes up, the skin is pushed back, and the glans appears very clean.

R: So the clamp takes care of that part?

G: The clamp is used but the pushing back is done by hand. The pushing back of the inner membrane with the thumbnail is not done that way any more. It is taken care of in a more modern way. Mezizah has been abandoned a long time ago because of the dangers involved. I think it was the only thing they knew how to do to stop the bleeding. Some fanatics will still observe the old time ways.

R: How is the mohel trained?

G: Religiously it is combined with the training for a Rabbi, but he also goes to a hospital to get experience with circumcision. In times past one mohel would simply teach the other.

R: Do you believe that circumcision traumatizes the baby or causes any lasting psychological ill effects?

G: Well, I believe the human race is a little bit more sturdy than this. There are traumatic experiences, but I think it's a rather wild assumption. I don't agree in many aspects with psychiatrists. We have a tendency to go haywire and we should stick to realities. If you want to get into culmination and imagination, there's no end to it.

R: You really don't believe that it has any ill effects?

G: No. I argued vividly with the psychologist that tried to bring that theory up in the presence of other doctors. The doctors agreed with me and so did the nurses. This was at a very good hospital.

R: I've certainly talked with other people who feel quite a bit differently about that!

G: Yes, but they are usually leaning toward psychiatry or psychoanalysis. They are not what I would call practical physicians. You also give the baby a little slap when it is born.

R: That isn't usually done any more.

G: But I don't think that causes any trauma. Those things are forgotten. There is no proof that such things really affect the future of the babies. They forget it, just like the bleeding stops. I don't believe it. You are entitled to your opinion and so am I.

Psychiatrists ... what would they have to do if they wouldn't bother with such things? They would be standing idly around.

R: I have known some Jewish couples who have had their baby circumcised in the hospital by a doctor to save money. Their insurance would cover it in the hospital but not for a mohel to do it. But then later they had a "Baby Naming Ceremony."

G: Then they didn't perform according to Jewish tradition! For traditional Jews the circumcision cannot be varied! I do not insist when I convert a person of full age to Judaism that a circumcision be performed, because I think it's a major surgical involvement which causes pain and sometimes people cannot afford. If a child is converted with the parents I will draw one drop of blood from the foreskin which is not a traumatic shock. I personally regard the sensitivities of the child at this age (past the newborn age) very important. If it can be a traumatic experience I will not practice it.

Now those Reform Jews who have the baby circumcised in the hospital by a doctor and then name the baby in the Temple ... they are not very firmly grounded in the Jewish tradition. It's a matter of convenience rather than sacrifice which you have to bring for every idea you believe in. They don't comply! You can eat matzoh with ham on it! I can't keep you from it if you are Jewish! But it's not according to the Jewish law.

R: If the baby has been circumcised as a hospital procedure that's considered not really circumcised according to Jewish tradition?

G: Then it's a medical performance rather than the real tradition. All the paraphernalia and all the reciting are part of it. It has to be by a certain ritual.

R: What if some people were a practicing Jewish couple and they had a baby boy and they didn't want him circumcised. What would the Temple do?

G: If it's Reform, the Temple would not react. They would accept their judgment. If it's any other like Conservative or Orthodox, you are not considered a Jew because this is one of the main things which brings you into the covenant ... the Brith. You cannot say "I subscribe to the American constitution, but when it doesn't fit me I don't do it." Unfortunately this is done and that's why we have such a restless society. This has its advantages and great disadvantages. The Jewish people have always been encouraged to ask questions and arrive at answers. That's why we have a Talmud, where opinions of opponents are also written down.

R: Are you Orthodox?

G: No, I'm Conservative.

R: I understand that in Russia and in some other parts of the world even Jewish people don't circumcise.

G: I don't know about that. I'm sure that the Jews do it in secret. They have done it over the centuries for thousands of years, even when they were threatened with death. So you speak about expenses, it might cost a few more dollars to have a Rabbi do it in a ceremony than to have a doctor do it in the hospital. But this was not a sacrifice that comes to dollars … but life!!

R: Do you have any idea how circumcision came to be popular in American hospitals as a medical procedure? Until the turn of the century most non-Jewish people in this society did not practice circumcision.

G: We were considered brutes! It was thrown into our faces, "You are Barbarians!!" But finally hypocrisy and prejudice gave way to reason. Even if you don't believe in it as a covenant, as the Jews do, it is still subscribed to from the medical point of view. I think if he is not circumcised, the baby gets into trouble later on when he grows up.

R: There are many Jewish doctors in the United States. Do you think that their influence could have anything to do with the popularity of circumcision in the United States today?

G: I doubt it. We keep our ceremonies to ourselves. We have no missionaries.

R: If an adult man converts to Judaism and is not circumcised, does he have to have it done?

G: In the Orthodox way, if an adult wants to convert to Judaism he has to be circumcised. The Reform don't insist. The Conservatives are flexible because we consider what is involved. It's a major surgical step. Some Rabbis would perform the circumcision after the person departs.

R: If an adult man did become circumcised when he joined the Jewish religion, would they do a ceremony for him the same way?

G: Yes. This is considered indeed a great sacrifice. The person is practically considered a holy man.

R: Do the Jews still have to circumcise a dead baby before burial?

G: Yes. The ceremony is limited. The joy is not there. If the baby didn't live thirty days it doesn't have to be done. But there's no harm done in bringing it into the covenant post-mortem.

R: Could a non-Jewish couple take their baby to a mohel to be circumcised?

G: No. The Rabbi has no right to perform a circumcision for a non-Jewish baby. I have a right to perform for Jewish people only. Otherwise I would compete with physicians. I am not permitted by state law.

R: How do you personally feel about doing circumcisions?

G: I feel all right. My personal experiences have been fine.

R: Have you had any bad experiences with it?

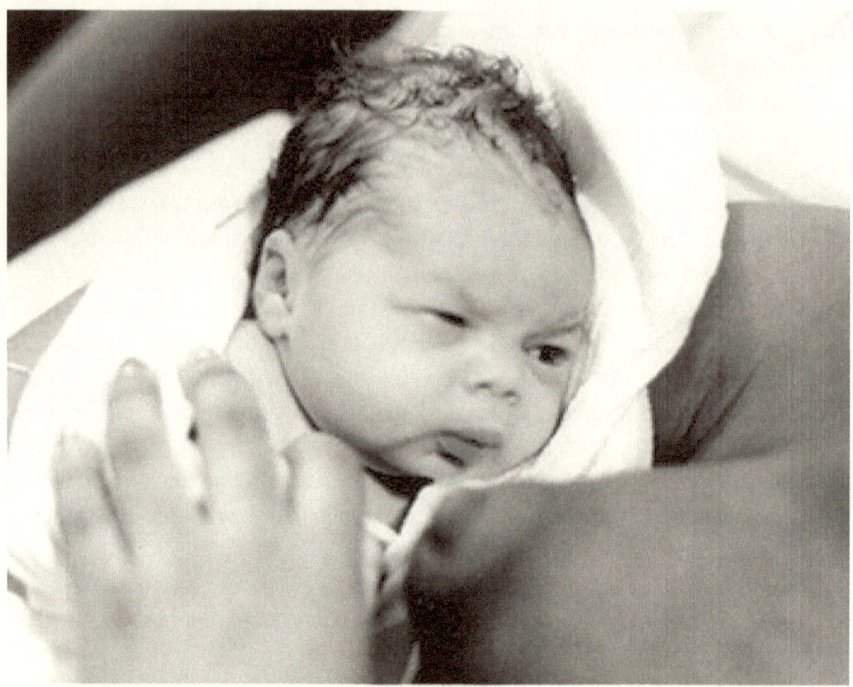

© Suzanne Arms

G: I had some in which I was apprehensive because the baby had difficulties immediately after birth. The blood wasn't okay. They had to drain the blood out and replace it with new blood. *[He was probably referring to the RH factor. – R.R.]*

But the circumcision went okay. I was watching for hours to see if there was any bleeding.

R: Why couldn't God have just made penises that way in the first place? If he didn't want males to have foreskins, why did He put them there in the first place?

G: It's a speculation. Why did God not create all men perfect? He could have. God is almighty! Why do we have to have crooks? Why do we have to straighten out people? They could have been born ideal. Some people would tell you that God made them that way because God wanted the Jews to prove themselves and take upon themselves some obligations and sacrifices. Not sacrifices in the sense that we sacrifice the foreskin, but sacrificing from pain or discomfort. But this question ... you could just as well ask why is a person not born smart and fully developed? Why does he have to be a baby and grow?

3.12 Interview with Elizabeth & Marsh Pickard-Ginsberg

(Young Jewish parents from Bellingham, Washington)

Marsh: I grew up in a very traditional Jewish family. For the last few years I have lived as an artist. I teach Tai Chi. For the last two years we have been in Iowa City, Iowa. Elizabeth and I have just moved to Bellingham (Washington state).

Rosemary: You had a home birth. What were your feelings and plans for that choice?

M: We were living in San Francisco and we were considering an alternative to hospital birth.

Elizabeth: We didn't have much education about pregnancy or birth. We moved to Iowa in November 1976. Jesse was born in February 1977. I hadn't had any prenatal checks (by November) but I knew I felt healthy. I went to a women's clinic and started exploring alternatives to a regular hospital birth. Hospitals were so foreign to me that I didn't feel that would be the best place where I could open up and relax. Everything I'd read about giving birth said that where it feels most comfortable is safest. We were frightened by the idea of home birth, too. There was so much we didn't know.

R: I think every expectant couple has some fears.

E: We had a strong feeling that there wouldn't be any problems with the birth.

R: And it was a normal birth?

E: We considered going to the hospital. I went into labor on a Friday and Jesse was born the following Monday. During that time the labor would stop. It was actually a lot of pre-labor.

R: I'm sure that must be terribly discouraging.

E: I had a lot of anxiety about wanting to get labor over with before I was really ready.

R: It's hard to deal with. You just feel like the baby's never going to come.

E: From Sunday about 3 p.m. to Monday 3 p.m. when he was born, there was hard labor. It was a good thing it was at home. Had I been in a hospital that 24 hour period might have really been ... I feel ... a lot more difficult.

R: They might have induced you to speed it up.

E: I might have ended up with a Caesarian because I wasn't dilating.

R: It can be normal for a first time mother to go slow like that.

E: It was good being with people who had the consciousness that they saw birth as a natural process. During transition, it was not one of these "blissful births." I was screaming "Knock me out!! Take the baby out!! Do anything to me, just get it over with!!" But somehow I got through it! Second stage labor (pushing) was 10 minutes. I pushed him right out!

R: And the baby was fine and beautiful after he was born.

E: Yes. Before the birth we'd talked a lot about circumcision, but we hadn't made a decision by the birth. It's embarrassing to admit, but I had hardly ever heard the word or thought about what it meant. I had never seen an uncircumcised man. I really didn't know what circumcision versus non-circumcision was.

R: A lot of American people are in the same situation. Some people have never seen an intact penis before until they have a baby boy of their own.

E: Neither of us knew much. We read some articles by Ina May Gaskin (*The Farm*, Tenn.) We respected her natural views on birth. I read that she had circumcised her son herself because of infections. That made me think that maybe circumcision wasn't such a bad thing. We also asked a few people and all they said about circumcision was "Well, they cry a few minutes, it doesn't hurt that much." My image was that they took a little bit of skin off the end of the penis and it was quick and painless. But I still kept saying to Marsh "Why tamper with the body? Why not just leave the body the way it is?" Then I turned the issue over to Marsh. He had more of a conflict because of his parents.

M: It was a conflict for me because I grew up in a very traditional Jewish family in which there was no question about it. If you have a baby boy you have him circumcised. When we asked questions it was "What is a circumcision? What happens?" We basically understood that there was *no pain*.

E: His parents sent us a check for the Bris after Jesse was born.

M: Looking back ... it seems like something very *cannibalistic* to me, *barbaric*, as to what a Bris is, because it's supposed to be something that binds all the Jews together. Bris means "covenant" between man and God. It was a conflict for me because I was just beginning to enter into a new consciousness of how much care and responsibility you have when you have a new person. Coming from a background and tradition in which you don't question circumcision, I wasn't questioning it as deeply as I could have. I don't feel good that we made that decision. We were told by the urologist who was Jewish and who did the circumcision, that there was a possibility that if we hadn't had a circumcision, Jesse might have had kidney problems when he was 10 or 11 because his foreskin was so tight. Now I question that.

E: Our midwife questioned it also. Statistics show that sometimes it takes three years or more to loosen.

R: It's normal for the foreskin of a newborn to be tight and have a tiny opening.

M: I remember the confrontation with the urologist and that I wasn't satisfied with his response.

E: Before the baby was born I kept bringing up the issue of circumcision. It was bothering me. I was pretty sure that it was a baby boy. Marsh was avoiding the issue

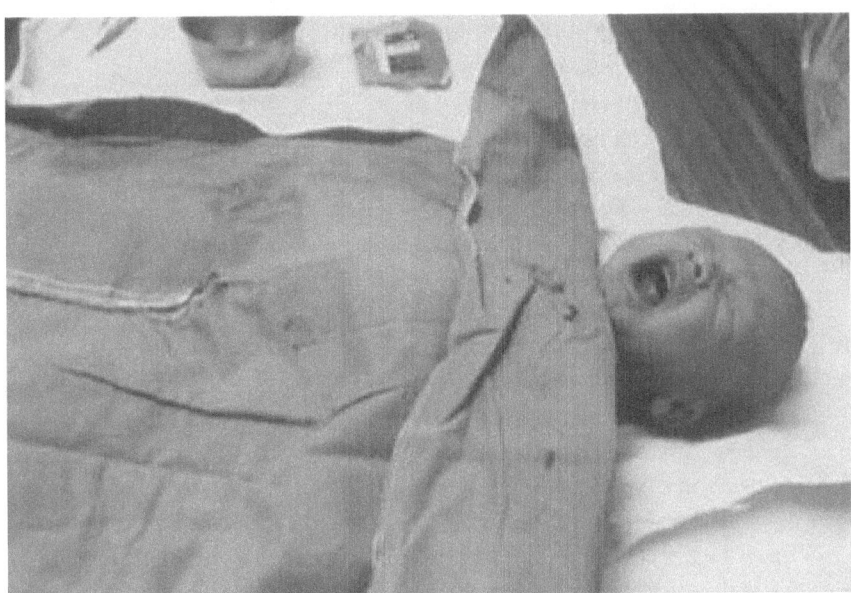

Reprinted with permission from The Saturday Evening Post Company © 1981.

because it was so disturbing for him. One day I said "Look, we have to make a decision about this!" We took all the facts that we had gathered at that time and sat down to make a decision. I said that I preferred not to have him circumcised, but I felt that since he was the father, there would be a strong identification there between father and son. It was very important for him to feel comfortable with the decision.

R: A lot of fathers feel that way. Even when he's not Jewish, often a father thinks that if he is circumcised, then his son should be also.

E: We had a very emotional conversation and at the end Marsh finally threw up his hands and said "I won't be able to relate to my son! I'll be exiled from my family if he were not circumcised!!" That was the big thing ... that there would be a lack of acceptance between father and son. That somehow Marsh would feel ... that he wouldn't be able to relate to Jesse because he wasn't circumcised. Also that his family would not take Jesse into their hearts. So at that point we felt that he would be circumcised. The issue was still hovering. Four days after his birth we went to a Jewish pediatrician for his check up. We asked him about circumcision. The pediatrician got very pale and stern and said he didn't do circumcisions any more!! He was upset!

M: He was a very conservative type of guy who looked like nothing could touch him, but he got really upset when we mentioned circumcision.

E: The upsetness showed by his becoming very tight.

M: It was like it was so upsetting to him that he couldn't even approach the subject.

E: When we pressured him to talk more about circumcision, he didn't want to talk about it. He did tell us that there was no medical reason for it, and I guess we knew that. We were looking for someone to tell us what to do. It's such a hard decision. But he wasn't able to. Finally, somehow, we were just going ahead with it. We'd contacted this Jewish urologist to come to our home to do the circumcision. We felt that it would be too alienating in a hospital. We might not have done it if we hadn't found anybody to do it at home.

R: Did you have a Rabbi there for the ceremony?

E: Marsh read the Hebrew from the Rabbi's book. We did the ceremony. The Rabbi was out of town. Our midwife and her assistant who had helped with Jesse's birth were there. Traditionally there's food prepared and we drank wine. The baby is given wine on a cloth.

M: I think that whole concept of "a ceremony" and having something to eat afterwards is totally barbaric! When I started to really feel that idea of cutting up this kid's body and considering it to be what the Jews call a "mitzvah," a "good deed," and then everybody is all smiles and laughs and has wine and cake is just ...

R: Do you still practice the Jewish faith?

M: Friday night is Sabbath for us and we light the candles and make the blessing over the bread and wine. We recognize the Sabbath as being separate from the rest of the week. We celebrate major holidays like Passover.

R: Do you go to Temple?

M: Not any more. I went to Hebrew school until I was 17 or 18. I went to Synagogue or Temple and I was confirmed when I was 15.

R: You had a Bar Mitzvah?

M: Yes. There was a great deal of Jewishness in my family. It was conservative. My father was brought up Orthodox. It was a Kosher household with two sets of dishes for meat and milk and two sinks. But since my going to college and basically living and opening up to what life is all about, I began to have a strong feeling that what goes on in the Synagogue is contradictory to what Judaism to me really is. I feel a lot of lip service is given in the synagogues and temples.

R: I've seen a lot of the same thing in Christian churches. Is Elizabeth Jewish?

M: Technically she is. Her mother is Jewish, but she didn't practice Judaism. Her father is Episcopalian.

R: Are you Jewish now?

E: Being Jewish is a part of me. I feel a tie there in my being. I feel like myself and that's a part of myself.

M: I feel strongly that by making people believe in and do something without feeling ... you're forcing something on them. Then what happens is two things ... one is fear and the other is hate. That is what I fear is happening now. There's a lot of Jewish things that are done on fear! Like fear of God, because you don't have an inner feeling of what God is.

E: And He's going to know that you're not doing this and not doing that!!

R: Do you mean a fear of your parents? Or the community? Or fear of God?

M: There's a connection there that in a sense my father is God. That's unconsciously tied into the Jewish religion. Also there is a fear of losing love and losing family.

E: It's a matter of approval or disapproval if you gain or lose ... not love.

M: Exactly. A banishment. That's what happened with Hagar and Ishmael. Sarah said, "Get out of here!" and they went like that!

E: Marsh and I have gone over and over the actual ceremony in our minds. When the urologist and our two friends arrived, the doctor said, "Let's put Jesse on the kitchen table." And we said, "No, we want to hold him! We want him to have contact!" So our midwife held Jesse, sitting on the bed that he was born in. The urologist was facing Jesse. I was facing Jesse and Marsh was sitting on the bed holding Jesse's hand and ... Did you have to hold him down? Was I holding down his legs?

M: The only thing I remember is his hand holding my thumb.

E: And shrieking!! He was just clinging to Marsh's thumb!! He had one of my thumbs too. I was holding a washcloth with wine on it that he was supposed to suck on. I can still remember all the wine dripping down on him. He was wearing a T-shirt that Marsh's sister had embroidered with a mandala on it – a very beautiful, special T-shirt. When the doctor opened up the instruments and I saw them I just pushed away any feelings that I could stop the circumcision. I don't know why!! All I could have said was "I've changed my mind." or "I absolutely won't allow this!" But I was in shock!!

M: I went into shock as soon as I saw the instruments!

E: He cut and held a hemostat on the cut. The foreskin wasn't retractible. They couldn't just use a bell.

R: That's what is normally done. They clamp it first with a hemostat to stop any bleeding and leave it on for a few minutes, completely pinching off the blood vessels. Then they snip it, making the slit large enough to put the bell in. It is normal for the foreskin of a newborn to be tight.

E: He made it sound to us that this was just because his foreskin was so tight.

R: He made you feel that it was abnormal?

E: Abnormal. Right. That was why he had to ... he gave us this word "dorsal slit." So Jesse was shrieking and I had tears streaming down my face. Marsh turned

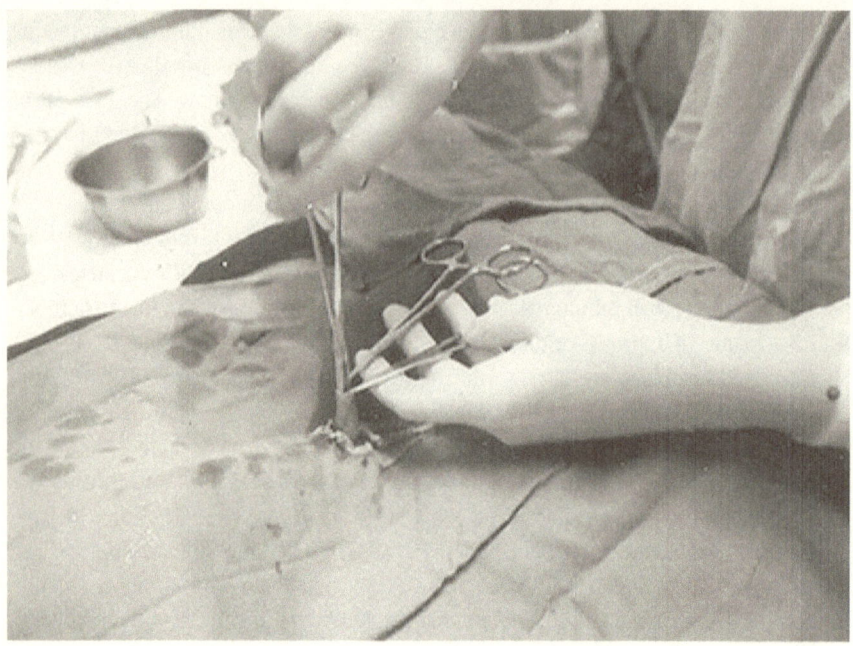

Reprinted with permission from The Saturday Evening Post Company © 1981.

gray yellow – a very odd color!! He looked like he was about to pass out. I can remember his face being in shock!!

M: It seemed like I was here and I was somewhere else. I get sick just thinking about it! Right now I just feel sick!! I also go into a rage!! If I had been in touch with my feelings at all I would have killed the guy!!

E: Or stopped it!! You would have stopped it.

M: Yeah, I would have stopped it!

E: Both of us cut off our feelings and allowed this thing to happen in our own house to our own baby because of all this ... cultural stuff. We were feeling like incompetent children ... as opposed to: "This is *our baby*. We can make a decision and a choice!! We can stop this!! We can answer his cries!! He was screaming and there was no doubt in his scream that he wanted mother, or a mothering figure to come and protect him from this pain!!

M: I know I went into shock as soon as he uncovered all the medical instruments. I saw all these stainless steel sharp numbers ...

E: Razors and scalpels.

M: I just had no awareness that this was going to be *surgery!!*

E: We thought it was going to be just a little tiny piece of skin!

3 – Circumcision and Judaism

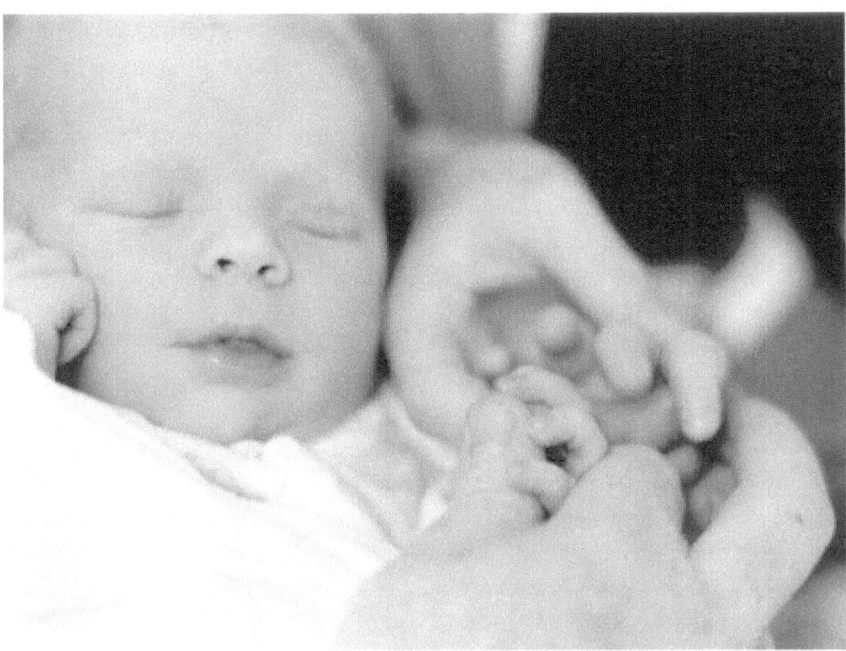

© Suzanne Arms

M: From my tradition I had always heard "Everybody's going to a Bris, and oh what a great thing it is!" so there was never in my mind any awareness of this being surgery! I had heard that they put a clamp on the end of the foreskin and snap it off like that! When I was going to Hebrew school I had a teacher who did circumcisions and that's the way he described it ... that they put a clamp on the tip of the penis and in a second it's over. But this circumcision took 25 minutes!

R: Why did he take so long? Normally it should only take a few minutes.

E: He said it was because the foreskin was so tight and because he held the hemostat a lot. I guess he was just being extremely cautious. And I couldn't believe it, he just kept pulling back this skin and pulling it back, and finally he said "Ah, we're finally getting to the tip of the penis!" And here's this *liver-colored, bloody* thing being exposed that definitely looked like an internal organ. I thought you just cut off this little piece of skin and there's the tip of the penis and that's that. I didn't know you had to pull back and cut off ... do so *much cutting!* And I didn't realize the tip of the penis was so *obviously* meant to be covered!!

R: In the intact individual the glans looks very much different. In the circumcised person it looks like the rest of his skin. In the intact person it's like the inside of our vaginas or the inside of the mouth. It's a totally different type of skin.

129

Circumcision – The Painful Dilemma

E: This is one thing Marsh also heard about circumcision. In Israeli war tribes they said circumcision helped the tip of the penis develop and made him grow into manhood faster.

R: People have all sorts of ideas. I don't believe that there's any truth to it.

M: I've never heard that idea since, but it seemed possible that circumcising the male makes the genital area grow faster, so that in time of war this was something that they needed. The Israelis are constantly in conflicts.

E: *(To Marsh)* You were talking about the circumcision ... You always want to go into the history and Biblical aspects of it. I keep wanting to hear more about your personal feelings. It makes me realize how much pain is still there. I didn't realize that there was that much pain still with you.

M: There's still a lot of pain there!

R: You had described the part where the doctor had been pulling the foreskin back. Did he use a clamp then?

E: He used a steel metal ball. It was a round clamp that he placed on it. At that point Jesse screamed so loud that all of a sudden there was no sound! I've never heard anything like it! He was screaming and it went up and then there was no sound and his mouth was just open and his face was full of pain!!

M: He had been crying up to that point and then it was too much.

E: I remember something happened inside me ... the intensity of it was like blowing a fuse! It was too much. We knew something was over. I don't feel that it ever really healed. At a certain point things metamorphosize when there's too much pain, and we'd gone beyond!!

R: It has been over two years since it happened and you're still recovering from it.

E: I don't think I can recover from it. It's a scar. I've put a lot of energy into trying to recover. I did some crying and we did some therapy. There's still a lot of feeling that's blocked off. It was too intense.

R: What was the immediate aftermath, right after the circumcision?

E: Jesse went into a coma-like sleep. And Marsh picked up his diapers.

M: Elizabeth was nursing Jesse. I picked up his diapers and they were just bloody!! I was crying! I just wept!

E: He put his head on the floor and just shook!!

M: I don't think I've ever cried like that before.

R: Were the doctor or any of the other people there aware of your feelings?

E: They were gone.

M: They were there for about 15 minutes afterwards.

E: They had cake and wine.

M: And we were left alone after that.

E: I remember Marsh ... how you felt that something terrible had happened that could never be redeemed. It was like the fall from the Garden of Eden. We had this beautiful baby boy and seven beautiful days and this beautiful rhythm starting, and it was like something had been shattered!

M: It was a very, very strange feeling.

E: Something we could not take back. Remorse! Deep, horrible remorse!

M: Things had been really beautiful. There was a certain cadence that we had to our lives and we were pretty much alone. All of a sudden something snatched the essence of what was ever there and damaged it! It couldn't just be given back. It's something that I had never experienced before with anything that I can remember. It's even hard remembering the circumcision. I get a glimpse for a split second and then it fragments.

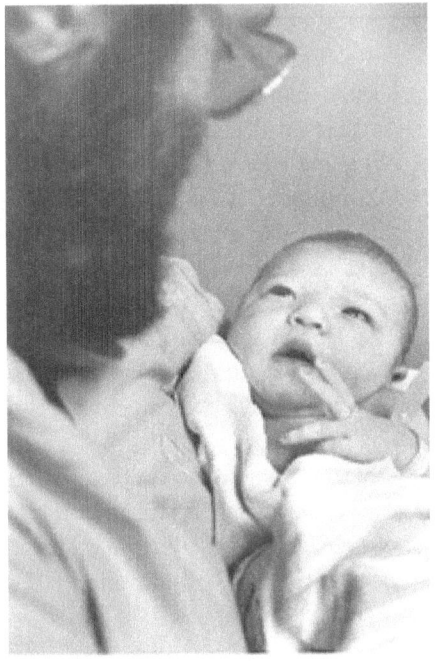

© Suzanne Arms

R: Didn't you say that you were up all night with Jesse?

E: When Jesse woke up and we changed his diaper for the first time, he started bleeding a lot, and I *panicked!!* I got hysterical! Marsh got on the phone. We couldn't reach the doctor. Jesse was *shrieking!!* I thought I was going to have the baby hemorrhage to death right in front of me!!

M: Then I called the pediatrician. He said "If you want I'll come over." He was really great. He said "Put a thick dab of Vaseline on it and don't diaper him." I think we did that for the next day. I held him all night. We didn't sleep most of the night. He fell asleep with his back to my chest. When he peed he just peed.

E: We left the diaper off and sat up all night holding him and dozing off and waking up with his peeing in my face and all over himself and then crying because of it. We couldn't put the diaper on him because he was so sore, he would just shriek! Then the next day we could diaper him real loosely. It was starting to heal. It was all scabby and blistery.

M: That's the last of anything I remember about it. It took apparently the usual amount of time that it takes to heal. After it healed it didn't seem to bother Jesse, but I can't imagine that something like that can happen and not affect the child. We've been very lucky. Nothing really awful has happened to him since then. But I know from my experience when I went into therapy and re-experienced my own circumcision, I could barely touch that.

R: What kind of therapy did you have?

M: Bio-energetics. It was a re-experiencing type of thing. When I was in therapy I went through a sort of visualization, a re-experiencing of my own circumcision. I can't remember clearly what it was, but I know it was pretty awful. I felt at the time that I was just barely touching the surface of what it was that I experienced. Just think of being a man or a boy who is a little bit older and somebody holding you down and taking the end of your penis off. It's no different. Some people have a crazy idea that babies feel less and experience less than somebody who is older!!

E: If anything it hurts more, if you just see it.

M: It's a feeling of rage and anger that came out. if you just close your eyes and think of yourself as being a child, a baby, and you can't talk, and you can't express your feelings, and you're being tortured ...

E: Murdered!! It's like being murdered, for a baby!!

M: Tying down your legs and arms ... There is total rage there! I know that as a man, if somebody were to come at Jesse or Elizabeth with that kind of intention, I would probably kill the f---------!! Or cause him a lot of bodily harm!! There would be no question!! Of course I have the power to reason, so I could say, "Look, I don't want you to do that!"

E: We let our baby boy be cut up by some stranger!

M: I didn't want Elizabeth to go to the hospital to have Jesse, even though at times it was very difficult. But when it came time for his circumcision, I just went into this other world.

E: There was a detachment between me and Jesse. So my therapist said "Next time you're nursing him, put him into bed and breathe with him ... often your breathing goes with a state of mind. If your breathing is shallow, you're cutting off feelings." I started this as he was going to sleep and I started crying and I got in touch with the real basic animal kind of feeling that ... when he was first born there was a tie with my young one, my newborn.

R: You had that immediate bonding.

E: And when the circumcision happened, in order to allow it I had cut off the bond. I had to cut off my natural instincts, and in doing so I cut off a lot of feelings towards Jesse. I cut it off to repress the pain and to repress the natural instinct to stop the circumcision. What I got in touch with was a feeling of "This is *my baby!*" and "You're not going to hurt *my baby!*" I would get glimpses of how much

I had repressed and cut off. *(At this point Elizabeth's voice is starting to break and choke and she is on the verge of crying.)*

R: How do you feel towards Jesse now?

E: I feel that there's an element of detachment there. I didn't ever really get through that pain. It was too intense.

R: What do you think it will be like when you have another child, either a girl or a boy who is left intact? Do you think you'll have a better relationship with that child?

E: I don't know. I don't know how to compare. Jesse seems like a pretty happy kid. I don't focus on the idea that I should be feeling any different.

R: *(To Marsh)* What about your relationship with Jesse?

M: We're very close. Jesse slept on my chest for the first couple of night during his life on this planet. I miss him when I'm not around.

R: Do you feel resolved about his circumcision now?

M: No. It's somewhere inside me. I don't know that I ever will get through it.

E: We've just tried to really love him and go beyond.

M: There are still a lot of people that when you talk to them about your experience they block that up. I had a friend in Berkeley. He and his wife were both Jewish, and they were going to have their baby circumcised. He seemed to feel it was a good thing to do. He was totally avoiding the idea that his baby was going to be feeling a lot of pain! Judaism has done a lot of brainwashing to people.

R: And the medical profession too.

M: I think if we have another baby boy we'll just have the Bris without the circumcision. We'll have some kind of ceremony.

E: I'm not interested. I don't think you need a ceremony to say there's a "covenant with God." By the fact that he was alive and healthy ... the "covenant" to me is by his birth.

M: Basically what I'm saying is that I think the idea of a circumcision ... a Bris is something that is internal. Jews have this propensity to want to externalize how they feel inside by doing a lot of different things. Unfortunately it has taken people a long way from the center of Judaism. We should share with people from the heart rather than by material things.

(Elizabeth and Marsh have since divorced. Elizabeth has since given birth to another son, Eli, who has been left intact.)

3.13   A Letter From a Jewish Mother

The subject of circumcision renewed itself for me recently as a Jewish friend was preparing to birth. In 1970 when I was pregnant with my son I gave the matter much thought. My husband is Jewish and I am too. The son in my womb – and I knew he was a he, having had a vision of him even before conception – brought up the question of circumcision. By tuning in to my deepest maternal feelings I knew that I would not violate my boy and my own maternity by inflicting willful pain on him and me. My mother-in-law was hurt by my rejection of the ancient practice. I myself was not pleased that my son would differ from his father in his masculinity, but I decided that this is an age of change and it was time to end a bad practice. My husband supported me and my mother-in-law finally accepted my decision also.

When my pregnant friend and I talked about circumcising newborn infants my old rage flared up again. She told me that her husband really wanted it done, in the traditional way, by a mohel, as a means of upholding the symbolism of a united Jewish family. I thought that a worthy goal, but suggested that if he was indeed so insistent on the tradition, that he take his child by the hand, after 7 years of age, and lead him to the surgery himself. It occurred to me that the main reason the rite is performed at birth is that at birth the mother is the main recipient of the pain – that in this paternalistic society it is better for the mother to be violated than for the father to take on the pain of a practice he upholds.

The story has a happy ending. When my friend's husband saw his son born he decided that God had made him to perfection – nothing need be added or subtracted.

Stella Fein
Boulder Creek, CA

3.14   Informational Resources

- A New Guide to Intact Jewish Welcoming: Book Review:
  jewishbusinessnews.com/2016/04/26/a-new-guide-to-intact-jewish-welcoming-book-review
- A Non-Traditional "Circumcision" Ceremony: noharmm.org/nontrad.htm
- A Woman's View of Circumcision *(neutral, some faulty ideas, but interesting insights):*
  lilith.org/articles/a-womans-view-of-circumcision
- Abraham, Moses and circumcision, the conundrum of the three Covenants: (Gn. 15, Gn. 17 & Ex. 20):
  academia.edu/2095572
- American Circumcision and Brit Milah in 2003: britshalom.info/reiss2.html
- Ancient Origins of Jewish Ritual Circumcision In Modern Society:
  web.archive.org/web/20150717231348/http://www.gnosticliberationfront.com/

ancient_origins_of_jewish_ritual_circumcision.htm
- Answers from the Bible to Questions about Circumcision: cirp.org/pages/cultural/glass2
- Anti-circumcision protests are a bizarre stunt, say Jewish campaigners:
  hooded2016.wordpress.com/2016/04/11/uk-the-jewish-chronicle-online-anti-circumcision-protests-are-a-bizarre-stunt-say-jewish-campaigners
- Anti-Semitism and Opposition:
  peacefulbeginningsrosemary.wordpress.com/circ-information/anti-semitism-and-opposition
- As a rabbi, I want to know why a Florida man insists on circumcising his son: washingtonpost.com/news/acts-of-faith/wp/2015/05/28/as-a-rabbi-i-want-to-know-why-a-florida-man-insists-on-circumcising-his-son
- Beyond Anti-Semitism: jewishcircumcision.org/beyondas.htm
- Beyond the Bris: beyondthebris.com
- Birth Rate *(negative, scary perspective of the father)*: cirp.org/pages/cultural/hammerman
- Bris Shalom Ceremony: cirp.org/pages/cultural/bris_shalom.html
- Brit Milah or Periah?: covenantcircumcision.info/milah_vs_Periah.html
- Brit Shalom – Covenant of Wholeness: nocirc.org/religion/Naming_ceremony.php
- Brit Shalom Information: britshalom.info
- Challenging Circumcision: A Jewish Perspective: nocirc.org/symposia/fourth/goodman.html
- Circumcision ... my position *(Mark D. Reiss)*: britshalom.info/reiss1.html
- Circumcision and Its Relationship to Attachment Impairment: jewishcircumcision.org/spectator.htm#19
- Circumcision Publications and Organizations: fathermag.com/health/circ/organizations
- Circumcision: A Source of Jewish Pain: jewishcircumcision.org/spectator.htm
- Circumcision: Identity, Gender And Power: huffpost.com/entry/1132896
- Circumcision: Motivational Changes in the Meaning of the Word of God:
  salem-news.com/articles/july022011/circ-motivators-rm.php
- Circumcision: Then and Now: cirp.org/library/history/peron2
- Circumstitions Ritual Myths 2: Abraham transforms sacrifice of firstborn to sacrifice of penis blood, Moses mimics Egyptians: hooded2016.wordpress.com/circumstitions-ritual-myths-2-abraham
- Circumstitions Ritual Myths 3: Joshua at Gilgal, The Mound of Foreskins:
  hooded2016.wordpress.com/circumstitions-ritual-myths-3-joshua
- Circumstitions Ritual Myths 4: Shechem and Dinah, Dinah's Brideprice of Foreskins:
  hooded2016.wordpress.com/circumstitions-ritual-myths-4-shechem-and-dinah
- Circumstitions Ritual Myths 5 David and Michal's Brideprice of Philistine Foreskins, Other mentions:
  hooded2016.wordpress.com/circumstitions-ritual-myths-5-david-and-michals-brideprice
- Comixio Religionis: Circumcision NOT Jerusalemic:
  salem-news.com/articles/july242011/comixio-religionis-rm.php
- Emotional Care of Hospitalized Children: An Environmental Approach: amazon.com/dp/0397543433
- Ending Circumcision in the Jewish Community?: pool.intactiwiki.org/wiki/File:Rothenberg.pdf
- Even in Israel, More and More Parents Choose Not to Circumcise Their Sons:
  haaretz.com/even-in-israel-more-and-more-parents-choose-not-to-circumcise-1.5178506

- Faith Considerations on Circumcision: www.drmomma.org/2011/01/faith-considerations-on-circumcision.html
- Female Genital Mutilation: What It Does To A Woman:
    npr.org/sections/goatsandsoda/2017/05/06/526766230/female-genital-mutilation-what-it-does-to-a-woman
- Greek influence and persecution: aish.com/jl/h/cc/48939692.html
- History of Circumcision: cirp.org/library/history
- How 11 New York City Babies Contracted Herpes Through Circumcision *(mezizah)*:
    healthland.time.com/2012/06/07/how-11-new-york-city-babies-contracted-herpes-through-circumcision
- Humanistic Judaism and anti-circumcision Intactivism:
    jewishbusinessnews.com/2016/04/06/humanistic-judaism-and-anti-circumcision-intactivism
- Intact and Jewish: naturalparentsnetwork.com/intact-and-jewish
- Israeli Health Ministry Recommends Against Direct 'Metzitzah B'Peh':
    jewishpress.com/news/israeli-health-ministry-recommends-against-direct-metzitzah-bpeh/2016/03/02
- It's 2017. Time to Talk About Circumcision:
    haaretz.com/opinion/.premium-its-2017-time-to-talk-about-circumcision-1.5445192
- Jehovah, His Cousin, Allah, and Sexual Mutilations: nocirc.org/symposia/fourth/aldeeb.html
- Jesse's Circumcision: peacefulbeginningsrosemary.wordpress.com/circ-information/jesses-circumcision
- Jewish Brit Shalom: peacefulbeginningsrosemary.wordpress.com/circ-information/jewish-brit-shalom
- Jewish Celebrities Make A Vocal Case For Intactivism:
    jewishbusinessnews.com/2016/04/18/jewish-celebrities-make-a-vocal-case-for-intactivism
- Jewish Father's Letter to His Son: www.drmomma.org/2009/12/jewish-fathers-letter-to-his-son.html
- Jewish Welcoming: peacefulbeginningsrosemary.wordpress.com/circ-information/jewish-welcoming
- Judaism & Circumcision Resources *(long list of resources)*:
    www.drmomma.org/2009/06/circumcision-jewish-fathers-making.html
- Kickstarter Judaism: A Book Review of Celebrating Brit Shalom:
    tikkun.org/kickstarter-judaism-a-book-review-of-celebrating-brit-shalom
- 'Make home circumcision illegal' (UK 2012):
    hooded2016.wordpress.com/2016/04/19/uk-2012-make-home-circumcision-illegal
- Mayor de Blasio and Rabbis Near Accord on New Circumcision Rule *(infections from mezizah)*:
    nytimes.com/2015/01/15/nyregion/mayor-de-blasio-and-rabbis-near-accord-on-new-circumcision-rule.html
- Men's Oppression: Being Rational About Circumcision and Jewish Observance:
    cirp.org/pages/cultural/rothenberg.html
- More than 130 Rabbis Offer 'Brit Shalom' for Intact Jewish Sons:
    jewishbusinessnews.com/2016/04/14/more-than-130-rabbis-offer-brit-shalom-for-intact-jewish-sons
- My Story of Ritual Abuse: www.drmomma.org/2009/12/my-story-of-ritual-abuse.html
- Name Shield for Mohel Who Gave Herpes to Baby:
    hooded2016.wordpress.com/2016/04/03/name-shield-for-mohel-who-gave-herpes-to-baby
- 'No circumcision for my son – it's not moral': ynetnews.com/articles/0,7340,L-4714002,00.html
- One Rabbis' Thoughts on Circumcision:
    web.archive.org/web/20190510184251/http://www.rabbinathan.com/writings/circum.shtml

- Open Letter From Dr. Jenny Goodman: cirp.org/pages/cultural/goodman.html
- Orthodox Jews, NYC officials negotiate over 'oral suction' circumcision after herpes cases: foxnews.com/us/orthodox-jews-nyc-officials-negotiate-over-oral-suction-circumcision-after-herpes-cases
- Peaceful Beginnings *(the author's website)*: peacefulbeginningsrosemary.wordpress.com
- Rabbis, Cantors, and Other Jewish Leaders Perform New Type of Welcoming Rituals: jewishbusinessnews.com/2016/03/08/rabbis-cantors-and-other-jewish-leaders-perform-new-type-of-welcoming-rituals
- Religious Traditions and Circumcision *(ancient origins and tales, good pictures / Larue)*: come-and-hear.com/editor/br-circum-history/index.html
- Religions and circumcision *(overview of publications)*: univ-paris8.academia.edu/MBertauxNavoiseau/Religions-and-circumcision
- Should religious circumcision be banned?: telegraph.co.uk/health-fitness/body/should-religious-circumcision-be-banned
- Song For an Intact Jewish Baby Naming Ceremony: nocirc.org/religion/song.php
- Surgical operation vs. traditional practice: 15square.org.uk/surgical-operation-vs-traditional-practice-2
- Talking Jewish Circumcision (Especially When You Aren't Jewish): www.savingsons.org/2014/06/talking-jewish-circumcision-especially.html
- The Case for Brit without Milah: circumstitions.com/Jewish.html
- The Circumcision Ceremony: The Brit Milah (Bris) Step by Step: chabad.org/library/article_cdo/aid/1472861/jewish/The-Circumcision-Ceremony-in-a-Nutshell.htm
- The culture war against circumcision: spiked-online.com/2014/02/06/the-culture-war-against-circumcision
- The First Amendment *(Wikipedia)*: en.wikipedia.org/wiki/Freedom_of_religion_in_the_United_States#The_First_Amendment
- The Guide of the Perplexed (by Moses Maimonides): cirp.org/library/cultural/maimonides
- The history of circumcision (Dunsmuir / good pictures): cirp.org/library/history/dunsmuir1
- The Jewish Roots of Anti-Circumcision Arguments: pool.intactiwiki.org/wiki/File:Moss.pdf
- The Many Jews Who Oppose Circumcision: thewholenetwork.org/twn-news/the-many-jews-who-oppose-circumcision
- The Other Side Of The Circumcision Debate: huffpost.com/entry/circumcision-debate-other-side_n_895132
- To Mutilate in the Name of Jehovah or Allah: Legitimization of Male and Female Circumcision: pubmed.ncbi.nlm.nih.gov/7731348
- Video testimonies of harm: circumcisionharm.org/testimony.htm
- Zipporah at the inn *(Wikipedia)*: en.wikipedia.org/wiki/Zipporah_at_the_inn

Videos:
- Circumcision "much of the pain of the world": youtu.be/7wd9A28JqXo
- Circumcision *(Joseph Campbell)*: youtu.be/5kh1JEb94as
- Culture is Changing *(Eliyahu Ungar-Sargon)*: youtu.be/13mvKdv65BQ
- Jewish American Scholar Leonard Glick – Circumcision: youtu.be/c4UEbsg-k5Y

- Jewish AND Uncircumcised – Intact Jew, member and accpeted in Jewish Community and Family: youtu.be/tv1opEu78fQ
- Jewish Mother – Intact Son *(Laurie Evans):* youtu.be/tn3ZHwpL-E0
- Jewish Mother Disturbed by Circumcision Policy: youtu.be/EfOXYL0hZOI
- Jews and Circumcision – Get over it! *(Tina Kimmel):* youtu.be/aqgCeAFkHIM
- Jews who choose not to circumcise: small but growing number of Israelis shun ancient rite: youtu.be/oW1Ndxg-iTw
- Proud Jewish Woman Has an Intact Grandson: youtu.be/tTCE-Waf8CY
- rabbi says being intact with a foeskin does not affect your jewishness: youtu.be/Q5o6VgBOpFQ
- Ronald Goldman testifies on circumcision trauma at historic PACE hearing: youtu.be/Ec92eRrnWdY
- Whose Body, Whose Rights? *(Morris Sorrells, 1995):* youtu.be/5JsieythZvU&t=1953s

4 Circumcision and Christianity

The Old Testament, which is the basis of Judaism, is the foundation of Christianity. Circumcision has played a central role in the Jewish religion. What relevance does this ancient operation have within Christianity? What significance does circumcision have for today's American Christian who faces the choice of having one's son's foreskin cut off by a doctor?

Little has been written about circumcision as it pertains to Christianity. My own brother, a Methodist minister with a Ph.D. in theology has communicated:

> "I don't know much about the subject of 'circumcision.' I don't remember the subject ever being discussed in any class of theology, or Bible courses, or psychology ... From the standpoint of Christianity, it does not appear to have ever been practiced for religious purposes and therefore, circumcision is not an issue, theologically or morally for Christians." [1]

4.1 Circumcision and the History of Christianity

In the early days of the Christian Church, many old laws came into question. As frequently happens within established religion, some people wanted to adhere strictly to the established rules and traditions, while lacking an inward spirit of loving and caring. Centuries earlier the prophet Jeremiah spoke of a metaphorical "circumcision of the heart," emphasizing that the physical act of circumcision alone was not sufficient if that person lacked love and commitment to God.

Jesus made little mention, at least in the scriptures, of circumcision. The covenant of Abraham was already ancient by the time of Christ. During the formation of the Christian religion, many of the early Christian leaders, particularly St. Paul, questioned the relevance of the operation. There are several references in the New Testament where St. Paul clearly states that circumcision is not necessary for the Christian:

GALATIANS: CH. 5:
1 STAND FAST, THEREFORE, IN THE LIBERTY WHEREWITH CHRIST HAS MADE US FREE, AND BE NOT ENTANGLED AGAIN WITH THE YOKE OF BONDAGE.
2 BEHOLD, I PAUL SAY UNTO YOU, THAT IF YE BE CIRCUMCISED, CHRIST SHALL PROFIT YOU NOTHING.
3 FOR I TESTIFY AGAIN TO EVERY MAN THAT IS CIRCUMCISED, THAT HE IS A DEBTOR TO DO THE WHOLE LAW [...]

---

1 The Rev. T.E. Romberg (brother of the author; personal correspondence).

6 FOR IN JESUS CHRIST NEITHER CIRCUMCISION AVAILETH ANY THING, NOR UNCIRCUMCISION, BUT FAITH WHICH WORKETH BY LOVE.[2]

It is plain that according to Paul, spirituality and Christian love are not to be found in an operation, a cutting of a part of the body, but in the inspiration, caring and love that exist in one's heart. Therefore the operation is meaningless in regards to whether or not one is a follower of Christ.

In Philippians, Paul denounces circumcision more strongly:

PHILIPPIANS: CH. 3:
2 BEWARE OF DOGS, BEWARE OF EVIL WORKERS, BEWARE OF THE CONCISION.[3]
3 FOR WE ARE THE CIRCUMCISION, WHICH WORSHIP GOD IN THE SPIRIT, AND REJOICE IN CHRIST JESUS AND HAVE NO CONFIDENCE IN THE FLESH.[4]

One writer paraphrases Paul and comments on the meaning of the above passage:

> "Those who want to show off and brag about external matters are the ones who are trying to force you to be circumcised. Even those who practice circumcision do not obey the Law; they want you to get circumcised so they can boast that you submitted to this physical ceremony ... It does not matter at all whether or not one is circumcised. What does matter is being a new creature." [5]

In Philippians, Paul is essentially saying:

> " 'Watch out for those who do evil things, those dogs, men who insist on cutting the body ...' This is a very strong denunciation of the ancient operation, for in the Bible the dog was considered a base, unclean animal – a scavenger that ate of corpses and carrion." [5]

Circumcision was a bitter source of contention in Christianity during the New Testament period. The early Christian leaders who were Jews, were themselves circumcised. Aside from spiritual considerations, circumcision was undoubtedly denounced for simple, practical reasons. For Christianity was not to be confined to the Hebraic peoples. The new religion was to spread to all peoples throughout the earth. Therefore, imposing circumcision on converts was imposing a practice that was foreign and repugnant to most peoples, as well as painful and dangerous during an age which

---
2 Galatians: Ch. 5: 1-3, 6.
3 Concision – in archaic terminology meaning "a cuttingup or off."
4 Philippians: Ch. 3: 2-3.
5 Runyan Hous "Thus Spake St. Paul" (... on circumcision) (unpublished).

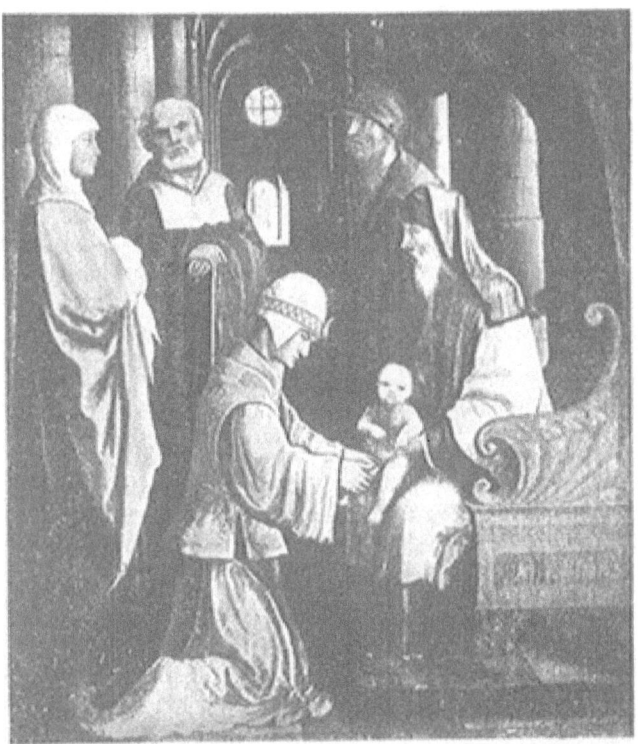

***CIRCUMCISION OF CHRIST** after Meister A. B. – XVI. CENTURY)*
From Bryk F. *Sex & Circumcision: A Study of Phallic Worship and Mutilation in Men and Women.* North Hollywood, CA: Brandon House; 1967: 24.

lacked anesthetics and modern surgical techniques. Requiring circumcision of converts to Christianity would undoubtedly have been a hindrance to the establishment of the new religion.

Some writers have suggested that the ancient rite of circumcision was replaced by Christian baptism. Is baptism for Christians what circumcision is for Jews? Baptism varies in significance among different denominations of Christianity. Some Christian denominations baptize infants. Others baptize adults. Some sprinkle a few drops of water on the head. Others practice total immersion.

There are differences between the significance of the two rituals, for in most churches baptism "makes" one a Christian, while a Jew is a Jew by birth. Both male and female Christians undergo baptism, but only Jewish males are circumcised. Circumcision does not make one a Jew. A male Jew who is left intact is still Jewish. The difference may lie in the fact that Christianity is primarily a religion shared by people from a wide variety of cultural backgrounds, while Judaism is *both* a religion and an ethnic heritage.

While it does not appear that Christian baptism was specifically intended to be a replacement for Hebraic circumcision, the two rituals may share common ancient origins. Circumcision finds its primitive origins in adolescent initiation rites, and was often part of a blood sacrifice ritual. The primitive rites were sometimes accompanied by priests smearing themselves with blood from circumcision or other sacrifice, or washing themselves with the sacrificial blood mixed with water. Some historians speculate that baptism finds its origins in the same ancient practices.[6]

Blood taboos predominated among the ancient Hebrews. Circumcision may have been connected to these blood taboos. Other blood taboos involved menstruating and recently delivered women, and draining the blood from freshly killed animals so that the blood was not consumed (i.e., "koshering" of meat). The significance of blood changed drastically with Christianity when Jesus presented his disciples with bread and wine that was to be consumed as His body and blood. The "Last Supper" (Eucharist) ritual is observed as "Mass" by Catholics and "Communion" by Protestants. Blood was believed to contain the life or soul of the being. This was the basis for the Hebraic blood taboos. It is possible that Christian Mass/Communion replaced Judaic circumcision, not with that specific intent, but by the drastic change in the significance of blood brought about by the new ritual.

4.2   Jesus' Circumcision

> ST. LUKE: CH. 2:
>
> 21 AND WHEN EIGHT DAYS WERE ACCOMPLISHED FOR THE CIRCUMCISING OF THE CHILD, HIS NAME WAS CALLED JESUS, WHICH WAS SO NAMED OF THE ANGEL BEFORE HE WAS CONCEIVED IN THE WOMB.[7]

Most Americans know very little about circumcision. However, most are aware that it is mentioned in the Bible, and that the infant Jesus was circumcised. Many people deduce, perhaps subconsciously, that whatever circumcision is, it must be a beneficial thing because it was done to Jesus.

Christians consider Jesus the most perfect being to have ever existed. Yet His foreskin was cut off. Therefore, many conclude that the amputation of the foreskin must be a "perfecting" of the body, rather than a detraction or mutilation.

---

6   Wrana P. Historical review – circumcision. *Arch Pediatr.* 1939; 56: 387.
7   St. Luke: Ch. 2: 15-21.

During the Middle Ages and Renaissance many works of art depicted the circumcision of the infant Jesus. Some Christian churches, primarily the Catholics, have observed the circumcision of Christ on the first day of January.[8]

One writer comments on the observance of this event during the early days of Christianity: "Half smiling and half philosophing, the grand old fathers of the Church were pitying the Christ infant for that torture He had to suffer, and it is still to be revealed whether such a celebration is to commemorate a happy event in the life of Christ, or rather His introduction to martyrdom!" [9]

Foley, in his vehement attack on neonatal circumcision states: "Certain Christian clergymen [...] are quick to point out that Jesus Christ submitted to circumcision. They are not so quick to point out that Jesus also submitted to crucifixion." [10]

Perhaps we should consider Jesus' crucifixion *and* the circumcision of helpless infants both as examples of innocent beings being tortured ... except that His crucifixion had a clearer purpose.

Jesus' circumcision does challenge the speculations that have been made about the traumatic operation's ultimate effect on the character of the individual. One can argue that most of the great spiritual leaders within Judaeo-Christian history, including most of the Old Testament patriarchs and prophets, John the Baptist, Jesus, most of the apostles and early saints were circumcised as infants in accordance with the Abrahamic covenant. Certainly today there are many men who are spiritual leaders or are in other ways commendable people, who also happen to have been subjected to circumcision in infancy. No one has ever done any controlled study concerning the percentage of circumcised penises among criminals and vagrants compared to that among highly accomplished people of exemplary character. *(Nor would most people consider any such effort of value. – R.R.)* It is doubtful that circumcision, or any other painful medical procedure is going to "turn anyone into a criminal or a terrible person." That is not the focus of today's anti-circumcision movement. The operation *is* painful and traumatic. It *is* depriving the individual of a valuable, protective and sensate part of his body. It *is* unnecessary. These are our major concerns.

Perhaps the parent who has already had a son circumcised and now feels remorse can find some solace in the fact that the most celebrated infant to have ever been born was also a circumcised baby. However, for those who have yet to make the decision, no modern day Christian should have himself or his son circumcised simply

---

8 In recent years the Catholic church has changed the focus and the name of this observance. Today January 1st – the eighth day after Christmas – is celebrated as a mass in honor of the "maternity of Mary." I have been told that Catholic authorities and Sunday school teachers decided that the subject of circumcision was too difficult and painful to explain to children. – R.R.
9 D'Alba A. *Circumcision, the savagery of the cradle.* Galen Medical Publications; 1979: 8.
10 Foley JM. The Unkindest Cut of All. *Fact.* 1966-07/08; 3(4): 6.

because Jesus' foreskin was cut off. Mary and Joseph were not modern day American parents who made a decision "should we or shouldn't we have the baby circumcised?" In ancient Israel, at the time of Jesus' birth, new parents had little or no *choice* about circumcision. Virtually *all* infant boys born to the ancient Hebrews were circumcised. Jesus was hardly in a position to be the exception. It was "against the law" not to have it done. Today's young parents, who must decide whether or not to have a doctor amputate their baby's foreskin, are in an entirely different situation.

4.3   An Ancient Holy Relic – The Prepuce of Christ

A bizarre sidelight in the history of circumcision concerns the amputated prepuce of the infant Jesus.

During the Middle Ages there was a craze of religious fetishism involving "holy relics" including "bones of the Saints" and "splinters from the Holy Cross of Jesus." Most of these "relics" were frauds which came from racketeers. This was made obvious by the fact that more "relics" existed than Saints or the Cross. This was another example of religious followers focusing on superficiality rather than true spirituality.

One of these "holy relics" was the "prepuce of the infant Jesus."

Bryk relates:

"… When the worship of relics was in full bloom, the question was heard, what really happened to the holy foreskin of Christ? Where is it being kept?

A holy legend was recalled according to which the mother of God had carried the foreskin of her Son about with her all her life like a precious jewel, in order that she might again accept Christ on the Day of Judgment … the Madonna was supposed to have entrusted this treasure to Saint John; … (or) to the holy Magdalen. The latter left the holy relic to the apostles, who left it to their successors. It was then hidden, until finally an angel from the land of the Unbelievers brought it to Charlemagne at Aix-la-Chapelle, who presented it to his only bride, the Sancta Ecclesia Romana. During the siege of Rome by Charles V in the year 1527, a soldier had stolen the relic, but it was evidently found again, as Gumbalungo relates in detail. The BLISSFUL WONDERFUL ODOR which met the nostrils of the women of Roman aristocracy (who were present when the find was opened and who ardently concerned themselves with the matter) is pictured as a miracle. This treasure was brought over to Calcata, where the relic is adorned every year by a complete indulgence (Muller).

Soon the foreskin of Christ emerged in other places, so that finally more than twelve abbeys could show this relic. According to Kessler, at Charroux this relic was 'set in silver and shown to pregnant women in order that they might be less painfully confined.' The common people of the region have quite corrupted the name of the preputium and made 'le Saint Repuce' out of it. Even a queen of Sicily, who suffered from an incurable disease, made a pilgrimage to one of the abbeys and returned healthy ...

These doings probably became too much for the prudent church fathers. For purely doctrinary reasons, however, they first began to doubt the genuineness of these relics, in that they assumed that Christ had taken His foreskin with Him into Heaven. From that ensued a scholastic debate which centered around the point: HAS CHRIST A FORESKIN IN HEAVEN, OR HAS HE NOT?" [11]

Most people today would find the history of Jesus' prepuce ridiculous. Let us hope that the infant Jesus' prepuce was buried in sand, as was the custom, decomposed normally, and ceased to exist. It seems bizarre that people would attach importance to a shriveled piece of tissue, regardless of its authenticity.

4.4   The Meaning of Circumcision for Today's Christian

ST. MATTHEW: CH. 6:
19 LAY NOT UP FOR YOURSELVES TREASURES UPON EARTH, WHERE MOTH AND RUST DOTH CORRUPT, AND WHERE THIEVES BREAK THROUGH AND STEAL:
20 BUT LAY UP FOR YOURSELVES TREASURES IN HEAVEN, WHERE NEITHER MOTH NOR RUST DOTH CORRUPT, AND WHERE THIEVES DO NOT BREAK THROUGH NOR STEAL.
21 FOR WHERE YOUR TREASURE IS, THERE WILL YOUR HEART BE ALSO.[12]

These words have many meanings for the Christian. One can only speculate if Jesus was foreseeing today's department stores, modern gadgets and rampant consumerism.

The admonishment to attach central importance to spiritual, rather than material, physical things, is one of the basic messages of Christianity. This is undoubtedly one of the reasons that St. Paul declared circumcision irrelevant to the Christian.

The American Christian male today probably had his foreskin cut off in infancy. Most American Christian parents allow doctors to circumcise their baby boys. However, few Christians consciously think of medical circumcision as relating to their religion.

---

11 Bryk F. *Sex & Circumcision: A Study of Phallic Worship and Mutilation in Men and Women*. North Hollywood, CA: Brandon House; 1967: 23-6.
12 St. Matthew: Ch. 6: 19-21.

Circumcision – The Painful Dilemma

The only exceptions are the Abyssinian and Coptic Christians who circumcise infants and young boys as part of their religious rites. Apparently this practice is derived from a cultural heritage which predates their adoption of Christianity. Additionally, some Messianic Jews, i.e. Jews who believe that Jesus is the Messiah, yet continue to embrace their Jewish faith and culture, do circumcise their baby boys.

Except for these, none of the Christian churches has any ritual related to infant circumcision. The operation is not performed in Christian churches. No Christian ministers or priests are expected to circumcise babies.

From the time of St. Paul and the beginning of the Christian church until the last few decades in the United States – a time span of almost two millennia – Christians were rarely circumcised. However, when routine circumcision of infants became a medical fad during the early part of the 20th century, American Christians have (perhaps subconsciously) accepted the practice more readily, because of its Biblical origins, than they might have otherwise.

Today there is an upsurge of Christian Fundamentalism. Some Christians today have decided that they should observe certain Old Testament laws, despite the fact that these were all rescinded in the New Testament. For example, some Christians refuse to eat pork. Similarly, others have enthusiastically accepted circumcision of their infant sons. Perhaps they have read some of the medical claims about cancer or hygiene, and decided that God must have commanded circumcision for "health" reasons.

The Christian is urged to learn the facts. The medical and "hygienic" arguments which have been posed for circumcision are not valid. Circumcision was declared unnecessary for Christians very early in the Church's formation:

I CORINTHIANS: CH. 7:
19 CIRCUMCISION IS NOTHING AND UNCIRCUMCISION IS NOTHING, BUT THE KEEPING OF THE COMMANDMENTS OF GOD. [13]

Although many Mormons[14] have their children circumcised, Mormon doctrine specifically states: "Mormon received this revelation: 'Little children are whole, for they are not capable of committing sin; wherefore the curse of Adam is taken away from them in me, that it hath no power over them; and *the law of circumcision is done away in me.*'" (Moro. 8.)[15]

Our medical profession has become for many a false religion. Some would readily call it an idolatry. Doctors are perceived as "holy men" and medical procedures are

---

[13] I Corinthians: Ch. 7: 19.
[14] I am well aware that many "mainstream" Christian denominations do not consider Mormonism true Christianity. However, any attempt to address such a theological issue would digress from the purpose of this book. – R.R.
[15] McConkie BR. Mormon Doctrine, pp. 143-4.

followed like "religious rituals." Infant circumcision is but one of the medical rituals that we have accepted in a manner *not unlike that of religious faith.*

Certainly the medical profession provides a needed function, but we must seriously re-evaluate its role. Except for those who choose to use only spiritual or other alternative means of healing, all people make use of the medical profession for treatment of diseases and injuries. But the foreskin is neither a disease nor an injury! By signing circumcision permission papers, perhaps the Christian parent is ascribing to a false religious rite. For if God made a "covenant" with the ancient Hebrew patriarchs, He made no such "covenant" with the "patriarchs" of our medical profession.

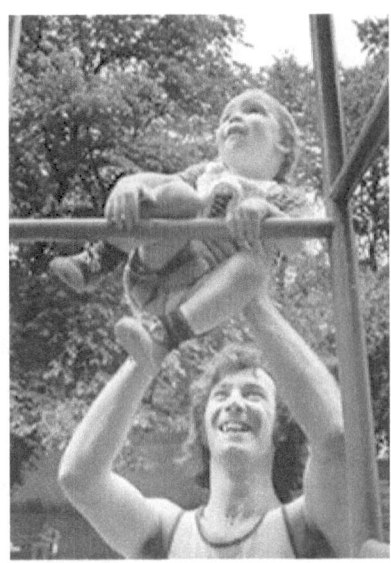
© *Suzanne Arms*

In I Corinthians St. Paul states:

I CORINTHIANS: CH. 7:

18 IS ANY MAN CALLED BEING CIRCUMCISED? LET HIM NOT BECOME UNCIRCUMCISED; *IS ANY CALLED IN UNCIRCUMCISION? LET HIM NOT BECOME CIRCUMCISED.*[16]

Paul was addressing this to prospective converts of his day. However, the modern Christian should consider this passage as it relates to infants. For the child who is born to Christian parents is in a sense "called" in that he will be raised as a Christian. And the infant male is born with his foreskin. Therefore, isn't the infant male "called in uncircumcision?" Perhaps the Christian parent is specifically going *against* this Biblical edict by having his son circumcised! Therefore, should not the Christian churches take a stand *against* circumcision for Christian babies?

Since attributes such as love, kindness, and caring are essential to the Christian character, the Christian should accept that a baby's entrance into life should be as peaceful and loving as possible, and that he should have the right to keep all parts of his body. With a Christian spirit of love, the Christian parent should spare his son the trauma of foreskin amputation.

---

16   I Corinthians: Ch. 7: 18. (Italics mine – R.R.)

However, within any religion or cause, there is the problem of individuals becoming self-righteous, judgmental, and condemnatory towards others. Christians too often make this mistake, thereby defeating the purpose of Christian love for others. Natural childbirth enthusiasts similarly often become narrow-minded about other people's choices concerning birth or breastfeeding. Some activists in the anti-circumcision cause also come across as angry, threatening and condemnatory towards others who have chosen circumcision for their sons. While intactivists do strongly hold that circumcision of non-consenting infants and children is child abuse, we are cautioned to be gentle and understanding about this matter when presenting our information to the uninformed public – however painful or damaging foreskin amputation may be, and however justified our feelings are on the matter. Our purpose is not intended to anger others and turn people *away* from this cause – only to inspire people to think. Those who have been enlightened enough to leave their son(s) intact, must remember that others who have chosen circumcision are either devout Jews who believe that they must do this for religious reasons, or are people who have been misled to believe the common medical or "social" arguments for foreskin amputation. Many anti-circumcision activists are parents of circumcised sons, doctors who have performed or nurses who have assisted with circumcisions in the past, or are circumcised males themselves, and therefore *realize* that the operation is only done out of misinformation, or religious convictions, not from conscious intent to harm the child. *All* parents make mistakes with their children.

The Christian should remember Jesus' words in St. Matthew:

ST. MATTHEW: CH. 7:
1 JUDGE NOT, THAT YE BE NOT JUDGED.
2 FOR WITH WHAT JUDGMENT YE JUDGE, YE SHALL BE JUDGED; AND WITH WHAT MEASURE YE METE, IT SHALL BE MEASURED TO YOU AGAIN. [17]

Author's note: The chapters for this book were originally written during the late 70's and early 80's. At that time my spiritual orientation was more "open-ended" than it is today. I was raised a Christian, primarily in Methodist and Lutheran churches, but in early adulthood perceived Christianity largely as a philosophy and a system of ethics. Like so many of us, I had little comprehension of the underlying spirituality involved centered in a relationship with God through Jesus Christ. During the mid-80's I underwent some profound spiritual changes in my life.

I have since written two other articles which explore infant circumcision and the Christian faith in greater depth. One is quite lengthy, describing my own life experience in detail and exploring additional writings on the subject to a greater extent.

---
17 St. Matthew: Ch. 7: 1-2.

The second is much shorter and is an extract of the first one, designed for use as a handout for new and/or expectant parents. Rather than rewrite the above chapter, I wish to recommend that interested readers check out the following article for further information: (My Website) "The Christian Parent" article.[18]

4.5   Informational Resources

- 1 Corinthians 7: 18-19: biblegateway.com/passage/?search=1+Corinthians+7%3A18-19%3B&version=KJV
- After Condom Remarks, Vatican Confirms Shift *(Catholic ok for condom use for aids prevention)*:
    nytimes.com/2010/11/24/world/europe/24pope.html
- Ambrose of Milan on circumcision *(letter to Clementianus)*:
    i2researchhub.org/articles/ambrose-of-milan-on-circumcision-letter-to-clementianus
- An Open Letter to the Physicians of The Catholic Medical Association: cirp.org/library/cultural/fadel1
- Answers from the Bible to Questions about Circumcision: cirp.org/pages/cultural/glass2
- Biblical Circumcision Information: www.drmomma.org/2010/07/biblical-circumcision-information.html
- Bipolar Christianity: How Torturing "Sinful" Children Produced Holy Wars:
    psychohistory.com/books/the-origins-of-war-in-child-abuse/chapter-9-bipolar-%20christianity-how-torturing-sinful-children-produced-holy-wars
- Catholic Church and HIV/AIDS *(Wikipedia):* en.wikipedia.org/wiki/Catholic_Church_and_HIV/AIDS
- Catholics Against Circumcision: catholicsagainstcircumcision.org
- Christian Parents and the Circumcision Issue: cirp.org/pages/cultural/peron1
- Christianity & Circumcision Resources: www.drmomma.org/2009/06/information-on-circumcision-for.html
- Christianity and Circumcision: cirp.org/pages/cultural/lewis1
- Christians and Infant Circumcision: Where Should I Stand?:
    mirandamamma.blogspot.com/2014/03/christians-and-infant-circumcision.html
- Christians For Holeness: acts15.net
- Christians: Baptism, Not Circumcision: www.drmomma.org/2010/02/christians-baptism-not-circumcision.html
- Circumcision *(Fish Eaters):* fisheaters.com/circumcision.html
- Circumcision and the Copts: britishorthodox.org/glastonburyreview/issue-122-circumcision-and-the-copts
- Circumstitions Ritual Myths 6: Jesus, The Holy Prepuce:
    hooded2016.wordpress.com/circumstitions-ritual-myths-6-jesus-the-holy-prepuce
- Comixio Religionis: Circumcision NOT Jerusalemic:
    salem-news.com/articles/july242011/comixio-religionis-rm.php
- Debates about FGM in Africa, the Middle East & Far East: religioustolerance.org/fem_cirm.htm
- Does a Biblical view of the body allow for circumcision?:
    littleimages.org/blog/does-a-biblical-view-of-the-body-allow-for-infant-circumcision
- "every multi-orgasmic man she dated, was intact":
    littleimages.org/blog/10-things-christian-men-know-about-sex/#comment-169

---

18   http://peacefulbeginningsrosemary.wordpress.com/circ-information/christian-parent/

- Faith Considerations on Circumcision: www.drmomma.org/2011/01/faith-considerations-on-circumcision.html
- Galatians 5:2: biblegateway.com/passage/?search=Galatians+5%3A2%3B&version=KJV
- Is circumcision a requirement for salvation for Christian males?:
  christiananswers.net/q-eden/circumcision.html
- Jack Black and Circumcision in Antiquity: www.drmomma.org/2009/11/jack-black-on-circumcision.html
- Little Images: Help us save babies from unnecessary cutting: littleimages.org
- Might as well jump?: littleimages.org/blog/might-as-well-jump-parenting-and-circumcision
- Mormonism and Circumcision: coloradonocirc.org/files/handouts/Mormonism_and_Circumcision.pdf
- My Biblical Journey to Intactivism: www.savingsons.org/2012/11/my-biblical-journey-to-intactivism.html
- Question Circumcision: Religion: questioncircumcision.com/religion.html
- Religious Traditions and Circumcision *(ancient origins and tales, good pictures / Larue)*:
  come-and-hear.com/editor/br-circum-history/index.html
- Religions and circumcision *(overview of publications)*:
  univ-paris8.academia.edu/MBertauxNavoiseau/Religions-and-circumcision
- Religious Reasons Not To Circumcise: organiclifestylemagazine.com/religious-reasons-not-to-circumcise
- Respect for Bodily Integrity: A Catholic Perspective on Circumcision in Catholic Hospitals:
  cirp.org/library/cultural/fadel2
- The AAP is not God: littleimages.org/blog/the-aap-is-not-god
- The Bible persuaded me not to circumcise my son:
  insuremekevin.com/the-bible-persuaded-me-not-to-circumcise-my-son
- The Book of Mormon on Circumcision: www.drmomma.org/2010/07/book-of-mormon-on-circumcision.html
- The Council of Florence (A.D. 1438-1445) From Cantate Domino – Papal Bull of Pope Eugene IV:
  catholicism.org/cantate-domino.html
- The First Amendment *(Wikipedia)*:
  en.wikipedia.org/wiki/Freedom_of_religion_in_the_United_States#The_First_Amendment
- The history of circumcision *(Dunsmuir / good pictures)*: cirp.org/library/history/dunsmuir1
- The Holy Bible, Circumcision, False Prophets, and Christian Parents: cirp.org/pages/cultural/christian.html
- The Morality of Circumcision: cirp.org/library/cultural/dietzen1
- The Morality of Circumcision According to the Catholic Church:
  www.drmomma.org/2010/03/morality-of-circumcision-according-to.html
- The Roman Catholic Church and Non-therapeutic Circumcision: cirp.org/library/cultural/catholic
- The Truth About Circumcision Within Christianity:
  www.drmomma.org/2007/11/the-truth-about-circumcision-within.html
- Why Catholics Don't Circumcise: web.archive.org/web/20170707062621/http://guggiedaly.blogspot.com/2014/05/why-catholics-dont-circumcise.html
- Why Christians need not be circumcised: circumstitions.com/Xy.html

Video:

- God Hates the Tips of Little Babies' Dicks (Trevor Moore): youtu.be/sw8nc48agJk

5 Infant Male Circumcision As a Medical Practice In 20th/21st Century USA

Foreskins have been cut off in tribal initiation rites since prehistoric times. Jewish infants have undergone ritual circumcision for thousands of years. But until the late 1800s, few non-Jewish people of Western civilization have ever practiced this rite. Within the past century, circumcision of newborn males has become a popular practice in American hospitals, and to a lesser extent in other English-speaking countries that have come under our influence. Today, most adult American males lack their foreskins.

Circumcision has no part of the ancestral heritage of the Caucasian, European backgrounds of most *white*, non-Jewish, non-Moslem middle class Americans. Some Americans of African, Middle Eastern, or Polynesian descent may have had a tradition of ritual circumcision among their predecessors. However, the medical procedure performed on their infants today bears no relationship to any tribal initiation rite that their ancestors may have practiced. Most non-Jewish and non-Moslem Americans had grandfathers or great-grandfathers who had intact penises.

How and *why* did the amputation of infant foreskins become a popular practice among our medical profession? The answers have been difficult to find. Most medical textbooks and medically oriented books for lay people give only vague, brief information on the subject. Most doctors can easily cite the common pro and con arguments for the operation. Many are experts at *doing* circumcisions. But few know any more than the average lay person about *how* neonatal circumcision became a popular medical practice today.

5.1 The Recent History of Infant Circumcision

Puritanism has been described as "The haunting fear that someone, somewhere, might be having a good time!" Americans have a strong Puritanical heritage. Included in this is an obsessive fear of masturbation.

An 18th century writer describes the common beliefs about masturbation during his time:

> "... One of two men who indulged in excessive masturbation became insane; the other dried out his brain so prodigiously that it could be heard rattling in his skull ... The effects of masturbation range from impotence to epilepsy, and include 'consumption, blindness, imbecility, insanity, rheumatism, gonorrhea,

priapism (painful continuous erection due to disease), tumors, constipation, hemorrhoids, female homosexuality, and finally lead to death.' " [1]

However, until the mid-1800s, treatments for the "evils" of masturbation were mild, basically consisting of dietary measures and baths.[1]

During the latter half of the 19th century, more surgical, punitive, sadistic, and bizarre anti-masturbatory therapies came into being:

"By about 1880 the individual ... might wish [to] ... tie, chain, or infibulate sexually active children ... to adorn them with grotesque appliances, encase them in plaster, leather, or rubber, to frighten or even castrate them ... masturbation insanity was now real enough – it was affecting the medical profession." [2]

The medical profession at that time believed that the unnatural loss of semen weakened both mind and body, thereby leading to the above-described disorders.

Another writer also comments on the barbaric methods used to prevent this:

"Some doctors recommend covering the penis with plaster of Paris, leather, or rubber, cauterization, making boys wear chastity belts or spiked rings, and in extreme cases, castration." [3]

Circumcision of males as a medical procedure originated as yet another of these measures to cure or prevent masturbation.

"In 1891, James Hutchinson, president of the Royal College of Surgeons (in Great Britain), published a paper 'On Circumcision as Preventative of Masturbation'. In it he not only advocated circumcision for the treatment and prevention of this 'shameful habit,' but proposed that '... if public opinion permitted their adoption ... measures more radical than circumcision would ... be a true kindness.' (Dr. Hutchinson's paper is generally credited as being the instigator in British and American routine infant circumcision.)" [4]

In 1893:

---

1   Marcus IM, Francis JJ. *Masturbation: From Infancy to Senescence.* New York: International Universities Press; 1975: 386-7.
2   Excerpt from an underground newsletter (Bud Berkeley).
3   Paige KE. The Ritual of Circumcision. *Hum Nat.* 1978-05; 40, 42.
4   Excerpt from an underground newsletter (Bud Berkeley).

"... Another British doctor wrote 'Circumcision: Its Advantages and How to Perform It,' which listed the reasons for removing the "vestigial prepuce." Evidently the foreskin could cause 'nocturnal incontinence,' hysteria, epilepsy, and irritation that might 'give rise to erotic stimulation and consequently masturbation.' " [3]

"Until its 1940 edition, one of the standard American textbooks on Pediatrics, Holts' *Diseases of Infancy and Childhood*, condemns the practice of masturbation as medically harmful. In earlier editions, the treatment recommended is mechanical restraint, corporal punishment in the very young, circumcision in boys ... *because of the moral effect of the operation.*" [4]

The same book similarly states: "... advocated female circumcision, cauterization of the clitoris, and even blistering of the vulva and prepuce for recalcitrant (female) masturbators." [3]

In 1891, Dr. P.C. Remondino, M.D. published a detailed textbook entitled *History of Circumcision from the Earliest Times to the Present: Moral and Physical Reasons for its Performance*. His title lists:

"Member of the American Medical Association, of the American Public Health Association, of the San Diego County Medical Society, of the State Board of Health of California, and of the Board of Health of the City of San Diego; Vice-President of California State Medical Society and of Southern California Medical Society [...]" [5]

Despite his impressive title and position, his writing is hardly rational or scientific. His phobia of foreskins is summed up as follows:

"... The prepuce seems to exercise a malign influence in the most distant and apparently unconnected manner; where, like some of the evil genii or sprites in the Arabian tales, it can reach from afar the object of its malignity, striking him down unawares in the most unaccountable manner; making him a victim to all manner of ills, sufferings, and tribulations; unfitting him for marriage or the cares of business; making him miserable and an object of continual scolding in childhood, through its worriments and nocturnal enuresis; later on beginning to affect him with all kinds of physical distortions and ailments, nocturnal pollutions, and other conditions calculated to weaken him physically, mentally, and morally, to land him, perchance, in the jail, or even in a lunatic asylum. Man's whole life is

---

5   Remondino PC. *History of Circumcision from the Earliest Times to the Present*. NY: Ams Press; 1974: 1 (original edition, F.A. Davis Co.; 1891).

Circumcision – The Painful Dilemma

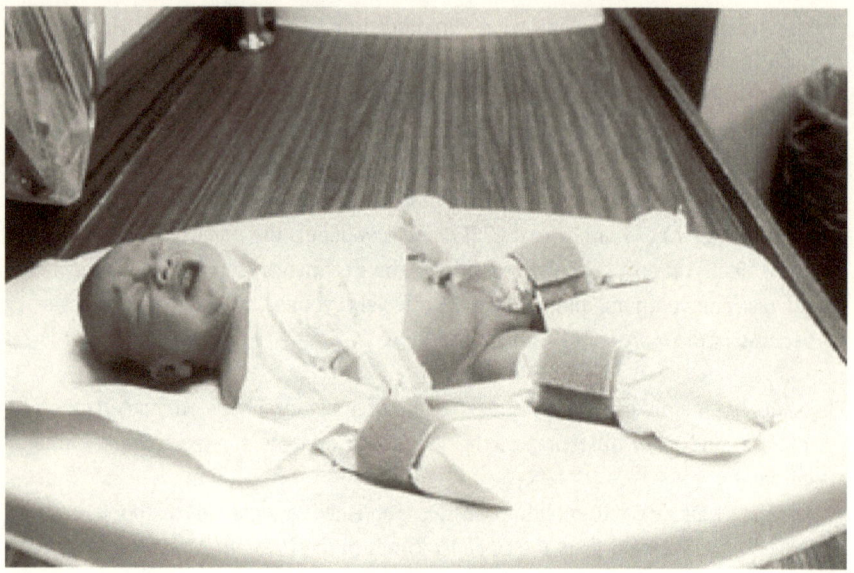

Reprinted with permission from The Saturday Evening Post Company © 1981.

subject to the capricious dispensations and whims of this Job's-comforts-dispensing enemy of man." [6]

Remondino echoed the anti-masturbation beliefs of his time, blaming this abomination on the "evils" of the prepuce. He advocated circumcision, not only as a cure for masturbation but as a preventive measure for all infant males:

> "There is not much doubt but that, if one of the cases reported by Dr. Price had not been circumcised, the expressionless, listless infant would have grown, in time, into a masturbating, feeble-minded, idiotic creature as many others so situated, have done before it." [7]

One section of Remondino's book covers the history of castration and other genital mutilations. He favors some of these other practices with enthusiasm similar to that he exhibits for male circumcision.

For example, his comments on the Australian practice of subincision. (Although in truth subincised males can and do father children, and there is no evidence in

---

6   Ibid., pp. 254-5.
7   Ibid., p. 269.

historical sources that the practice was ever intended to be a birth control measure, Remondino believed that was its purpose):

> "... It is certainly an operation of the highest merit, and it should be introduced, by all means, in the United States ... Whenever the writer sees the poor anemic, broken down victim of many miscarriages, he cannot help but feel that if the laws of the Damiantina River savages were enforced on their husbands, it would be a blessing to the poor women without materially injuring their husbands ..." [8]

Elsewhere he describes and advocates a horrifying practice that took place in Soudan:

> "... The very peculiar and unmistakably painful gait was due to the fact that each woman carried a bamboo stick, about eight inches in length, three inches or more being inserted in the vagina so as to effectually fill the opening, the balance projecting beyond, between the thighs of the person; this bamboo stick, or guardian of female virtue, was held in place by a strap with a shield that covered the vulva, the whole being held in an undisplaceable position by a padlock. This was affixed to the woman whenever she was allowed outside the harem ground, being placed in position by the eunuch, who carried the key at his girdle. In such a harness virtue can be perfectly safe; ... In Soudan there are no divorce courts, hence the probable necessity of the apparatus, and, as the woman is not obliged to wear it unless she chooses to go out unattended, *it can hardly be considered as a compulsory barbarity. In the United States such a practice might do away with considerable divorce proceedings*" [9]

Remondino also, in all seriousness, advocated the ancient practice of employing eunuchs:

> "... I have alluded to the very appropriate arrangement which formerly existed when music teachers were eunuchs, ... our higher circles of society would do well to employ eunuchized coachmen, especially if possessed of susceptible and elopable daughters..." [10]

---

8   Ibid., p. 59.
9   Ibid., pp. 52-3. [emphasis mine – R.R.]
10 Ibid., pp. 102-3.

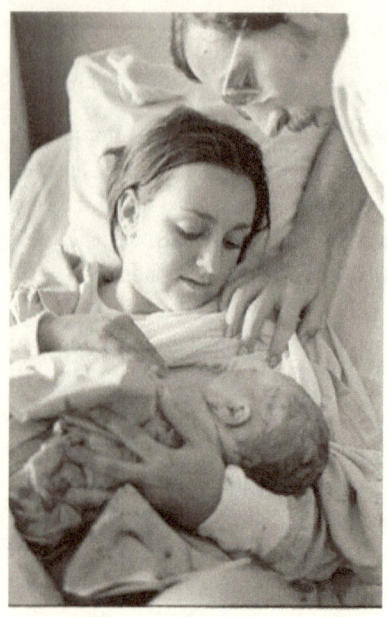

© Suzanne Arms

Fortunately few others took up Remondino's other suggestions. But, *this is the same type of mentality from which our current medical practice of infant circumcision originated!*

There is a certain "mystique" about surgery. Some people do take a certain masochistic enjoyment out of being medical patients, gladly suffering the pain involved for the attention received. Of course, what is *choice* for an adult becomes *victimization* for infants and children.

It has only been within the past little more than a century that surgery could be done with antisepsis and anesthetic. Modern surgery is truly a new art. The field of medicine has struggled with growing pains, and trial and error adoption of new procedures. New ideas and techniques are constantly presented. Many later become disproven or outdated. Types of surgery and other medical treatments have often been fads. Carter comments:

> "With the discovery of anesthesia in 1846 and a new antiseptic method of treatment about 21 years later, the whole face of medicine was changed. The hazardous and painful undertaking of surgery became fashionable, and large numbers of beginners poured into the medical schools to study surgical methods... As time went on, more courage, better facilities and better trained staffs, plus more comfort, safety and operative skill contributed to the surgeon's art ... it became exceedingly easy, for the first time in history, for patients to have an operation ... fashions in surgery began to develop ... Unfortunately, the public often adopts a surgical craze and runs with it, as it were, the result being that insistent patients rush to the surgeon's door demanding an operation rather than simply asking for advice about a medical problem ..." [11]

While infant circumcision as a medical practice began during the late 1800s, it became increasingly widespread during the earlier part of the 20th century. The practice went hand in hand with another phenomenon – routine hospitalization of all births.

---

[11] Carter N. *Routine Circumcision: The Tragic Myth.* London, England: Londinium Press; 1979: 29.

In 1900 less than 5 percent of American women delivered in hospitals. By the 1920s between 30-50% of births in most larger U.S. cities took place in hospitals. By the early 1930s between 60 and 75% of the births in various cities were in hospitals.

In *Lying-In*, a revealing book on the history of childbearing customs in the United States, Wertz & Wertz comment:

> "Some commentators have suggested that doctors sought to centralize all medical care in hospitals because of the model of industry, which had taught them that control of a work space would make them a new elite, like the 'captains of industry.' Perhaps doctors were aware that institutionalizing medicine would bring them power and prestige, [as well as having] immediate practical reasons for centralizing care." [12]

It is no *coincidence* that routine circumcision of infants became widespread during the same time that nearly all normal births, for the first time in history, took place in hospitals. Parents who have given birth at home – whether in previous ages when this was the accepted norm, or today for the few who choose this as a "radical" alternative – have had to *think* about whether or not to take their infant to a doctor to have his foreskin cut off. But the new mother who is recovering from birth at one end of a hospital maternity ward, and the father who is outside in the waiting room, have had little awareness of what is being done to their infant who is hidden away in the hospital nursery.

Unfortunately, "progress" in the form of medical advances in obstetrics, has been gained at the expense of the emotional well-being of parents and infants. Wertz & Wertz comment:

> "Hospital delivery had become for many a time of alienation – from the body, from family and friends, from the community, and even from life itself. The safe efficiencies had become a kind of industrial production far removed from the comforts of social childbirth or the sympathies of the proverbial doctor-patient relation. A woman was powerless in the experience of birth and unable to find meaning in it, for her participation in it and even her consciousness of it were minimal. She was isolated during birth from family and friends, and even from other women having the same experiences. She had to think of herself instrumentally, not as a woman feeling love and fear or sharing in a creative event, but as a body-machine being manipulated by others for her ultimate welfare. She played a social role of passive dependence and obedience." [13]

---

12 Wertz RW, Wertz DC. *Lying-In; A History of Childbirth in* America. NY: Schocken Books. 1979:132,159-160.
13 Ibid., p. 173.

Within recent years we have striven to re-humanize birth. Childbirth Education classes have endeavored to familiarize expectant parents with the birth experience and their choices. The movement has brought about such things as father participation and rooming in within hospitals. Alternative birth centers and services for home births have been made available. Unfortunately through the decade of the '70s and into the '80s and the ensuing decades, birth has become a battlefield. Professionals have often been reluctant to change or listen to lay people. Factions within childbirth education have different ideas. Expectant parents have been caught in the middle. Medical practices which surround birth and babies have been questioned and attacked. Among these have been fetal heart monitors, unnecessary Caesarian deliveries, episiotomies, enemas, pubic shaves, and routine separation of mothers and infants. Somehow, circumcision of infant boys has been one of the last things for us to question.

Infant circumcision was also a concurrent trend with some peculiar and uncompassionate practices in other aspects of infant care. Although virtually all mothers have nursed their babies since the beginning of human existence until the past few decades, suddenly during the 1920s and '30s mothers were being told that artificial formula was "best" for their infants.

Breastfeeding went "out of style." Mothers were told to feed their infants with "scientific" rigidity, following 3 or 4 hour schedules with total disregard for the infant's needs or hungers. Mothers were admonished "not to give in," "let him cry it out," "crying is good exercise for their lungs," or "let him know that you are the boss and not him." Parents were admonished not to cuddle or rock their babies, or handle them any more than necessary for fear of "spoiling" the child.

While the turn of the century advocates of circumcision did express concern over the obvious pain felt by infants undergoing this operation, later, as neonatal circumcision became increasingly widespread and routine within hospitals, the belief that infants feel no pain took over. Soon doctors became no more concerned about strapping the infant down, and clamping and slicing off his foreskin, than they were about cutting the umbilical cord.

During recent years parents have been striving to "relearn" the "art" of breastfeeding, and "relearn" such things as rocking and cuddling their babies, and answering their hungers and emotional needs. (It seems absurd that such things should even be questioned or that there have to be organizations devoted to this!) It is now time to view infant circumcision as yet another vestige from an era that totally disregarded the needs and feelings of babies.

Like other trends, circumcision has followed social and economic class lines. During the early decades of the 20th century, upper and middle class parents were usually the first to have their babies in hospitals, to bottle feed their babies, and to have their infant sons circumcised. Soon only the poorer, less educated people were not following these practices. Therefore "stigmas" became attached to the "old" ways. Birth at home became "uncivilized," breastfeeding "old fashioned," and foreskins "dirty." Soon the lower classes became aware of the "stigmas" and also followed the trends. Paradoxically, today parents with more education and higher incomes have been more likely to choose breastfeeding, to take classes in natural childbirth, to give birth at home or in alternative settings, and to leave their sons intact. The college educated young mother may nurse her baby while her neighbor who never finished high school bottle feeds with the idea that only "ignorant" people breastfeed! The 1970s saw a reawakening to natural childbirth, father participation in birth, birth alternatives, and breastfeeding. Hopefully in the future we will see a similar reawakening to leaving our sons as they came into this world.

5.2 Are the Jews to Blame?

Until neonatal circumcision became a common medical practice in the United States, Jews were one of the few peoples who circumcised infants. In other times and places this has brought ridicule and persecution upon the Jews. In the United States today, the Jew does not stand out as different for having a circumcised penis.

Have Jews been the cause, directly or indirectly, of the widespread popularity of routine infant circumcision in the United States? There *are* many Jewish doctors in the U.S. Has there been a conscious Jewish plot to deprive the rest of America of their foreskins? To make Gentile males "match" Jews? Or to "give" non-Jewish males the supposed benefits of circumcision?

In an article on anti-Semitism a psychiatric patient is quoted as saying:

> " 'I can't understand why so many Gentiles are circumcised. That's what the Jews did to America. Their mission is to circumcise every Christian in the country ... The Jews try to judeify the Gentiles ...' [There is a] belief that a defective person is defective because someone has taken something back from him; hence defective people will retaliate by trying to get back what has been taken from them. This fantasy is another in a series of such projections onto the Jews of the anti- Semite's own feelings and desires." [14]

The writers who advocated neonatal circumcision during the late 1800s, such as Remondino and Hutchinson, were not Jewish. Remondino, however, does expound at length about the high moral character and generally good health enjoyed by Jews,

---

[14] Glenn J. Circumcision and Anti-Semitism. *Psychoanal Q.* 1960; 29: 395-7.

compared to other peoples, somehow concluding that all this is related to their lack of prepuces:

> "There is ... a less tendency to criminality, debauchery, and intemperance in the race; this, can in a measure be ascribed to their family influence ... Crimes against the person or property committed by Jews are rare. They likewise do not figure in either police courts or penitentiary records; they are not inmates of our poorhouses, but, what is also singular, they are never accused of many silly [!] crimes such as indecent exposures, assaults on young girls ..." [15]

> "The weight of testimony is evidently convincing that the Jew has a greater longevity and stronger resistance to disease, as well as a less liability to physical ills, than other races; that all these exemptions or benefits are not altogether due to social customs is evident; how much circumcision may have to do with inducing these favorable conditions can be better appreciated by a consideration of how circumcision affects those of other races, and more particularly how its performance works changes in the individual in his general health and condition, and in doing away with many physical ailments that the individual was previously subjected to. So that the Jew cannot be said to be a loser by his observance of this rite, and he and his race have been well repaid for all the sufferings and persecutions that its observance has subjected them to." [16]

If the Jews indeed have been a healthier, longer-lived people than their Gentile counterparts, it seems more plausible that this could be attributed to their highly moral, regulated, and family oriented lifestyle, and their careful inspection of meats, rather than their lack of foreskins. It is also possible that a "survival of the fittest" principle has operated with Jews, since they have endured many centuries of hardships, starvation, suffering and persecution.

There is no evidence that Jews have *deliberately* conspired to take away the foreskins of their Gentile brothers. However, circumcision's Biblical origins have caused it to be more readily accepted by non-Jewish people. If infant circumcision had not been a part of our Judaeo-Christian heritage, it is highly doubtful that it would have ever been presented as a medical procedure. If suggested, the operation would have seemed strange and abhorrent.

Once the practice was established, it is certainly understandable that most Jewish physicians would be in favor of routine infant circumcision. The Jewish doctor has been likely to conclude "God was right all along, and the medical profession just

---

[15] Remondino, p. 2.
[16] Ibid., p. 181.

learned what our people knew for centuries!" (However, there are some Jewish doctors who oppose routine circumcision – realizing that ritual justification is very much different from the purported medical reasons.)

The Jewish practice of infant circumcision has been an *indirect* influence on the widespread medical fad. However, *there has been no organized "Jewish conspiracy" to amputate the foreskins of the rest of America.*

5.3   The Medical Profession as a "Pseudo-Religion"

> "What more resembles an esoteric religious ritual than an operation? It's done behind closed doors, with the anxious relatives waiting in an anteroom until the surgeon, still wearing his robes of office, comes out and shakes his head sadly or beams wisely before he says, 'Well, we've done what we could.'?" [17]

We have made a false religion out of the medical profession. We treat hospitals like "sacred temples" and have turned doctors into false "gods." Medical people, institutions, and practices are more difficult for us to question or defy than are other aspects of society. Lay and medical people alike must become aware of this "false religion," for it strongly affects the way we interrelate with all facets of our health care system. Doctors, however much they may enjoy their elevated status, must awaken and seek to change this as well. For much of the anger and attacks that have been leveled against doctors and medical practices stem from people's realization of the truth, that doctors are *not* infallible gods, but are people who can make mistakes. Medical procedures are *not* sacred rituals, but are often trial-and-error fads which frequently do fall into disfavor.

In primitive societies the role of healer and priest was usually the same. Attending the sick involved calling upon the gods, as well as dispensing medicines and treatments. Probably health, curing of diseases, and worship are *meant* to be interconnected. People naturally place in awe those who have the knowledge and skills to cure disease, save lives, perform surgery, assist with birth, or deal with death. Perhaps the artificial separation of the institutions of religion and medicine in our complex society, with its resultant fragmentation and compartmentalization of different areas of life, is the *real* problem, rather than our tendency to revere doctors.

Just as many people believe that birth *has* to take place in a hospital, we have come to believe that the newborn infant must go through a number of rituals and ablutions to be "official" and survive in society. Weighing, measuring, putting ointment in the eyes, washing the baby, putting on identification bands, putting him in a spe-

---

17 Tushnet L. (quoted in) Isenberg S, Elting LM. *The Consumer's Guide to Successful Surgery.* NY: St. Martin's Press; 1976: introductory page (quote orig. printed in *The Medicine Men,* NY: St. Martin's Press).

cial warming crib, bundling him in blankets, and keeping him in the hospital nursery are all hospital rituals imposed upon the newborn. How different are we from the primitive who believes that his illness will be cured from his shaman shaking rattles and dancing? In this respect, infant circumcision in hospitals has become a "ritual" of its own accord – a product of our tendency to regard all medical practices as "sacred."

In his extensive study of the history of circumcision Bryk observed: "... We have found no circumcision that was not performed amid special rites." [18]

Is medical circumcision the exception, or is it too a "special rite"?

Paige comments: "The practice developed differently in modern industrial nations than it did in pre-industrial societies. But circumcision was no less a ritual for all its scientific trappings." [19]

A doctor adds:

"I cannot accept that the parent is primarily responsible for their performance [of circumcision]. The prime mover is the physician, who has come to be regarded in modern society almost as a high priest, Flower's superior, or revered person. The natural inclination of the parent is to defer to the judgment or his or her medical advisor ... [Routine infant circumcision] became overlaid with mystical rites as a means of ensuring its observance. The original reasons have been forgotten and the meaning transferred to the actual rite, this applying in a modern civilized society like a primitive one ..." [20]

The point is best made in the following anthropological satire. (Reversing the spellings of "Nacirema" and "latipso" reveals the identity of the people described):

"The fundamental belief underlying the whole system appears to be that the human body is ugly and that its natural tendency is to debility and disease. Incarcerated in such a body, man's only hope is to avert these characteristics through the use of the powerful influences of ritual and ceremony. Every household has one or more shrines devoted to this purpose. The more powerful individuals in the society have several shrines in their houses and, in fact, the opulence of a house is often referred to in terms of the number of such ritual centers it possesses.

The focal point of the shrine is a box or chest which is built into the wall. In this chest are kept the many charms and magical potions without which no native believes he could live. These preparations are secured from the medicine men,

---

18 Bryk F. *Sex & Circumcision: A Study of Phallic Worship and Mutilation in Men and Women.* North Hollywood, CA: Brandon House; 1967: 157.
19 Paige, p. 41.
20 St. John-Hunt D. Circumcision and Tonsillectomy (letter to the editor). *N Engl J Med.* 1969-09-11; 281(11): 621.

whose assistance must be rewarded with substantial gifts. However, the medicine men do not provide the curative potions for their clients, but decide what the ingredients should be and then write them down in an ancient and secret language. This writing is understood only by the medicine men and by the herbalists who, for another gift, provide the required charm ...

The medicine men have an imposing temple, or 'latipso,' in every community of any size. The more elaborate ceremonies required to treat very sick patients can only be performed at this temple. These ceremonies involve not only the thaumaturge [working of magic] but a permanent group of vestal maidens who move sedately about the temple chambers in distinctive costume and headdress.

The latipso ceremonies are so harsh that it is phenomenal that a fair proportion of the really sick natives who enter the temple ever recover. Small children whose indoctrination is still incomplete have been known to resist attempts to take them to the temple because 'that is where you go to die.' Despite this fact, sick adults are not only willing but eager to undergo the protracted ritual purification, if they can afford to do so. No matter how ill the supplicant or how grave the emergency, the guardians of many temples will not admit a client if he cannot give a rich gift to the custodian. Even after one has gained admission and survived the ceremonies, the guardians will not permit the neophyte to leave until he makes still another gift ...

... Excretory functions are ritualized, routinized, and relegated to secrecy. Natural reproductive functions are similarly distorted. Intercourse is taboo as a topic and scheduled as an act. Efforts are made to avoid pregnancy by use of magical materials or by limiting intercourse to certain phases of the moon. Conception is actually infrequent. When pregnant, women dress so as to hide their condition. Parturition takes place in secret, without friends or relatives to assist, and the majority of women do not nurse their infants." [21]

5.4 The Perspective of Medical Professionals

Although infant circumcision was introduced as a medical procedure during the late 1800s and became widespread during the 1920s and '30s, relatively little was written about it until the late 1940s. In the 1950s a number of articles, most favoring circumcision, appeared in medical publications. In the 1960s a veritable barrage of letters and articles on the subject were published in medical journals. Some condemned the procedure. Others defended it. Some were quite emotional. Others were neutral and weary of the subject. As examples:

---

21 Miner H. Body Ritual Among the Nacirema. In: Lessa WA, Vogt EZ. *Reader in Comparative Religion*. 2nd ed. NY: Harper & Row. 1965: 414-6.

One doctor denounces it:

> "It's high time we stopped performing the mutilating operation known as circumcision... It is a leftover from the barbarous ages. It is a custom. It is not a medical need. It is a traumatic procedure usually done without anesthetic, on helpless newborn babies. Done at the parents' request or the doctor's insistence, for no disease or deformity, with no informed consent, it is truly unique among surgical procedures." [22]

Another doctor defends it:

> "With so many advantages to the operation it is difficult to understand why so many doctors in this country work themselves up into such an emotional frenzy at the mention of the word circumcision. Our medical world generally favor [sic] the operation, yet the anti-circumcision school would have us believe that doctors in these countries are all either barbaric savages or sordid money grubbers." [23]

Dr. Foley, an avid anti-circumcision crusader, states:

> "Circumcision provides a convenient and socially acceptable outlet for the perverted component of the circumciser's libido. I have had personal experience with the psychopathology that underlies the wish to circumcise. The pitiful wails of the suffering infant are all too often the background for lewd and obscene commentary by the obstetrician to his audience of nurses." [24]

Yet another doctor cites its supposed advantages:

> "Many wise physicians having performed routine newborn circumcisions have saved innumerable young men countless hours of having to perform the constant task of retracting their foreskins and extracting their smegma. Perhaps some of these young men have used this time in more profitable and pleasurable pursuits!" [25]

This is a tiny sampling of the numerous articles and letters on the subject. Few of these expressed any concern about the feelings of the helpless baby undergoing the operation. Fewer still expressed any awareness of the basic human right of keeping

---

22 Fitzgerald WD. Circumcision is Barbarous. *Northwest Med.* 1971-10; 70: 681-2.
23 Newill R. Circumcision (letter to the editor). *BMJ.* 1965-08-14: 41.
24 Foley JM. The Unkindest Cut of All. *Fact.* 1966-07/08; 3(4): 6.
25 Freedman LD. Circumcision (Letter to the Editor). *JAMA.* 1970-12-21; 214(12): 2194.

all parts of one's body – the lack of choice and therefore victimization of the infant who loses his foreskin. None expressed any concern or awareness of the sensual or protective function of the foreskin itself. Rarely did any of these articles reach lay people, especially expectant parents. Yet most doctors continued to circumcise babies, claiming that parents insist upon it. Rarely have doctors given parents any intelligent information about the decision. Do they forget that young parents do not usually read medical journals?

Some doctors refuse to circumcise babies. Some strongly oppose the operation. Others have strong feelings that all baby boys should be circumcised, and will attempt to talk any reluctant parent into it. Most doctors fall within the range of "neutral," with attitudes varying from "I think circumcision should be done, but if you really don't want it I won't do it," to "I don't believe in it, but if you really want your son circumcised, I will do it." Most doctors want to go along with what their patients want. (Of course circumcision is *not* what their *little* patients want!) Probably some fear that they will lose business if they refuse to circumcise babies.

Most give the operation very little thought, even though they circumcise babies regularly. Virtually no doctor *specializes* in doing circumcisions. The operation is easy to perform, usually takes only a few minutes, and is but a sidelight in his or her knowledge and skills. Most medical professionals develop a certain amount of callousness to the pain and suffering that surrounds them. Much of this is necessary for their own mental health, because they have to deal with so much trauma. From their perspective, as they regularly deal with serious surgery, fatal diseases, and severe injuries, infant circumcision seems trifling. While most lay people react with shock and horror upon witnessing or hearing detailed descriptions of infant circumcision, doctors perform this operation regularly without a second thought.

There has been a tendency for pediatricians to be less in favor of infant circumcision and for obstetricians to favor it. Technically the obstetrician is "finished" with the baby once it is born, yet he is often the one who performs circumcisions.

Perhaps because of their choice of specialty, pediatricians are more likely to have compassion for infants. Or perhaps pediatricians favor it less because they are usually the ones who see and treat the complications of the operation. In 1971 and 1975 the American Academy of Pediatrics officially announced that routine circumcision of the newborn infant lacks medical justification. The American College of Obstetricians and Gynecologists, at that time declined to endorse that statement.[26] Later, in 1978, they chose to support the position of the American Academy of Pediatrics' Ad Hoc Task Force on Circumcision that "There is no absolute medical indication for routine circumcision of the newborn." This statement, however, was only released in

---

26 Grimes DA. Routine Circumcision of the Newborn Infant: A Reappraisal. *AJOG.* 1978-01-15; 130(2): 125.

the ACOG Newsletter. It was not made known to the public until it appeared in Edward Wallerstein's book *Circumcision: An American Health Fallacy* in 1980.[27]

(Sadly, in more recent years the AAP has backtracked on their declaration of the non-necessity of infant circumcision. While they have refrained from recommending it for all newborn males, they have adopted the vague, waffling stance of declaring that infant circumcision has "benefits as well as disadvantages and risks." Perhaps they have perceived their position of elitism and authority as threatened by the many outside of their medical circle who have sought to educate and enlighten others. Also the billions of financial returns from use of infant foreskins in the cosmetic and other industries has been far too great of allure away from medical honesty. This scandal is thoroughly discussed in Chapter 21 "Use of Infant Foreskins in Cosmetics, Skin Grafts and Other Industries".)

Routine circumcision of infants was a well-established practice before almost all of today's doctors entered medical school. Most male American doctors themselves have been circumcised and therefore are likely to want to believe that the circumcised state has some benefits. All of us – doctors, parents, and babies – have found ourselves caught up in a process that none of us created.

5.5 Is Profit an Important Motive?

When my own sons were circumcised as infants, the operation cost around $30. Today *[ed. note: 1985]*, the fee for the procedure is usually over $100. (More recently I've heard of circumcision charges of as much as $3,000.) This is for a procedure that is simple to learn, can be done with relatively little skill, and normally takes only about 5-10 minutes. Circumcising babies *does* give doctors extra "pocket money." For example, if a doctor were to circumcise 100 baby boys in one year, at $75 each (both low estimates), this would add $7,500 to his annual income. Doctors have been repeatedly accused of promoting infant circumcision out of "profit hungry" motives.

Editor's addendum: In 2021, you still find various prices for circumcision in the USA which in general are lower for newborns and increase as they go up. There is e.g. an outpatient clinic in California that charges $250 for a newborn, $350 for an infant older than 29 days and about $1,600 for adults. In the hospitals, they charge much more, but bill insurance, wherever they can.[28] A clinic in Dallas charges §385 for an infant and as much as $1,875 for an adult.[29] It seems the costs can go all over the map, especially because of the insurance fiasco in which hospitals or clinics will try to charge more if they can get away with it than if a family pays out of pocket.

---

27 Wallerstein E. *Circumcision; An American Health* Fallacy. NY: Springer; 1980: 218.
28 gentlecircumcision.com/contents/pricing
29 gentleproceduresdallas.com/circumcision/cost-how-much-2

While a family may find a bargain price in a local clinic of $150 or so out of the pocket, that seems to be rare and more typical $400 or more out of pocket for the uninsured.[30]

One writer states:

"Chronic remunerative surgery, although a declining specialty, still plays a role in the economic life of many of the medical profession. In this specialty, before an operation can qualify as suitable for inclusion in the established repertoire, certain criteria have to be fulfilled. Firstly, it should require a minimum of skill; secondly, it should have few immediate complications – delayed complications can always be attributed to other factors; and lastly, and above all, there should be a fee attached. Circumcision, while certainly not the answer to a maiden's prayer, is the procedure par excellence for the chronic remunerative surgeon." [31]

It would be preposterous to say that routine neonatal circumcision *deliberately* began simply as a scheme to generate extra money for doctors. Nor are all doctors *intentionally* promoting circumcisions out of greed. Most doctors are "drifting along with the tide" in their willingness to perform this established medical procedure. Nonetheless, the factor of extra income cannot be overlooked. The doctor who *does* believe that infant circumcision is wrong, who will not perform the operation, and attempts to talk new parents out of it (often only to see them turn to another doctor for the operation!) is certainly an individual with strong principles and admirable character. Such a doctor is forfeiting *several thousand dollars* per year for the sake of his convictions.

From a different perspective, another doctor points out that the costs, time and effort presently being put into infant circumcision, represent money and personnel taken away from more health-essential areas of medicine.

"Routine newborn circumcision constitutes a health program of large proportions, for newborn circumcision is probably the most frequently performed operation in the United States. With the assumption that 80 percent of the 1,608,326 male infants born in 1973 were circumcised, approximately 1,287,000 newborn foreskins were excised during that year …

With a physician's fee of $25 and an instrument fee of $15 per case, the cost of circumcising 1,287,000 babies would be approximately 51 million dollars.

---

30 health.costhelper.com/circumcision.html
31 Morgan WKC. Penile Plunder. *Med J Aust.* 1967-05-27; 1: 1102.

... Mass campaigns such as wholesale circumcision, draw money and personnel away from other areas of medicine; if these other areas of medicine are more important, then the campaign has a negative effect on the public's health... At a time when health care resources are limited and demands are great, investment each decade of a half a billion dollars to trim foreskins appears injudicious." [32]

(Again, today further monetary reimbursements from cosmetic and other industries have greatly increased the financial temptation to continue recommending circumcision.)

Neonatal circumcision used to be popular in Great Britain for many of the same reasons as in the United States. However, during the 1970s the rate of infant circumcision in that country reached nearly zero.[33, 34] The change has come about with England's switch to socialized medicine. With the absence of a profit factor, British doctors apparently lost their motive to circumcise babies.

"Routine circumcision of English boys remained rampant until the start of the Second World War, when it is estimated that 85% of the upper class was circumcised and 50% of the working class was circumcised. During the first three decades of this century anti-masturbation was medical excuse enough for the mass destruction of British prepuces. In the thirties the medical profession began to search for other excuses to continue cutting away at English cocks, which, after all, provided them with a financial bonus! Then came the blitz, loss of Empire, socialized medicine, and the end of the financial bonus. Routine circumcision became 'officially discouraged' in 1941, and soon after the war it waned." [29]

5.6 The Factor of Insurance Coverage

Many insurance companies pay for infant circumcision. Their choice to cover this procedure, but not other types of medical procedures is curious. When our second and third sons were born we had insurance that mainly paid for treatment of accidents and surgery. It did not pay for prenatal care, or any other hospital expenses associated with birth, nor did it pay for routine immunizations, well baby care, prescriptions, or medical treatments for illnesses. It did, however, pay for two of my sons' circumcisions. Why do insurance companies pay for this provenly unnecessary operation when they do not cover other services which offer greater medical value?

---

[32] Excerpt from an Underground Newsletter (Bud Berkeley).
[33] Jolly H. Circumcision. *Practitioner.* 1964-02; 192: 257.
[34] Bernal JF, Richards MPM, Brackbill Y. Early Behavioral Differences: Gender or Circumcision? *Dev Psychobiol.* 9(1): 91.

I wrote to a well-known insurance company which had re-evaluated its policies and chose to continue covering routine neonatal circumcision:

> "Babies *have* become severely retarded from undetected PKU. Babies *have* had severe bleeding problems that could have been prevented by vitamin K. People *can* die from diseases such as polio and diphtheria that are preventable through immunizations. But nobody has ever died or become severely retarded from having a foreskin! Why do you consider circumcision worth paying for when it is at best 'cosmetic surgery?' I'm sure you do not pay for ear piercing or body tattooing ..." [35]

Their reply:

> "... Routine neonatal circumcision had been considered, but rejected, as a procedure of questionable usefulness ...
>
> The analogy you attempt to draw between routine immunization services and routine neonatal circumcision is an interesting one. Basically ... the position in regard to these services is dictated by our contracts. Immunizations and well baby care are generally outpatient services, which are seldom, if ever, covered under the terms of our agreements. Additionally these are unequivocally preventative in nature. Alternatively, circumcision is a surgical service, which is covered under most agreements. Its need is controversial among the medical authorities.
>
> [We do] not attempt to dictate the nature of services rendered to a patient. That is a matter best left to the patient and the physician. On the other hand, it is our responsibility to establish the level of benefits and services to be covered under the terms of our agreements. Although these issues may appear to be merely alternative sides of the same coin, please be assured that they are, in fact, quite different." [36]

They must have considered me "some kind of a nut" for they obviously did not answer my questions accurately. For PKU tests, vitamin K shots, and other routine hospital nursery procedures are also clearly "in-patient" services. Conversely, my third son's circumcision took place in a doctor's office, and therefore was definitely an "out-patient" service. Thus the location of the service rendered is not the criterion. Furthermore, if their choice is to pay for surgery, then they should also pay for the mother's episiotomy which has more medical justification than infant circumcision.

---

35 Romberg R. Personal correspondence to an insurance company.
36 Insurance company (identity withheld) personal correspondence.

Obviously insurance companies do not provide services for what is going to save lives or protect the health of their clients, so much as for what is going to sell insurance. Individual insurance companies undoubtedly fear that if they drop coverage for infant circumcision, they will lose business. (In actuality, I seriously doubt that many people give consideration to infant circumcision when purchasing insurance coverage.)

Meanwhile a "vicious circle" has been created. The naive expectant or new parent, upon learning that their insurance pays for infant circumcision, is less likely to question the operation than they would if they had to pay for it themselves. Insurance companies continue to cover circumcision because they claim that parents insist upon it. Unknowledgeable new parents conclude "It must be important to the baby's health because our insurance covers it." If more parents and doctors questioned the procedure, insurance companies would be more likely to drop coverage. On the other hand, if insurance companies were to cease coverage for circumcision, more doctors and parents would question the operation.

5.7 Delivery Room Circumcision

The flurry of debate over the optimum time to perform infant circumcision has been a controversy within a controversy. When circumcision first began as a medical practice, young boys and infants of all ages were brought to doctors for the operation. When the hospital became the standard place for birth and newborn circumcision became routine, foreskins were usually cut off a few days after birth. During the 1940s and '50s "delivery room" circumcision became popular. This came about due to shortages of medical personnel brought about by the "post-war baby boom."

The rationale used to justify immediate newborn circumcision are incredible:

> "Safety ... healing ... by the time the mother takes her child home there is no dressing on the penis, healing is well advanced, and the dangers of infection negligible ... Convenience ... the obstetrician finishes his [?] episiotomy, walks across the hall and circumcises the infant, and is finished with the whole business [!] ... Observation in the nursery, redressing, and the handling of any complication that might develop are easily expedited in the hospital ... Sterility – at birth the newborn is as near to absolute sterility as he will ever be ... Stimulation of the baby – Frequently following a general anesthetic the newborn is depressed and various stimulants are employed; circumcision unfailingly produces an excellent response in a sleepy baby [!] ... Physiology – hemoglobin averages between 19 and 23 gm, and maternal antibodies are present in fetal serum which are soon lost. This suggests less possibility of infection and hemorrhage ... Although

the pain sense is present at birth, it is much less intense than in later infancy ..." [37]

The writer of that article assumes that an infant will get more attention and care in a hospital nursery by the impartial nurses than he will at home by his own mother. He assumes that there is less danger of infection in the notoriously germ-ridden hospital than there would be at home. He cites the all-too-common, but unfounded opinion that newborn infants feel less pain. The reference to the obstetrician being "finished with the whole business" upon repairing "his" [!] episiotomy and doing the circumcision reflects the impersonal approach too often taken by the medical profession. And slicing off the foreskin to awaken a sleepy baby is an attitude nothing short of incredible! Is this how the men of today experienced their entrance into this world? ... arriving in an anesthetized stupor to awake into consciousness by having their penises tortured?! Could there be a connection between this and the fact that so many people today have serious problems related to drugs and sex?

Within recent years there has been a trend away from delivery room circumcision. During the 1970s articles discouraging this practice have appeared in medical journals. The main objection was that the infants became chilled due to their longer stay in the delivery room.

> "This statistical study of 1,047 infants in 1968 indicates that the percentage of chilled infants in the circumcised group was significantly greater than in the uncircumcised group.
>
> 'The following is the routine care given to infants in the delivery room: An infant who is born in this hospital is received from the delivery table by a nurse who carries him wrapped in a dry towel, to the resuscitation unit where he is wrapped in a warmed cotton blanket and resuscitated. Infants who are not to be circumcised are then taken to the regular nursery. Infants who are to be circumcised remain in the resuscitation unit until the obstetrician finishes with the mother; the infant then is placed on the circumcision table, still covered except for the genital region, and is circumcised. He is then carried to the nursery. There is a warmer beneath the infant in the resuscitation unit but none on the circumcision table. On arrival in the nursery the infant's rectal temperature is taken immediately and recorded.'" [38]

---

37 Miller RL, Snyder DC. Immediate Circumcision of the Newborn Male. *AJOG*. 1953-01; 65(1).
38 Spence GR. Chilling of Newborn Infants: Its Relation to Circumcision Immediately Following Birth. *SMJ*. 1970-03; 63: 309.

The article concluded that some circumcised infants were arriving in the nursery with low temperatures, and they recommended that circumcision be delayed until the baby's body temperature was better established.

The Report of the Ad Hoc Task Force on Circumcision by the American Academy of Pediatrics includes:

> "The procedure is also contraindicated in the immediate neonatal period or until complete neonatal physical adaptation has occurred (usually 12 to 24 hours.) The avoidance of circumcision in the delivery room immediately after birth is particularly important because neonatal disease is not always apparent at birth. In addition it entails protracted exposure of infants to significant cold stress." [39]

It is true that newborns do experience a rapid loss of body heat at the time of birth. They should be quickly dried off and warmed. Over-chilling of a newborn can be dangerous. Hospital delivery rooms are commonly kept at around 65 degrees F. Most hospitals have sophisticated, expensive baby warming equipment in which babies are placed after birth. Mothers who have pleaded with the doctors that they might nurse, hold, and touch their babies immediately after birth have been countered with the argument that the baby will get chilled unless he is quickly taken to the nursery and put in a baby warmer. Today, many hospital personnel are learning that the mother's body is an excellent "baby warmer" and the baby's body temperature is usually easily maintained by immediate, uninterrupted contact with the mother.

It is highly debatable whether immediate circumcision or circumcision a few days later is more traumatic for the baby. Those of us who are concerned about the baby's emotional well-being usually suggest waiting a few days to allow the baby to adjust to life in this world before circumcising him, (if circumcision must be done). But probably the operation is equally painful regardless of the time in relation to birth. Immediate circumcision is unquestionably *totally* disregarding of the infant's feelings during his introduction into this world. It constitutes the absolute antithesis of non-violent birth. However, welcoming the baby into the world with non-violent birthing techniques, only to subject him to circumcision a few days later, is nothing but hypocritical!

The current rationale against immediate circumcision is unfortunately too typical of the medical profession's non- emotional, "scientific" approach. The risk of loss of body temperature or undetected medical problems are the *only* issues they find worthy of consideration. They express NO concern for the baby's feelings. They apparently have no awareness of how the operation, not to mention his subsequent stay

---

39 American Academy of Pediatrics, Committee on Fetus and Newborn. *Report of the Ad HocTask Force on Circumcision Pediatrics.* 1975-10; 56(4): 610.

in the nursery, will affect the mother-infant bond! Also, the need for resuscitation of infants at birth is a curious reminder of a largely bygone era when parturient mothers were often heavily anesthetized during labor and birth.

5.8 Coercion and Unauthorized Circumcision

In the past parents who desired natural birth often had to plead with doctors and fight with nurses who wished to give medication during labor. Mothers desiring to breastfeed have often been given erroneous information persuading them to bottle feed. Despite mothers' protests, nursing babies have been given bottles of formula in hospital nurseries. In a system geared for medicated births and bottle feeding, parents giving birth naturally and breastfed babies were often "oddities" that inconvenienced the hospital staff. Today much of this has changed. But in similar fashion, sometimes new parents have had to fight the system in order to leave the hospital with an intact baby boy. Usually mothers in labor upon admittance to the hospital are bombarded with many routine procedures. Amid haste and excitement she signs a number of papers, including a consent form for circumcision. Sometimes consent for circumcision of newborn boys is written into the general admission form. Usually she signs it without thinking. The fact that a consent form is required makes obvious the fact that parents have the right to refuse the operation. However parents have frequently been harassed when they have decided against circumcision.

> "When my wife was pregnant the OB-GYN would not listen to her when she insisted that if it were a boy we would not tolerate his being circumcised under any circumstances. The doctor stopped badgering her only when I spoke to him and told him that I would take him to court and sue him if there were the slightest 'slip-up' and he were 'accidentally' to be circumcised. When she was admitted to the hospital I wrote boldly on the admission slip that I would sue the hospital if my child were a boy and they permitted him to be circumcised. My child was a girl ..." [40]

Another father writes:

> "I was circumcised in the service and I didn't want my son to go through life without a complete organ as I am doing. When we realized that it might be a boy, I told the doctor that I forbade circumcision. He just laughed and said, 'Don't you want him to be like other boys?' I kept reminding him but I don't think he took me seriously. Then I told him that if my son came home circumcised he would

---

40 W. C., New Jersey, "What They Say", INTACT Educational Foundation – reprint, Wilbraham, MA.

have a lawsuit on his hands. Even that didn't seem to bother him, so we changed doctors just in time. Now my son is going through life with a beautifully formed foreskin ... a pleasure of which I have been deprived." [41]

A less fortunate father reports:

"Prior to our son's birth his European-born mother and I discussed the question of his circumcision if we had a male child. We decided that if it were not necessary the child would not be circumcised. I was planning to tell the doctor when he asked me. My wife was also prepared to tell him 'no circumcision.' The question was never asked. Because of complications during childbirth, my son's mother was confined to bed for two weeks after his birth. I was the first to change his diapers and was shocked to see the circumcision clamp on his penis. I confronted his mother who told me she never authorized it. I confronted the doctor. He told me it was 'routine' at that hospital." [42]

A similar experience:

"I told the doctor that if the baby was a boy I would refuse to permit a circumcision. Yet when the child came home he was circumcised. When I confronted the doctor he made all kinds of excuses, including that the delivery section was so busy they couldn't be bothered. He agreed to take the cost of circumcision off our bill." [41]

An unauthorized circumcision *is* grounds for a lawsuit. Court settlements have taken place for this reason.

The U.S. Army's "Military Law Review" describes a case in which the Army paid the parents a compensation of $500 for the unauthorized circumcision of their baby. This was not a botched or later infected circumcision, but simply a case in which the parents were opposed to unnecessary circumcision and had withheld the required consent to have the baby subjected to such trauma.[43]

In 1979 an Orthodox Jewish couple gave birth to a baby boy in a Los Angeles Hospital. Because they had planned a Bris, they did not want a hospital circumcision.

"... Hospital employees had tried 'at least twice' to get her to sign consent forms allowing a circumcision there, but she refused. Just after the last request, she

---

41 Excerpt from an Underground Newsletter (Bud Berkeley).
42 Ibid.
43 U.S. Army "Military Law Review", Vol. 75, (Dept. of Army, Pamphlet 27-100-75.)

learned that the child had already been circumcised ... The family had made arrangements to have a Bris ceremony for the child, but the Mohel, upon finding that the child had already been medically circumcised, refused to perform the ritual ... Since there was no permission, the mother considers the circumcision an assault and hopes that her lawsuit will help prevent the same thing ever happening again to another Jewish child." [44]

5.9 The Perspective of Expectant and New Parents

Most expectant parents, especially those having their first babies, are extremely naive about *everything* concerning pregnancy, birth and babies. Even highly educated, sophisticated people usually have to learn their new calling from the beginning. Some expectant parents make commendable attempts to read and learn as much as they can, while others drift along with very little preparation, trusting the medical profession to make their decisions for them. But even parents who have sought to inform themselves in every possible way are still incredibly "green" when faced with the reality of birth and the new baby.

Our highly mobile, affluent society is largely to blame for the discontinuity in the education of young parents. In primitive societies a young girl grew up caring for younger siblings, nieces and nephews. When she bore her first child she had extensive personal experience in infant care and the constant companionship of her own female relatives. Commonly a woman would bear her last children after becoming a grandmother.

The small families, delayed age of childbearing, isolation, mobility, and constantly changing values and beliefs of today's society have virtually obliterated such continuity between generations. Twenty to thirty years may span the time between the birth of a woman's youngest child and that of her first grandchild. Styles and philosophies change and the grandmother may have little knowledge or help to give to her daughter or daughter-in-law.

The expectant mother of today may have never been around another pregnant woman. She may never have seen another woman breastfeed. Perhaps she has never seen or held a newborn baby.

Books, childbirth classes, La Leche League groups, doctors, and midwives have all served as attempts to fill this gap. Women's heritage, the art of birth and infant care passed from mother to daughter from time immemorial, has now fallen into the hands of substitutes.

Expectant and new parents are bombarded with advertisements for products. Babies and birth is a lucrative consumer industry. Toys, gimmicks, furniture, photo-

---

44 Policzer M. Jewish Parents Sue Hospital Over Circumcision. *Los Angeles Herald Examiner.* 1979-03-18.

graphs, insurance, etc. – some useful, most harmless, some damaging, most unnecessary – all exploit new parents' naivete and desperate desire to do what is best for their infant. Infant circumcision is, in a sense, yet another of these "products" that new parents are being sold.

The conflicting viewpoints and well-meaning advice with which expectant parents are barraged is enough to drive anyone to distraction! "Breastfeeding might tie me down. Bottle feeding is unnatural and will give the baby allergies. Cloth diapers might give the baby a rash. Disposable diapers are a threat to the environment. Commercial baby food is full of additives. Homemade baby food might spoil. Natural childbirth might hurt too much. Medication during birth might harm the baby. If I go back to work I'll be neglecting the baby. If I stay home I might stagnate. The hospital seems impersonal. Home birth seems dangerous. Start solids early or late? Follow a feeding schedule so he'll be 'regulated?' Feed him on demand to 'answer his needs?' Pick him up whenever he cries and risk 'spoiling' him? Let him cry it out and be a cruel mother? ... aaggh!!!"

It is little wonder that concern about circumcision has been shoved to the background. Despite all that has recently been written and said about parents' choices, most parents trust their doctors about medically related matters. Perhaps the "dilemmas" over cloth versus disposable diapers or homemade versus commercial baby foods are confusing enough to the expectant parent, without even attempting to question medical issues!

The 'medical world' is usually a mystery to first-time expectant parents. They have probably been healthy all their lives and have never before had to visit a doctor on a regular basis or be a hospital patient. Often common obstetrical terms such as "Caesarian," "placenta," "episiotomy," or "meconium" are foreign even to the educated lay person.

Classes, books and articles have been of immense value to expectant and new parents. Parents learn exercises, relaxation and breathing techniques for comfort during pregnancy and use in labor. They are taught what to expect during the hospital stay, and are usually given information about nutrition, breastfeeding, and infant care.

But circumcision has rarely been mentioned. Most books on infant care say nothing. A few give brief, neutral, usually forgotten advice. Most childbirth instructors have not informed expectant parents about circumcision. Doctors also rarely advise people about the operation. Usually expectant mothers are simply asked by their doctors whether or not they want the baby circumcised – without discussion. That is the total amount of attention given to the subject.

Some have called this a "conspiracy of silence" in not informing parents about the painful and unnecessary operation that is being performed on babies. But in fact,

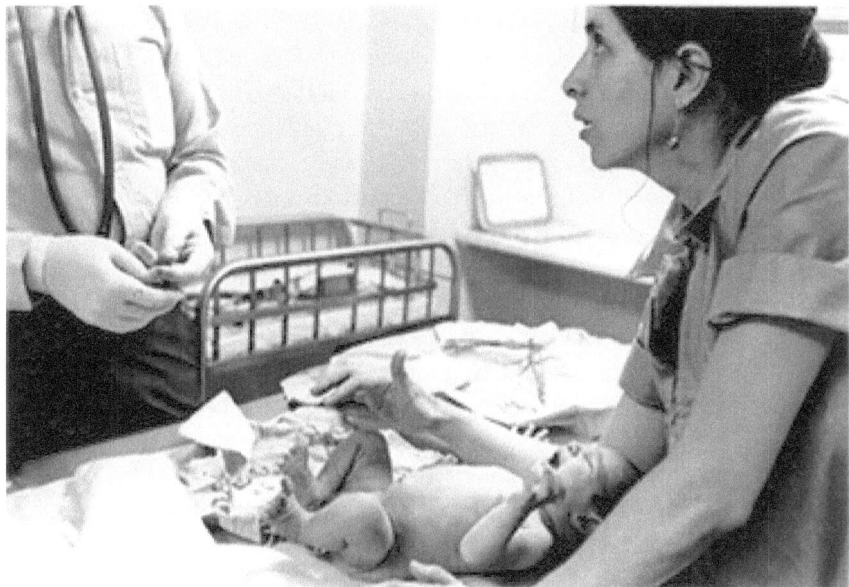

© Suzanne Arms

childbirth educators, and even doctors have rarely known any more than parents about this matter. The childbirth education movement is still young. Too many other concerns have had to be aired, such as medication during birth, father participation, breastfeeding, and maternal-infant bonding before we could get around to questioning circumcision.

A significant number of expectant parents, especially mothers, are not familiar with the term "circumcision," or if they know the word, have no comprehension of what it means.

Wynder and Licklider's study, investigating the alleged relationship between circumcision and cervical cancer, questioned men about their own circumcision status and women about their husbands' circumcision status. Among the female patients, 36% of those in Los Angeles and 38% of those in New York, either did not understand the term "circumcision" or did not know the circumcision status of their husbands. Of the men, 5% in Los Angeles and 17% in New York did not understand the term circumcision. 14% of the men in Los Angeles and 6% of those in New York stated that they were circumcised but upon examination by a doctor it was learned that they were not.[45]

Amidst a barrage of hospital admittance procedures mothers in labor are handed permission slips for circumcision. If the above study is representative, it is possible

---

45 Wynder EL, Licklider SD. The Question of Circumcision. *Cancer.* 1960-05/06; 13(3): 442-3.

that one out of three of these mothers has no idea what circumcision even means. Other slightly more informed mothers, who do know the difference between the circumcised and the intact penis and understand that the foreskin is cut off, are not much more knowledgeable, yet they sign away their sons' foreskins without thinking. They are naive and anxious to please their doctor and go along with all the hospital's practices on the belief that they are doing what is best for their baby. Medical patients are in such a position of passivity, cooperation, and gullibility, that most would accept *any* medical practice that their doctor suggests. It would be an interesting experiment for someone to make up a medically sounding name for a non-existent procedure and present it to a sampling of hospital patients. It is my guess that over half would unquestioningly agree to it.

Who is insisting upon circumcision? Accusations have been hurled in many directions. Parents claim that doctors push them into it. Doctors claim that parents demand it. And despite women's *proven* naivete about the matter, men have accused women of wanting to perpetuate it. In the *Journal of the American Medical Association* in 1965 Dr. W.K.C. Morgan posed:

> "Perhaps not the least of the reasons why American mothers seem to endorse the operation with such enthusiasm is the fact that it is one way an intensely matriarchal society can permanently influence the physical characteristics of its males." [46]

The statement is ludicrous, if not infuriating, for the medical profession is unquestionably a *male* dominated establishment. Few of us "matriarchs" even read the Journal of the American Medical Association!

Suzanne Arms has expounded upon the routine, unnatural, dehumanizing, and potentially dangerous practices within our *male* dominated medical establishment:

> "It was man who moved in on normal birth to baptize the baby and mother that he himself may have damaged; man who spread disease, man who cured disease, man who institutionalized birth in the hospital. Man placed woman on her back in labor, then devised metal tools to pull her baby out, then knocked her senseless with anesthesia. And it was man who, throughout history, did it all in the name of 'saving' woman from her own body, from the curse of her gender, from the 'pain' of her travail, and from her own ignorance. Today the male obstetrician with his kindly paternalism comforts woman by advising her to leave everything to him, to simply place herself in his hands and abide by the procedures of his institution,

---

46 Morgan WKC. The Rape of the Phallus. *JAMA*. 1965-07-19; 193(3).

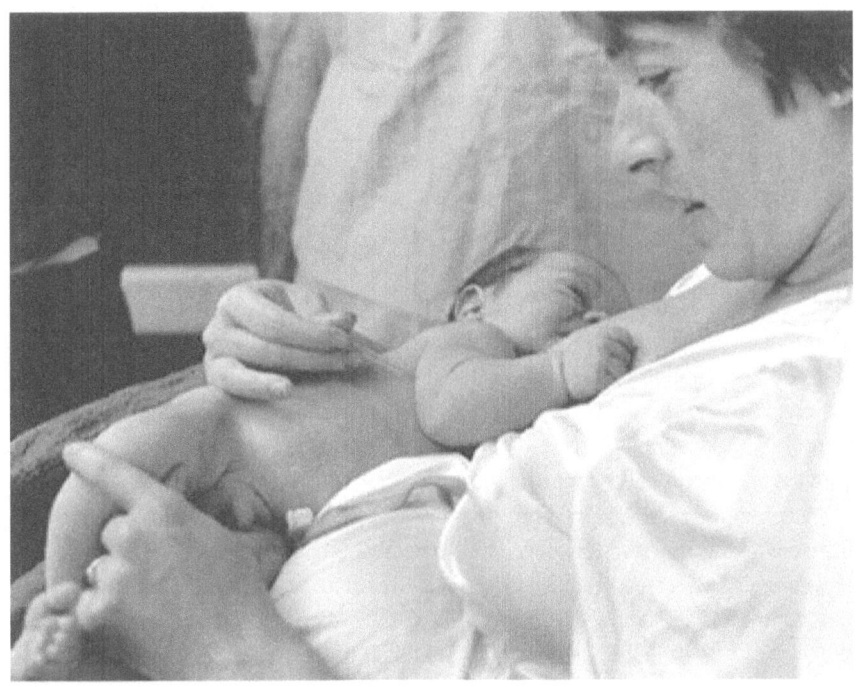

© *Suzanne Arms*

the hospital. And woman, that docile, ignorant, cursed, weak, and dependent victim of deception, willingly agrees." [47]

Today's mother does not make an *intelligent* decision to have her son's foreskin amputated any more than she makes an intelligent, rational decision to have her own pubic hair shaved, an I.V. stuck in her arm, a fetal heart monitor wired to her body, or to be confined to a labor bed, to deliver on a delivery table, or to have her baby separated from her after birth. Circumcision is but one more routine, questionable hospital procedure to which she passively, unthinkingly agrees.

Many men appear not to realize that most women simply have not seen very many penises. The male organ is not normally on view in public. Males, of course, grow up seeing each others' bodies in restrooms and locker rooms. Therefore, most are aware of foreskins or the lack of them. But unless a woman has either worked in a hospital, lived among nudists, or had a large number of male lovers, she has probably not seen very many penises. Therefore the American woman assumes that the

---

47 Arms S. *Immaculate Deception.* San Francisco, CA: Houghton Mifflin; 1975: 22.

appearance of the circumcised penis with the "head" exposed is the way they are "supposed" to look and has no awareness that something was ever cut off.

If parents *do* think about circumcision, their concerns may be as follows:

Most young American fathers today have been circumcised. Frequently, perhaps for want of any other reasons, fathers decide that their sons should "match them" in this respect. (How come our intact grandfathers and great grandfathers didn't worry about their sons matching" them?)

If new parents do see their infant son's penis before he is circumcised (and in many cases they do not!) this may be the first time that at least the mother has ever seen an intact penis. To American middle-class eyes, the long pointed foreskin may tend to look "strange." Nurses are sometimes asked to explain why the baby's penis looks so "funny." Looks are in the eye of the beholder. Americans often perceive the foreskin as "something that needs to be cut off." Perhaps there is some confusion with the concept of cutting the umbilical cord.

A common "reason" given for circumcision is concern that their son will "look different" from his peers or other family members, if he keeps his foreskin. Today, however, as increasing numbers of parents are choosing to leave their sons intact, this concern is lessening. Parents readily explain to their children the anatomical differences between children and adults, and males and females. If he is circumcised, they may have to explain to him why his foreskin was cut off. Furthermore, "styles" of circumcisions vary because some doctors take off more skin than others. Therefore, circumcised brothers or friends may still "not match." Most children give the entire matter very little concern. Explaining to an intact boy why he has his foreskin is not normally a difficult problem.

People have been led to believe that circumcision somehow makes a male cleaner – although few could explain how. Some people have the idea that smegma must be a horrible substance. They think of circumcision in the same light as routine immunizations. Shots prevent the baby from getting polio, diphtheria, measles, etc., and circumcision keeps him from having "smegma" which must be just as bad!! Who would want a baby that had "smegma!" The new mother probably does not realize that she regularly washes smegma out of her own genitals, and if she has a baby girl will clean it out of her labia. Additionally, circumcised males do have smegma, although to a lesser extent than their intact peers. Smegma is simply a build-up of dead skin cells that tends to stay moist because it is in a closed space. In contrast to the dirty diapers, spit up, and "snotty" noses that parents will attend to, smegma is an extremely trivial concern.

The new mother sometimes chooses circumcision for her son, fearing that otherwise she would have to handle her son's penis while retracting his foreskin. However, she will quickly learn, usually with the first dirty diaper that she changes, that she must handle and wash all parts of her baby regardless. She soon matter-of-factly accepts all parts of her child's body. Besides, retraction of the foreskin should not be done during infancy.

Parents usually have no idea how the operation is done. Rarely have they ever actually seen it. If they think of it at all, they imagine a momentary trimming of a little piece of skin (perhaps like some strange little membrane). Perhaps they have been told that it is painless. Or it may occur to them that it might hurt the baby – but then shots and many other medical procedures are painful – so what? During pregnancy "the baby" is an abstract concept to most expectant parents. He is not yet a person that they have grown to love. Rarely have parents ever been presented with the idea that circumcision might *not* be a good idea.

An oft-cited belief is that it is "so much more painful" if circumcision is done to an adult. This is refuted in many other places in this book, so it will not be expounded here. But where did we ever get the idea that "Circumcision is so painful that a grown man cannot take it, so inflict it on a helpless newborn baby instead?!"

An additional consideration is that a woman who has just given birth has been through a major emotional and physical upheaval. She usually has been through hours of challenging labor contractions. She is probably sore from an episiotomy or Caesarian incision. She may be having painful after-contractions as her uterus involutes. Her nipples may be sore from her first attempts to breastfeed. In other words, *her own body is in a state of great pain and trauma!* The new mother perceives of her baby as an extension of herself. So if she thinks about her baby being cut and his genitals being sore, it may not seem inappropriate. It is not hostility to the child, but simply a sense of "everything is blood, soreness, and pain right now and what's a little bit more?" She has not yet begun to think of him as a separate individual.

The general appearance of the newborn baby is usually surprising if not alarming to new parents. The baby's head may be molded from birth. His skin may appear quite red or blotchy. He usually has skinny little arms and legs with his head and body seeming strangely large in proportion. The umbilical stump is almost always a startling experience for new parents – a strange, sticky, bluish piece of tissue, later becoming shriveled, hardened, and brownish before it falls off. In addition to all this, their baby boy's penis may be reddish around the end or may have a plastic clamp around it. Upon being confronted with so many unfamiliar things about their new baby, the appearance of the newly circumcised penis may not stand out as any more alarming or unusual than these other features.

One of the most important factors in the widespread acceptance of routine neonatal circumcision has been the delaying and hampering of the bonding process between parents and babies. The traditional routine in hospitals has been to take newborn babies to the nursery immediately after birth, and bring them to their mothers several hours later. In the past many mothers were unconscious during delivery and learned about their babies several hours after birth. Mothers who were conscious or even unmedicated for birth often got only a brief glimpse of their babies before they were whisked off to the nursery. Even in "progressive" hospitals, where mothers have been "allowed" to hold their babies in the delivery room, the baby is almost always wrapped in blankets before he is given to her. The lack of skin-to-skin contact is definitely an impediment in the bonding process even if the baby is held by the mother right away. Usually when babies are brought to mothers for feeding they are bundled up in blankets and mothers are not allowed to unwrap their own babies. The only part of her baby that the mother is able to see or touch is his head. Rarely is the newly delivered mother in a hospital given the opportunity to explore all parts of her baby's body.

Therefore, if her baby is circumcised, she will probably not ever see his penis before his foreskin is cut off. She also may not see it immediately after the operation when it is freshly red and sore. By the time she takes him home and is changing his diapers his circumcision wound is nearly healed. For the amount of involvement the mother is given in the event, the baby boy may as well have been born circumcised. (My own mother, who gave birth to four children, had never before seen an umbilical stump until she stayed with me after my first son's birth!.)

When a mother has immediate, skin-to-skin contact with her baby at birth and as few interruptions as possible thereafter, she develops stronger feelings of *attachment* and *protectiveness* towards her baby. Mothers have known from the beginnings of time that we should not be separated from our babies at the time of birth. But in recent times our voices have not been heard. It took two male doctors, Marshall H. Klaus and John H. Kennell, to convince the medical profession of the importance of bonding. They have researched and made in-depth observations of the interactions between mothers and their infants, and have taught us much about the emotional bond that is formed and how it is affected by separation and other interferences. They state:

> "This attachment is crucial to the survival and development of the infant ... after birth [the mother] insures his survival while he is utterly dependent on her. The power of this attachment is so great that it enables the mother or father to make the unusual sacrifices necessary for the care of their infant day after day, night after night changing dirty diapers, attending to his cry, *protecting him from danger* [emphasis mine], and giving feedings in the middle of the night despite a desperate need to sleep ... This original mother-infant bond is the wellspring for all the infant's subsequent attachments and is the formative relationship in the course of which the child develops a sense of himself. Throughout his lifetime

the strength and character of this attachment will influence the quality of all future bonds to other individuals." [48]

In a traditional hospital birth setting, the parents have not yet developed feelings of intense love or attachment towards their baby. Therefore, they are likely to be unconcerned about the prospect of his foreskin being cut off. *If* parents were truly in control of birth, or *if* the medical custom were to circumcise babies at a later time in their lives, few parents would choose to have it done. Maternal and paternal protective instincts would intervene to prevent such pain from befalling their baby! So who is responsible? Roger Saquet summed it up by saying:

> "... Mothers blame the doctors for advising them to circumcise ... doctors complained that the mothers insisted on having the operation done! To the reader it may sound like a pair of criminals caught red-handed, each one accusing the other of coercion. It would seem most probable that both groups share equal responsibility.
>
> Point of fact: no doctor is obligated to perform an operation which he deems unnecessary. He is at liberty to refuse to operate and have the parents go to another doctor. Point of fact: virtually all hospitals require the written permission of at least one parent in order to circumcise the child. The buck must stop right here." [49]

It is true, however, that infant circumcision would not take place *if* hospitals did not have the equipment for the operation and *if* doctors were not trained and willing to perform the operation.

5.10 Circumcision Techniques: Gomco and Plastibell

5.10.1 The Gomco technique

1. Stretch the preputial ring.
2. Break preputial adhesions so that the foreskin is completely retractile. (A)
3. Retract the foreskin until you can see the corona. Check the glans for any hidden adhesions. If the entire preputial space is not free, you stand a good chance of pinching the glans on the bell or clamp, or of leaving adhesions behind.
4. Apply a small amount of lubricant such as petroleum jelly to the glans so that it won't stick to the inside of the bell.

---

48 Saquet R. Circumcision in Social Perspective. Reprinted from "The Country Lady's Daybook," 1976-03.
49 Topp S. Why Not to Circumcise Your Baby Boy. *Mothering.* 1978-01; 6: 69.

5. Apply the bell-shaped plunger over the glans. The bell should fit easily over the glans so that it covers the corona. Too small a bell may injure the glans and fail to protect the corona, If stretching the preputial ring does not allow the bell to be inserted in the preputial space and entirely cover the glans, a dorsal slit may be necessary. (B)
6. Pull the prepuce up over the bell. The foreskin should not be stretched or pulled too snugly over the bell. If it's pulled up too tightly, it's possible to remove too much shaft skin or to pull the urethra up so you get a tangential cut through the urethra as well as the skin. (C)
7. Judge the amount of the shaft skin left below the corona; the skin should be relaxed and supple.
8. After you're sure of the dimensions, apply the plate of the clamp at the level of the corona. (D)

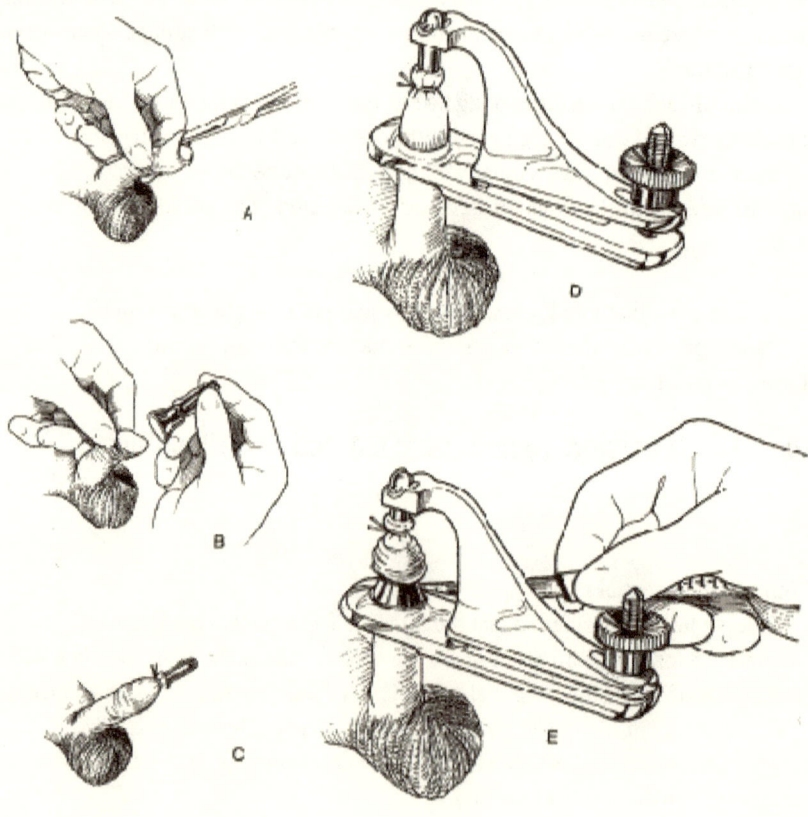

The Gomco technique. © *Patient Care, March 15, 1978, p. 82-83.*

9. With everything in proper alignment, tighten the clamp. This squeezes the prepuce between the bell and the clamp to make it blood-free. Be sure the weight of the clamp doesn't distort the anatomy so there isn't the proper amount of skin in the clamp.
10. Make a circumferential incision with a cold knife, not an electrosurgical instrument. (E)
11. Leave the clamp in place at least five minutes to allow clotting and coaptation to occur.
12. Remove the clamp and apply antiseptic ointment (Betadine) to the crush line. Apply a light dressing or loin cloth arrangement to keep the ointment from rubbing off.
13. If you remove the clamp prematurely, the crushed edges may separate and bleeding will occur. When this occurs, suture the mucocutaneous margin, being careful to avoid deep sutures that might penetrate the urethra. If the whole edge separates, treat as a freehand circumcision. placing quadrant sutures and sewing between them with fine stitches.
14. Have the baby watched overnight for any sign of bleeding.
15. If late separation occurs, it's best to keep the wound clean and let it heal secondarily rather than to try to suture it and risk development of stricture or fistula. Skin of this area tends to re-epithelialize rapidly.

5.10.2 The Plastibell technique

1. Stretch the preputial ring.
2. Break preputial adhesions with a probe or closed forceps.
3. Make a small dorsal slit of 0.5 to 1.0 cm in the prepuce. Keep the initial slit short; it can always be extended. To minimize bleeding, previously crush the line of incision with artery forceps for one minute. Take particular care not to place forceps or scissors in the urethral meatus; before cutting or crushing, lift the prepuce away from the glans and visualize the meatus. (A, B)
4. Separate the edges of the slit with a pair of artery forceps to reveal the glans. If necessary, extend the cut to expose the coronal sulcus. (C)
5. Free any remaining adhesions and lay the prepuce back (inside out) to expose the entire glans.
6. Slip the Plastibell of appropriate size over the glans as far as the coronal sulcus. It should slip over the glans easily; too small a bell may injure the glans.
7. Place the prepuce over the bell to hold it in place. (D)
8. Tie the ligature as tightly as possible around the prepuce on the ridge of the bell; oozing will occur if the ligature is loose.

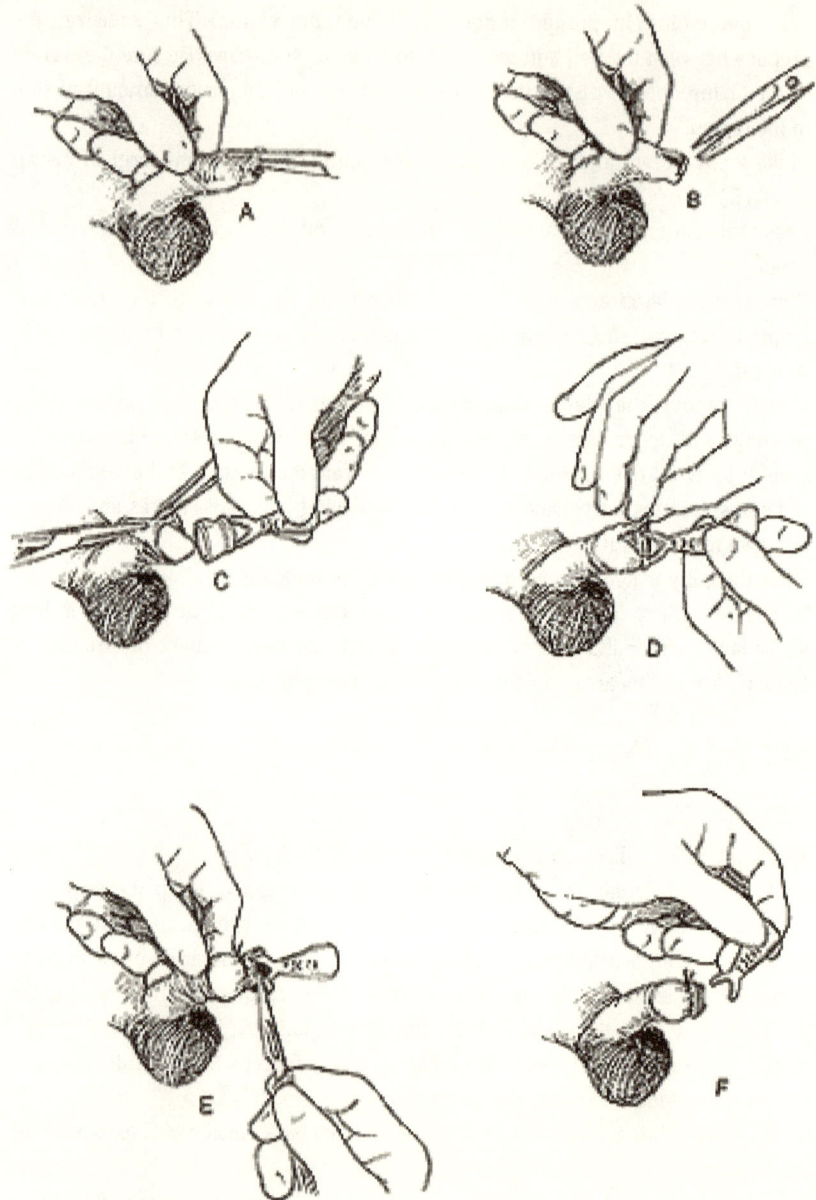

The Plastibell technic. © Patient Care, March 15, 1978, p. 84-85.

9. After 1-2 minutes to allow for crush, trim off the prepuce at the distal edge of the ligature, using a knife or scissors. Trim as much tissue as possible to reduce the amount of necrotic tissue and possibility of infection. (E)
10. Snap off the handle of the bell, leaving the bell and ligature in place. You should be able to see an unobstructed urethral meatus. (F)
11. No dressing is necessary; the baby may be bathed normally; the rim of tissue under and distal to the ligature will become necrotic and will separate with the bell in 5-10 days.
12. Complications are unusual with this technique. Occasionally, however, edema will trap the plastic ring on the shaft of the penis. In this case, it's usually necessary to cut off the ring, using a guide and ring cutter, although application of ice will sometimes reduce edema enough to remove the ring.

5.11   Conclusion

Parents rarely read medical publications. Few parents have ever seen circumcision performed. Most have no idea how circumcision is done. Little information has appeared in publications that reach lay people. However doctors have *ample* opportunity to read medical publications. They know *full well* how the operation is done. They *should be expected* to be knowledgeable about the matter. Yet rarely do they inform expectant parents about it. Too few doctors have been willing to take a stand against infant circumcision, even when they have personal feelings opposing it. Most doctors today agree that infant circumcision is *unnecessary*. The next step is to deem it *unethical*. (For example, if a parent wanted his baby's ears cut off – no doctor would do it. Will the foreskin ever be given equal consideration?) Some parents who have looked for medical leadership about circumcision have received mere passivity from their doctors ("The decision is up to you."). Many parents of intact sons owe the decision to the advice of their doctors.

Doctors have more influence on the matter than anyone else. Sylvia Topp quotes the results of a study by Patel (in Canada), which revealed that

> "… doctors opposed to circumcision performed the operation on only twenty percent of their male patients, those who felt the decision was up to the parents circumcised fifty percent of their male patients, while those doctors who believed circumcision was necessary managed to convince one hundred percent of their parents." [49]

Circumcision – The Painful Dilemma

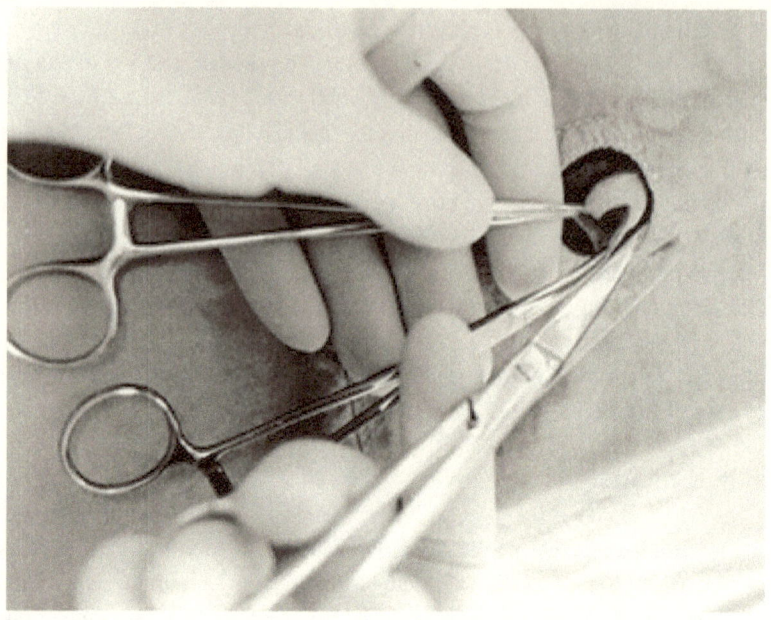

1. The dorsal slit. © Suzanne Arms

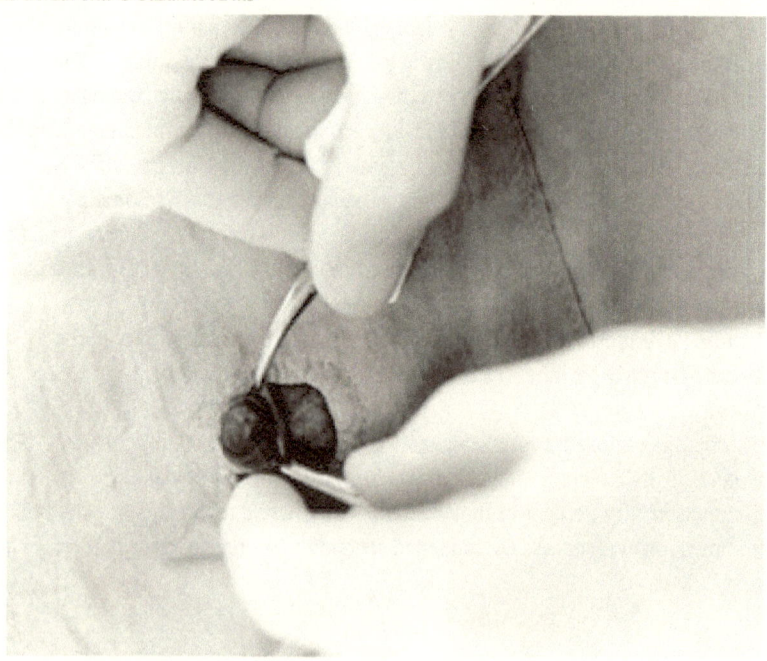

2. Foreskin retracted, glans exposed. © Suzanne Arms

5 – Infant Male Circumcision As a Medical Practice In 20th/21st Century USA

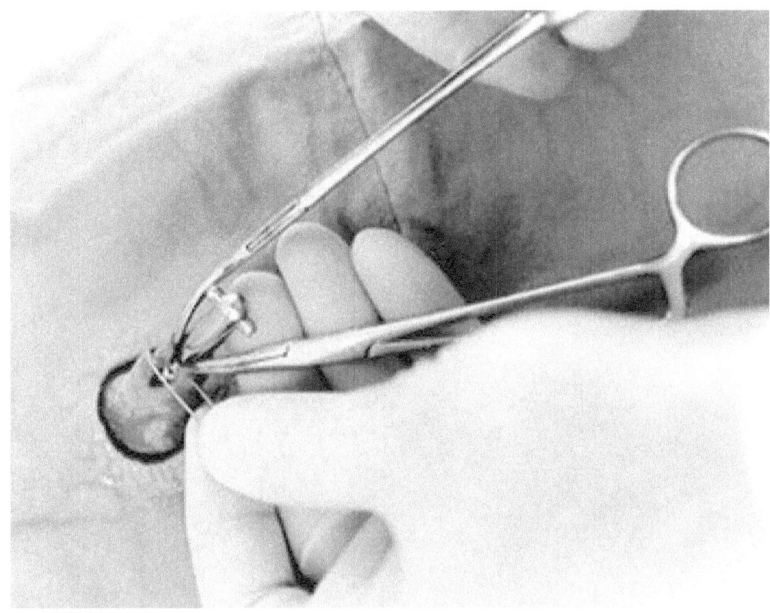

3. The "bell" inserted © Suzanne Arms

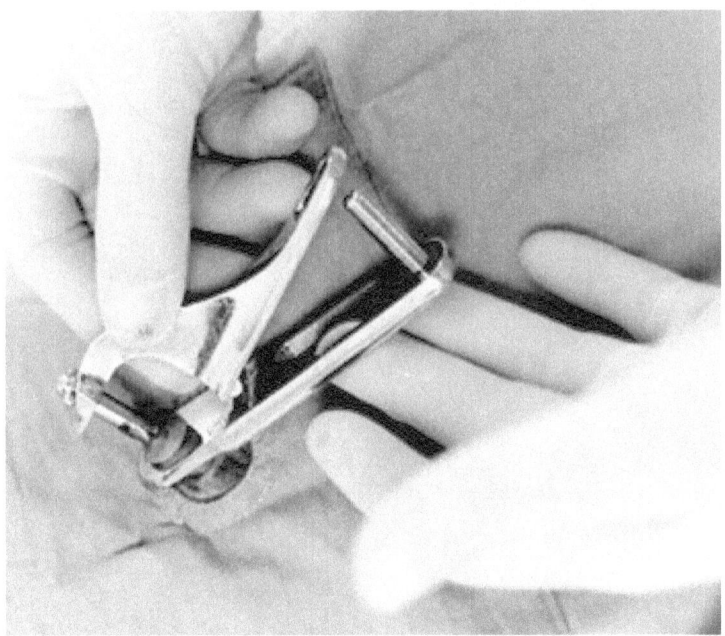

4. The clamp applied. © Suzanne Arms

Circumcision – The Painful Dilemma

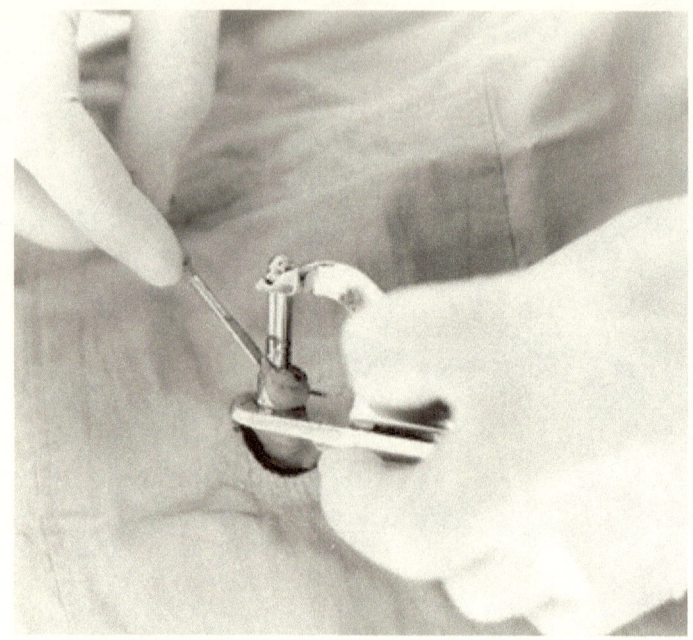

5. The foreskin sliced off. © Suzanne Arms

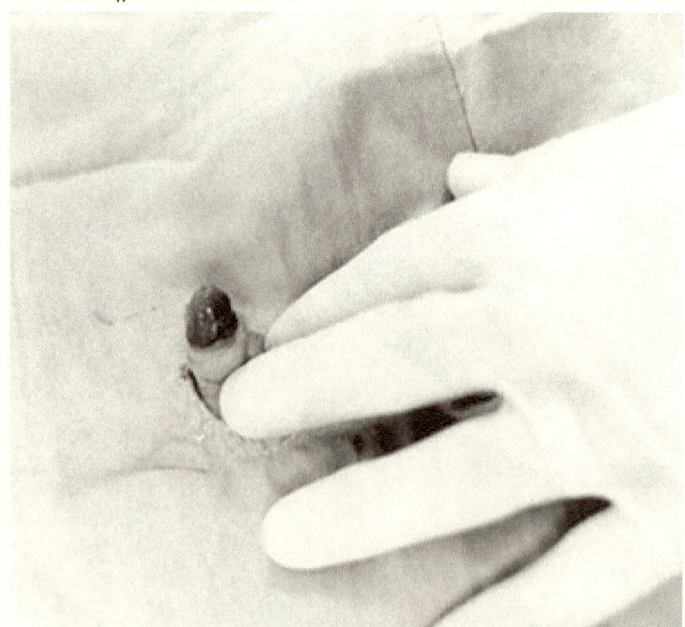

6. The freshly circumcised infant penis. The newly exposed glans is bright red. © Suzanne Arms

5 – Infant Male Circumcision As a Medical Practice In 20th/21st Century USA

She adds, "Two thirds of the mothers I interviewed said they would not have had their sons circumcised, if their doctor had advised against it. So please, at least give it a try." [49]

Doctors must become open to the importance of the *human* factors involved in birth and health care. Too often the medical approach seems akin to that of auto mechanics working on engines of cars. There truly are many doctors who are warm, understanding human beings. It is the *structure* of the entire system, not the *individuals*, wherein the real problem lies.

Parents *must* take a position of responsibility about *every* type of medical procedure – surgery, medication, injection, heart monitoring, etc. – that may be done to themselves or their babies. They must become informed about the matter, and if the procedure in question is not beneficial they should refuse it. For the medical world is not a sacred institution with unbreakable taboos and rituals. It is supposed to be a

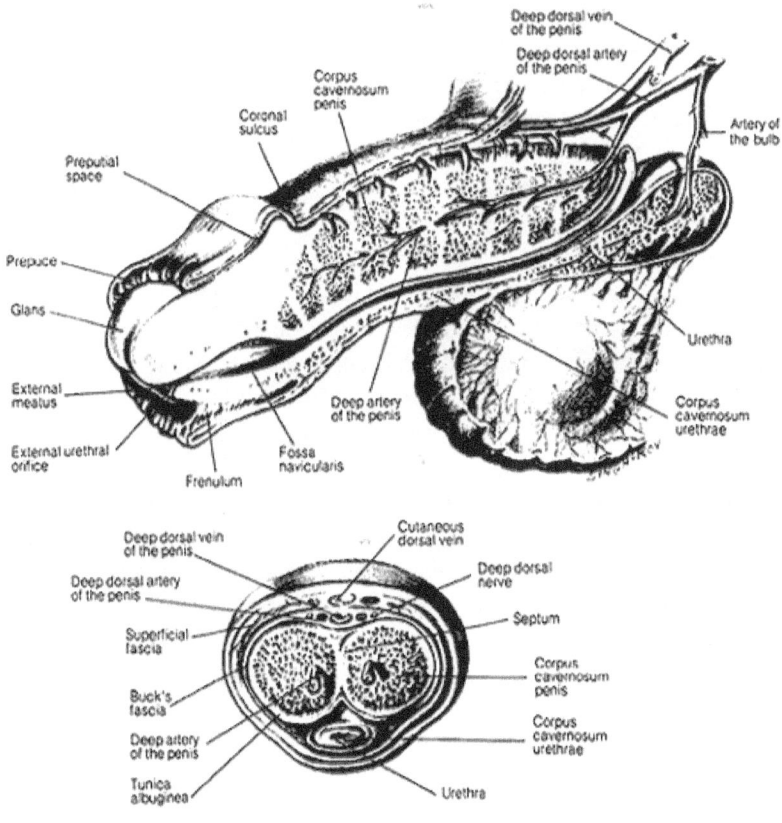

© *Patient Care 1978-03-15: 84-5.*

service to the public. New medical practices are constantly introduced, tried out for some time, and then, more frequently than not abandoned when found inadvisable. Unfortunately this is usually at the pain and expense of the consumer. Therefore it is *extremely dangerous* to one's health and well-being to passively, unquestioningly accept whatever medical practices are currently in vogue.

5.12 Interview with Dr. Howard Marchbanks, M.D.

Dr. Marchbanks is a natural childbirth oriented doctor. He has delivered thousands of babies at home. At the time of this interview he was practicing in a birth center in Orange County, California. He passed away in 1995 at age 75.

Dr. Marchbanks: I have had so much experience doing circumcisions that I consider myself an expert. I have circumcised almost all of the baby boys that I have delivered until the last few years. Since 1976 I have begun to question it. I discovered that some people were having their babies circumcised because they thought it was the law! So I started explaining to people that there's no law that says you have to be delivered by a doctor, and there's no law that says the baby has to be circumcised. My feeling is that it is a traumatic experience and I am opposed to traumatizing the baby. I'm also opposed to inflicting an operation on an individual without his permission.

Rosemary: Yet you've done this so many times.

M: Yes, and I continue to do it. I tried to stop by pricing myself out of the market. I raised the price from $35 to $125. The parents objected. They still said, "I want my baby circumcised!" So I said, "All right, I will circumcise him, but it takes $125 to salve my conscience."

(Author's note: This interview took place in 1977, thus it reflects the appropriate prices of that time.)

R: Often insurance pays for it so the cost doesn't matter. What do you tell parents about circumcision?

M: I try to explain to them that it is not something that has to be done. I feel that if you want to have little boys circumcised, then we should circumcise little girls too. They have foreskins!

I know that the circumcisions that I have done, without exception, have been painful for the baby. In medical school I was taught that the baby's nervous system is not developed sufficiently to be aware of the pain of circumcision. But my experience in doing it and observing the baby's reactions tells me otherwise. My feelings became more concrete when I talked to Dr. Leboyer and saw his birth film. It seemed so incongruous to have a non-violent birth and then immediately do violence to the baby by circumcising him. Anyone who has a foregone conclusion that it was not painful for the baby and therefore one should not hesitate to do it only has to listen to the baby while it is being done!

R: What method of circumcision do you use?

M: I have used the Gomco clamp. For the past ten years I have been using the Plastibell. You have to stretch the foreskin and break the adhesions between the foreskin and the head of the penis. You make a dorsal slit. With the Plastibell you slip the little bell inside and tie a string around it. The tying of the string is extremely painful! This method is probably more painful than the other methods because it stays on for several days. It is also possible to get a mild infection around the area where the string is. But I believe it is much safer as far as hemorrhage is concerned. About one in fifty to one in seventy-five babies will hemorrhage following circumcision by the Gomco clamp. That is because it just depends on the tissue cement. The edges are cut and you put a piece of Vaseline gauze around it. The only thing that's holding it together is the faith and hope that those little tissues will hold.

R: Why do they sometimes have to take stitches?

M: Maybe the baby had an erection. That could cause it to come apart. If it pulls apart then the doctor would have to sew those two edges together.

R: Do you use any kind of anesthesia for it?

M: No. Since it is a *circum*cision, a circular thing, in order to anesthetize the penis you would have to inject novocaine or xylocaine into the foreskin all around the penis. This would be more traumatic than just doing the cutting.

R: What about a topical anesthetic to numb it?

M: But the most painful part of circumcision is when you break the adhesions to free the foreskin from the head of the penis. There isn't any way to anesthetize that. You can't spray it down in there. What I prefer is to let the baby nurse while the circumcision is being done.

R: How do you go about that?

M: It's very difficult. You have to have the mother hold the baby's legs and bend over and get her boob in the baby's mouth. The mother is crying and the baby is crying. It doesn't work out too well.

R: If a boy or man needs to be circumcised he is given anesthesia for the operation. Why can't they give babies this consideration?

M: Because they're not big enough to complain about it or do anything about it. If they had to be anesthetized the doctor would certainly think twice about doing it. It's a very inhumane thing to do without an anesthetic. But it only takes a few minutes. They heal quickly. There's no way to know whether they remember it or not.

R: What do you think about waiting until the child is older so that it can be done under an anesthesia?

M: I feel that you should wait until the child has an awareness and you can explain it to him – maybe when he is twelve years old. This is another concern. If an individual has never been circumcised, when he gets older, if he doesn't like it he can always choose to be circumcised. But the person who has been circumcised in infancy, if he decides when he is older that he doesn't want to be circumcised … it's too late. There's no way of putting it back on.

I have nothing against circumcision, but I think the individual should have a say in the decision.

5.13   Interview with Paula Coleman, R.N., Camarillo, CA

Mrs. Coleman worked as an obstetrical nurse for five years prior to the birth of her first child. She now teaches classes for the American Academy of Husband-Coached Childbirth (Bradley Method). She and her husband, Bernie, have two daughters, Shelly (Rachel) and Becky (Rebecca). Their second child was born at home.

Paula: In the hospital where I worked circumcisions took place in the nursery on the first, second, or third day of the baby's life. The babies were put on a "circi" board in which their arms and legs were restrained with little Velcro strips. The baby was awake, not anesthetized. We'd put a sterile drape over his body exposing only the penis which we would spray with Merthiolate. The doctor would pick up the foreskin with a little "mosquito" hemostat and clamp down at the "12 o'clock" position. The hemostat has little teeth-like grooves which clamp down completely and smash the foreskin. The doctor leaves that on for about one or two minutes. When he takes it off the skin is flattened out and he snips it with scissors. It bleeds very little because all the blood has been smashed out of the foreskin. In my experience, the Gomco clamp was always used. It has a base. It has a part that screws down. There's the bell that covers and protects the glans. The base has a ring on it and you pull the baby's skin between that and the bell. Then the top part helps tighten up the bell against the hole in the base by screwing it down. The Gomco clamp comes in different sizes for different sized babies. There's a very small size that is used for tiny, premature babies.

Rosemary: I didn't know they would circumcise a preemie.

P: Sure, they can circumcise a preemie. They don't do it until he's out of trouble. Usually when babies reach 5 pounds they can go home and 5 pounds is still very tiny.

5 – Infant Male Circumcision As a Medical Practice In 20th/21st Century USA

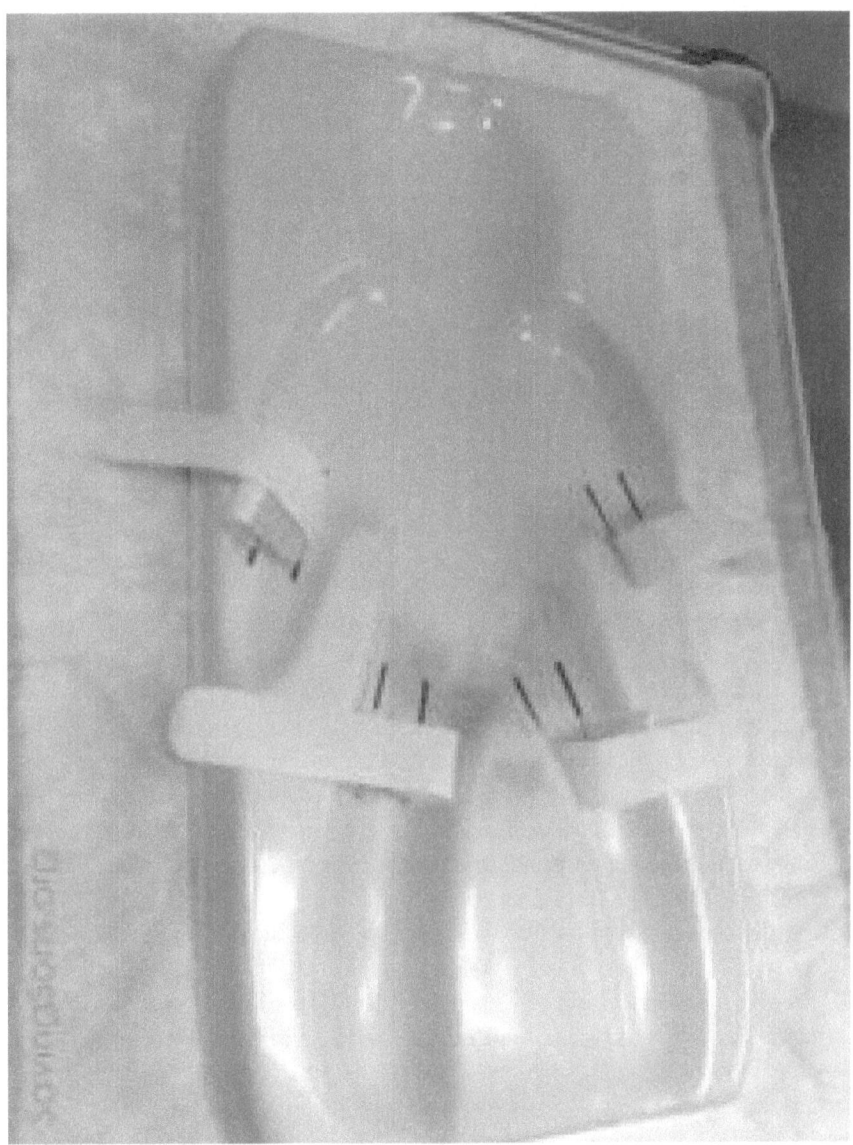

Stained Circumstraint, by permission from DrMomma.org / SavingSons.org

Back to the procedure, they tighten the screw of the clamp so that the foreskin between the base and the bell is completely smashed and clamped off all the way around. The doctor waits about five minutes and then takes a scalpel around where the foreskin is up on the Gomco clamp and cuts it off. Then he unscrews

Circumcision – The Painful Dilemma

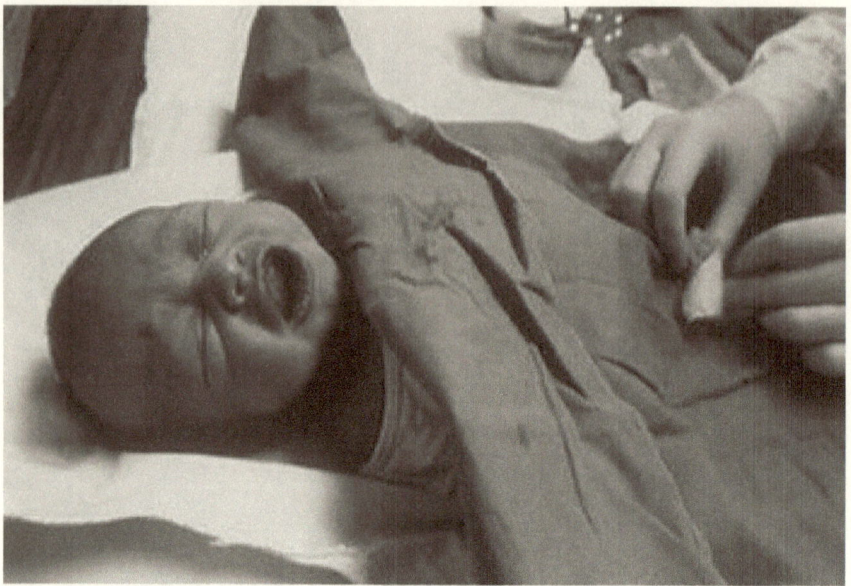

Reprinted with permission from the Saturday Evening Post Company 1981

the clamp and releases it. There's usually not any bleeding at all. It makes for a neat, even circumcision.

R: What have been your observations about the babies being traumatized?

P: Some babies appear to be traumatized the minute you put them on the board. You strap their legs and arms down and they start crying and complaining. There are some babies that don't cry until the doctor actually starts doing the circumcision. And some babies don't cry at all.

Now I've only seen the Plastibell procedure a few times. They still have to slit the foreskin to make room to get the bell on. Then this plastic, bell-shaped gadget fits over the glans. Instead of a clamp they tie a piece of string around the bottom of the bell. There's a little handle on the end of the bell that they use to place it on. They break this off and the baby goes home with this plastic ring in place over his penis. *[Also, some of the foreskin in front of the ring is trimmed away – R.R.]* It's a matter of waiting for the foreskin to atrophy and drop off. If a baby has an extra finger or toe they tie it off with a piece of string and it will go gangrenous and drop off. The Plastibell is based on the same idea. With the Plastibell there's no problem of bleeding, while with the Gomco clamp occasionally a circumcision will bleed. Sometimes too much of the foreskin gets pulled through and taken off so that the cut area is down on the shaft of the penis. That can result in a lot of

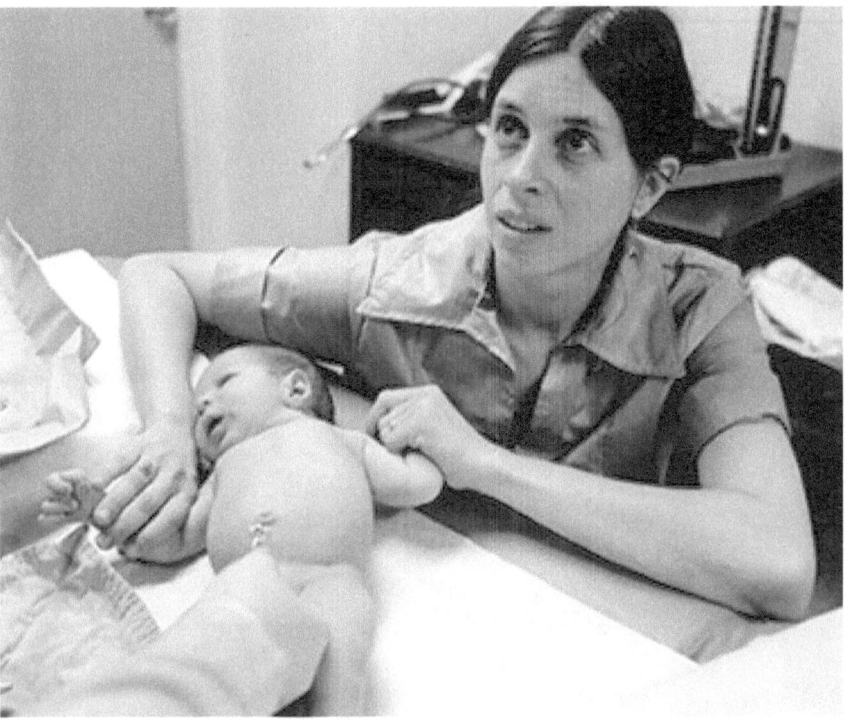

© *Suzanne Arms*

bleeding. Sometimes they either put a silver nitrate stick to it, or cauterize it, or put a hemostatic gel foam on it.

R: Have you seen any bad complications from circumcisions?

P: I've seen some that have bled quite a bit. These have been ones that were done far down on the shaft of the penis or on the rim where the glans meets the shaft. Some doctors take off more skin than others. I've heard of cases that have gone to court because the tip of the baby's glans got cut off. The bell is supposed to protect the glans from being injured. Possibly the bell and base don't fit properly. If several Gomco clamps were washed and sterilized and then the right bell doesn't get back with the right clamp then the bell doesn't fit into the hole. That wouldn't be the doctor's fault. That would be the fault of whoever was working in central supply and washing up the instruments.

R: What are some other methods of doing circumcisions?

P: One of the older methods is to take the foreskin and stretch it up over the glans and clamp a hemostat down on it and then wait for about five minutes and then cut along that line where the skin has been smashed. Then they would pull the

Circumcision – The Painful Dilemma

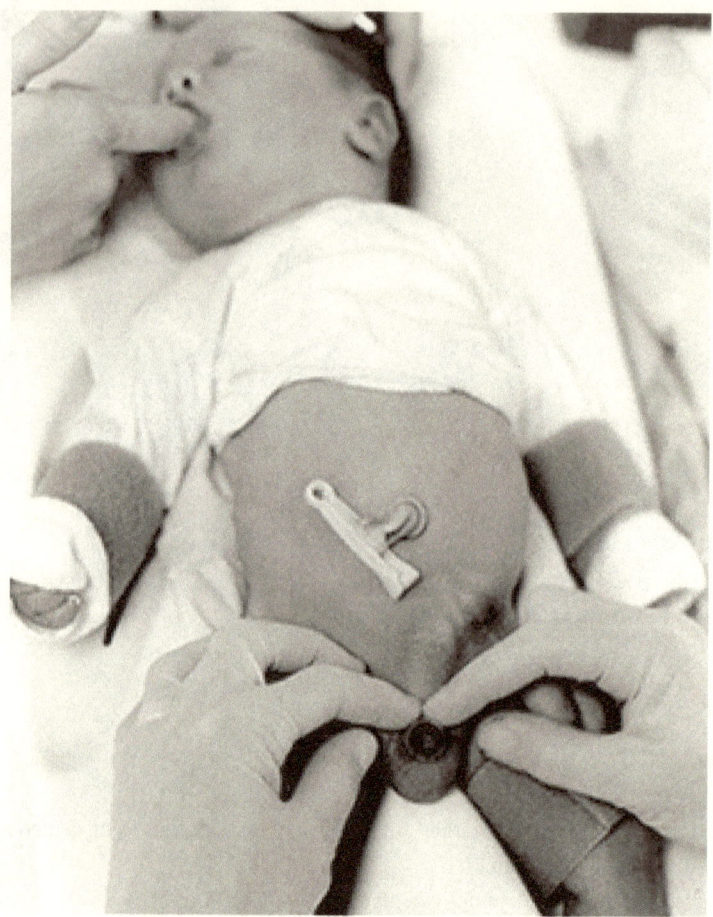

© *Suzanne Arms*

    remainder of the foreskin back under the glans and sometimes suture underneath to hold it back.
- **R:** How traumatizing do you think circumcision is to the baby?
- **P:** Most of the babies that I've seen cry for the first five to ten minutes. They cry more if you just put them back in their beds. If you take them out to the mother, it seemed that they cried less. I used to always take the babies out to the mothers regardless of what time it was. If it was visiting hours I'd have the mother come into the nursery. Usually the babies were circumcised before feeding times. It's a good idea for his stomach to be empty before the operation so that he won't

vomit. Usually the doctors would come in in the mornings and do them around discharge time. The operation usually only takes about 10 minutes.

R: Would they tell the parents when the circumcision was going to be done?

P: They didn't make a point of telling the mother exactly when they were going to do it. We'd tell the mother in the delivery room that they would do the circumcision before the baby went home. Of course they knew after we brought the baby out to them and explained that the baby was circumcised. The doctors just did it, charted it, and left. They left it up to the nurses to tell the mothers.

R: Did the hospital where you worked have rooming in so that the mothers were changing diapers?

P: We had both rooming in and regular schedules. When a baby was circumcised, even with rooming in, we'd check every ten minutes for the first hour to make sure that there was no bleeding.

R: Circumcision and other routine hospital procedures have become a big concern when parents want to have a Leboyer birth and have everything be right for the baby.

P: It doesn't make much sense, does it?! I've heard doctors mention that. Parents are so concerned about silver nitrate burning the baby's eyes or a vitamin K shot being uncomfortable and then they turn around and circumcise the baby!

R: Parents have been kept ignorant about circumcision. They are rarely able to make an informed decision about it. What is the rationale for not using any medication when circumcising a newborn?

P: The old theory was that babies didn't feel very much pain. Also it's not good to give anesthesia to a newborn who may have already gotten some during labor and delivery.

R: I think that the trauma is more than just pain. It's the trauma of being strapped down and worked over.

P: It's scary. It's an emotional thing.

R: What reasons did the doctors you worked with usually give for circumcision?

P: Most of the doctors have said it really doesn't matter. It's a matter of personal preference on the part of the parents. The older reasons were out of cleanliness.

R: Did almost all parents have it done?

P: Mexican-American parents almost never chose it. Among the *"white"* parents, approximately 75% chose circumcision. I think that rate is lower today because people are becoming aware of the fact that it is a trauma for the baby. We are seeing fewer parents choosing circumcision.

R: What can you tell me about caring for the infant's foreskin?

P: If the baby isn't circumcised it's important to know that they're not going to be able to retract the foreskin during the first year *[or often longer – R.R.]* One doctor where I worked insisted, for every baby under his care that wasn't circumcised, from birth on he instructed the parents to retract and loosen the foreskin every day ... Now talk about *trauma!!* That was more traumatic for the baby than a circumcision!! And you have to do that every day! The foreskin is very tight on a newborn and the opening is just a tiny little hole! When that baby got his foreskin pulled back he howled! Sometimes it took more than just five minutes to work on it and get it to go back!

R: Parents and doctors have to learn to leave it alone.

P: Back to circumcisions ... mothers are always so sensitive to their babies' cries that when you have a situation like that happening mothers will get very, very upset. We used to have mothers who would come and look through the examining room window. We didn't tell them to come look, but sometimes they would see it because it was right there across from the postpartum rooms. Sometimes I saw very scared looks on their faces.

R: There are a lot of couples in which the father wants it done, probably because he thinks his son should match him, but the mother doesn't want it done. It can cause real conflicts.

P: I am glad that we had girls. I'm certain that we would have had that conflict too.

R: If you ever have a boy would you have him circumcised?

P: That's a bridge that we never crossed.

R: Did you talk it over?

P: Sort of. Since he was, he thought it would be a good idea if our boy would be also. I think if he ever saw one done it might change his mind. He just figures "Well, I don't remember anything! I had it done when I was a baby and it didn't hurt me any!"

R: They are finding now that people do have these subconscious memories about early traumas.

P: I think the worst trauma would be to circumcise the baby in the delivery room. That used to be pretty common. They figured they could get it over with all at once. It's convenient and they're in a sterile room. But the child has just had so much trauma from just being born. His circulatory system is changing and his lungs have to start working. Do you have to do a number on the kid's penis too?!! Welcome to the world!! What a welcoming committee!! Doctors really seem cruel-hearted sometimes.

R: I'm sure doctors and nurses see so many things that are much worse than circumcision. They see people that are dying or have been mangled up in accidents.

P: Sometimes when you get into your everyday work at a hospital you don't look upon anything as traumatic. You see so much that you get calloused to it all. You forget that patients are not exposed to hospital routine every day the way we are.

R: So when you saw babies being circumcised you sometimes would tune it out and not think about it?

P: Well I still used to feel sorry for them when they cried. There ain't nothin' like a baby's cry to turn your heart over! I used to pacify them with a nipple or pat their heads or stroke them. Some of them would respond by calming down, but with some there was nothing you could do but take them out to the mothers and let them nurse. One thing I never did was to turn the babies on their stomachs after being circumcised. I always laid them on one side. I always thought, boy I'd sure hate to lie on that!!

But you do get into a rut when you work in a hospital, especially if there's a lot of hurriedness. You get so busy with the whole darn system trying to get it to work. You get new babies being admitted to the nursery and discharges and feedings and keeping recordings and chartings of everything. It can be very hectic. Sometimes you just don't have time.

5.14 Interview with Nancy & Frank Ring (young parents)

Nancy and Frank are the parents of Joshua, Jason, and Gabriel, who were all born at home and subsequently circumcised in doctors' offices. Nancy is an instructor for the Association for Childbirth at Home, International. Nancy was present at my first home birth when my third son was born. The Rings lived in Thousand Oaks, California at the time of this interview.

Rosemary: What motivated you to have your babies at home?

Frank: I guess we both figured "Why not?" We'd both seen a lot of animals giving birth without difficulty. We were in tune with each other. We thought it would be nice if we were at home, quiet and still, just to lie down and have the baby. We were living simply and raising a lot of our own food. When Nancy was in early pregnancy we went to the clinic of a nearby medical school. We got put through this big procedure, orientations and meetings, and different rooms for labor and delivery.

Nancy: You'd get a little credit card that you used.

R: You felt like you were being processed on an assembly line.

F: It was the opposite of the way we liked to live.

R: You had Joshua by yourselves, didn't you?

N: Yes. We had a good doctor but we didn't want him to deliver our baby. We were very naive! We had a long labor. It went really well. There were things we did wrong. I ended up hyperventilating. I got overwhelmed by pain. We just sort of endured it. I pushed very hard. The baby crowned and the next thing I knew he

Circumcision – The Painful Dilemma

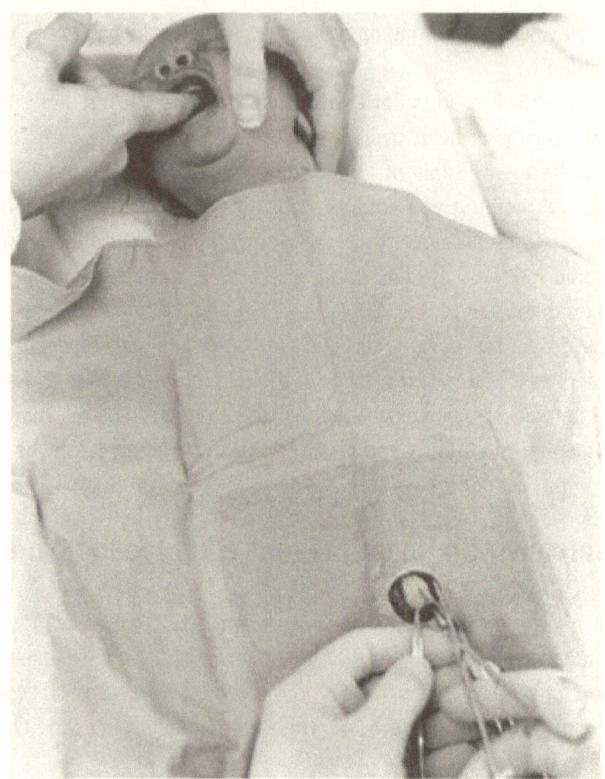

© *Suzanne Arms*

was out to his knees and Frank caught him! I tore very badly. But the baby was healthy with good coloring, beautiful, clean, eyes open and looking around. He nursed really well.

R: After Joshua was born you had him circumcised. How old was he when you took him to the doctor?

N: He was eight days old. The only guideline we had was the Bible. We didn't know when people ordinarily did it. That seemed just about right. It was the first time we'd taken him out. We asked the doctor "How necessary is this?"

F: He explained that he was not circumcised, nor were his sons. He asked us to think about it.

N: That was the first time we'd ever heard of anybody who wasn't circumcised. We hadn't given it much thought. It seemed like all boys should be. I don't think we even realized we had a choice in the matter.

5 – Infant Male Circumcision As a Medical Practice In 20th/21st Century USA

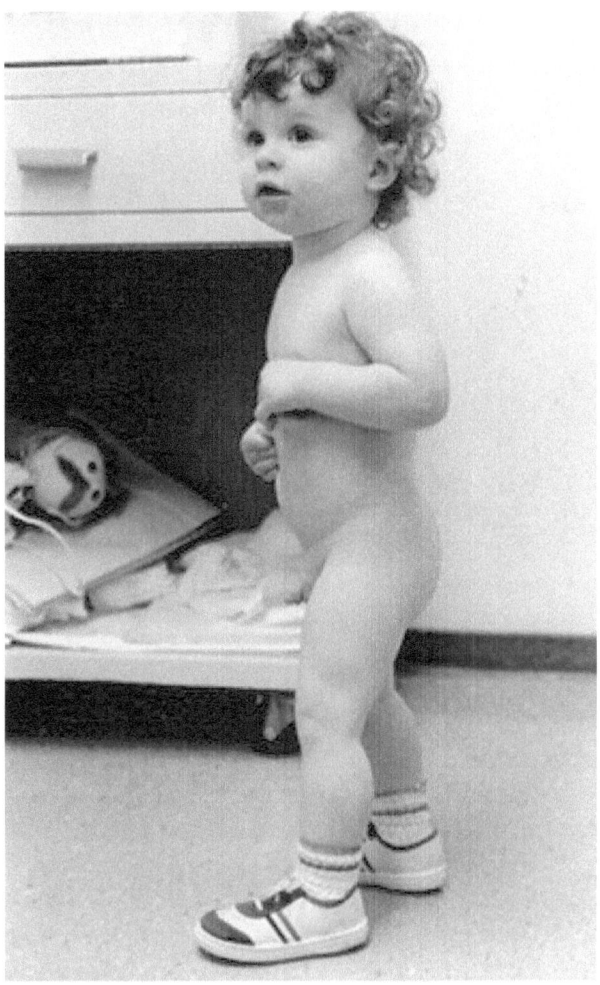

© *Suzanne Arms*

F: I thought about him growing up, his first encounter in junior high school, taking a shower with the other guys. I thought it might be a social stigma (not to be circumcised). It seemed to be a good healthy thing to do. It seemed to make sense the way it was described in the Bible. We went along with it. And it turned out to be extremely painful for the kids. It was hard for us. The doctor let me hold Josh and he took his time. He took a little metal round piece of doweling and went in and loosened the skin over the penis.

N: First he sprayed it with antiseptic.

Circumcision – The Painful Dilemma

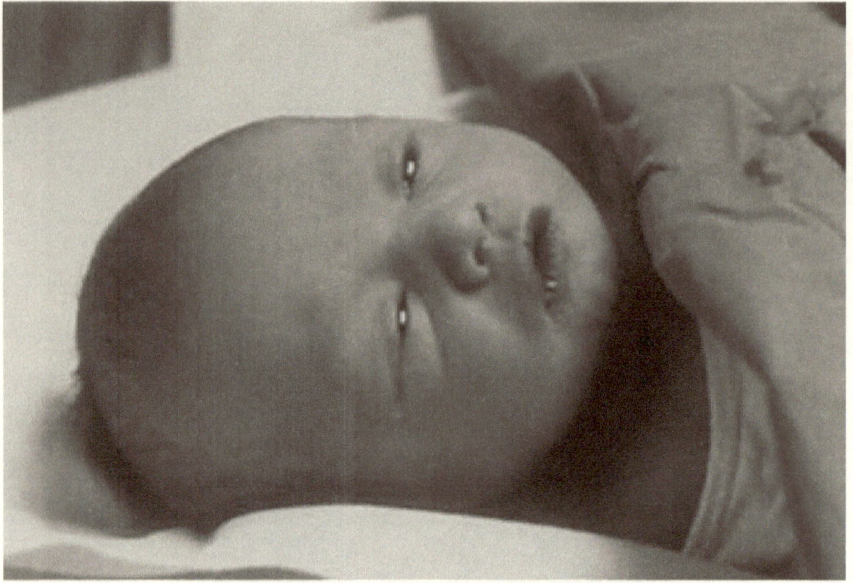

Reprinted with permission from the Saturday Evening Post Company 1981

F: And then he took a plastic cap and inserted it to protect the head of the penis, and cut off the skin.

R: How did the baby react to it?

F: He screamed. But after he was cut he stopped screaming. It seemed like that was pretty much it.

N: He covered it with gauze and petroleum jelly and handed him to me without diapering him. I nursed him right there. The gauze fell off with the first diaper change and we never heard a whimper from him. It did not seem to us to be that traumatic.

R: Then you had Jason a year and a half later. You had him at home but with a doctor.

N: Jason was born very quickly. He was a little bit distressed when he was born. He was sort of gray-blue, but he turned pink right away. The cord was wrapped once around his arm and once around his neck. But he was fine.

R: When did you have him circumcised?

N: I think it was the 12th day.

F: He used the string method instead. He took a plastic cap and a string and tied it. He said that in a few days it would all fall off.

N: And that method *was* traumatic and distressful for him! Any position that I put him in for the next two days, he screamed a very high-pitched "ouch!" He wouldn't move his legs or move around. You could tell that it really hurt him.

Again this time we had asked the doctor "Just how necessary is this?" He gave us an answer that we weren't totally satisfied with, but I think ... because we'd done it with Joshua, we figured we should do it with Jason too.

F: It seemed that what we had experienced with Josh hadn't been that traumatic. It seemed that we should have Jason circumcised also because they would always be taking baths together. I'd hate to have Josh, being the older one, use it against Jason, and make him feel that he was different.

R: Then two years later you had Gabriel at home with a midwife.

F: I thought it was the best birth experience of all. It was nice for me because she was there to take the responsibility of delivering the baby. I could just be with Nancy and enjoy it. Things happened fast. We all just sat there with the baby on Nancy's stomach. About a half hour after the birth the placenta was delivered.

R: It was a peaceful birth.

N: It was really casual. It was two o'clock in the afternoon. The weather was nice. I felt fine. I put Gabriel to the breast about ten minutes after he was born and he nursed for an hour. He was very alert.

F: By six o'clock that night we had all our friends and folks over for a barbecue and to see our new baby.

R: Did it seem that you should have your third son circumcised? How much did you think about it?

N: I knew that it wasn't necessary. I had bad feelings because of the experience with Jason. I didn't know which way to go so I left the decision up to Frank. Our pediatrician had retired so we had to find a new doctor to do the job. We found a man and we talked to him about it. We didn't have bad feelings about him, but we didn't have good feelings about him either. I remember the morning when we took him in, I felt like this wasn't right. He was 14 days old. I was really nervous about it. The other two times it had seemed right. But this time I felt like the only reason we were doing it was because the other two were. At the time I felt that I was the one who wouldn't be able to deal with it.

R: You mean if Gabriel had not been circumcised?

N: Yes. I didn't feel that I had the strength at that point. I still felt that there was something basically unclean about an uncircumcised male. The only way I can explain it was that I didn't feel brave enough not to circumcise.

R: Even though you could have your babies at home?

N: I felt wrong about it because it was my hang-up and not the baby's. It was for social reasons, and I knew those weren't strong enough for the way that we live our lives. The only thing that tipped the scales was that the other boys were and we didn't feel that Gabriel should be different. So we went to the doctor expecting that Frank would hold the baby again. But the doctor said, "Absolutely not!" He not only did not want Frank to hold the baby, he did not want us in the room!!

F: I told him I had held the other two boys and that I'd like to hold Gabriel too, and he just said, "No, this is the way I do it."

R: So you waited in the waiting room while he operated on him?

N: Yes. That's not like us to accept something like that being done to our child and then have us excluded.

F: I didn't know what to think. Gabriel was in there and was laid on the table and the doctor was ready to do it and ... I didn't have enough time to make a decision. He had a problem with Gabriel bleeding. The doctor had to cauterize him. He had to burn him to stop the bleeding. The baby screamed for about 30 minutes!!

N: In the waiting room we could hear the baby screaming far more traumatically than the other boys had! After about 40 minutes the doctor came out and explained that there was one spot that would not stop bleeding. He said this was normal, a lot of babies hemorrhage. We weren't aware that there could be complications. The doctor had to get a cauterizing iron and cauterize one spot. By this time there was no doubt in our minds that this was wrong ... knowing that it wasn't necessary in the first place ... especially since he had not, from the very moment of his birth, ever experienced any kind of trauma. We totally meet our babies' needs, we don't put them on schedules or anything.

R: You said that you were crying by this time?

N: I was crying! Frank was swearing! All we wanted was to get the baby and run!! The doctor cauterized it. He stitched it. He put this black, tarry substance over the head of the penis.

F: It looked like the end of a cigar.

N: It was really swollen. We couldn't even see what he had done because of all the black stuff that was on it. It must have been just torture for him. By this time my whole being was pushing into the room! I couldn't stay out any longer. And all they were concerned about was scrubbing him up. He had been screaming for 45 minutes. They wanted to get a diaper on him. They wanted to wash the blanket. They were being all cheery and happy like this was all quite normal. I was so upset that I took him in the bloody blanket and went out to the car to nurse him.

The doctor didn't even come out and talk to us! He didn't explain how to take care of it. He left the responsibility to his nurses and receptionist which just infuriated us! We paid them. They wanted us to bring him in in a few days but there was no way we were going to bring him back. We didn't know the extent of the damage that he had done. I made an appointment with another doctor as soon as I got home. I felt that the doctor had done something terribly wrong.

The day that Gabriel had been circumcised I didn't diaper him all day. He constantly cried and sniffled and went back to sleep and would wake up crying and sniffling ... this went on all day. I left the kids at the sitter's and I held Gabriel the whole day. I couldn't move him. I felt horrible. I felt like I had just killed him!! I can't explain the guilt that I felt! It was the most traumatic experience that I'd ever been through with my children. I was angry. I hurt all over for my baby! I knew that either I wouldn't have any more children because if I had another boy I'd die. Or if I did have another boy I would definitely not have him circumcised!

R: Did Gabriel heal right away?

N: It took him longer to heal. It was a week before it looked fairly normal. I took him to another doctor three days later. He didn't understand why the doctor had stitched it. He said it was a little bit infected. He cut the stitches out. He scrubbed it with Phiso-hex to get the rest of the black stuff off. Then he said, "It's okay and should heal fine."

R: It seems like Gabriel has been a good baby ever since. I'm sure the nursing and comforting you gave him made a lot of difference.

N: I honestly don't know how the trauma affected him. One of the reasons that we have chosen home birth was because it would be the least traumatic for the baby. It was important to us who caught the baby and how he was handled right after the birth. The way that babies are handled after birth in the hospital is very much wrong ... to have the baby separated from you, taken off to a nursery and weighed and measured and put in an incubator ... that's repugnant to us! So having all that be so important to us, we really wondered how the trauma of his circumcision would affect him. We just don't know.

R: So both of you have decided that if you should ever have another son you will definitely not have him circumcised.

N: Unless there was a true medical justification for it, I would definitely be against it.

F: I would be willing to take the time to deal with the problems that he might have with the other children, about not being circumcised and being different.

N: I think I would be able to explain to his brothers the reason why he was different. Just because his penis would look different from our other sons', I don't think it would bother me.

(Nancy and Frank have since had a fourth son, Seth, born in November 1979, three years after Gabriel's birth, He has been left intact.)

5.15 Letters from Parents of Circumcised Sons

Our son Kristopher Andrew was circumcised. It was something we debated about all through my pregnancy. We even hoped we'd have a girl so we wouldn't have to make the decision. Our doctor doesn't do them routinely. When Andy was born we still hadn't decided. I guess we basically figured we would not. When Andy was four days old my husband said he really felt he wanted their penises to look the same. He felt it was important for Andy's identification with him. I felt, not being male, maybe it was important for them. He is both of ours and even though I had decided it was not necessary, Rick had a say. Even if we would have decided before his birth, we would never have had it done when he was born. Birth is traumatic enough.

On the eighth day we met the doctor at the emergency room. We stayed with Andy the whole time. They strapped him down which I hated. I had asked if I could hold him! We massaged his head, stroked him, and talked to him the whole time. It seemed to only really hurt him a couple of times. He was more upset about being exposed and strapped down. My husband said it was the most awful thing he'd ever seen or done. It was gross! How and why did this barbaric custom have to start? As soon as it was finished I put Andy to the breast and he was fine. He seemed to have handled it really well.

My feelings now are, if we ever have a second boy, then all the males should look alike. But how do I know I'll stay with Rick and not be with a man who isn't circumcised?! Now that I think about it, identification was a lousy reason.

I guess we were trying to do what we thought was best for his entire life.

Paula and Richard Sloun, Trinidad, CA

◆

My husband and I decided to have a home birth. We read stacks of books about birth and babies but never found any information about circumcision. We asked my doctor and he said circumcision decreased the incidence of disease and infection later in life. I didn't believe him but didn't argue either. We questioned our male friends and found that almost all were circumcised. The few who weren't never had any complications. Everybody liked the way he was. We decided to go ahead with circumcision because we didn't want our son to be laughed at in the school locker room because he was different from the other boys.

Five days after Ben was born we took him to the doctor's office to be circumcised. My husband held the baby to the table while the doctor performed the operation. I found the screams unbearable and retreated to a chair in the waiting room. The

5 – Infant Male Circumcision As a Medical Practice In 20th/21st Century USA

doctor told my husband that at that age a baby's penis isn't that sensitive and he was screaming out of fright and not pain.

Immediately after Ben was bandaged and dressed, the nurse left the three of us alone so I could nurse him. Nursing was the only thing that would quiet his cries (and mine). We left the office with instructions to soak the bandage off in his bath the next day and bring him back in two weeks for a check-up.

When we took Ben in two weeks later we discovered he had an adhesion. His (remaining) foreskin had grown over the head of his penis. The doctor tried to pry the foreskin away with a metal instrument. One small section wouldn't come apart so he had to cut the skin. I nearly fainted from the sight and sound of my son screaming! The doctor told us the whole problem could have been avoided if I had retracted the foreskin every time I changed him. I didn't know this was necessary. Everything I had read about circumcision had said to leave it alone.

Within a few weeks my son's penis healed completely. There is still a scar to remind me of the incident. We realize now that we made the wrong decision and our reasoning was ridiculous. I feel even worse for putting Ben through it twice. Any other male children born to us will not be circumcised.

Maggie and David Seastrom, Morgantown, IN

♦

My fathers, brothers, nephews, and husband were all circumcised. As far as I knew, every man *had* to be circumcised. When I was in labor with my first baby they brought me the paper to sign to have it done and without a second thought I signed it. The baby was a girl. With my second baby the same thing happened. This baby was a boy. When he was born the doctor called it some name and then said he just didn't have enough skin to be circumcised.[50]

You cannot imagine all the things that went through my head! I thought he was deformed! I thought he wouldn't be able to have sex when he grew up. I asked, "Couldn't it be done later?" Everyone I knew must have felt the same way because they were feeling sorry for him. One guy told my husband it was terrible not having it done because the Bible said a man was unclean if he wasn't circumcised.[51]

On our first visit to the pediatrician the doctor took an instrument that looked like a crochet needle and pushed his foreskin back. He screamed and cried and it bled and looked horrible. The doctor also snipped the skin under his tongue because he was

---
[50] This condition of having a naturally short foreskin is known as aposthia. There has been speculation that circumcision may have originated in prehistoric times because some highly revered leader had this condition.
[51] The Bible says nothing about circumcision being important for cleanliness.

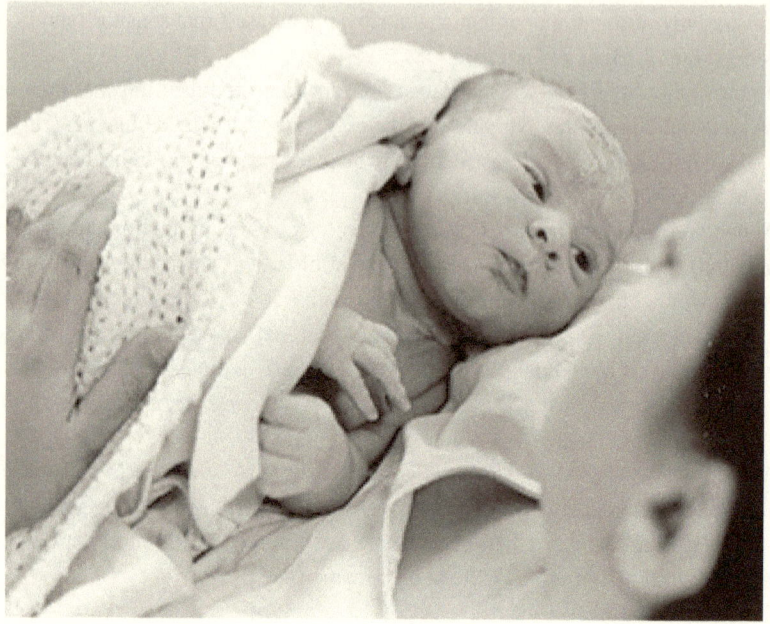
© Suzanne Arms

almost tongue tied. I wonder if that visit left a mark on my son which he will never get over!! The doctor said to be sure to keep the foreskin pushed back every day. I tried to do what the "good" doctor said to do. If I let it go for a day, the skin would try to heal back up and then I would have to break it loose again! My baby would cry every time I did this to him. He has just turned two and when I try to push it back he says "No! Hurts!" and cries until I quit! I don't do it as often now, but I'm still afraid that since the foreskin has been pushed back already, I may cause harm by not keeping it up.

I have since read some articles about circumcision and now my husband and I have decided against ever having it done. During the past four years my husband and I have been "getting back to nature." I am also a member of La Leche League. My oldest is four and she nursed through my second pregnancy and is still nursing along with the baby who just turned two. I want only the best for them. Now I believe circumcisions are unnatural and I will *never, never* have one of my sons circumcised nor let another doctor push the foreskin back unless it's absolutely necessary.

Carolyn Miller, Lakeland, FL

◆

While pregnant, my husband and I discussed circumcision quite often. We knew very little about it and wanted to do the best thing. There was no reference to circumcision in any of the books I read, save *Spiritual Midwifery* by the Tennessee Farm Midwives. They told their reasons for doing it. We respected the opinions of these folks so we decided to have our little boy circumcised.

The morning after he was born in the hospital, a nurse came in and asked me if I wanted him circumcised and if so to sign this piece of paper. Later that night when my obstetrician came to see me I asked him if they'd done it yet. I was going home in the morning and wanted to make sure everything was in order. He said no, but that he would do it before leaving after making rounds and then have Jacob brought to me.

About 20 minutes later I heard the nurse coming with my little bundle who was wailing louder than I'd ever heard him! She gave him to me and assured me that it was "only his feelings that were hurt." I tried to nurse him, to calm him, but he'd have no part of it. I still remember how the only way I could keep him from crying was to hold his head right up to my heart beat, very closely, and rock back and forth. I told him how very sorry I was that he'd been hurt like that, and that I thought it was for him I did it, and that no one would ever mess with him like that again. The sound of my voice seemed to ease his tense little body. I kept talking to him, rocking him, and holding him close to my heart. I felt very good that he was able to be with me right after instead of stashed back in the nursery where there wouldn't be anyone to love him and make him feel better. I never wanted the nurse to come back and take him away. I wanted to go home and be with my husband where the three of us could begin our life together and let our love for this new little one grow. That must have been the beginnings of my motherly feelings toward this small creature.

We did go home the next day. I've learned not to regret the decision I made. That only gets one in trouble. I wouldn't have this operation performed again should I ever have another boy and possibly wouldn't have with Jacob if there had been more information on the subject.

Emydee Hannon, Bowling Green, KY

♦

Willy was circumcised three days after birth. I stood outside the door while they were doing it to him and listened to him scream and cry. That's the first time I really began to wonder what the hell I had let them do to my baby. Since then I have asked myself that a million times. Everything was all right until he was one year old when he developed a cyst on his penis where he had been circumcised. The urologist said

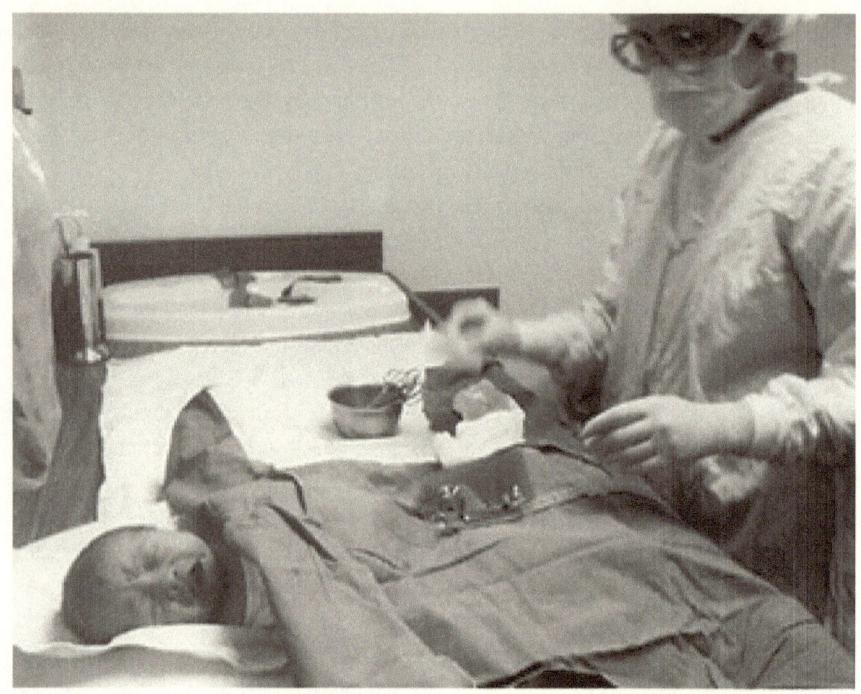

Reprinted with permission from the Saturday Evening Post Company © 1981

that the cyst[52] was caused by the circumcision. He also said that cysts such as this were quite common.

So Willy had to go to the hospital. At least they gave him anesthesia this time. What the doctor did was re-circumcise half the penis where the cyst was. I'm sorry I did it in the first place. I hope Willy has no more trouble because of it.

The strange thing about circumcision is that it's supposed to make things better. If Willy hadn't been circumcised, he wouldn't have had any trouble at all.

Jacque Dyer, Oakhurst, CA

◆

I have three children. Our first is a son whom I did have circumcised. Before his birth I had worked in a nursing home and saw problems the uncircumcised men had.[53] I decided that any of my boys would be circumcised to avoid these problems

---

52 Please see Chapter 11 "Complications of Circumcision" for discussion of this occurrence.

in later life. My husband (who is intact) only went along with me because of my insistence. I was very stubborn.

Our son was born in 1976. On the second day in the hospital the other three women in my room had their babies brought to them, but they did not bring mine. When I asked the nurse why, she said, "Oh, he was circumcised this morning." I was so upset. It was me who had requested it be done but I wanted to be with him. When I went up to the nursery to get him I was told he couldn't leave. He had to be under observation. I felt so bad for him, but I didn't think I could press them into giving me my baby.

For his first five months Derek cried almost continuously. During his first two years he was very dependent on me. His sleep and emotional patterns had no real pattern at all.

My next two babies, both girls, were very peaceful, happy, and content. Our second baby was born in a hospital, but we stayed only 12 hours and were only separated a short time. With our third we had a beautiful home birth. People tell me that my second and third babies were content because I was more experienced and because they were girls. I believe it was because they developed a sense of trust and security from the beginning, whereas Derek's first day of security was shattered by his second day of circumcision. It has taken him a long time to feel safe again.

No son of mine will ever again go through the torture of being tied down and having his body cut (and of course it hurts more than we can imagine!) and then being placed in a huge, noisy room in a plastic box for hours to be observed like someone in a cage. I realize now that when those men in the nursing home were circumcised they didn't go through half the agony that a tiny babe does.

Deana and Steve Ives, Fulton, NY

♦

My son Aaron was born in April 1976. His penis was so small that the doctor said he couldn't circumcise him at birth. He was a normal sized baby, but had a lot of fat around that area which prevented his penis from coming out like it normally does.

---

53 Elderly, senile individuals sometimes become unable to care for even their most basic personal needs. If and when this happens they usually have difficulties with *many* parts of their bodies. Still, the wisdom of routine amputative surgery to prevent eventual foreskin problems must be questioned. Similar arguments could be offered for permanent amputation of fingernails at birth to prevent lifelong need for cleaning and attending to one's fingernails, or routine amputation of toes to prevent lifelong need to clean out the dirt between one's toes. The "difficulty" lies in people's squeamishness about genitals that they rarely have for other body parts. A hospital attendant probably would have no difficulty cleaning the fingernails or brushing the teeth of a patient unable to do this, but may have qualms about similarly attending to the patient's genitals. – R.R.

Circumcision – The Painful Dilemma

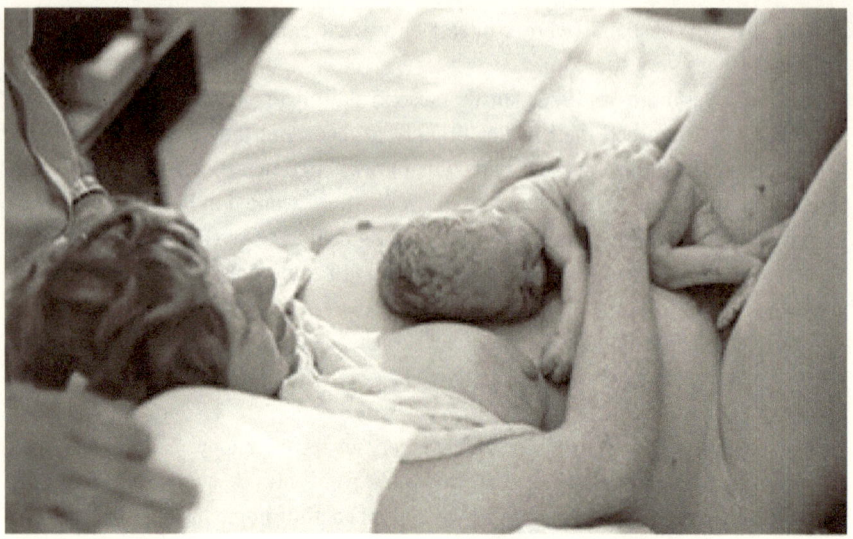

© *Suzanne Arms*

My husband is Jewish and I am not. I always thought circumcision was a necessary health advantage. Now I am sorry I ever had it done. If I have another son I do not want him circumcised.

Aaron was circumcised at age 2 months. I can still remember his chilling screams!! My husband had to hold me back. How could I ever have let them do that to my poor defenseless child?! Every mother tries to do her best for her child, and I thought I was doing the best thing. If I had thought more about it I would have realized it [the foreskin] was there for a reason. I don't think God intended for us to mutilate our children this way! I pray that Aaron will understand when he grows up that I didn't mean for him to be hurt.

Aaron was so small that the skin grew back over his penis. He had to be re-circumcised at age 4 months. This time they put him in the hospital and used anesthesia. I was a nervous wreck. I was nursing Aaron and he got comfort only from this.

Some of Aaron's skin has still grown to the penis. The doctors said to keep the skin pulled back 2 times a day and put petroleum jelly on it. I don't know if I'm doing the right thing. I grew up thinking the doctor's word was law, and am finding out most don't know half the time and guess the other half. I know several wonderful doctors who are trying their best to do right but they are few and far between.

I have talked to other people and they were as in the dark as I was before I had Aaron circumcised. We all just believed our doctors who said circumcision was right.

I hope more doctors and lay people start speaking out that this operation is unnecessary and inhumane!!

I just hope my realization is not too late for my son. I realize I have made a decision that should have been his when he is old enough to make it. The doctor did not make me aware of all the facts. I should have asked more questions. I think my doctor would have suggested I not circumcise him had he not known I wanted it done.

Sheila Soslow, Dallas, TX

♦

During pregnancy we had planned a home birth, but as labor began my doctor and midwife realized that my son was breech. Neither felt good about helping us at home, so after traveling to two hospitals (because the first would only perform a Caesarian for a breech baby) I delivered in the latter. I was advised to stay 24 hours after the birth. As I was preparing to leave the next morning a doctor came in and said my son hadn't urinated since birth and because his foreskin was long, he needed a circumcision. Earlier, when he was six hours old they had asked whether I would have the operation done and I said no. No mention was made at this time about anything being wrong with his penis. But now they said he needed it because he hadn't urinated and this was very dangerous.[54] So I said okay. I went to be with him, but was told I couldn't be there. I did hear him scream. After this the nurse who was there when my son was born came on duty. She told me he had urinated as he was being born. I am so sorry now for not knowing better.

Ann Conceicao, St. Petersburg, FL

♦

We had our first son cut because the doctor said it was "medically necessary" and so he wouldn't "look different." He used a Plastibell on him and got it on crooked and now the end of Matthew's penis is slightly deformed (so he "looks different!"). He stands in front of a tree to pee and misses the tree to the left. He has to stand slightly sideways to hit the tree.

We had our second son done because we were still ignorant. He was born in a labor bed 10 minutes after I crawled up on it. I picked him up, birthed the placenta, wrapped up the baby and came home. We weren't admitted to the hospital. We were

---

[54] During prenatal development a fetus regularly swallows amniotic fluid and urinates into it. If he were not able to do so he would not survive to term. Any medical person should know this.

never separated and the bonding was absolutely *beautiful*. Five days later I took him back for the PKU and circumcision. When I walked in carrying him and my purse I requested to get the papers signed and payments made before the procedure so I could just concentrate on the baby afterward. A nurse said, "Here, let me hold him for you while you sign the papers." So I gave him to her, and at that instant he looked at me, and *he knew* he was about to be sacrificed. He said with his eyes "Why are you betraying me? I trusted you ..." I turned back to sign the papers and write out a check and when I turned around to get him, the nurse was gone with him. At that moment I heard a blood-curdling scream and knew it was Michael getting cut. I dropped my purse and *ran* back to the delivery room (that's where they did it) and was fully prepared to kill whoever was hurting my baby. A male nurse stopped me at the door and told me to wait outside, that I was not allowed in during the surgery. I had tears running down my face, listening to the screams of someone who was being murdered coming from the delivery room. The nurse escorted me outside the hospital where I sobbed and sobbed until it was over. Then they brought Michael to me. His little face and eyes were red and closed to the world. The doctor said, 'See, that didn't hurt ... he's asleep.'

When we got home, Michael "woke up" and looked at me with pain and betrayal in his face. He forgave me when he nursed, but I have never forgiven myself.

Julie Butler, Lewis, KS

(Julie has since given birth to another son, Joseph, who was born at home in December 1980 and has been left intact. She has provided the following update:)

I am convinced that baby boys' penises are not completely developed at birth. Joey's penis was so tiny when he was born, and now that he is 9 months old it has grown much bigger. If we had him circumcised after birth I think it would have been traumatic not only for the usual reasons, but also because he wouldn't have had much to work with. Also, the surgeon might have cut too much off so he would have had trouble as he grew. That is what I am afraid has happened to our oldest boy. He is almost 9 years old and there is so little skin on the penile shaft that as it grows it is pulling the glans downward and to the left.

Joey's foreskin does not retract yet at 9 months but I don't expect it to. We've had no problems whatsoever with it. It stays clean and the hole in the end gets bigger as he grows. If only I'd known – famous last words!

◆

I have three sons who have all been circumcised. With our first son, Ian, circumcision was the only way to go. He was two days old and everything was fine.

With our second son, Joshua, the minute he was born the doctor asked me if I wanted him circumcised. I said yes, and he circumcised him right there! I didn't realize he was going to do it right then! I was upset about the fact that it was done so soon after birth, but it was done before I had a chance to say anything.

When they brought him to me I noticed that his penis looked a mess! It looked like they cut too much of the foreskin off. As he got older the skin loosened up but it was still tight just under the penis. The doctor kept saying it was fine until he was a year old and he said it did look kind of tight. The doctor also said that if his penis bent pointing down when he had an erection then they would have to operate. Can you imagine that?!

When he was eighteen months old I took him back to the doctor, still concerned. He had erections but not real strong. The penis did not bend at all, so there was no need to operate. I am still concerned but I think he will be all right.

With my third pregnancy I was hoping it would be a girl and I wouldn't have to worry about circumcision. Well, it was a boy, and there was the question ... should I or shouldn't I? My sons are close in age and I was afraid he might feel different from his brothers if he weren't circumcised, so I had it done. I made sure to let the doctor know about Joshua's problems. Nathan was one day old and the circumcision was fine but it was very painful for him.

If I had a chance to start all over again I wouldn't have had any of them circumcised. If I ever have another son he will *not* be circumcised. I don't think I could stand to have him go through the ordeal my other sons went through.

I chose circumcision because I felt it would be easier to keep clean and avoid infection. Also, at the time, as a typical American woman I thought an uncircumcised penis was funny looking. My husband Larry was circumcised and preferred that our sons be circumcised. However, he is very flexible and would agree not to have any more of our sons circumcised.

If I have any more children they will be home births. When I gave birth in the hospital they stressed circumcision so I went right along with it. If I had been given a chance to see both sides I could have made a decision with my eyes open.

Linda Pellegrin, Sylmar, CA

♦

When my first son was born in October of 1980 I was apprehensive about circumcision. I sought advice from my obstetrician, my family-practitioner, and my family.

Circumcision – The Painful Dilemma

Though no one was insistent about its necessity, no one advised against having it done. My family doctor admitted it was not a medical necessity but thought it should be performed so that the boy would "be like his father." My in-laws said that it should be done for medical reasons (?) and for cleanliness. I was hesitant but gave in to the opinions of others.

Whether I did something wrong or the surgeon did something incompletely I do not know. My little boy's foreskin became adhered to the rest of his penis and healed up thoroughly. My family doctor and I discussed the situation and he advised me that when Curt was about two years old he would need surgery again. He said that it was now worse than if he had never been circumcised.

In June of 1982 the doctor decided it was time to take care of the foreskin adhesion. My sister accompanied us and the doctor instructed my sister and me to each pin down one of Curt's arms and legs. He then – *using no anesthesia* – tore the foreskin from all around the glans. It was minutes of horror!! Perhaps it was worse than his original circumcision, for now he could recognize exactly what was happening. Here were three adults, two of them close love-figures, restraining him and putting him through this agony!! He screamed, "Mamma, Daddy, Lola ... I'm sorry, I'm sorry ... Mamma ..." over and over again. My poor baby, sorry for what!? I was the

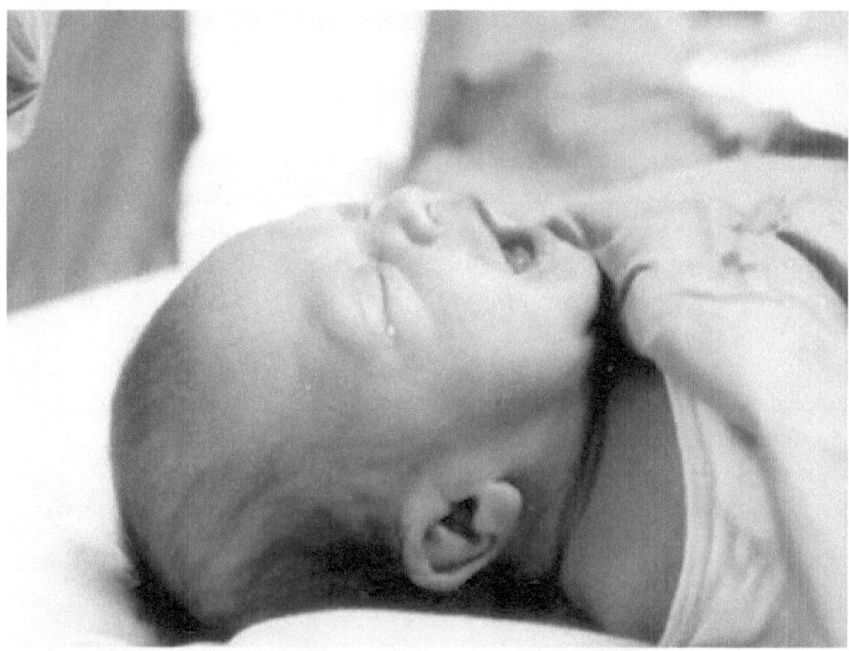

Reprinted with permission from the Saturday Evening Post Company © 1981

one to be sorry. I cannot express how I feel that I put my precious baby through that torture.

After the doctor was done with Curt he had us put ointment on the wound until it healed. This took two adults just to pin him down again to get the ointment on. For weeks after this ordeal Curt wouldn't allow anyone near his penis.

When our second son Alex was born in July of 1982 my husband and I decided to forego a circumcision. I considered that this boy would not "be like his father" or his older brother. I think I will be able to explain this to him when he is older.

I am glad that there is now more information available about circumcision. I hope that more and more people will break out of their ignorance and see what they are doing to the ones they love so much.

Rebecca Conrad, San Rafael, CA

5.16 Informational Resources

- Circumcision Statistics: mgmbill.org/statistics.html
- Fast Facts About Circumcision: chp.edu/our-services/urology/patient-procedures/circumcision
- Should I Circumcise? The Pros and Cons of Infant Circumcision:
  www.savingsons.org/2011/01/neonatal-circumcision-video-for.html
- The Circumcision Debate: Beyond Benefits and Risks:
  pediatrics.aappublications.org/content/early/2016/04/04/peds.2016-0594

6 Circumcision and Sexuality

The presence or absence of the foreskin constitutes a dramatic difference in the appearance and nature of the male genital organ. Therefore, circumcision must have *some*, if not considerable, effect on human sexuality. How does the foreskin or lack of it affect the subjective sexual experience of the male? How does his "style" of penis affect his body image? Does it make a difference for his female partner? Does circumcision contribute to homosexuality? Does the pain inflicted upon the infant's penis have any long lasting effect upon his attitudes about sex?

In its primitive origins, some peoples believed that circumcision was a necessary prerequisite for sexual life, that it increased fertility, and that it enhanced sexuality. Other peoples considered circumcision to be a "civilizing" influence which was deliberately intended to decrease sexual sensation.

The people of the New Hebrides had the following myth about the origins of circumcision:

"... A man went into the jungle with his sister. She climbed a breadfruit tree to cut down the ripe fruit with a bamboo. When she had finished she threw down the bamboo which accidentally cut the man's foreskin. After the man recovered, he had intercourse with a woman, who found it so good that she told another woman; soon this man was in great demand, to the fury of the other men; but their women sneer at them and say they need to be like that one. So they pay him to tell the secret. He tells, and they have in such wise cut their children ever after." [1]

(It is not clear *how* the cut supposedly made intercourse better, nor whether his foreskin was cut *off* or merely cut.)

In contrast, the ancient scholar, Philo Judaeus of Alexandria:

"... regards circumcision as a symbol of the excision of pleasures which bewitch the mind, and the legislators thought good to dock the organ to signify not only the excision of excessive pleasures, but 'that a man should know himself and banish from the soul the grievous malady of conceit'." [2]

Similarly, in the 13th century Rabbi Moses Maimonides wrote:

---

1 Bettelheim B. Symbolic Wounds. In: Lessa WA, Vogt EZ (ed.) *Reader in Comparative Religion*. 2nd ed. NY: Harper & Row; 1965: 235-6.
2 James T. Philo on Circumcision – History of Medicine. *SAMJ*. 1976-08-21; 50(36): 1409-12.

> "As regards circumcision, I think that one of its objects is to limit sexual intercourse, and to weaken the organ of generation as far as possible, and thus cause man to be moderate. Some people believe that circumcision is to remove a defect in man's formation, but every one can easily reply: How can products of nature be deficient so as to require external completion, especially as the use of the foreskin to that organ is evident. This commandment has not been enjoyed as a complement to a deficient physical creation, but as a means for perfecting man's moral shortcomings. The bodily injury caused to that organ is exactly that which is desired. It does not interrupt any vital function, nor does it destroy the power of generation. Circumcision simply counteracts excessive lust; for there is no doubt that circumcision weakens the power of sexual excitement, and sometimes lessens the natural enjoyment; the organ necessarily becomes weak when it loses blood and is deprived of its covering from the beginning. Our Sages (Beresh. Rabba, c. 80) say distinctly: It is hard for a woman, with whom an uncircumcised had sexual intercourse, to separate from him. This is, as I believe, the best reason for the commandment concerning." [3]

It is questionable that anything as subjective and individual as sexual sensation can be measured or analyzed. However, Masters and Johnson attempted a study of this:

> "Thirty five uncircumcised males were matched at random with circumcised study subjects of similar ages. Routine neurologic testing for exteroceptive and light tactile discrimination were conducted on the ventral and dorsal surfaces of the penile body, with particular attention directed toward the glans. No clinically significant difference could be established between the circumcised and uncircumcised glans during these examinations." [4]

Many others refute Masters' and Johnson's findings, however, claiming that much sensitivity is lost when the glans is deprived of its protective covering.

Among Dr. Foley's findings:

> "During a boy's growth, the foreskin protects the sensitive glans. Normally the surface of the glans is composed of a smooth, glistening membrane only a few cells in thickness. The surface cells are alive, and naked nerve-endings are distributed among these cells. After circumcision when the glans is exposed to soiled diapers and rough clothing, this membrane becomes 10 times thicker, and the free

---

3 Maimonides M. *Guide for the Perplexed.* NY: Dover Publications. 1956: 378.
4 Masters WH, Johnson VE. *Human Sexual Response.* London: J & A Churchill. 1966: 189-91.

nerve-endings disappear. The surface becomes covered with an adherent layer of dead cells, rough, dry, and insensitive." [5]

According to Dr. Morgan:

"The subcutaneous tissue of the glans is provided with special sensory receptors that are concerned with appreciating pleasurable sensations occurring during coitus. They are stimulated normally only when the glans is exposed. In the circumcised subject, these receptors are constantly stimulated and lose their sensitivity." [6]

Also the foreskin itself is an erogenous zone, of which the circumcised male is deprived. In a technical article on the subject, Dr. Winkelmann writes:

"The specific type of erogenous zone is found in the mucocutaneous regions of the body. Such specific sites of acute sensation in the body are the genital regions, including the *prepuce*, penis, clitoris, and external genitalia of the female, and the perianal skin, lip, nipple and conjunctiva. It is the special anatomy of these regions that requires the use of the term 'specific' when one speaks of erotic sensations originating in the skin. This anatomy favors acute perception." [7]

Personal experiences of men who underwent circumcision during adulthood and were able to compare their "before and after" sexual sensations, are quite revealing:

"For thirty years, my penis was as it came, uncircumcised. After thirty years in the natural state I allowed myself to be persuaded by a physician to have the foreskin removed – not because of any problems at the time, but because, in the physician's view, there might be problems in the future. That was five years ago and I am sorry I had it done from my standpoint and from what my female sex partners have told me.

For myself, the sensitivity in the glans has been reduced by at least 50 percent. There it is unprotected, constantly rubbing against the fabric of whatever I am wearing. In a sense, it has become calloused. Intercourse is now (as we used to say about the older, heavier condoms) like washing your hands with your gloves on. Masturbation for me has lost many of the dimensions it once had. With the foreskin over the glans I could masturbate to orgasm at a leisurely pace, or I could

---

5 Foley JM. The Unkindest Cut of All. *Fact.* 1966-07/08; 3(4): 3-9.
6 Morgan WK. Penile Plunder. *Med J Aust.* 1967-05-27; 1: 1102.
7 Winkelmann RK. The Erogenous Zones; Their Nerve Supply and its Significance. *Proceedings of the Staff Meetings of The Mayo Clinic* (Rochester, MN). 1959-01-21; 34(2): 39.

pull back the foreskin and, using the natural lubricant which had seeped out, speed up the process. It was also handy to be able to catch the come in the foreskin.

The same was true regarding manual manipulation of my penis by my female partners. Now they can't do as much. The options in fellatio are also sharply reduced. I seem to have a relatively unresponsive stick where I once had a sexual organ." [8]

In contrast to this, a doctor who underwent circumcision during adulthood reported improved sexual satisfaction:

"The overpowering erotic sensation has been dulled, and with it some of the immediate pleasurable sensation. Initial excitement has decreased ... Friction and therefore sensation are diminished, and this in turn is a retarding factor in ejaculation ... The factor of penis sensation has been greatly altered by circumcision. If one's objective is an intense, overpowering sensation on intromission and rapid ejaculation, circumcision is undesirable. But if one is willing to sacrifice some sharp sensation for a more prolonged experience, for enjoyment of more foreplay, and for a situation where each thrust of the penis is not likely to result in that fluid termination of the act, circumcision is a great help. It amazes me how 'tough' my penis has become and how light pressure stimulation does not bring intercourse to the plateau phase." [9]

Apparently this man had difficulty with premature ejaculation, which was helped by circumcision. The dramatic contrast between these two experiences reinforces the case for *individual choice* which infants and children are not afforded if circumcised.

A woman writes of a ruined relationship resulting from her boyfriend's circumcision at her insistence:

"I became obsessed with the idea that my boyfriend should be circumcised. We were very happy together, had much in common, and, best of all, we were very compatible in bed. But I refused to get married until he was circumcised – and he gave in.

That little operation completely destroyed our life together. Before he had fabulous staying power, but after the operation he would have an orgasm in five minutes and leave me high and dry.

---

8   Anonymous. The Unkindest Cut of All. *Playgirl.* 1979-07; 108, 111.
9   Valentine RJ (pseudonym). Adult Circumcision: A Personal Report. *Med Aspects Hum Sex.* 1974-01; 8: 33.

To make things worse, sex became very painful for me. Twice I had to see a doctor due to minor infections from the chafing. Our beautiful sexual togetherness became a laborious nightmare of staying creams, lubricants, and frustrations.

He says he will never forgive me, and we no longer speak to each other. I am now dating a French boy with a lovely long foreskin, and my sex life is back to normal, but I cannot forget what a stupid mistake I made that altered the life of a lovely person. Should I give birth to a son after I'm married, believe me he will stay natural." [10]

Much speculation and debate has centered over whether the intact or the circumcised male has better "staying power" or fewer problems with premature ejaculation. The two totally opposite experiences previously cited, suggest that the ability to last during intercourse is a highly individual matter based primarily on psychological factors rather than the presence or absence of the foreskin.

Still another aspect of the foreskin's function relates to facilitating insertion with resultant greater ease in sexual penetration. According to Morgan:

"During the act of coitus, the uncircumcised phallus penetrates smoothly and without friction, the prepuce gradually retracting as the organ advances. In contrast, when the circumcised organ is introduced during coitus, friction develops between the glans and the vaginal mucosa. Penetration by the circumcised man has been compared to thrusting the foot into a sock held open at the top while on the other hand, penetration by his intact counterpart has been likened to slipping the foot into a sock that has been previously rolled up." [6]

Ritter adds:

"With the loss of the foreskin the male loses a natural gliding mechanism helpful with the sex act. With a foreskin it's possible for the erectile body of the shaft to move back and forth within the loose outer skin ... The lubrication by the mucous membrane of an uncircumcised penis is extremely helpful in coitus, especially for men who have sex with older women, who may experience a dryness of the vagina in later years. With the foreskin covering all or part of the glans, a man can insert his penis and move the erect shaft against the outer skin without irritating the dry vagina." [11]

---

10 La Roc C. Circumcision Not for Everyone. *Playgirl.* 1975-02; 11(9).
11 Conaway T. The First Rip-Off – Report on Circumcision. *Hustler.* 1979-05: 94-5.

In the previous chapter considerable discussion was given to the anti-masturbation hysteria of the late 1800s, with circumcision being one of the many "cures" or "preventatives" for this "malady." Today most people agree that masturbation is harmless. Virtually all males, and probably most females, do masturbate, at least occasionally. Some proclaim the practice as beneficial – a harmless avenue for sexual release for people too young for marriage or responsible relationships, or for people who must be separated from their mates. Probably most couples practice mutual masturbation as part of sexual foreplay or as an occasional alternative to intercourse. Even those who disapprove of masturbation must realize that circumcised males certainly do masturbate. The operation is not justified as a deterrent. However, with the lack of a foreskin, much technique is lost. The circumcised individual obviously has less skin with which to perform the act and therefore he is not afforded many subtleties and variations.

The foreskin or lack of it can have an effect on the individual's body image. In the USA, since the circumcised penis has been the norm, most circumcised males do not question their lack of foreskin. Sometimes the intact individual feels like an "oddity." On the other hand, many intact males have been proud of their "individuality," feeling a sense of "completeness" that other males lack. Some circumcised males feel a sense of deprivation and incompleteness over their missing foreskins. In other countries where circumcision is not practiced, the intact male would simply feel normal, and the circumcised male would feel pronouncedly at a loss, similar to a person who is missing a finger. How the individual feels about his intact or circumcised penis will affect his body image, which will in turn affect his sexual performance. However, for someone who is dissatisfied and prefers a change, the foreskin *can* be easily cut off but *cannot* truly be replaced.

If it is any reassurance to the male who feels inadequate over his "style" of penis, most American women are abysmally ignorant about this matter. Most are familiar only with the circumcised penis and have no awareness that it should be any different. However, with the growing trend for parents to leave their sons intact, our daughters will certainly have more awareness. Sometimes women from foreign countries express dissatisfaction over American men's lack of foreskins.

A Swedish woman writes:

"I have been in the United States nearly five years, since leaving my native Sweden. When I first started dating here, I was surprised, confused, shocked, and disappointed because almost all of the men here are circumcised. I have always regarded circumcision as barbaric and ugly. There are many American ways I still do not understand. Perhaps I am still experiencing culture shock, but a whole penis can't be *that* bad, can it?" [12]

Among women who are aware of the difference or have experienced sex with both intact and circumcised males, some have different preferences, at least over its appearance. According to Comfort in *The Joy of Sex:* "Some find the circumcised glans 'neater' ... while others love the sense of discovery which goes with retraction. If you are uncircumcised and if she prefers the other, retract it – if vice versa, you've had it." [13]

In an article in the NOCIRC Annual Report, Jeannine Parvati Baker has shared the following:

"I have had both intact and circumcised lovers and find the intact to embody the difference between a symphony and monotone. However, when one is in love with a circumcised man, that monotone can be like a Tibetan bell – holding all the sounds of the universe in a single tone." [14]

A mature and loving relationship should transcend superficial, physical attributes. Which type of penis the man has is definitely secondary to such things as gentleness, caring, kindness, and a sense of humor. However, if a man is intact, it is highly doubtful that circumcision will improve his sexual experience, for in most cases the opposite has proven true. And most importantly, if parents allow their son to grow up with his penis intact, it appears he will have advantages sexually by having a complete organ.

6.1 The Question of Homosexuality

Does the presence or absence of the foreskin have any influence upon the individual's eventual hetero- or homosexual orientation?

Authorities cannot agree on the many purported causes of male homosexuality. Theories include the absence of a father figure during childhood (or an unsatisfactory father-son relationship), a domineering mother, genetic predisposition, "mis-incarnation" – a female spirit imprisoned in a male body, and developmental arrest. Is homosexuality a "disease", "a symptom of a sick society" – or is it a potentially beneficial variation of the sex drive which enables individuals to concentrate productivity in ways that do not include having and raising children? While no answer will satisfy

---
12 Playgirl Answers. *Playgirl.* March 1974.
13 Comfort A. *The Joy of Sex.* Simon & Schuster; 1972: 65.
14 Baker JP. Excerpt. *NOCIRC Annual Report.* 2000/Spring: 4.

everyone, there has been a marked trend among psychologists in recent years to regard homosexuality simply as a matter of preference – "no big deal" as long as the individual accepts it as an innate part of his being.

I have been told that most homosexual males (in the U.S.) have been circumcised and prefer circumcised males. Their literature depicts almost exclusively circumcised penises, although they have ample access to foreign material with intact males.

Dr. Foley commented on a study of admissions to a large Naval hospital: "Of all admissions, 32% had been circumcised. Of all admissions of 'overt homosexuality,' 100% had been circumcised." [5]

One writer, responding to a newsletter's article about circumcision, informs us: "As a connoisseur of penises – I'm gay – I prefer the nice round head of a circumcised penis. So do almost all of my friends." [15]

Male homosexuality does exist in Europe and in other parts of the world where circumcision is rarely practiced. Therefore the lack of foreskin could not be a sole factor. The question is raised as to *why* the homosexual male would prefer the circumcised penis. And if the absence of foreskin contributes to male homosexuality, *why* is this so? Dr. Alfred Kinsey intended to investigate the relationship between circumcision and homosexuality before his death. It is hoped that in the future someone will do an objective study about this.

It has been noted that there are some men who are otherwise heterosexual – perhaps they are married and have children, perhaps they have never had an overt homosexual encounter, but who have been circumcised and have an unusual interest in other men's foreskins. Possibly "foreskin envy", these strong feelings of missing something, is the basis of some men's homosexuality, and certainly in many more cases, the homosexual aspect of bisexuality. Some pose the theory that the original trauma of circumcision, and the resultant resentment over the lack of foreskin brings about a castration anxiety.

Patricia Nicholas, a primal therapist, writes:

> "One patient, a homosexual, had a circumcision primal after which it became evident to him why he had been unable to have sexual relations with a woman. Each time he had tried to enter a woman he had experienced excruciating pain, the same pain he experienced when he relived the operation. Obviously this is not to say that circumcision invariably leads to homosexuality but merely that the experience on its own, or compounded with earlier or later trauma, can contribute to neurosis." [16]

---

15 Ryan B. (letter to ed.) *Moneysworth*. 1976-03-29.
16 Nicholas P. The Lasting Impact. In: Ward C & F: *The Home Birth Book. Washington:* Inscape. 1976: 82-3.

Circumcision – The Painful Dilemma

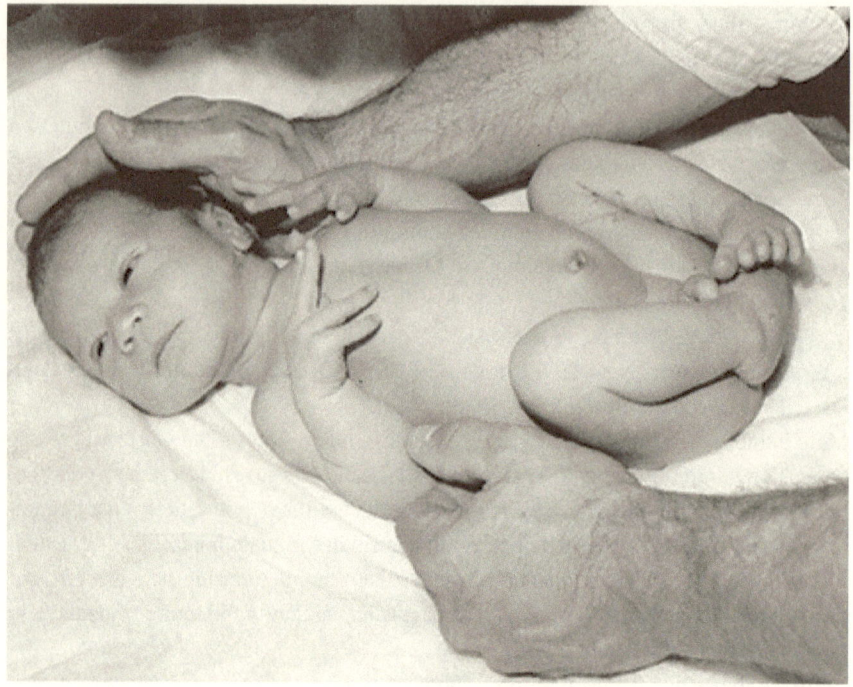

© *Suzanne Arms*

We are now learning that the newborn is a sensitive, aware human being. Certainly pain inflicted upon his penis during the first days of his life must have *some* impact upon his ultimate sexuality. There is evidence that the newborn infant experiences a certain degree of sexual arousal:

> "The more obvious forms of sexuality also begin very early. Dr. Rene A. Spitz, of the University of Colorado School of Medicine, who is a pioneer in the detailed study of the behavior of infants, has noted the signs of sexual arousal in newborn babies during the REM (rapid eye movement) stages of sleep. Dr. Charles Sarnoff, child psychiatrist and author of *Latency*, a recent book on childhood sexuality, visited hospital delivery rooms and observed what just-borns do with their hands. In the first few minutes of life, he noted, a child's hands move at random, now touching the covers, now touching different parts of the body. Within a half hour the first bit of sex learning takes place. The infants discover which parts of the body are most pleasant to touch. Some babies return again and again to the mouth, others to the ear, and many others return to the genitals." [17]

---

17 Safran C. How Children Feel About Their Bodies. *Redbook*. 1979-06: 140.

In the light of this – what is the ultimate effect if the baby's first sensations in his penis are not pleasure but instead extreme pain?

6.2 Author's Addendum

During my years of activism I have received countless phone calls from all over the world. On two separate occasions I have had lengthy conversations from men who were intact, had always given the matter little concern, and had married women who had experienced sexual relationships with many other men. In both cases their wives had selected them as husbands because of their intact foreskins. In each case the woman had discovered, out of her personal experiences and comparisons, that her intact partner gave her greater sexual satisfaction. In one of these instances, the woman was the daughter of an Orthodox rabbi!

I firmly believe that the emotional/spiritual connections in a romantic relationship vastly outweigh the importance of any physical characteristic. (I admit, however, that had I ever had a sexual relationship with an intact man, I would undoubtedly have some different insights on the matter. I am now a middle-aged woman, married to a circumcised man, and despite having been young during the 60's, still embrace relatively conventional values, so did not include that in my "research!")

6.3 Informational Resources

- 5 Insane Ways Fear of Masturbation Shaped the Modern World:
  cracked.com/article_19520_5-insane-ways-fear-masturbation-shaped-modern-world.html
- 8 Negative Effects of Male Circumcision on Female Sexuality:
  endalldisease.com/8-negative-effects-of-male-circumcision-on-female-sexuality
- A Change in How Intercourse Works: www.drmomma.org/2009/10/change-in-how-intercourse-works.html
- A preliminary poll: 82% of circumcised men ignore the serial anejaculatory mini-orgasms, 91% of intacts enjoy them: academia.edu/5812258
- Adding Insult to Injury: Acquisition of Erectile Dysfunction from Circumcision:
  researchgate.net/publication/322056383
- Adult Circumcision Outcomes Study: Effect On Erectile Function, Penile Sensitivity, Sexual Activity and Satisfaction: cirp.org/library/sex_function/fink1
- Adult male circumcision: effects on sexual function and sexual satisfaction in Kisumu, Kenya[18]:
  pubmed.ncbi.nlm.nih.gov/18761593

---

18 This study by Krieger is included in a meta-analysis, without declaring conflict of interest by Krieger being co-author of the meta analysis. Something I found interesting in Krieger is that both the circumcised and uncircumcised group reported improvement on satisfaction during the study. It's difficult to understand why the uncircumcised group would have an improvement if they were not treated, and it's important to recognize that there could be a bias since the men who were circumcised wanted to be circumcised. – R.R.

- Advances in Sexual Medicine: scirp.org/journal/asm
- Adverse Sexual and Psychological Effects of Male Infant Circumcision: cirp.org/library/psych/boyle5
- Alexithymia and Circumcision Trauma: A Preliminary Investigation: researchgate.net/publication/270190401
- An erogenous lip, protective of erogeneity and the tool of autosexuality, the foreskin is a sexual organ; its ablation is mutilation: academia.edu/2274700
- Author's Response to: Does sexual function survey in Denmark offer any support for male circumcision having an adverse effect?: ije.oxfordjournals.org/content/41/1/312.full.pdf
- Cereal 'killer' Dr. Kellog Created Cornflakes To Crush Sex Drive:
  web.archive.org/web/20150220024159/http://yournewswire.com/cereal-killer-dr-kellog-created-cornflakes-to-crush-sex-drive
- Circumcised Penis's Elongated Thrusting Stroke Dries Out Vaginal Lubrication:
  sexasnatureintendedit.com/10F/3lube_loss.html
- Circumcising cuts off the best part...: circumstitions.com/Images/sorrellsvm&j-poster.pdf
- Circumcision and feminicide, honour crime, stoning, excision, rape, harems, polygamy, forced marriage, forced obesity, dry sex, veil, causality and correlation: academia.edu/3086663
- Circumcision in the United States: Prevalence, Prophylactic Effects, and Sexual Practice:
  cirp.org/library/general/laumann
- Circumcision makes the penis smaller: wisewomanwayofbirth.com/circumcision-makes-the-penis-smaller
- Circumcision: Social, Sexual, Psychological Realities:
  psychologytoday.com/intl/blog/moral-landscapes/201109/circumcision-social-sexual-psychological-realities
- Clinical presentation and pathophysiology of meatal stenosis following circumcision:
  cirp.org/library/complications/persad
- Dicks (uncut): dailycal.org/2016/04/12/352616
- Discourses on sexual pleasure after genital modifications: the fallacy of genital determinism *(a response to J. Steven Svoboda)*: tandfonline.com/doi/abs/10.1080/23269995.2013.805530
- Does Circumcision Cause Erectile Dysfunction?:
  thewholenetwork.org/twn-news/does-circumcision-cause-erectile-dysfunction
- Does circumcision cause erectile dysfunction? *(Dr. Gifford-Jones)*:
  www.drmomma.org/2010/03/does-circumcision-cause-erectile.html
- Does Circumcision Hurt Sexual Pleasure? Study Draws Fire:
  livescience.com/27769-does-circumcision-reduce-sexual-pleasure.html
- Does Male Circumcision Adversely Affect Sexual Sensation, Function, or Satisfaction? Critical Comment on Morris and Krieger: scirp.org/journal/paperinformation.aspx?paperid=55256
- Does male circumcision affect sexual function, sensitivity, or satisfaction? – a systematic review *(Brian Morris' meta-analysis where he rates many studies as "low quality")*: pubmed.ncbi.nlm.nih.gov/23937309
- Effects of circumcision on male sexual functions: a systematic review and meta-analysis:
  ncbi.nlm.nih.gov/pmc/articles/PMC3881635
- Effects of male circumcision on female arousal and orgasm: academia.edu/11851529
- Erectile function evaluation after adult circumcision: pubmed.ncbi.nlm.nih.gov/14979200

- "every multi-orgasmic man she dated, was intact":

    littleimages.org/blog/10-things-christian-men-know-about-sex/#comment-169
- Factors Associated With Early Deaths Following Neonatal Male Circumcision in the United States, 2001-10:

    researchgate.net/publication/326040454
- Feminine and masculine sexual mutilation, the greatest crime against humanity: academia.edu/2095540
- Fine-touch pressure thresholds in the adult penis: pubmed.ncbi.nlm.nih.gov/17378847
- Fine-touch pressure thresholds in the adult penis *(Hugh Young compares Sorrells to Master & Johnson):*

    pubmed.ncbi.nlm.nih.gov/17669150
- Fine-touch Pressure Thresholds In the Adult Penis *(rebuttal to Morris):*

    bjui-journals.onlinelibrary.wiley.com/doi/abs/10.1111/j.1464-410X.2007.07072_1.x
- Fine-touch Pressure Thresholds In the Adult Penis *(written by Brian Morris – a notorious pro-circ advocate):*

    bjui-journals.onlinelibrary.wiley.com/doi/abs/10.1111/j.1464-410X.2007.06970_6.x
- Foreskin Sexual Function/Circumcision Sexual Dysfunction: cirp.org/library/sex_function
- Frisch's response to Brian Morris: circumstitions.com/Docs/morris-2013-ann.pdf
- Global Survey of Circumcision Harm: circumcisionharm.org/research.htm
- Here are 5 American sex norms Europeans think are crazy:

    web.archive.org/web/20151220185434/https://www.rawstory.com/2015/07/here-are-5-american-sex-norms-europeans-think-are-crazy
- How Circumcision May Be Affecting Your Love Life: boystoo.com/medical/conversion.htm
- How Male Circumcision Harms Women: circumcision.org/how-male-circumcision-harms-women
- Human prepuce: some aspects of structure and function: cirp.org/library/anatomy/lakshmanan
- I LOVE foreskin: restoringtally.com/blog/2011/03/i-love-foreskin
- Information on circumcision: to cut or not to cut, that is the question:

    existere.wordpress.com/2012/02/10/information-on-circumcision-to-cut-or-not-to-cut-that-is-the-question
- Intact or Circumcised: A Significant Difference in the Adult Penis:

    www.drmomma.org/2011/08/intact-or-circumcised-significant.html
- Introduction to the natural, intact penis *(photo gallery, graphic):* circumcisionharm.org/gallery%20intact.htm
- Is Circumcision Why We Need Viagra?: canadafreepress.com/medical/urology030302.htm
- Keratinization: noharmm.org/IDcirc.htm#keratinization
- Lifelong premature ejaculation: from authority-based to evidence-based medicine:

    bjui-journals.onlinelibrary.wiley.com/doi/full/10.1111/j.1464-410X.2004.4886d.x
- Long-Term Adverse Effects of Circumcision:

    i2researchhub.org/articles/ch-6-long-term-adverse-effects-of-circumcision-doc-genital-integrity-statement
- male circumcision and sexual difficulties for men and female partners:

    circumstitions.com/news/news41.html#denmark
- Male circumcision and sexual function in men and women: a survey-based, cross-sectional study in Denmark: pubmed.ncbi.nlm.nih.gov/21672947
- Male Circumcision and Women's Sexual Health:

    www.drmomma.org/2009/07/how-male-circumcision-impacts-women.html

- Male circumcision decreases penile sensitivity as measured in a large cohort: pubmed.ncbi.nlm.nih.gov/23374102
- Male circumcision leads to a bad sex life: sciencenordic.com/denmark-gender-hiv/male-circumcision-leads-to-a-bad-sex-life/1371590
- Male Circumcision: Mothers, Don't Mutilate Your Boys: dodsonandross.com/sexfeature/male-circumcision-mothers-don%e2%80%99t-mutilate-your-boys
- 'Manhood: The Bare Reality': 100 Men Had Their Penises Photographed To Explore Masculinity: huffingtonpost.co.uk/entry/manhood-the-bare-reality_uk_59357df5e4b0fa3f6ae63d01
- Meet James Ketter: yourwholebaby.org/meet-james-ketter
- Men Do Complain (The Effect of Male Circumcision on the Enjoyment of the Female Partner): mendocomplain.com
- New study: male circumcision and sexual difficulties for men and female partners: web.archive.org/web/20130312091702/http://www.examiner.com/article/new-study-male-circumcision-and-sexual-difficulties-for-men-and-female-partners
- Not Just Skin: notjustskin.org
- Pamphlets and Handouts: coloradonocirc.org/pamphlets.php
- Pfizer Reports Fourth-Quarter and Full-Year 2008 Results and 2009 Financial Guidance: pfizer.com/news/press-release/press-release-detail/pfizer_reports_fourth_quarter_and_full_year_2008_results_and_2009_financial_guidance
- Plain Facts for Old and Young *(Kellogg – sexual repression)*: books.google.de/books?id=pubVzCbD_DMC&dq=infant+circumcision+kellogg&pg=PA383&hl=en&redir_esc=y#v=onepage&q=circumcision&f=true
- Response to Ej Dickson: A Plea for Reason from a Jewish Man to a Jewish Woman: dbalablog.blogspot.com/2017/06/response-to-ej-dickson-plea-for-reason.html
- Sensation and sexual arousal in circumcised and uncircumcised men: pubmed.ncbi.nlm.nih.gov/17419812
- Sex As Nature Intended It: sexasnatureintendedit.com
- Sex as Nature Intended It: The Most Important Thing You Need to Know about Making Love, but No One Could Tell You Until Now: amazon.com/dp/0970044216
- Studies on Circumcision: circumcision.org/studies-on-circumcision
- Study: Circumcision Doesn't Reduce Sexual Sensation: abcnews.go.com/Health/Sex/story?id=3436936
- Study: Circumcision Removes Most Sensitive Parts: livescience.com/1624-study-circumcision-removes-sensitive-parts.html
- Terminal innervation of the male genitalia, cutaneous sensory receptors of the male foreskin *(Martin-Alguacil basically supports the 1996-1999 findings of John Taylor)*: onlinelibrary.wiley.com/doi/10.1002/ca.22501
- The Circumcision Complex: Fundamentals: circumcisioncomplex.com/fundamentals
- The Cutaneous Innervation of Human Newborn Prepuce: cirp.org/library/anatomy/winkelmann2
- The Difference Between Intact & Cut: momsnotbombs.blogspot.com/2012/03/difference-between-intact-cut.html
- The effect of male circumcision on sexuality: pubmed.ncbi.nlm.nih.gov/17155977

- The effect of male circumcision on the sexual enjoyment of the female partner: cirp.org/library/anatomy/ohara
- The Erogenous Zones: Their Nerve Supply and Siognificance: cirp.org/library/anatomy/winkelmann
- The Frenular Delta: A New Preputial Structure: cirp.org/library/anatomy/mcgrath1
- The Global Survey of Circumcision Harm is a groundbreaking exploration into the effects of infant circumcision on adult men: pool.intactiwiki.org/images/Circumcision_Harm_Survey-1.pdf
- The Guide of the Perplexed *(by Moses Maimonides)*: cirp.org/library/cultural/maimonides
- The Joy of Uncircumcising!: Exploring Circumcision: History, Myths, Psychology, Restoration, Sexual Pleasure, and Human Rights: amazon.com/dp/093406122X
- The prepuce: Specialized mucosa of the penis and its loss to circumcision: cirp.org/library/anatomy/taylor
- The purpose of circumcision is to ruin male sexuality: web.archive.org/web/20140220180919/http://www.moralogous.com/2012/04/29/the-purpose-of-circumcision-is-to-ruin-male-sexuality
- The Rise of Viagra: How the Little Blue Pill Changed Sex in America (Sociology): amazon.com/dp/081475211X
- The Sexual Effects of Circumcision: www.drmomma.org/2009/07/sexual-effects-of-circumcision.html
- The troubled history of the foreskin: arstechnica.com/science/2015/02/the-troubled-history-of-the-foreskin
- What exactly is circumcision and what is it not? *(Not a study, but an essay at CIRP. It's actually a great paper, but I don't think it has ever been published. The "triple whammy" really says it all)*: cirp.org/library/anatomy/garcia
- What is lost due to circumcision?: norm.org/lost.html
- What were the original motivations behind routine infant circumcision in the West?: cirp.org/pages/whycirc.html

Videos:
- Circumcision and Sexual Function Difficulties: youtu.be/yfGkZZ-KzpU
- The Penis – Sex Education 101: youtu.be/BgoTRMKrJo4

7   Circumcision and the Military Service

Some people believe that circumcision is a requirement for entrance into the military service. Just as military recruits must wear uniforms and standard short haircuts, some people have the idea that there are similar military rules about "standard equipment" for penises. Undoubtedly some military authorities have wished that this were so, but in truth, there are no requirements in any branch of American (or any other) military service that an intact recruit must forfeit his foreskin upon enlistment.

Nonetheless, some new parents have their infant sons circumcised for this reason. (How did people get the idea that the operation is *less* painful for an innocent, freshly born, exquisitely sensitive infant than for a rigorously trained, battle-hardened soldier?!)

One recent medical source cites a rate of 0.3% circumcision among the Armed Forces.[1] Therefore, it appears that stories about military men undergoing circumcision must be exaggerated.

According to one military authority:

"I am sure that no medical military personnel are oblivious of ANY circumcision. After all the purpose of the military is to protect the nation, not to defend the sacred American rite of circumcision. I am also certain that no branch of the service has ever had a policy of concerted circumcision. However, there is a high incidence of circumcision in the military. In most cases, these circumcisions appear to be more on an individual doctor-patient level rather than unit-wide. Military doctors have the duty to keep the men under their authority combat-ready, health-wise. Some of these doctors, obviously, have been conditioned to think all foreskins are health-hazards, just as do some civilian doctors. Some military doctors have been circumcision zealots, as have some civilian doctors. Most doctors probably couldn't care less whether a man is cut or uncut." [2]

The following are several accounts of men who have either witnessed or experienced circumcision or pressure to have circumcision while in the military service:

"In the midst of sex in Saigon I got just a short slit in the foreskin ... had to go to the infirmary on account of the bleeding ... I was very close to being discharged and the Army dogs said that it had to be circumcised, otherwise it would hold me up from going home. I protested vigorously, but you know who won the battle! The circumcision kept me out of action for about 5 weeks. Losing the foreskin

---

1   Group Health Cooperative of Puget Sound. Circumcision (information brochure).
2   Berkeley B. Excerpts from an Underground Newsletter.

was a traumatic experience sort of like losing a limb, or for a woman, a breast. I have gotten used to it now, but it was many degrees more pleasurable with foreskin, sensations were more intense. The army was sure adamant about cutting and I often wonder if it was really necessary. I can't believe it was in my case. But their attitude gave me the feeling that they had a 'thing' about it." [2]

"I was born in the USA but grew up in the Ukraine during the Nazis' occupation. During that time all circumcised men in Carpantho, Ukraine, were arbitrarily deported to extermination camps by the Germans. When I returned to America I immediately joined the Armed Forces and only then did I realize that most American men are circumcised. Once they almost did it to me against my better judgment. I finally agreed to circumcision and was already prepped and enemaed when I backed out. My foreskin is loose and gives me no hassle so I told them to go to hell." [2]

"I entered the Army and at age 20 was relocated overseas. I developed tonsillitis and the doctor advised tonsillectomy. I had no objection. I woke up in the recovery room with a sore throat *and* a sore penis! The doctor was standing by me admiring his butchery and said 'While you were under, I noticed you hadn't been circumcised, so I gave you a freebie.' I called him a son of a bitch and his reply was, 'You ought to be thanking me, I made a man out of you!' " [2]

"Army Signal Corps stationed in Germany, on duty/kidney stone attack. Doctor wants me to sign surgical release. Under 'Operation to be Performed': Circumcision and removal of kidney stones. I refused to sign and was told this was disobeying an officer (the doctor). I asked to see the chief doctor. ... (I) meantime called the company X.O. (uncut) and asked for his help. He got Cp., C.O., & Chaplain to call Chief Orderly at hospital. The word 'circumcision' was removed from the release. Operation Success." [2]

"During the Vietnam war I joined the Navy. We had routine short arm inspection every few weeks. This is a real experience because the doctor has everyone milk them. The 10% or so who are not cut have to peel back their foreskins and bare the head as well as go through the milking routine. I never had any trouble at these inspections until a new doctor showed up. He seemed to be particularly interested in my cock and made me skin it several times. Then he told me to report to him in Sick Bay, and I wondered what was up.

I think the creep just hated guys who had not been cut as babies or maybe he was some kind of kooky closet queen who was envious of me. Anyway he said

I had to report for a circumcision. I told him I never had any V.D., I never had any trouble with coming, I kept myself clean, and I just didn't want to go around minus my foreskin and with a scar on my prick, and I wouldn't report. The M.F. said, 'OK, sailor, then it's a court martial and a general discharge for you.' Well, I didn't want that on my record and I knew I couldn't beat the system.

So now I have a cock like all other poor bastards whose folks didn't have enough sense to say 'NO WAY' when the doctor asked them if they wanted to have the baby cut ... If somebody's religion says 'get cut' OK, but why the hell should 90% of the male babies in America have to sacrifice their foreskins because of a lot of bloodthirsty doctors? Someday the men of this country will put an end to all this mutilation and cocks will be like nature made them and like mine used to be." [2]

"It was during the Korean war that I almost got circumcised. There was a long lull in the fighting and the medical corps was idle. They called for a short arm inspection of uncircumcised personnel and as about half of my company seemed to be uncut that involved a lot of men. As I was waiting in line I noticed that some of the men were released after inspection but others were referred to another lineup. We all began to put two and two together and realized that these guys detailed were going to get clipped. As I got closer I realized that the presence of smegma was their main criteria for circumcision. I always produced a lot of it. I asked permission to go to the urinal, but instead peeled it back quick and cleaned myself out. It saved my foreskin!" [2]

"I was in the Navy during WW II, spending months on end cooped up on a miserable ship. With nothing else to do, some of us formed an initiation club. The doc, with nothing else to do, was into circumcising. Usually he had gone through every foreskin on the ship, including mine. My club was made up of ex-uncut men who were graduates of the doc. Whenever 'new cocks' were transferred to our ship, the doc would let us know which ones were uncut. We went to work on them – 'Going to let the doc take care of that buddy?', 'About time you join the U.S. Navy, isn't it buddy?', 'Ready to get that thing clipped, buddy?', 'Just think, buddy, this time next week, you'll be a regular circumcised American sailor.' We usually got them to sign quick and we made a big thing of initiation ceremonies as we watched the doc clip off another dick. Shit! What a lousy way to spend a war!" [2]

"I was attending a military academy during my teens. My foreskin and I had a running battle with the doctor who appeared monthly at the school to give each cadet a physical. After each check-up he would invariably give me a sealed note to take home to my parents. Intuitively, I knew the notes recommended circumcision and I hid them. Each month he would make me push my foreskin back and forth (which at 15 was embarrassing as hell to do in front of an adult) and then he would write his little note. Maybe he felt sorry for me because I was just about the only uncut boy at the academy. One day my mother asked me about the notes and I made a flimsy excuse. A few weeks later I ended up in the office of our family doctor who, after examining me, asked me right out whether or not I wanted to be circumcised. I said NO and he said there was no reason for it. That was that!" [2]

"I know of a Navy doctor who always circumcised on Saturday night so he could use foreskins for bait when he fished on Sunday." [2]

"A doctor on my ship fed foreskins to his pet piranha fish." [2]

"In my battalion (Seabees, WW II) the doctor did his damndest to 'sweet-talk,' coerce, and 'politic' us uncuts into allowing him to add our foreskins to his 1/2-gallon jar of alcohol-pickled foreskins." [2]

"I was one of the last Vietnam draftees. We had about two weeks of orientation before training started. At the end of the first week a few guys were called to a special session after supper. Some Medical Sargent showed us a slide show and gave us a talk on circumcision especially in Vietnam (because of V.D. and fungus infection). He answered some questions and then told us to sign some papers. We were all pushed into signing without being given time to think about what was going on. The next morning we were called to Regiment Headquarters and loaded on a mini-bus and sent to the base hospital. There were eight guys in my ward and when they stripped us and we got on beds as instructed, I realized that none of us were clipped. Then two young doctors and two male nurses examined each of us between the legs. One doctor told us that there were no complications and that we would have easy circumcisions that afternoon. They got some tranquilizers for us and we calmed down. One by one we were wheeled out. Some guys jerked off for the last time with skins. I was the last to go. Two men were already back and were feeling no pain so I wasn't worried. I looked at them but couldn't tell much because of the bloody gauze bandage. When I got on the operating table they put a screen up so I couldn't see what they did but I could feel an injection. After the injection I was numb but could sense them pulling the skin, cleaning it, and putting a clamp on. I could tell what they cut and when. It was like a tearing feeling. They put stitches around the cut, sprayed it with something, and bandaged it up. About three hours later in the ward the pain hit all the guys. It was like a bad burn. Most of' the guys got hypos and the aids put ice packs on their crotches. Nobody said much for the next two days. We never made it to 'Nam' ... the war was over before we left training." [2]

Dr. Mendelsohn comments:

"In the past, the U.S. Armed Forces advocated circumcision perhaps because it gave an opportunity for young surgeons to practice, there was an excess of available hospital beds, the procedure presumably promoted cleanliness, and, in their view, it prevented venereal disease.[3] Circumcision was also felt to promote discipline: I presume as a result of the young recruit's learning what the Army could do to him at the outset he might be influenced to behave himself during the rest of his tour of duty. Possibly because of this conditioning, many people think that circumcision is mandated by state law." [4]

The type of situations described, of being overwhelmed by pressures of authority, is not at all unlike the experience of new parents, overwhelmed by hospital authority when they sign away their sons' foreskins. Within the hospital institution, whether upon giving birth or in the military service, people have often had to be strong, assertive, and unafraid of being different in order to keep this piece of skin. Passivity and cooperation will more likely lead to loss of the foreskin.

Jeffrey R. Wood has suggested a possible military "advantage" of circumcision. Perhaps the circumcised recruit would be more willing to risk injury or death in battle because his body has *already* been injured with the loss of his foreskin.[5]

For some military authorities and other people, revulsion to foreskins may be akin to the intense hatred for beards, mustaches, and longer hair on men that was so prevalent in past decades, especially during the 1960s. The public needed at least a decade to learn that society is not going to fall apart as a result of longer hair or facial hair. Hopefully in the future we can become equally relaxed about foreskins.

Sylvia Topp relates: "An American doctor in Vietnam claims that many man-hours of active duty were lost by uncircumcised men who acquired balanitis (infection of the foreskin) and had to be hospitalized and later cured or circumcised." [6]

---

[3] Author's note: Circumcision is not a preventative against "sexually transmitted disease." Please refer to Chapter 14 "Sexually Transmitted Infection" of this book for further discussion. – R.R.
[4] Mendelsohn RA. Circumcision Views Solicited. *People's Doctor* (newspaper column). Hayward CA. 1978.
[5] Wood, JR. Personal correspondence.
[6] Topp S. Why Not to Circumcise Your Baby Boy. *Mothering.* 1978; 6: 76.

From a different perspective, perhaps some men, experiencing fatigue or hysteria from active combat have welcomed circumcision as the "lesser of two evils." The operation would keep one out of battle for several weeks, and was at government expense. And since a considerably higher percentage of men die in battle than as a result of circumcision – perhaps the operation saved some men's lives.

However, top priority for medical services, especially during wartime, must be directed towards healing and saving the lives of those injured in battle. One must hope that supplies and energies given to circumcision "mania" has not stolen needed medical attention from others with more crucial, life preserving needs.

Ms. Topp adds: "If you intend your son to be a soldier fighting in hot countries, perhaps you should circumcise him now, although you might leave both decisions up to him." [6]

It must be emphasized that circumcision within the military service has been an American practice peculiar to World War II, the Korean War, and the war in Vietnam. World War I, the Civil War, the Revolutionary War and most other previous wars throughout history were fought (apparently) effectively by men whose foreskins were intact. These wars took place during a time when bathing facilities and opportunities were vastly inferior to what we have had in the 20th century.

Obviously the practice of circumcising our own soldiers has been one that was doctor *constructed* rather than based on true need.

No one can predict the future. We do not know when or whether our country will be at war again. No parent can know whether his son, if circumcised today, will someday be thankful that it was over and done within infancy, or will resent the fact that he was deprived of his foreskin. Nor does any parent know whether or not his son will want to be a part of the military service. Hopefully in the future the intact penis will be considerably more acceptable than it is today. Soldiers in other countries who do not practice circumcision apparently function without problems. By the time a child born today is old enough to enlist in the military service, perhaps medical circumcision will be confined to those who exhibit true need or desire for it. Routine amputation of the foreskin will no longer be advocated out of mere conformity or supposed "preventative" medicine.

8   The Circumcision of a Three-year Old

Chris Thomas, Port Hueneme, CA

(Mrs. Thomas is the mother of Sonny who was circumcised shortly after his third birthday. She has a stepson, Christopher, also age three at the time of this interview. Mrs. Thomas was expecting another baby when this interview took place.)

I conducted this interview when my research on circumcision was just beginning, so unfortunately did not have the knowledge to advise Mrs. Thomas about her son's unfortunate situation, since conferred with informed medical sources about Sonny Thomas' condition. This experience should not be viewed as an argument in favor of immediate infant circumcision. His condition developed due to incorrect care of his foreskin during infancy and early childhood. The condition could have been corrected without surgery.

It is normal *for a baby's foreskin to be tight and adhered to the glans. If left alone it will gradually loosen of its own accord and become fully retractable. This can take several months, or sometimes years. The infant's foreskin should be left entirely alone. Frequent, over vigorous retraction of the child's foreskin is what* caused *Sonny's condition. When an infant's foreskin is forced back when it is still naturally adhered to the glans, this breaks the natural adhesions. When the foreskin is replaced, these adhesions heal back together. Sonny's condition in which his foreskin "grew back to the head of the penis" is known as "acquired phimosis." Unfortunately many parents are given incorrect advice about the care of an intact baby. Had Mrs. Thomas left her son's foreskin alone his condition would not have developed.*

Rosemary: Why did you choose not to have Sonny circumcised when he was born?
Chris: The baby's father was not circumcised. Before that I had always felt that if God had meant for man to be circumcised, he would be born that way. There's a reason for the foreskin to be there and it was to be left alone! If I had a boy it was just not going to be done. Then when Sonny was a year and a half old, he started having problems with it. He was having difficulty urinating. He would get two streams coming from the end of his penis.
R: How did you care for his foreskin when he was an infant?
C: It was drawn all the way back over the head. It took time to work it back all the way because it was naturally sealed up. But by the time he was two months old I could get it completely drawn back. I would wash it with soapy water with every bath. It was also cleaned every time his diapers were changed. Then when he was about a year and a half old it started growing back to the head of the penis. So the

doctor decided it would have to be surgically removed. It was almost completely growing shut and he could barely even urinate through it.

R: Was it painful for him?

C: During the last three months before he had the surgery he started complaining of pain. But most of the time it was just annoying. So I took him to the hospital and they did the surgery. I didn't see the operation and I'm not sure how they went about it. They put him out completely. The doctor said he used a scalpel to surgically remove the foreskin. It was like coring an apple. Then the skin was drawn back and cut off. He had 14 stitches. He still (5 months later) hasn't completely healed from it. After a bath when he is being dried off with a towel it hurts. The surgery was a very traumatic experience for him.

R: Even though he was put out for the operation?

C: Yes. He still talks about it. He talks about the knife that the doctor used to cut him and how the doctor fixed it, but it hurt when he fixed it. He was at the age where he was old enough to understand what was happening, but not old enough to be able to fully understand why it had to be done.

R: Was he potty trained?

C: He was trained, but still having accidents. Now after they completed the surgery, the doctor wrapped the incision with gauze and told me that when Sonny started urinating it would be very painful for him. The first potty afterwards didn't bother him at all. They took the wrapping off the next day and that's when urination started being painful. What I learned with Sonny going through this kind of surgery ... my new baby, if it's a boy, he will be circumcised immediately. I won't take any chances of having my child go through something like that again.

R: It's a big trauma for a newborn too. They heal very fast, but with a newborn they don't use anesthesia. Could you imagine, with your son, if they had just strapped him down and started cutting on him without anesthesia?

C: No. I couldn't imagine that!

R: But that's how it's done for a newborn. And the feelings in a new baby are just as strong.

C: It really is hard to make a decision.

Now when Sonny was taken in for surgery the doctor told me that it would be a couple of hours before the baby would be back in the recovery room. The doctor said that Sonny would probably want to sleep for the rest of the day and wouldn't want to eat. But when they brought him back into his room, I couldn't believe it! He was standing up in his crib jumping up and down as they were bringing him down the hallway! He was screaming, "I want breakfast!! I'm hungry!!" The nurse suggested starting him out with a little bit of ice water, and Sonny didn't want to hear about the ice water. He wanted food! When they brought him his food he ate a complete breakfast!

R: Did you take him home that day?

C: No, we spent another three days in the hospital, so the doctor could watch him. I stayed with Sonny from the time he was admitted until the time he was released. I never left his side except for when they were doing the surgery.

R: Do you wish that you had him circumcised as a newborn, so you wouldn't have gone through that?

C: I don't know. I really don't know which is worse ... circumcision for a newborn or for a child Sonny's age. It's a hard thing to decide. But it's something that I feel definitely has to be done at one time or another.

R: How common is a problem like Sonny's ... the foreskin growing back to the head of the penis?

C: As far as I know, it's not very common at all.

R: Did Sonny have an infection with it?

C: No. It was just his skin closing up. I guess it's just a freak thing.

R: You also have a stepson.

C: Right. My husband has a child from a previous marriage and we are raising him. Sonny is from my previous marriage. And the one that I am expecting now is ours together.

R: And your stepson was circumcised at birth.

C: Yes. I have no idea what the reasons were or how it went.

R: Since you are raising the two boys together do you feel that it is just as well that they are both circumcised?

C: I really haven't thought about it. But I have overheard the boys' conversations when they're in the bathtub together. Shortly after Sonny's operation when the boys were taking a bath, Christopher made a comment about it. "Oh, it's different now!" and Sonny said, "Yeah, the doctor fixed it. It's just like yours now! They work just alike now!" I'm not sure what was going through their little minds but they knew that there was a big change made.

R: They had not understood the difference before Sonny was circumcised?

C: Right. Now they know that Sonny's penis has been "fixed" and the doctor made it better.

R: Was Sonny really frightened about the operation?

C: No, because we had talked about the operation with him. He basically understood what was happening.

R: So it may or may not have been as traumatic as having a newborn circumcised.

C: I'm sure it must be a terrible experience for a newborn to go through without any medication to kill the pain at the time that it's done. But with Sonny, it was almost

8 – The Circumcision of a Three-year Old

six weeks before the stitches were gone. With a newborn baby I don't believe that there are any stitches.

R: Not normally. Not unless there's a problem.

C: I didn't think that there was. Sonny had 14 stitches and it took six weeks for them to go away.

R: Did the stitches bother him?

C: Yes, they really did. They'd start drying out and get itchy.

R: Couldn't you have just pulled them out?

C: No. They were self-dissolving stitches. If I pulled any of them out it could cause it to break back open again and lead to infection. They gave me a prescription for some cream to use on it and we used it several times a day. But the stitches would get dry and break in between where the actual knot was made. They'd scratch and stick out and snag on his underwear and it would pull. Sometimes it pulled just enough to draw a little bit of blood and then his underwear would get stuck to that spot and when he'd pull them down to go to the bathroom it would break at that point. He was having a pretty difficult time with it. He didn't do that much complaining. At three years old they try to be pretty tough! But I know it was a lot harder for him than he wanted Mommy to think. I really think, if this baby is a boy, we'll have it done right away. I just want to get it over with and not have to worry about it. I'm glad Sonny's problem doesn't happen that often. I'd hate to know of other children having to go through something like that. It's a horrible thing. It's got to be the most sensitive part of the male body and to have it cut on ...

R: Why are you planning to have this baby at home?

C: I had a horrible hospital experience when Sonny was born. I was 18 years old and knew nothing about having babies. I didn't do any reading on the subject and didn't take any classes. I accepted everything that the hospital did. I got an enema and I was shaved. If anybody tries to give me an enema with this baby they're going to have a fight on their hands! The enema caused my contractions to become much harder and I panicked. I was sitting on the commode and all I could think of was "My God, what if I had my baby right here!" I didn't like being shaved because of the irritation when the hair started growing back.

When I was in the labor bed I gave birth to the baby's head. Then they moved me over onto a gurney with the baby's head out. They took me into the delivery room and put me on the delivery table and strapped my legs up into the stirrups. Now the only thing left was to let the rest of my baby's body come out. They were telling me to hold it, not to let the baby come out, and I did what they were telling me to do. Then the doctor came into the delivery room. When he saw that the baby's head had been born, he said, "Somebody put her up in the stirrups too soon." So they took me out of the stirrups, rolled me over on my side, gave me a spinal, rolled me back over onto my back, and put my legs back up in the stirrups. Then he gave me an episiotomy ... after the baby's head had been born!! I didn't know anything!! I thought that was the way it was supposed to be!! Then he delivered the rest of the baby's body with forceps. The baby was six weeks old before the bruises went away!

R: Were his shoulders stuck?

C: No. That was just the only way that the doctor knew how to deliver a baby. If I had just been allowed to relax and let go, the baby would have come right out!!

R: He just figured he had to give you all the standard equipment.

C: I don't want to go through that with this baby. When Sonny was born, the doctor asked me what we wanted. I said "A boy." And he said, "Well, you have it!" He held him up for a few seconds and then handed the baby to the nurse and then he was gone. The baby was born at 9:44 a.m. and it was about 7 p.m. when they first brought him to me. I didn't get to nurse on the delivery table or even touch him. By the time they brought him to me, the baby was very unconcerned. He was totally uninterested in me.

R: I went through the same thing with my first baby.

C: After the nurse left, Sonny passed his first stool. I didn't want my baby lying in that! So I proceeded to unwrap him and take off his dirty diaper and was ready to clean him up. The nurse came back and saw me with this unwrapped baby, and she read me a riot act! You'd think I had committed first degree murder! She told me that I had absolutely no right to unwrap MY baby! And change MY baby's pants!! I said "If I'm not supposed to do it, then who is?" And she said, "You're supposed to ring for a nurse to come in and take the baby back to the nursery, change him, and then he will be brought back to you." I thought, "That's crazy! Who has a better right to change her own child than the mother herself?"

R: They worry about germs and infection.

C: I understand the hospital is the best place to get an infection. I'm really looking forward to having this baby at home. It's going to be perfect!

Chris' new baby was a girl, so fortunately the question of circumcision did not arise. She had a hospital birth due to prolonged rupture of the membranes, but had a positive birth experience in the hospital.

9   The Circumcision of an Adult

Johannes Peglow, Chatsworth, CA

Johannes: I had the circumcision because of medical reasons. I had warts on my foreskin. The doctor said it was the easiest way to remove the warts. He said he could burn them out, but they could come back. This way was a better guarantee. So I said okay.

Rosemary: How old were you when you had the operation?

J: I was 22. I thought it was a good idea. So I went to the hospital at 7 o'clock in the morning. They assigned me to a bed. They gave me some pills. I don't know what they were, but they put me out. After the operation I was lying around for another two hours. They have to check it to see whether you bleed. I got out by 11 a.m. I walked out of the hospital. I had a bandage about the thickness of my arm here.

R: Wasn't that embarrassing?

J: Not really. I had some very big pants on. I got home and then the "fun" started. It started hurting. It wasn't real hurting ... more like burning. It's really weird. It was just uncomfortable, like the irritation if you had your whole skin scraped off. It didn't really hurt. And going to the bathroom was a bummer, because I had stitches around it and if it scratches. That hurts a little bit.

R: Did you have to take your own bandage off?

J: No. They put it on in a way so that I could still urinate. I had to leave it on for the first week. When I had to go to the bathroom, I put a plastic bag around the bandage because I wasn't supposed to get it wet. I had to go back to the doctor to change the bandage.

R: Did the doctor have to remove the stitches?

J: No, they were self-dissolving. The problem is, if you're not circumcised, you're much more sensitive. So I stayed home about two days and then I went back to work. When you walk, it rubs. The thing that bugged me was that I'd start to get half erections, and then it started to pull against the stitches and it hurt and then it went down again. I was driving a truck at that time and that vibrates. So it was "up and down, up and down" and it was hurting a lot. I was going around with the bandage on for two weeks and then it was taken off. Then trying to have sex after that, I had to wait another week because the first time I tried it it hurt too much. I just couldn't do it. Then after the third week I tried it again. It felt completely different. It was good. The only thing was, the moment I was going to come it started hurting so much that I couldn't the first few times.

R: Your experience reminds me very much of what a woman goes through if she has an episiotomy or tearing after she's had a baby.

J: I don't know. But the whole thing ... it's nothing very difficult. For the first two days it was hard. I didn't know which way to sleep and it always seemed to touch something. But after that it's just a slight irritation. It's nothing very bothersome.

R: You were not circumcised as an infant because you were born in Germany.

J: In Germany they don't do it. It never bothered me, not being circumcised.

R: They put you out for the operation. When a newborn is circumcised, he is awake and feels all of it. Would you have allowed them to do the operation to you without anesthesia like that?

J: NO!! Oh No!!!!!

R: Yet that's the way it's done to babies!! Their feelings are just as strong and important at that age.

J: Well, I really don't think that it's necessary to have it done. I see no reason for [infant] circumcision apart from ritual. My parents brought me up, teaching me that I have to clean under there, and I was clean. So I don't know why they do circumcision to babies. I don't think it's unhealthy.

R: You and your wife are expecting a baby. If your baby is a boy, will you have him circumcised?

J: No, I don't want to do it. If he wants to have it done as an adult, or younger like at age 14 or 15, I think he can make the decision.

R: It is more expensive.

J: Yeah, it cost $600. I was lucky because I was insured through my work and I could give it as a medical reason. I don't know how it is if somebody does it for so-called "beauty" reasons! I don't think insurance would pay for it. But $600 is a lot of money and that was in 1974. Today I don't know how much it would cost.

R: So if you have a son you will be able to teach him how to clean under his foreskin.

J: I think he's going to wash every day anyway. That's just another part of your body. He can pull the foreskin back and wash under it. It's just like blowing your nose or brushing your teeth.

R: Do you wish that you had been circumcised as an infant so that you would never have gone through it at age 22?

J: No, not at all. It was just a slight irritation. It was nothing that bad.

R: You were an adult and could understand what was happening to you.

J: Yes.

R: Babies are little and cannot understand what is happening to them.

J: I'm sure that it hurts. It's funny, because in Germany you never even hear about it because nobody is circumcised.

Johannes was a very "together" person who was equally content with his intact and circumcised conditions. He was not traumatized by the operation, nor was he embarrassed about this interview.

I find his experience an excellent challenge to the popular belief that "newborn babies should be circumcised because it is 'so much more painful' when it is done to an adult."

In the United States doctors tend to consider the foreskin as something "dispensable". A wart on an ear is not corrected by cutting off the entire ear, nor is a wart on a finger cured by amputation of the finger. Had Johannes been living in Germany when he developed this condition, his doctor would probably not have cut off the entire foreskin to get rid of the warts.

It is difficult to ascertain the true percentage of actual need for adult circumcision among intact males. In a circumcision-oriented society such as ours many doctors prescribe the operation for conditions which could be resolved, often easily, without resort to surgery. In other countries where male circumcision is not the norm, few, if any, males ever undergo circumcision, regardless of the condition of their foreskins. European, African, or Asian foreskins are not inherently different from American foreskins. This suggests that cultural influences rather than true medical need have caused many American doctors to recommend circumcision.

Additionally, some American men elect to be circumcised for "personal" (i.e., conformity) reasons. As a rule, insurance companies will pay for adult circumcision if it is medically prescribed, but will not pay if it is merely a "cosmetic" procedure. Therefore, many doctors will list a "medical" reason for circumcision on the patient's charts so that insurance will be collected. This practice obviously distorts the data on the actual necessity of adult circumcision.

Regardless of the likelihood or unlikelihood of eventual circumcision if it is not done in infancy, the argument that all infant males should be foreskin-deprived because some may need it later in life is analogous to a similar proposal to cut off the breasts of all women because some may eventually need mastectomies.

10 Foreskin Restoration

I was born in 1940 in an Army hospital. A circumcision was performed approximately six hours after birth.

I cannot pinpoint the exact time when the realization came that I was damaged, incomplete. My early recollection around the age of 4 years was that something was missing, and with it an intense feeling of loss coupled with a complete lack of understanding as to what had happened. The overwhelming feeling was not that I was simply different, but that something was *terribly wrong*. During grade school years I can remember the depression I felt when I realized that the scar signified amputation. Something had been cut off of me that other boys had. Why me? Did I do something wrong? Was this a punishment? If other boys had foreskins why didn't I have mine? They could appear circumcised by simply retracting their foreskins, but there was no way that I could gather enough skin to cover the head of my penis to look non-circumcised. My circumcision was exceedingly tight. Some three-quarters of the shaft skin had been amputated. I was literally "scalped." In addition, I had curious "bumps" along the scar line which were painful to the touch and the glans was often painfully abraded even to the point of bleeding, by the rubbing of underwear. Also there were "holes" in several places around the scar lines with one particularly large hole created by an unhealed flap of skin where the frenulum had been severed about ¼ inch from the glans. Thirty years later, I learned that the "bumps" were granulomas just under the skin surface involved in nerve damage and that the flaps were left over from sutures and uneven healing.

One particularly vivid memory as a first grader is an afternoon spent trying to pull enough skin over the glans to create a foreskin and keep it in place with a band aid. Using six year old logic, I thought that this would allow the skin to "grow out." That afternoon was a study in frustration, pain, panic and inadequacy. Even so, I remember trying other ways during the next few years – adhesive tape, clay, cardboard – anything I could think of which might force the stump of skin to cover the head.

By the time I was in high school, my masculine identity had been established as one of every other male being better than I was. If he was uncircumcised, he was complete and therefore better. If he was circumcised, he was *also* better than me because (apparently) he was not troubled by it as I was.

When I was in high school I began some preliminary research into circumcision, the medical reasons which were given at the time and the religious issues. Although there was precious little written dissent from medical authorities, I began to have more and more difficulty with the basic logic of such surgery. Over the years as isolated bits of research would debunk one more of the "reasons," I became more and more angry and dissatisfied both with the fact of my circumcision and *especially* the manner of it, a real "hack job." I also began developing associated problems with overweight, depression, poor school adjustment and peer group social problems. The ability to focus on daily living was becoming increasingly difficult. And the worst of it was that there was *not one person, adult or peer, that I was able to talk to!!* A couple of initial attempts had been met with either complete amusement or total embarrassment. One learns very quickly to keep controversial problems a secret! Even so, I was unwilling to accept my circumcised state, especially considering the poor results and the continuing pain and abrasions.

By the time I entered college I had researched enough to know that many peoples of the world were never circumcised and the dire predictions of American physicians toward the uncircumcised seemed totally unrealistic. I concluded that circumcision was a ritual peculiar to only some peoples, and that in terms of medical practice, an amputation had been performed for *no reason* other than the obstetrician's faith in a medical practice currently in vogue. (How any rational person can honestly believe that the cutting off of a piece of skin will save him from disease or make him religious is still beyond me!)

In the more cosmopolitan atmosphere of college, I was able to share my thoughts with some peers without the devastating reactions of the earlier attempts. This provided a safety valve of sorts while I continued collecting data with the added facet of medical reports concerning surgical repairs. Very little was available, but what there was convinced me that there should be some way of, if not reconstructing a foreskin, at least alleviating my pain problems. I consulted a physician who could not conceive of anyone wanting a foreskin. He did not comprehend the pain I was having, but he did surgically remove in an office procedure under a local anesthetic the largest (and unsightliest) granuloma on the dorsal scar. The result was a little less pain in one spot and the beginning of an earnest search to find a doctor who could and would undertake to repair and reconstruct. A number of initial inquiries were met with such ridicule that it literally threw me back for long recovery periods until I would get up the courage to try again with the almost sure knowledge that I would be subjected to more ridicule. I tried the family doctor and while not ridiculed directly was given a pat on the head and an immediate appointment with a psychiatrist. This particular psychiatrist was such a complete fiasco and so filled with hostility that it took me several years to revive the courage to approach anyone again. I wrote letters to some plastic surgeons. When there was a reply it was judgmental, curt, and unemotional: "There is no reason to attempt this, and no way to do it!" I tried a local plastic surgeon who had the cruelest diagnosis of all: "Yes," he said, "It is possible to create a tube of skin surgically from a graft, *but under no circumstances would I do it!"* That rebuff took me another several years to reconcile. I wrote to Ann Landers and got a gentle admonishment to try a psychiatrist as quickly as possible. The inequity of the whole thing really depressed me. Here I found it acceptable, even encouraged, for any man to walk in off the street to any doctor and have a circumcision performed and be considered to have made an appropriate and laudable choice. On the other hand, let someone come along who wishes to be *uncircumcised* and he is immediately psychologically suspect! (One head of a psychiatric clinic once told me that *all men* who had a wish to be uncircumcised were paranoid, schizophrenic personalities!)

Some years later I tried the family doctor again and managed to convince him that I was in constant pain and irritation, and serious about repair. This time he made a medical referral which quickly led to a series of doctors. I finally met Dr. Don Greer of the University of Texas Medical School Plastic Surgery Department. He was the first to spend any amount of non-judgmental time and give any positive confirmation to the availability of surgical repair and reconstruction techniques. Although the idea of creating a foreskin was unique to him, he agreed to research medical and surgical angles for six months and I was to undergo some therapy as a pre-surgical requirement. If, in six months he found there was adequate plastic surgical technique available to produce the desired results *and* if I still wanted to gamble, then we would go ahead.

The empathy and perception of this man to be able to see through all the years of anger, pain, frustration and rejection was no less than a miracle.

The initial surgical procedure was completed in May of 1977. A double pedicle graft was raised from the lower scrotal area approximately 6" by 2" and imbedded into a complete circular incision over the original circumcision site. The residual membranes were turned over the glans creating a foreskin with about 4/5 coverage of the glans. The hospital stay was five days and a catheter was in place for some 12 days. Post-operative swelling was considerable but the complete graft "took" and in a second and third procedure, the two connective pedicles were cut free and the newly constructed foreskin was utilizing its own internally generated blood supply. Two subsequent operations a year later removed scar tissue and repositioned some of the pedicle closure areas. There is still some swelling as the lymphatic system slowly regenerates. There is a marked reduction in pain due to the excision of the granulomas. There is still extreme sensitivity of the glans to pain, however, the coverage of the glans renders it much less subject to the daily stresses of underwear abrasion. A vein system has grown across the surgical line and there is some return of gross feeling in the graft, although by no means is it the equivalent of a natural foreskin.

While I can understand the motive of the obstetrician in performing circumcisions according to the practices of his time, I can never forgive him the fact that he botched the procedure miserably. I have been subjected to an amputation for *no good reason*, without my consent (or my parents – they were *not* asked!) and to which I would *never* have agreed had I been consulted.

As of this writing, five restoration surgeries have been performed here. Three more are scheduled for the coming year. The number of surgical steps has been reduced as has the time between the steps.

Research has revealed that these procedures have been performed throughout history. In the United States currently there are a number of people who have had such repairs done.

Intensive psychiatric testing and evaluation has shown that there are no psychiatric reasons for withholding this type of surgery other than the physical and emotional inability to withstand surgical stress in itself.

People should realize that just because there is a repair procedure, one should not go ahead and cut a baby because it can be fixed later. It is far from easy and while the results are entirely satisfactory, it must be emphasized that this is *not* a *natural* foreskin and never will be. The sensitivity and some of the mechanical subtleties of the natural foreskin are lost forever.

John Strand, San Antonio, TX

10.1 Informational Resources

- 8 '-Ates' of Foreskin Restoration: apollotechonline.com/pdffiles/8-Ates_Of_Foreskin_Restoration.pdf
- A father's talk with his son about infant circumcision:
    restoringtally.com/blog/2010/03/fathers-talk-his-son-about-infant-circumcision
- A Successful Restoration Regimen: norm.org/regimen.html
- A Technique for Foreskin Reconstruction and Some Preliminary Results: cirp.org/library/restoration/greer1
- An Open Letter to the American Academy of Pediatrics:
    science20.com/crawler_superland/blog/open_letter_american_academy_pediatrics-93830
- Attention Cut Guys: Foreskin Regeneration Therapy Might Be On Its Way: towleroad.com/2015/02/foreskin
- Baby bottle nipple retainers: restoringtally.com/blog/2009/12/baby-bottle-nipple-retainers
- BC man's foreskin op a success *(repair of adult botched circumcision)*:
    nationalreviewofmedicine.com/issue/2006/06_30/3_patients_practice01_12.html
- Beginner's Guide to Foreskin Restoration: restoringforeskin.org/beginners-guide-foreskin-restoration
- Benefits of foreskin restoration – Part 1: Sensitivity:
    restoringtally.com/blog/2009/11/benefits-foreskin-restoration-part-1-sensitivity
- Benefits of foreskin restoration – Part 2: Newfound Well-being:
    restoringtally.com/blog/2009/11/benefits-foreskin-restoration-part-2-newfound-well-being
- Bloodstained Men & Their Friends: facebook.com/BloodstainedMenTheirFriends
- Boys and the Hood: pool.intactiwiki.org/wiki/File:Fs2301.pdf

- Boys and Their Hoods: westword.com/news/boys-and-their-hoods-5056869
- Category: Foreskin restoration *(IntactiWiki)*: en.intactiwiki.org/wiki/Category:Foreskin_restoration
- Circumcised as boys, thousands of men are restoring their foreskins: pool.intactiwiki.org/images/Fs14.pdf
- Circumcised Men Do Complain: facebook.com/circumcisedmencomplain
- Circumcised Men May Soon Be Able To Regrow Foreskin, Thanks To Science:
    199.188.247.58/post/circumcised-men-may-soon-be-able-regrow-foreskin-thanks-science
- Circumcised men may soon be able to REGROW their foreskin: New technique could help increasing number of men angry they were given the procedure: dailymail.co.uk/health/article-2958422
- Circumcision circumspection: Weigh the facts before making the call:
    cirp.org/news/chicagotribune2007-01-09/
- Circumcision Reversal Gains in Popularity: noharmm.org/reversal.htm
- Circumcision, Child Rights, and Sex Abuse:
    web.archive.org/web/20021012100726/http://www.angelfire.com/nm/helthe/childrights.html
- Coverage Index: How much foreskin do you have?: restoringforeskin.org/coverage-index/CI-chart.htm
- Each Year, over 1 million baby boys lose part of their body:
    facebook.com/photo.php?fbid=10203171066632303&set=p.10203171066632303
- Famous men who resent/ed being circumcised: circumstitions.com/resent-celebs.html
- Film Tube Foreskin Restoration Method:
    apollotechonline.com/pdffiles/Film%20Tube%20Foreskin%20Restoration.pdf
- For treating "Phimosis": pages.suddenlink.net/manual_methods/phimosis.html
- foregen: Regenerating the foreskin with its natural benefits and functions: foregen.org
- Foreskin and several years from now: salon.com/1999/12/17/tuggers
- Foreskin restoration: cirp.org/pages/restore.html
- Foreskin Restoration: foreskin.gc.bz/other_historical.php
- Foreskin Restoration – a growing movement: circumstitions.com/Restore.html
- Foreskin Restoration (Saving Our Sons): www.savingsons.org/2009/10/foreskin-restoration.html
- Foreskin Restoration FAQ:
    apollotechonline.com/pdffiles/Foreskin%20Restoration%20-%20Frequently%20Asked%20Questions.pdf
- Foreskin restoration growing in popularity in Australia:
    aussiepenis.com/2013/10/09/foreskin-restoration-growing-in-popularity-in-australia
- Foreskin Restoration Intactivist Network: foreskinrestoration.vbulletin.net
- Foreskin Restoration Intactivist Network – Forum: foreskinrestoration.vbulletin.net/forum
- Foreskin Restoration is a non-surgical process: apollotechonline.com
- Foreskin Restoration. Everything you need to know: facebook.com/notes/james-ketter/foreskin-restoration-everything-you-need-to-know-an-faq/1530401383879668
- Foreskin Restore: foreskinrestore.com
- Friendly Plastic for Foreskin Restoration:
    apollotechonline.com/pdffiles/Friendly%20Plastic%20Foreskin%20Restoration.pdf
- Getting Back What was Lost: A Journey to Foreskin Restoration:

- thewholenetwork.org/twn-news/a-journey-to-foreskin-restoration
- Gimme Some Skin: stylemens.typepad.com/details__details/2008/09/gimme-some-skin.html
- Greg's T-Tape Strips and Insert:
  www.restoringforeskin.org/images/greg_b-t-tape-strips-and-insert-Ilustrated.pdf
- How One Company Aims to Help Circumcised Men Grow Their Foreskin Back:
  vice.com/en/article/pgawqg/regrowing-foreskins-like-salamander-arms
- How to start restoring your foreskin: restoringtally.com/blog/2010/06/how-start-restoring-your-foreskin
- HyperRestore: hyperrestore.com
- I am circumcised and Hate it: facebook.com/IAmCircumcisedAndHateIt
- I AM NOT THANKFUL: facebook.com/IAmNotThankful
- I LOVE foreskin: restoringtally.com/blog/2011/03/i-love-foreskin
- I Survived Mutilation: facebook.com/ISurvivedMutilation
- I was circumcised and I want my foreskin back!: pool.intactiwiki.org/wiki/File:Fs34.pdf
- I'm circumcised – can my foreskin be restored? *(negative doctor response, denial of loss of sensitivity through circumcision)*:
  netdoctor.co.uk/ask-the-expert/sex-faqs/a11799/im-circumcised-8211-can-my-foreskin-be-restored
- In defense of the foreskin: salon.com/2012/12/24/in_defense_of_the_foreskin
- 'Intactivists' Seek to Undo A Long-Practiced Ritual: cirp.org/news/wsj12-28-00
- Is circumcision reversal possible?:
  jamaicaobserver.com/magazines/AllWoman/Is-circumcision-reversal-possible-_14620467
- Local men restoring their foreskins: pool.intactiwiki.org/wiki/File:Fs17.pdf
- Low Cost Device Using a Funnel: norm.org/funnel.html
- Manual restoration methods: pages.suddenlink.net/manual_methods/aboutmethods.html
- Manual tugging: restoringforeskin.org/category/public/foreskin-restoration-methods/manual-tugging
- Manual Tugging Squeeze-Stretch Technique:
  restoringforeskin.org/public/manual-tugging/squeeze-stretch-method
- Measuring foreskin restoration progress:
  restoringtally.com/blog/2009/12/measuring-foreskin-restoration-progress
- Meet the circumcised men who want their foreskins back:
  mamamia.com.au/meet-the-circumcised-men-who-want-their-foreskins-back
- Men Do Complain (The Effect of Male Circumcision on the Enjoyment of the Female Partner):
  mendocomplain.com
- Men Missing Foreskin Fume On Forums: huffpost.com/entry/4072048
- Men who resent being circumcised: circumstitions.com/Resent.html
- Mourning a Foreskin: tikkun.org/mourning-a-foreskin
- Multiple O-Rings for Foreskin Restoration: iomfats.org/resources/restoring/media/Multiple_o-ring_update.pdf
- My responses to a few Frequently Asked Questions about Non-Surgical Foreskin Restoration:
  iomfats.org/resources/restoring/media/restoring_faq.pdf
- Non-surgical Foreskin Restoration *(BUFF method)*: pool.intactiwiki.org/images/Fs01.pdf

- NORM: The National Organization of Restoring Men: norm.org
- "Parents love genital cutting more than they love their own children": Two "intactivists" tell Salon about foreskin restoration:
    salon.com/2015/01/31/%E2%80%9Cparents_love_genital_cutting_more_than_they_love_their_own_children%E2%80%9D_two_intactivists_tell_salon_about_foreskin_restoration
- People who regret genital cutting: circumstitions.com/regret.html
- Photos showing an average penis with an average infant circumcision in various kinds of restoration devices:
    web.archive.org/web/20120112153216/https://adult.eskimo.com/~gburlin/restore/image.html
- Pictures and videos of my restored foreskin *(an album full of statements from unhappily circumcised men)*:
    foreskinrestore.com/restored_foreskin.html
- Resources for Foreskin Restoration: iomfats.org/resources/restoring/resourcelist.html
- Restoration Archive and F.A.Q. (The Restoration Mailing List):
    web.archive.org/web/20070925085148/http://www.eskimo.com/~gburlin/restore/archivefaq2.htm
- Restoration Devices: norm.org/devices.html
- Restoration Product Comparison: norm-wi.org/compare.htm
- Restoring For Men: restoringforeskin.org
- S.T.O.R.M Foreskin Restoration (Staggered Tapered O-Ring Method):
    apollotechonline.com/pdffiles/STORM%20O-Ring%20Foreskin%20Restoration.pdf
- Second skin now an option: www.starobserver.com.au/news/second-skin-now-an-option/11
- Sensitivity Is the Rising Issue on Circumcision: cirp.org/library/restoration/pertot
- Sexology, Body Image, Foreskin Restoration, and Bisexual Status: jstor.org/stable/3812956
- Sore point: Circumcision – beloved by the Victorians, crucial to two of the world's great religions, arguably a health boon – can be a cause of great anguish: theguardian.com/society/2005/oct/29/health.religion
- Surgical methods of restoring the prepuce: cirp.org/library/restoration/brandes1
- Suspended Weights / GravityForeskin Restoration Method:
    apollotechonline.com/pdffiles/Suspended%20Weights%20Foreskin%20Restoration.pdf
- T-Tape Foreskin Restoration Method: apollotechonline.com/pdffiles/T-Tape%20Foreskin%20Restoration.pdf
- The Fantastic Foreskin: houstonpress.com/news/the-fantastic-foreskin-6575549
- The Foreskin Flap: chicagoreader.com/chicago/the-foreskin-flap/Content?oid=886868
- The Foreskin Renaissance: goodmenproject.com/health/the-foreskin-renaissance
- The Great Uncircumcision Debate: content.time.com/time/health/article/0,8599,1679981,00.html
- The Intact-ivists: narratively.com/the-intact-ivists
- The joy of uncircumcising: cirp.org/library/restoration/anonymous1
- The ManHood – Underwear for circumcised men:
    restoringtally.com/blog/2012/02/the-manhood-underwear-for-circumcised-men
- The men who want their foreskins back *(IntactiWiki)*: pool.intactiwiki.org/wiki/File:Fs37.pdf
- The Real Coverage Index – RCI: restoringforeskin.org/public/foreskin-restoration-real-coverage-index-rci
- There's A Movement For Men To Regrow Their Foreskin: buzzfeed.com/abagg/regrow-your-foreskin
- These men want their foreskins back: nbcnews.com/id/wbna3543481

- They took my foreskin and I want it back: independent.co.uk/life-style/health-and-families/health-news/health-they-took-my-foreskin-and-i-want-it-back-some-men-feel-their-circumcision-at-birth-was-an-assault-now-they-can-be-uncircumcised-without-surgery-writes-cherrill-hicks-1458890.html
- TLC Tugger *(foreskin restoration)*: tlctugger.com
- Transforming your penis *(graphic pictures, IntactiWiki)*:
  https://pool.intactiwiki.org/wiki/File:Fs4501.jpg + pool.intactiwiki.org/wiki/File:Fs4501.jpg
- Uncircumcised: Foreskin Restoration: pool.intactiwiki.org/images/Fs1305.pdf
- Uncircumcising: Undoing the Effects of an Ancient Practice in a Modern World:
  cirp.org/library/restoration/bigelow1
- Uncircumcision *(Tushmet)*: cirp.org/library/restoration/tushmet1
- Uncircumcision: A Historical Review of Preputial Restoration: cirp.org/library/restoration/schultheiss
- Uncutting: uncutting.tumblr.com/tagged/foreskin%20restoration
- What is Foreskin Restoration?: restoringtally.com/blog/2009/11/what-foreskin-restoration
- What Kind of Tape is the Best to Use?: norm.org/faq.html#Tape
- Why Should I Restore?: norm.org/whyrestore.html
- Willy Nilly: metroactive.com/papers/metro/01.27.00/foreskin-0004.html

Videos:

- I'm a victim of brit milah – the government should have protected me: youtu.be/GVO6YzROkZE
- My Circumcision *(Jewish man commenting on video of his own circ)*: youtu.be/VJ8Kt6Vu4oE

11 Complications of Circumcision

All medical procedures, especially those involving surgery, can and do result in complications. Circumcision is certainly no exception.

Parents rarely know even the simplest details about infant circumcision.

Much less often do they have any awareness that the operation can have complications. Even doctors are frequently unaware of the many complications that can result from circumcision. Commonly doctors pronounce infant circumcision a "simple operation with few risks." The procedure is easy to perform. However, the risks are many and can be devastating and tragic.

Many of the complications listed here are admittedly rare. Some are obscure enough to be medical curiosities. A doctor practicing over an entire lifetime, performing or seeing the results of thousands of circumcisions may never see or hear of some of these complications.

Meatal ulceration, the first condition discussed in this chapter, results from ammoniacal urine burns on the unprotected glans of the circumcised infant. This is extremely common among circumcised infants during the diaper wearing period. Possibly over half of all circumcised infants develop this.

The other listed complications are uncommon. All of these put together probably involve 5-10% of all circumcisions. (It is difficult to accurately document the precise rates of circumcision complications because some difficulties are either never reported or are never attributed to circumcision.) Therefore a parent having one's son circumcised can be assured of an approximate 90-95% chance that the wound will heal normally without undue bleeding or infection, and that the outcome will be a "normal" circumcised penis.

Some of the complications of circumcision are easily resolved. Others have resulted in disastrous consequences, pain, trauma, psychological ill effects, prolonged hospitalization, tremendous expenses, lifelong mutilation, and death. When viewed in terms of *percentages*, the fact that some of these complications occur in one out of several hundred or thousand infant circumcisions, the risks seem insignificant. But when viewed in terms of *individuals* and *families* involved in these tragic events – particularly when the operation is *unnecessary*, the risks are quite significant.

Parents who give birth in hospitals often do not change diapers or see their babies' bodies during the entire hospital stay. Therefore, the circumcision wound may be nearly healed by the time they see the baby's penis. Some complications arise during the first few days in the hospital of which the parents are never aware.

Sylvia Topp points out:

"One doctor says that on his daily hospital rounds in New York he frequently finds babies with ugly granulating wounds and others requiring surgical treatment to stop bleeding. Many of these results are remedied by the hospital staff without *ever* bringing them to the attention of the babies' parents." [1]

Interestingly, some doctors, upon reviewing the complications of circumcision, merely conclude by calling for greater skill and care upon operating rather than questioning this unnecessary operation. Perhaps they are too conditioned by society to think of foreskins as having any purpose other than being something to cut off. Or perhaps they feel that it would be overly idealistic to try to change the situation.

Upon reviewing the literature, nearly all from medical publications, I have discovered 28 different complications that can result from circumcision. Some of these interrelate or cause other complications. They are listed here in approximate order of frequency:

11.1 Meatal Ulceration

Many infants and toddlers in diapers develop "urine burns" from contact with ammonia in urine-soaked diapers. This is unquestionably painful for the child. The glans consists of sensitive, delicate tissue, and is intended to be protected by the thicker, less sensitive foreskin. The destruction of the foreskin creates an abnormal state in which the glans is exposed and in constant contact with outer clothing, and for the infant, with urine soaked diapers. Ammonia burns on the glans, especially around the urinary opening, called the meatus, can be a particularly troublesome problem for the circumcised male infant.

Two of my own three (circumcised) sons had this problem during infancy. When my second son was around 8 months old he developed blisters in his diaper area and a whitish, eroded area around the urinary opening of his glans. As time went on it became crusty. Several nurses at a local "well-baby-clinic" were unable to identify the condition. The doctor (who had delivered and circumcised him) gave it little concern, prescribed a topical ointment, and apparently was unaware that this was a complication of circumcision. Likewise, a relative who is a family doctor, when shown the condition, remarked that this was a fairly common problem that baby boys had, and had little concern or awareness about it. The problem persisted until my son was completely out of diapers. By the time he was three his glans was thick and leathery in appearance. This is skin which is supposed to be like the delicate tissue inside the mouth!

---

1 Topp S. The Argument Over Circumcision – The Case Against. *The Village Voice*. 1975-06-16: 9.

Later, my third son also developed meatal ulceration. His was not nearly as severe as Jason's had been. By this time the research for this book was underway and I readily recognized the condition.

Meatal ulceration is clinically described as follows:

"... The lesion manifests itself as a rather superficial ulceration about the meatus. From what we know about the development of similar ulcers in the diaper region due to the same cause, it is probably preceded by a vesicle [blister] ... At times the ulcer becomes deep and extensive, up to 2 mm. in depth and more than 5 mm. in width. Usually it is more or less covered by a crust which is very firmly attached over a considerable area. Surrounding the ulcer there is often an area of inflammation which involves both the adjacent surface of the glans and extends into the urethral opening with consequent narrowing. In the severer cases there are commonly present at the same time erythema [redness], vesication [blistering], and ulceration of the glans, scrotum, and the rest of the diaper region wherever the diaper is in intimate contact with the skin." [2]

"Many children have this ammoniacal diaper [condition] for weeks and months without any unpleasant symptoms. Usually it produces at least a local redness and subsequent desquamation of a large part of the diaper region. In severer cases there is scattered vesication and ulceration. These ulcers often remain denuded for a long time, often they heal over but remain as discrete nodules during the whole time that the ammoniacal condition persists. Often the exposed meatus is the only seat of a deeper lesion; rarely it escapes; as a rule, it is involved with the rest of the diaper region ... The male meatus is peculiarly [?] exposed to such contact, and the delicate mucous membrane is the most vulnerable spot; the female meatus is well protected and is apparently rarely if ever involved." [3]

The incidence of meatal ulceration among circumcised infants is very common. Kaplan estimates an incidence of between 8% and 31%.[4]

Mackenzie found an incidence of 20% meatal ulceration upon following up 140 infants whom he had circumcised, and then examined within the next few weeks. He commented that:

---

[2] Brennemann J. The Ulcerated Urethral Meatus in the Circumcised Child. *Am J Dis Child.* 1920; 21: 39.
[3] Ibid., p. 41.
[4] Kaplan GW. "Circumcision – An Overview" Current Problems. In: *Pediatrics Year Book.* Chicago, IL: Medical Publishers; 1977: 23-4.

11 – Complications of Circumcision

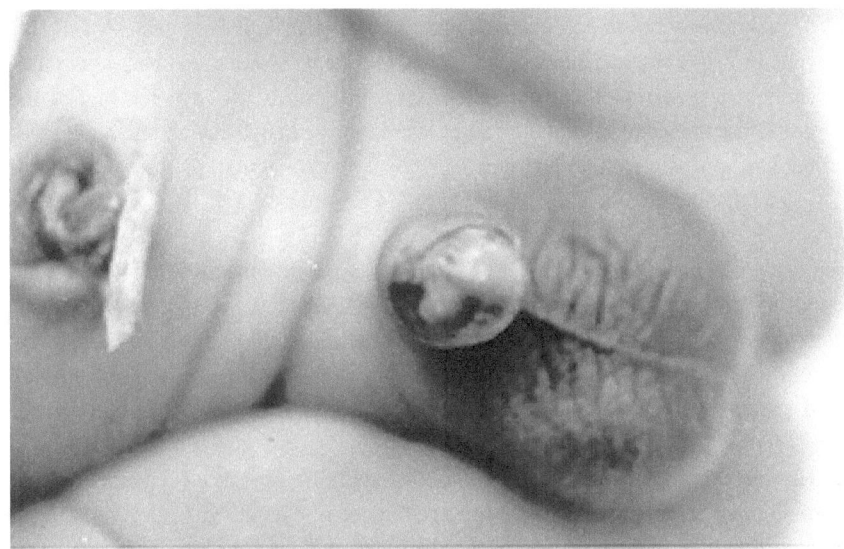

Meatal Ulceration. Photograph contributed by John C. Glaspey, MD.

"Several of the mothers whose infants were seen later reported that ulceration had been present and had healed. Such cases were not included since the ulceration had not been observed by me ..." [5]

The true incidence of meatal ulceration is undoubtedly much higher than reported. Many cases are undoubtedly treated by the parents with over-the-counter ointments and are never brought to the doctor's attention. Meatal ulceration appears to become more troublesome as the infant becomes older. The urine of a newborn, totally breastfed infant is quite mild, but as his diet becomes more varied more ammonia is produced. Older babies and toddlers are not taken to the doctor as frequently as are newborns. Additionally, some doctors see instances of meatal ulceration but fail to recognize or note the condition.

Since meatal ulceration usually does not manifest itself during the *immediate* aftermath of circumcision, many authorities have failed to recognize it as a complication of circumcision.

Mackenzie comments:

"Ulceration of the meatus is generally not recognized by obstetricians as a complication of neonatal circumcision. Speert failed to mention it in a series of 10,802. Hovsepian reported 1,844 circumcisions without tabulating the number

---

[5] MacKenzie AR. Meatal Ulceration Following Neonatal Circumcision. *Obstet Gynecol.* 1966-08; 28(2): 222.

of infants who developed meatal ulceration. Moeller and Moss evaluated the results in 2,400 circumcisions as uniformly excellent. Manson claimed no complications in a series of 387 circumcisions ... Pediatricians have recognized the greater incidence of meatal ulceration in circumcised boys than in uncircumcised, but have not related it to the immediate postoperative period, thereby more closely establishing circumcision as the cause." [5]

Ironically, parents upon contemplating circumcision are frequently warned about the supposed "problems" that the child will have if he keeps his foreskin and are given the erroneous advice that the penis of the circumcised child requires *no* care. Many doctors who regularly treat the sore, eroded, and encrusted glans of the circumcised child apparently lack awareness that the protective foreskin would have prevented this.

The foreskin of the intact infant can occasionally become reddened and swollen. Some doctors believe that this is an indication for immediate circumcision. Others believe that all infant males should be deprived of their foreskins to prevent this occurrence. In actuality the swollen, red foreskin is performing its function of protecting the sensitive glans from *more* painful and troublesome irritation.

Hutchings comments:

"Now this condition of a red swollen prepuce is, in fact, a very good reason for *not* having the operation done.

... One of the main constituents of urine is a substance known as urea. Certain germs from the bowel can alter urea to form ammonia, and the red area ... is a small burn caused by the action of ammonia ...

If circumcision is performed, the ammonia can now burn the meatus instead of the prepuce and thus produce a small ulcer. When this ulcer heals a tiny scar forms, resulting in a slight constriction at the meatus.

The logical treatment of such an ammonia burn is not to circumcise the child, but to attack the cause, i.e., the ammonia itself." [6]

Treatment for ammonia burns varies. The child's diet appears to contribute to the development of ammonia. Yet another advantage of breastfeeding is hereby discovered. According to Brenneman: "It is almost unknown in the nursing baby." [7] (I presume that he means the *totally* nursing baby. My two sons were both still nursing – although eating many other foods – when they developed meatal ulceration.)

---

6   Hutchings G. Notes on the Care of Uncircumcised Infants. (Originally printed in the *New Zealand Doctor*.) INTACT *Educational Foundation* reprint.
7   Brennemann, p. 42.

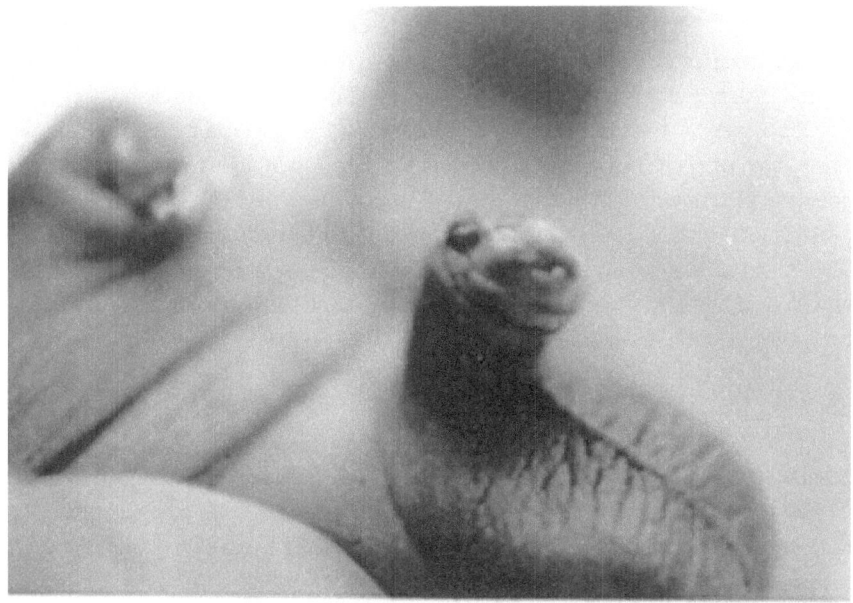

Meatal Ulceration. Photograph contributed by John C. Glaspey, M.D.

Brenneman cites the following theory:

"... based on the work of Keller and others that in certain nutritional disturbances due to the ingestion of cow's milk fat beyond the infant's tolerance there is produced a relative acidosis of enteric origin which manifests itself in the urine in the excretion of a hypernormal amount of ammonium salts ..." [8]

Mild topical ointments are usually recommended for meatal ulceration and other urine burns. Petroleum jelly, or petroleum-based germ killing substances containing antibiotics are often prescribed. The parent should consult their child's doctor about the appropriate ointment to use.

Some authorities emphasize careful washing of cloth diapers, as ammonia residues can build up in diapers if they are not thoroughly rinsed and washed. Boiling diapers, use of non-detergent soaps, several rinse cycles, and adding vinegar to the final rinse have all been advised.[9]

---

8 Ibid., p. 43.
9 Schlosberg C. Thirty Years of Ritual Circumcisions. *CLP*. 1971-04; 10(4): 208.

Frequent, conscientious diaper changing is especially important if the child is irritated by ammonia burns. However, if he takes long naps or sleeps through the night, his skin is still in contact with urine-soaked diapers for several hours.

Out of personal experience I have found that either disposable diapers or diaper liners, both of which draw urine away from the baby's skin, help to protect him from contact with ammonia.

(Author's update: Today use of cloth diapers is far less common than it was in the 1970's and 80's. I would be curious to know whether or not meatal ulceration and ammonia irritation is more or less common today with nearly universal use of disposable diapers in the United States. – R.R.)

11.2 Meatal Stricture

Meatal stricture results from prolonged or repeated episodes of meatal ulceration. The repeatedly irritated meatus becomes narrowed. This results in pain and difficulty with urination. In extreme cases this can result in infections and kidney problems.

Brenneman describes this:

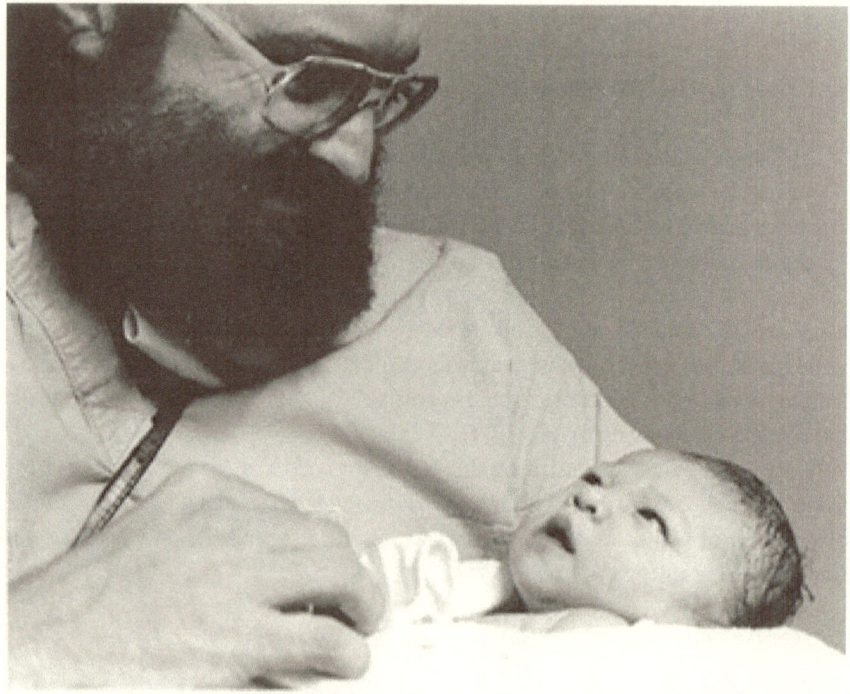

© Suzanne Arms

"The urethral opening is nearly always narrowed, often so much that the urinary stream is threadlike and the urine can be expelled only with evident effort ... [He describes a] scab that forms on the ulcerated area. This is very adherent and can hardly be removed without tearing and bleeding of the denuded and adjacent portion of the glans. This is practically always accompanied by a narrowing of the meatus, and it is at times impossible to tell whether the occlusion is due chiefly to the scab or to the narrowing of the urethra itself." [7]

One doctor claims that different types of circumcision devices result in varying degrees of "pinpoint meatus," stating that the Plastibell results in more incidence of narrowed meatus.[10]

Berry and Cross calibrated the urethral meatuses of 100 circumcised and 100 intact adult males, and did a similar study of 100 each of intact and circumcised infants. In both groups the urethral meatuses were significantly narrower among the circumcised individuals than among the intact individuals. Men undergoing circumcision early in life showed a higher incidence of meatal narrowing than did those circumcised later.

The results among infants were not as marked, indicating that narrowing of the meatus develops over time.[11]

The authors conclude:

"The results of this study suggest a relationship between meatal narrowing and circumcision, particularly when the procedure is done early in life. It is during that period that the meatus would be most vulnerable to irritation and trauma if not protected by the prepuce. A breakdown of the delicate mucosa of the urethral meatus, whether resulting from acute ulceration or low-grade inflammation, could result in eventual secondary stenosis of varying degree in many cases." [11]

Some authors believe meatal stricture to be hereditary, pointing to a familial pattern. What they may actually be observing is more likely a familial tradition of circumcised males.

Difficulty in urination is frequently a problem that results from urethral stricture. Campbell describes this:

"... straining to void, small stream, urination intermittent and painful. Mucoid discharge may be noted. Hernia may result from excessive straining. Enuresis

---

10 Graves J. Pinpoint Meatus: Iatrogenic? *Pediatrics*. 1968; 41: 1013.
11 Berry CD Jr, Cross RR Jr. Urethral Meatal Caliber in Circumcised and Uncircumcised Males. *AMA J Dis Child*. 1961-02; 107: 149.

[inability to control urine, bedwetting] may be present. Progressive renal [kidney] injury by urinary back-pressure with or without complicating infection, the systemic manifestations of urinary toxemia appear chiefly as gastrointestinal disturbances, anorexia [lack of appetite], or failure to grow. Hyperirritability or sluggishness may result from toxic effects on the central nervous system. With the advent of infection there may be a fever; the diagnosis of 'pyelitis' [kidney infection] is made." [12]

The most common treatment for the condition is "meatotomy" – a snipping of the urinary meatus to enlarge the opening.

Linshaw describes two infants who suffered from this condition:

"I have personally cared for two male infants under a year of age who had obstructive renal disease on the basis of meatal stenosis. One infant was irritable and fussy on urination, had occasional intermittency of his urinary stream, and had a palpable left kidney. The other infant presented with hematuria [blood in the urine]. Both infants had been circumcised and also had a tiny meatal opening ... A tiny pinpoint external meatus should warn the physician that obstructive renal disease is a real possibility." [13]

The incidence of enuresis (bedwetting, inability to control urine) caused by meatal stricture, resulting from the exposed, irritated glans due to lack of protective foreskin, is of particular interest in light of the earlier arguments given in favor of circumcision. Remondino and other turn-of-the-century writers listed enuresis among the alleged "dangers" of the foreskin. Evidence now indicates that the opposite is true. The *absence of foreskin* by exposing the glans to trauma and the urethra to stricture appears to be a *cause* of enuresis.

11.3   Hemorrhage

Hemorrhage is defined as excessive bleeding. It can result from any event that ruptures blood vessels, including any cut or surgical procedure. Hemorrhage is a fairly common complication of circumcision.

Shulman, Ben-Hur, & Newman list it as the most common (immediate) complication, and estimate that 2% of all circumcisions result in hemorrhage. They state

---

12 Campbell MF. Stricture of the Urethra in Children. *J Pediatr.* 1949; 35: 169.
13 Linshaw MA. Circumcision and Obstructive Renal Disease. *Pediatrics.* 1977-05; 59(5): 790.

that bleeding may be caused by inadequate hemostasis (compressing of blood vessels), by abnormalities of blood coagulation, or by anomalous vessels.[14]

The Plastibell device, in which a ring of plastic and remaining stump of foreskin are tied with a string, after which the foreskin atrophies and falls off, has been purported to prevent hemorrhage. However, one recent study evaluated 59 newborns who experienced hemorrhage following circumcision (out of 5,882 subjects) and noted that 29 of these had been circumcised with the Gomco clamp and 30 with the Plastibell. Apparently the Plastibell string was improperly tied.

Fortunately most cases of hemorrhage, if promptly treated, have been easily resolved. Treatments include application of adrenaline-soaked gauze sponge to the bleeding site, ligature (tying off) of a blood vessel, Gelfoam (chemical foam to stop bleeding), silver nitrate stick, or topically applied thrombin, retying of Plastibell string, and administration of cryoprecipitate.[15]

Occasionally babies have required blood transfusions as a result of post-circumcision hemorrhage. One doctor tells of his experience:

> "... I spent a considerable portion of one evening transfusing an infant circumcised by an expert Rabbi. The hemorrhage had to be controlled in the operating-room and the baby was hospitalized for two days ... I know of other cases needing transfusion under the same conditions and I have seen several babies considerably anemic owing to the insidious loss of blood which is easily overlooked for several hours." [16]

Modern clamp type devices seal the cut edges of skin. Normally infant circumcision is followed by very little bleeding. Today most doctors and mohelim use such devices. However, the Orthodox Jewish circumcisors do not use clamps. The incidences of hemorrhages resulting from such ritual circumcisions may be a result of not using a clamp device, rather than the skill of the operator.

Babies have died from post-circumcision hemorrhage. Since Biblical times the Jews have had a law that if two sons of the same mother bled to death following circumcision, any future sons were exempt from the ritual. This indicates that hemorrhage has *always* been a complication of circumcision. I have found no record of deaths from post-circumcision hemorrhage in the modern literature that I have reviewed. Obviously in past ages when blood transfusions and modern methods of treatment did not exist, such tragedies were more frequent.

---

14 Shulman J, Ben-Hur N, Neuman Z (Israel). Surgical Complications of Circumcision. *Am J Dis Child.* 1961-02; 107: 149.
15 Gee WF, Ansell JS. Neonatal Circumcision: A Ten-Year Overview. *Pediatrics.* 1976; 58: 827.
16 Banister PG. Circumcision. *Lancet.*

Finally, undetected hemophilia can produce drastic results if such an infant is circumcised. Occasionally hemophilia is discovered when the infant undergoes circumcision and subsequently hemorrhages:

> "Brian's birth ... was routine – until it came time for his circumcision. When it didn't heal properly, a hematologist was called in for consultation. Four days after Brian was born a physician told his parents [that he had hemophilia]." [17]

While it is hoped that in the future all parents will choose against circumcision, it must be emphasized that any parents who carry the genes for hemophilia should *definitely* not have their sons circumcised. Even parents who are convinced that their son's foreskin must be cut off, should have preliminary blood tests performed to rule out the defect. The hemophiliac infant *must* be left intact. The difference may mean life instead of death, or at least will prevent a drastic bleeding problem. Additionally the child's foreskin *must* be left alone until it is fully loosened of its own accord. Forceful retraction should not be done even to a normal child as it is painful and leads to problems. In the hemophiliac child this is especially important, because forceful retraction often results in slight bleeding, and even a slight injury can produce a severe hemorrhage for a hemophiliac.

11.4 Infection

Infection of the fresh circumcision wound has been a fairly common complication. I have found more reports of this incidence than of any other complication. Infection has occasionally been accompanied with disastrous results, including death. Some of the other complications described elsewhere in this chapter, such as loss of penile skin, have resulted from infection of the circumcision wound.

Any open area of skin is a potential avenue for infection. Because the freshly circumcised infant penis is in constant contact with wet and/or soiled diapers, this area cannot be kept sterile. Therefore it is unusually in danger of infection.

An infection would be accompanied by fever, pus, redness, and swelling.

Kaplan cites a post-circumcision infection rate as high as 8%.[18] While Rosner cites an extremely low rate of only one out of 10,802.[19] Gee & Ansell reported 23 infections out of 5,882 circumcised infants (0.4%).[15]

Of the 23 occurrences of post circumcision infection reported by Gee & Ansell, 4 followed use of the Gomco clamp and 19 followed use of the Plastibell. Critics of the

---

17 Gottschalk EC Jr. Living With Hemophilia. *Fam Circle*. 1979-04-24: 14.
18 Kaplan, p. 29.
19 Rosner F. Circumcision – Attempt at Clearer Understanding. *NY State J Med*. 1966-11-15: 2920-1.

Plastibell device often cite a greater possibility of infection. The remaining piece of foreskin tied to the plastic ring and left to dry up and fall off is in contact with wet diapers and therefore cannot be kept dry. Obviously this is a great potential site for infections.

Particularly antibiotic-resistant strains of bacteria and other infectious agents abound in hospitals. Newborn infants are not as able to resist infection as are older individuals who have built up more immunities. It is not uncommon for newborns in busy hospital nurseries to develop infections, particularly Staphylococcus-based. Sometimes babies do not manifest symptoms of infections until they are home from the hospital.

A 1960s study, investigating the effectiveness of hexachlorophene-based detergents in reducing infections, reported 3.15% of male infants and 1.38% of female infants experiencing staph infections. They cited the umbilical stump and the freshly circumcised penis as the major sites of highest concentrations of *Staphylococcus aureus* to be found, saying "the blood on the cord and the circumcised penis provide an excellent media for growing bacteria." [20]

A wide variety of different infections with the circumcision site as port of entry have been listed by different sources. Besides *Staphylococcus aureus*, other infections include *Staphylococcus epidemidis*, *Klebsiella pneumoniae*, *Escherichia coli*, and *Proteus mirabilis*.[15]

Scurlock and Pemberton report four cases of "fulminating neonatal sepsis with meningitis." In other words, infection of the circumcision site resulted in infection of the spinal cord and brain. Each case describes the infants as feverish, irritable, crying, with a swollen infected circumcision wound, lethargic, and not feeding. Further symptoms included pallor or cyanosis, "fits," apnea, bulging fontanelle, head retracted, and lumbar puncture revealing cloudy cerebral-spinal fluid containing the same bacteria present at the circumcision site. Two of the infants healed and recovered normally following treatment, one died, and one showed signs of cerebral palsy upon follow-up at 5 months.[21]

In another report Annunziato and Goldblum describe severe staphylococcus infections originating from the circumcision site which they call "scalded skin syndrome." They describe three cases of infants with skin red and peeling, pustules, circumcised area red, swollen, and covered with profuse thick, yellow-green exudate. The infants were feverish, lethargic, cyanotic, and had diarrhea. After administration of antibiotics, two infants healed normally and one died.[22]

20 Kravitz H, Murphy JB, Edadi K, Rosetti A, Ashraf H. Effects of Hexachlorophene-Detergent Baths in a Newborn Nursery with Emphasis on the Care of Circumcisions. *Ill Med J*. 1962-08; 122(2): 133-9.
21 Scurlock JM, Pemberton PJ. Neonatal Meningitis and Circumcision. *Med J Aust*. 1977-03-05; 332-3.
22 Annunziato D, Goldblum LM. Staphylococcal Scalded Skin Syndrome – A Complication of Circumcision. *Am J Dis Child*. 1978-12; 132: 1187-8.

Sussman, Schiller, and Shashikumar describe a type of infection which they call "Fournier's Syndrome." They describe three cases of this condition, one resulting from a burn, and two from infected neonatal circumcision. Their descriptions include extensive gangrenous ulcerations around the base of the scrotum, tip of the penis, and in the perineum, with the skin sloughing off. The infants healed following treatment with antibiotics, but scarring remained.[23]

Sauer reports a fatal staph infection following ritual circumcision. On the 13th day the infant exhibited fever, pallor, and lack of appetite. The circumcision blade had cut away a slight amount of the glans, which appeared to be the center of the infection. Antibiotics were given. On the 18th day of life several cc. of blood and mucus were vomited spontaneously and the infant expired before medical aid arrived. Autopsy revealed over 50 gray abscesses in the lungs. The infecting agent was *Staph Aureus*. The circumcision wound was nearly healed at the time of death.[24]

Kirkpatrick and Eitzman describe two cases involving premature infants who developed infections after being circumcised with the Plastibell device. In one case: "The circumcision site had frank pus around the plastic ring. Necrotic [dead] tissue was present in this area with incrustation of the glans and ulceration at the meatus." [25]

The infant healed normally following antibiotic therapy. In the other case:

"Pus was noted at the base of glans adjacent to the plastic ring. Gross hematuria [blood in the urine] was present. Blood transfusion was given. Condition remained critical until age two weeks ... Pneumonia and congestive heart failure which were major problems during the recovery period responded to medical management. Infant eventually recovered normally." [25]

Routine circumcision is often recommended because of the possibility of "infection." In truth *any* part of the body can become infected. Intact men and boys can develop infections of the foreskin. This type of infection is invariably mild and local in nature. It usually can be remedied easily with proper washing, without resort to any drastic measures. This minor type of infection does not begin to compare with the potentially disastrous consequences of an infection of a fresh circumcision wound. It appears that authorities have been concerned about the wrong kind of infection.

---

23 Sussman SJ, Schiller RP, Shashikumar VL. Fournier's Syndrome. *Am J Dis Child.* 1978-12; 132:1189-91.
24 Sauer LW. Fatal Staphylococcus Bronchopneumonia Following Ritual Circumcision. *AJOG.* 1943; 1(46): 583.
25 Kirkpatrick BV, Eitzman DV. Neonatal Septicemia After Circumcision. *CLP.* 1974-09; 13(9): 767-8.

11.5 Retention of Plastic Bell Ring

If a Plastibell device is used to circumcise a baby, the remaining foreskin should dry up and fall off with the ring within about 10 days after the operation. A complication peculiar to this device occurs when the ring fails to fall off and instead becomes buried under the skin along the shaft of the penis. A piece of plastic imbedded in the skin is undoubtedly painful to an infant, and leaves undesirable cosmetic results in the form of a permanent ridge or groove along the shaft of the penis.

Rubenstein and Bason report the following:

"Three infants, two aged 3 weeks and one aged 4 weeks respectively have returned to our outpatient clinic with the plastic ring at midshaft of the penis. In the first of these cases, the infant was brought to the clinic because he was 'always crying'; in the other two, the infant had no symptoms but the mother thought the penis 'didn't look right.' Although there was marked swelling both [above and below] the ring, in no case was there interference with the urinary stream, and in all three cases, the penis appeared normal within three weeks of the removal of the ring with a ring cutter ... Although in our series of three cases no serious sequallae were noted, it is certainly conceivable that infection or necrosis of the head of the penis, or both, as well as the recognized complications of urethral stenosis could result from such prolonged midshaft constriction." [26]

Datta and Zinner comment:

"Because the plastic material of the Plastibell has relatively rigid and sharp edges, there is compression damage and ulceration of the corona and portions of the proximal glans as well as that of the penile shaft. Edema and vascular congestion distal to the ring further complicate matters. All four infants [in their study] had extensive ulceration of the skin of the penile shaft ... Although we did not observe it, urinary retention and gangrene of the glans penis may occur and should be considered." [27]

Johnsonbaugh, Meyer and Catalano comment on the ridge often left behind by this occurrence: "Five days later [the infant] was again brought to the clinic with the

---

26 Rubenstein MM, Bason WM. Complication of Circumcision Done With a Plastic Bell Clamp. *Am J Dis Child.* 1968-10; 116: 381-2.
27 Datta NS, Zinner NR. Complication from Plastibell Circumcision Ring. *Urology.* 1977-01; 9(1): 57-8.

complaint that the ridge had not disappeared ... this constriction appears to be permanent." [28]

Lawton hypothesizes that: "... this complication is due to pushing the bell too far over the glans, perhaps further than the coronal sulcus, prior to tying the ligature." [29]

11.6   Concealed Penis

An unusual complication occurs when the penile shaft, following circumcision, retreats into the surrounding skin and fatty area and cannot be seen. This problem must be corrected by surgery, and often skin grafting, to produce a normal penis.

Drs. Shulman, et al. describe this occurrence:

> "... The penis is forced into a subcutaneous position by wound contraction following circumcision. This may be produced if there is a tendency of the penis to retract into the fatty mons pubis, and later the circular wound heals, contracts and holds the penis in a submerged position beneath the pubic skin." [30]

They describe the following case:

> "On exam, the penis was palpated deep in the subcutaneous tissue of the pubic region. Over the scrotum, only a tag of penile skin was visible, in the center of which there was a sinus through which the child passed urine. After careful dissection of the skin ring, it was possible to pull the penile shaft outwards. The shaft was normal but was denuded and it was necessary to cover it with a skin graft." [30]

Trier and Drach report two similar cases and offer their explanation for its occurrence:

"Failure to completely separate the inner surface of the prepuce from the glans penis. Circumcision, when correctly performed, eliminates the possibility of phimosis by excision of a sufficient portion of redundant prepuce in order to leave the glans penis exposed. Usually more of the inner preputial surface than the outer requires excision, so that very little penile skin need be discarded. If the inner surface of the prepuce is not adequately dissected from the surface of the glans penis, most or all of the inner surface of the prepuce remains. Penile skin is then pulled into the circumcision device and amputated immediately, or in a week's time in the case of

---

[28] Johnsonbaugh RE, Meyer BP, Catalano DJ. Complication of a Circumcision Performed With a Plastic Bell Clamp. *Am J Dis Child.* 1969-11; 118(5): 781.
[29] Lawton NM. Circumcision (letters to editor). *BMJ.* 1965-08-14; (2): 420.
[30] Shulman, et al., p. 152.

the plastic bell clamp. The circular wound contracts as it heals and confines the glans penis in a subcutaneous position." [31]

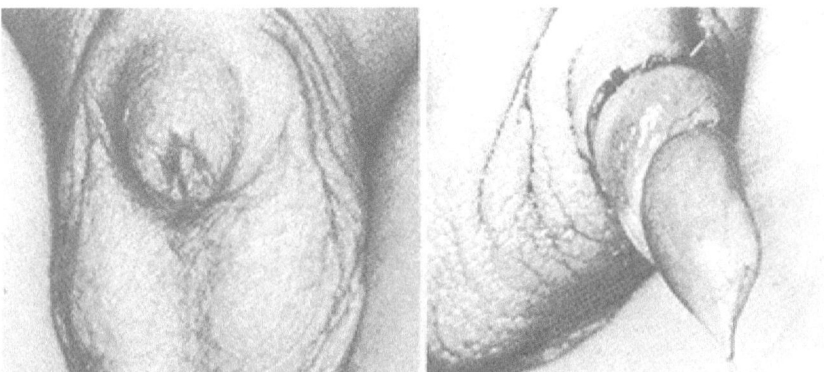

Left: Concealed penis. Bulge of glans is seen under skin.
Right: Glans exposed and held by traction suture. Suture line of inner surface prepuce and penile skin is visible.[31]

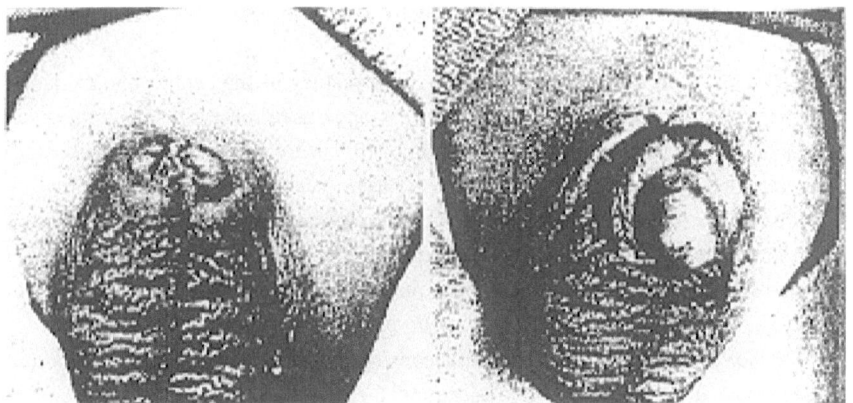

Left: Concealed penis prior to operative exposure.
Right: Penis after exposure of glans and suture of inner surface prepuce to skin.[31]

---

31 Trier WC, Drach GW. Concealed Penis. *Am J Dis Child.* 1973-02; 125: 276-7.

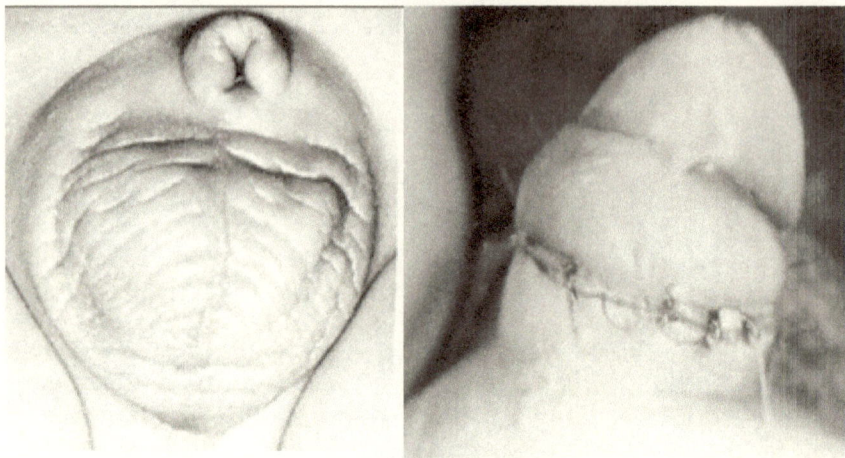

Concealed penis after circumcision.   *Repair of concealed penis. The inner preputial epithelium has been folded back to provide skin cover.*

Kaplan GW. Circumcision – An Overview. *Current Problems in Pediatrics*. 1977-03; 7(5): 18, 20.

Talarico and Jasaitis describe a similar case and conclude:

> "The most common accepted theory is the tendency of the penile shaft to retract into a deep prepubertal fat pad. This disappearance, although temporary, can become more permanent by the reaction of the newly formed circular mucocutaneous union with cicatrization [scarring]. The puckering scar tissue builds up, closes over the retracted penis and completely entombs it in a pseudosac with a pinpoint for the egress of urine. Fortunately the glans around the meatus is not involved in this scarring process ... We suggest a more adequate disruption of adhesions and more aggressive followup in the case of newborn circumcision ... *The mother should be instructed in cleansing the genital area and retracting the skin around the penis.*" [32] [emphasis mine]

These instructions are interesting because expectant and new mothers are often urged to consent to circumcision of their sons on the belief that the circumcised infant's penis "needs no particular care."

Today "concealed penis" can be resolved by modern surgical procedures. Certainly this complication has also occurred throughout ancient times. One shudders to

---

32 Talarico RD, Jasaitis JE. Concealed Penis: A Complication of Neonatal Circumcision. *J Urol*. 1973-12; 110: 732-3.

think of the lifelong difficulties suffered by such individuals in ages when surgical correction was not possible.

11.7 Urethral Fistula

A fistula is an abnormal opening in any part of the body. A urethral fistula is a hole going from the side of the male urethra to the outside of the penis. Usually the fistula occurs on the underside. This can develop as a result of circumcision. It results either from accidental crushing of the urethra by the circumcision clamp, an abnormality in the urethra, or from a stitch placed in the underside of the penis to control excessive bleeding at the site of the frenulum.

Kaplan comments:

> "This complication presumably occurs either because the urethra is pulled into and crushed by the Gomco clamp or because the urethra actually is incised, either with a knife or a suture placed for hemostasis. The prevention of this complication results from being able to visualize exactly what is being done in the course of the circumcision and ... can be accomplished by marking the level of skin to be excised and by completely freeing the preputial sac from the glans penis. Additionally, if any penile abnormality is uncovered in the course of freeing the preputial sac, I would strongly recommend desisting and referral at that point." [33]

Limaye and Hancock describe such a case, its repair, and its probable cause:

> "[A 7 year old child] voided in two streams ... One stream came from the tip of the penis and was directed forward; the other, a little larger, emerged from the underside of the penis and was directed downward. The child had undergone circumcision on the third day of life ... there was bleeding [after the circumcision] in the area of the frenulum. This was controlled with some difficulty with a suture. [The defect was repaired as follows:] A circular incision was made 3 mm. from the margin of the fistula and a skin cuff raised. The fistula was closed by inverting the margins of this incision ... [Subsequent healing was normal and the fistula closed.] ... Urethral injury seems more likely to occur when there is bleeding from the frenulum and an attempt is made to control it with a suture. A suture placed too deeply may strangulate a part of the urethral wall, thus leading to the formation of a fistula." [34]

---

[33] Kaplan, pp. 26-7.

Circumcision – The Painful Dilemma

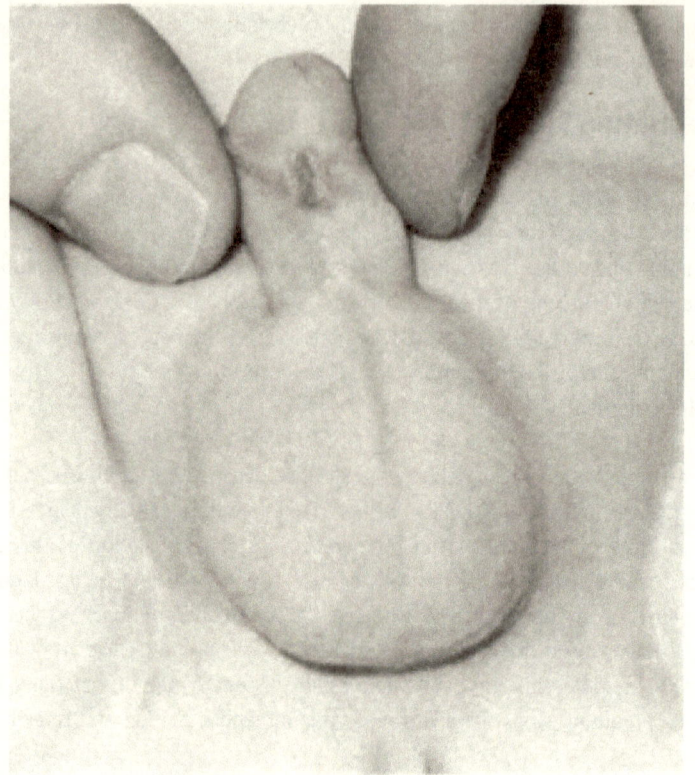

Urethrocutaneous fistula following circumcision.
Kaplan GW. Circumcision – An Overview. *Current Problems in Pediatrics.* 1977-03; 7(5): 27.

Byars & Trier describe a similar case:

> "... a 10 year old boy who was circumcised soon after birth: A complete segment of urethra was destroyed, resulting in a large defect of the urethra and chordee [painful downward curvature of the penis on erection] secondary to scar contracture. This was corrected by a two stage repair." [35]

Shiraki describes an unusual cause of such a fistula. A newborn baby boy was born with an abnormally enlarged urethra which instead of being a normal narrow tube, formed a "pocket" in the underside of his penis. This was termed "congenital mega-

---

34 Limaye RD, Hancock RA. Penile Urethral Fistula as a Complication of Circumcision. *J Pediatr.* 1968-01; 72(1): 106.
35 Byars LT, Trier WC. Some Complications of Circumcision and Their Surgical Repair. *AMA Arch Surg.* 1958-03; 76: 477-8.

lourethra." It became distended with urine and the condition was mistaken for phimosis with urine filling the preputial- glandular space. Circumcision was performed with a plastic bell clamp at age four days. Afterwards his urinary stream was poor with a tendency to spray. Circumcision had created a fistula on the underside of his penis where the large urethral pocket had been cut open. This was corrected by plastic surgery to close the hole and make a normal stream.[36]

11.8   Phimosis of Remaining Foreskin

Phimosis refers to any condition in which the foreskin cannot be retracted. This condition is normal in the intact infant, and *is not true phimosis*. Occasionally the older intact male may have a tight foreskin that is difficult to retract. This condition can usually be resolved by simple methods, and does not need to be corrected by circumcision. One of the purported arguments in favor of routine neonatal circumcision is that the operation will supposedly prevent phimosis. This is proven untrue, for occasionally the remaining piece of foreskin becomes tightly attached to the sides of the glans and the infant then must undergo a painful loosening procedure or possibly a second circumcision.

Browne describes this occurrence:

> "Removal of too little mucosa ... allows the circular wound to slip forwards over the end of the penis, where it contracts rapidly and completely, so that urination may be very difficult. The resultant problem is far from easy to solve if approached in the wrong way. The trick in untangling this is to make a circular cut through the skin just proximal to the ring of scar tissue and retract this so as to leave only mucosa covering the glans. This mucosa is then torn through cautiously with forceps and, once the corona is exposed, the situation is clear." [37]

Kaplan comments:

> "... Insufficient skin has been removed from the shaft of the penis and, in addition, insufficient inner preputial epithelium has been removed. As healing progresses there is contraction of the preputial ring so that true phimosis is produced. This can, at times, be quite severe and result in urinary obstruction. The prevention of this complication lies in the suggestion made to mark the area of the coronal sulcus on the shaft skin with ink and to be sure that the inner

---

36   Shiraki IW. Congenital Megalourethra with Urethrocutaneous Fistula Following Circumcision: A Case Report. *J Urol.* 1973-04; 109(4): 723-6.
37   Browne D. Fate of the Foreskin. *BMJ.* 1950-01-21: 181.

preputial epithelium has been completely freed from the underlying glans penis prior to removing the prepuce ... the treatment for this complication is a repeat circumcision." [38]

In *Mothering* magazine a young mother writes of her experience with her child who had this complication:

"I ... was unaware of what a horrible thing circumcision is, and allowed my son to be circumcised the same day he was born ... When he was 15 months old ... the doctor discovered that a half-inch of skin had grown back to the head of Jared's penis.

Our pediatrician referred us to a urologist who assured us that he could sedate Jared and simply 'pull' the adhesion apart; that there shouldn't be much discomfort to Jared.

Jared was given a sedative. He was then put on a table where a nurse held him down while the doctor pulled on the adhesion. Jared woke up crying immediately. The doctor injected a local anesthetic into Jared's penis to prepare it for surgery. Jared struggled with all he had to free himself from the nurse's hold.

As the nurse and doctor prepared the surgical room, I held and nursed my son. He was so upset that his little body convulsed with sobs the whole time he nursed. His penis had swollen to double its normal size!

I insisted on accompanying my son into the surgical room. Jared began to cry as soon as they laid him on the table. I held down the upper half of his body while the nurse held his lower half and kept his legs spread. Even though he was sedated, Jared was like a wild animal ... The doctor inserted the hemostat into one opening of the adhesion, and pushed it through to the other side, pulling up on the hemostat as he cut. After the cut was made, the doctor had to cauterize the wound to stop it from bleeding.

I was beyond myself, hearing and seeing my son scream for his life ... I am so sorry I was ignorant about circumcision. Had I witnessed a circumcision first, I never would have consented to having my son circumcised.

... If you decide to circumcise your son, prevent growth-back adhesions: bathe the baby and gently pull the skin back as he soaks in the water. Also apply Vaseline to the penis when you change him." [39]

(Yet mothers are usually told that circumcision will prevent "problems" and that the circumcised infant's penis needs no special care!)

---

[38] Kaplan, pp. 17-8.
[39] Sexty L. Jared's Ordeal. *Mothering*. 1979/Summer; 12: 84-5.

11.9 Urinary Retention

Occasionally a baby will not urinate for several hours following circumcision. Sometimes the cause is an overly tight bandage wrapped around the wound. In other instances the cause is less clear.

No special dressing was applied to my own babies' penises following circumcision except for a tiny, loosely applied petroleum jelly coated gauze strip. However, some operators, particularly ritual circumcisers, apply a tightly wrapped bandage around the end of the infant's freshly circumcised penis. Most doctors today would agree that this is not necessary.

A group of doctors report the following:

"Performers of ritual circumcision in Israel wrap the circumcised penis with a firm, circular bandage for hemostasis. The three newborn infants we saw were brought to the emergency room about a day after the procedure because of restlessness, refusal to eat and occasional vomiting. One of the mothers noticed blue discoloration of her child's legs. On examination, cyanosis of both lower extremities and a huge bladder were found in all three infants. In each case after removal of the bandage, a large quantity of urine was passed and the cyanosis disappeared. The babies became quiet and began to drink avidly. It is conceivable that the tight bandage constricted the urethra giving rise to a distended bladder. This in turn led to the discomfort and restlessness of the infant and caused compression of the iliac veins interfering with venous return from the legs and producing cyanosis.[40]

Horwitz, Schussheim, and Scalettar report a similar case:

"An 18 day old infant was brought to us with a ten hour history of mild, green, watery diarrhea and refusal to eat. There was no fever or vomiting, and on close questioning it was learned that he had been voiding normally. Over this period of time he refused to take any milk or liquids and it was this feature that had the parents particularly concerned.

On examination, he was found to be in a state of shock, mildly dehydrated, with grunting respiration, and with a hugely distended abdomen. There had been a ritual circumcision two days previously (somewhat delayed because of prematurity) and the penis was still covered by a tightly bound circular bandage. The tip of the penis was red and looked necrotic. While being examined he voided in a

---

[40] Frand M, Berant N, Brand N, Rotem Y. Complications of Ritual Circumcision in Israel. *Pediatrics*. 1974-10; 54(4): 521.

weak stream. After we released the bandage he voided a tremendous amount of urine ... The abnormal distention rapidly diminished and the grunting respiration improved but he was still obviously in shock. In fact, he appeared to be temporarily worse immediately after the release of the gauze.

Our impression was that he was in septic shock secondary to urinary obstruction and he was admitted immediately to a neonatal intensive care unit ... Escherichia coli was cultured from the blood, urine, throat, and tip of the penis ... A ventral meatotomy and urethral dilation were performed. The penis was intermittently soaked in warm saline for a few days, during which time improvement was seen ... The baby was also treated with antibiotics." [41]

Kaplan tells of another case of post-circumcision urinary retention by a different cause:

"I once was consulted about a 72-hour old male who had failed to void. He had been circumcised immediately following delivery. On examination, his bladder was distended and his glans penis was covered by a brownish film that obscured his urethral meatus. As this film was teased away from his meatus, he voided a full stream and had no further difficulties. Subsequently, it was learned that this film was dried tincture of benzoin used as a circumcision dressing." [42]

It is conceivable that similar urinary retention could result from an overly tight plastic bell ring. There have also been instances of infants failing to void for several hours following circumcision when no bandage or plastic ring was in place. This may be a psychological response on the infant's part to the trauma of the operation.

11.10 Glans Necrosis

"Necrosis" refers to the death of body tissue. This has happened to the glans following circumcision due to an overly tight bandage or a Plastibell ring that is too small.

Kaplan describes this occurrence:

"On occasion, in an attempt at hemostasis, the circulation to the glans penis may be compromised, resulting in either cyanosis or necrosis of the glans penis. I was asked to see a child with cyanosis of the glans penis one day following circum-

---

[41] Horwitz J, Schussheim A, Scalettar HE. Abdominal Distension Following Ritual Circumcision. *Pediatrics.* 1976-04; 57(4): 579.
[42] Kaplan, pp. 22-3.

cision. Many sutures were present. Additionally, an anaerobic streptococcus was cultured from the wound so that it was not clear whether the cyanosis was secondary to the sutures used or to an underlying infection. With removal of the sutures and use of antibiotics, this problem resolved without tissue loss." [43]

When a baby is (vaginally) born in breech position frequently the lower extremities become swollen from the pressures of birth. Rosefsky reports of a case of glans necrosis in a breech baby who was circumcised with a Plastibell:

"A breech baby was circumcised 12 hours after birth with a Plastibell. At age 24 hours, the baby was observed to have a moderately edematous scrotum, leg edema, and a black necrotic-appearing glans. The ligature and the plastic ring were removed ... following which the glans gradually became quite swollen and slightly moist over the following 12 hours. The urinary stream was narrow and forceful. By the 6th day the glans was moist and remained black. By day 7 the edema was almost gone. An outer black 'crust' of necrotic tissue, and part of the prepuce which had been distal to the ligature, began to slough. A reddish-purple, shiny glans underlay the old 'crust.' By the fifteenth hospital day the glans looked nearly normal. The patient was discharged and showed no evidence of urethral stenosis.

Breech delivery was almost certainly the cause of the edema of the legs and scrotum. The size of the plastic bell was satisfactory at age 12 hours, but 'became' insufficient, suggesting that the penis became more edematous, whether as a continuing process secondary to the breech delivery, or as a consequence of the circumcision method." [44]

11.11 Injury and Loss of Glans

Occasionally the glans can be injured or entirely cut off during circumcision. Usually a permanent deformity results. Both the Plastibell and the Gomco clamp employ the protective "bell" which covers the glans before the clamp or string is applied, thus precluding injury to the glans. Other methods not employing a "bell" pose greater risk of injuring the glans. The glans can also be injured before the bell is in place, during the dorsal slit procedure, or as the operator frees the foreskin from the glans.

Shulman, et al. describe two cases of injury to the glans during circumcision:

---

43 Ibid., p. 28.
44 Rosefsky JB. Glans Necrosis as a Complication of Circumcision. *Pediatrics.* 1967; 39: 744-5.

"[A two year old boy:] The glans was deformed in shape, divided by a deep transverse scar, and slightly edematous. The urethral meatus was not visible. There was also a post coronal stricture ... At operation, the clefts were excised and resutured, the stricture was opened, and the normal penile skin was rotated into the defect ...

A five year old boy sustained amputation of the glans penis during circumcision, with severe postoperative hemorrhage. Wound healing was uneventful but was followed by repeated urinary infection. On examination only a small part of the glans remained. The meatus was very small and the urinary stream exceedingly narrow ... meatotomy was performed and ... to produce a glans-like corona, a circumferential incision was made above the meatus, and the penile skin retracted proximally to give rise to a raw surface 1.5 cm. in width which was covered with split skin graft." [45]

McGowan describes a different type of injury:

"... surgically bivalving either the dorsal or ventral half of the glans penis. This is caused by inadvertent placement of one limb of the scissors into the urethra rather than between the foreskin and the glans prior to performing either the dorsal or ventral slit in the prepuce ... Once the incision is made, the glans penis is bivalved and the urethra laid open. In effect, a first degree hypospadias or epispadias has been produced." [46]

11.12 Excessive Skin Loss

A newborn baby's penis is very tiny. Usually only about one-half inch of skin is amputated during circumcision. Some operators tend to take off more than others, consequently there are many "varieties" of circumcised penises. Some males have no remaining foreskin while others have a sizable ring of skin left in place.

Considerable debate abounds over what is the "right" amount of foreskin to cut off. (Hopefully soon we will decide that the best answer is "none!") Taking off a small amount of skin can result in phimosis of the remaining foreskin with possible medical directive for repeat circumcision. However, devastating complications result from cutting off too much skin. The fact that the ultimate size of the penile shaft, proportionate to the foreskin, is not attained until later in life, further complicates the matter. A newborn's foreskin usually extends far beyond the glans. It may appear overly long, but as he matures he will in effect "grow into it." For this reason, some

---

[45] Shulman, et al., p. 151.
[46] McGowan AJ Jr. A Complication of Circumcision. *JAMA*. 1969-03-17; 207(11): 2104-5.

adult intact penises appear as if they have been circumcised. An advantage of delaying circumcision until adulthood (if desired or medically necessary) is that the individual has reached his full size and can have it "tailored to fit."

Excessive skin loss can result from the operator severing too much foreskin, from infection of the wound resulting in tissue death, or from a burn caused by an electrocautery device. Sometimes the entire penile shaft becomes denuded and skin grafting is necessary. Other times the results are less drastic and the wound heals, but as the individual grows older his penile skin becomes too tight, causing discomfort on erection.

Van Duyn & Warr state:

> "Reports of major losses of penile skin as a complication of circumcision are fairly common; the causes of such loss being usually either a complicating infection, the use of the electrocautery, or improper surgical technic [sic] ... when these defects are allowed to heal without grafting, there may be 'discomfort' during adulthood, and a shortening of the future functioning (erectile) length of the organ. Theoretically, even a minor inadequacy of penile skin in the shaft would tend to result in a holding back of the subcutaneous part of the penis against the abdominal wall." [47]

They describe the following case:

> "An infant male was circumcised on the third day of life with a Gomco clamp. The next morning the wound was pulled apart and it was apparent that an excess of penile skin had been removed leaving a gap of 1.0 cm underneath and 0.7 cm. above. Three days later plastic surgery was done. A split graft was cut from the left lower abdomen ... and wrapped around the defect in the penis and covered with fine mesh gauze. On the fourth post-operative day the dressings were removed and left off. The baby's hands and feet were restrained to keep him from disturbing the area. Ten days after the operation the patient was discharged from the hospital. The patient healed normally. The parents were told to look for evidence of constricting scar tissue at the juncture lines as this can result." [47]

Wilson & Wilson describe another case:

> "Child was circumcised one day after delivery. The guillotine method [!] of circumcision had been used and electrocautery employed. Mother and child left on the 6th day. One week later the physician examined the child and found the

---

47 Van Duyn J, Warr WS. Excessive Penile Skin Loss From Circumcision. *J Med Assoc Ga.* 1962-08;51:394-6.

entire penis to be black and gangrenous. Two days later it had apparently sloughed off completely and there remained only a small scarred area at the base ... At age three weeks, the first stage procedure was begun. Scar tissue was excised and after removing dense adhesions, a completely denuded penis was exposed. There was complete loss of the glans, but about two-thirds of the penile shaft was intact. Two horizontal incisions were made an inch apart in the scrotum and the intervening skin undermined to create a subcutaneous tunnel. The penis was inserted under this bridge of full thickness skin and the distal incision sutured around the end of the penis leaving the amputated end exposed.

The second stage was performed 6 weeks later (the baby being 9 weeks old). By this time the scrotal skin was adherent over the entire penis and the cut distal end of the penis completely epithelialized. The penis was freed from its subcutaneous bed along with adequate flaps of scrotal skin adherent to the sides and distal end. These three flaps were approximated without tension over the naked ventral surface and the scrotal incision closed vertically. A meatotomy was performed to insure an adequate urethral orifice. Recovery from this second procedure was also uneventful." [48]

11.13   Skin Bridge

"Skin bridge" can result from circumcision. It is a complication in healing of the wound, by which a piece of skin from the shaft of the penis has become attached to the glans, or another point along the shaft, forming a "bridge" that must be surgically corrected.

Klauber & Boyle describe this condition:

"A small portion of the circumference of the shaft skin is found to be continuous with the epithelium of the glans penis, producing a bridge over the coronal sulcus. Retraction of the shaft skin, or erection may cause deviation of the glans with respect to the shaft of the penis. Smegma may accumulate under the skin bridge, causing infection ... [It is caused by] damage to a small area of the glans penis during separation of the prepuce from the glans penis. Divided skin edge of the penile shaft skin must come in contact with the damaged area on the glans and become adherent. Subsequently, healing with epithelial bridging between the coronal sulcus from the glans to the shaft skin occurs." [49]

Kaplan comments:

---

48   Wilson CL & MC. Plastic Repair of the Denuded Penis. *SMJ.* 1959-03; 52: 288-90.
49   Klauber GT, Boyle J. Preputial Skin-Bridging – Complication of Circumcision. *Urology.* 1974-06; 3(6): 722-3.

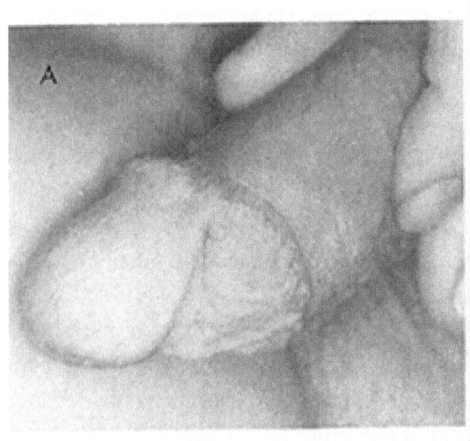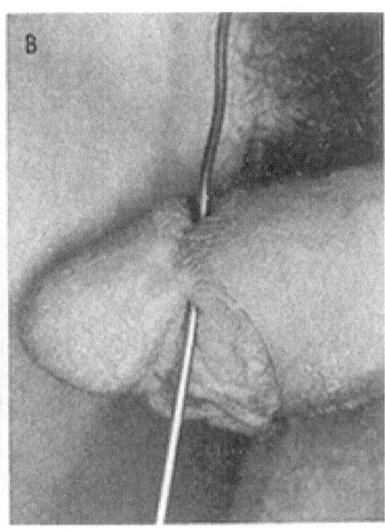

A. Patient with a skin bridge. – B. A probe has been passed under the bridge.
Kaplan GW. Circumcision – An Overview. *Current Problems in Pediatrics.* 1977-03; 7(5): 21.

"When present, these often result in accumulations of smegma or infection. Additionally, they tend to tether the erect penis, with resultant pain or curvature. Their treatment is simple surgical division. However, there must be preparation for hemostasis, as they often contain many vessels that can bleed vigorously. Some authors have stated that they arise by injury to the glans at the time of circumcision, with resultant fusion of the circumcision line thereto. It is my belief that there is yet another dimension in genesis; namely incomplete separation of the inner preputial epithelium at the time of circumcision. Consequently, there is firm fusion of skin, inner preputial epithelium and glans at this point, with later separation of the inner preputial epithelium from the glans, resulting in a skin bridge." [50]

11.14 Vomiting, Apneic Spells

Apnea (British spelling apnoea) means cessation of breathing, usually for a short period of time. Sometimes normal healthy infants have spells of apnea during sleep and it is of no consequence. However, sometimes this event can be life-threatening.

Fleiss and Douglass report:

---

50 Kaplan, p. 20.

"A healthy 1-week-old infant had a circumcision done by a well-trained and experienced physician without any anaesthetic. The infant tolerated the procedure well except for excessive crying, which began at the time of the operation. The mother, attempting to soothe her distressed infant, resumed breast feeding after the operation. An episode of vomiting followed the feeding. An apnoeic spell followed the emesis. The infant was taken to a local emergency room and subsequently transferred to [a children's hospital]. He received a complete septic workup, intravenous antibiotics and hospitalization for five days of observation until the cultures were negative and sepsis was ruled out. The infant was discharged from the hospital six days after circumcision doing very well.

Infants do feel the pain of the surgical removal of the foreskin performed without any anaesthetic, and they respond to the pain by crying. That crying may be excessive. Air may be swallowed. Mothers do soothe their infants by feeding them. Vomiting may follow the feeding. Apnoea may follow vomiting ..." [51]

11.15   Sewing of Penile Skin to the Glans

Stitches are not normally required following neonatal circumcision, so presumably this bizarre complication has resulted from circumcision performed on older individuals.

Browne mentions: "Sewing the skin edge to the glans, with consequent burying of the corona. This mistake arises from not retracting the mucosa fully. It entails a tedious little dissection." [37]

11.16   Laceration of Penile or Scrotal Skin

Circumcision jokes often center around "What if the knife slips?!" This feared event *has* happened.

Shulman, Ben-Hur, & Newman report:

"Accidental laceration of the penile skin and scrotum following circumcision has been seen in 2 cases ... [In one case] the Mohel slipped during the performance of the operation, and the knife opened the ventral surface of the penis and scrotum and exposed both testes. The skin was sutured under general anesthesia six hours after the accident and healing was uneventful." [52]

---

51 Fleiss PM, Douglass J. The Case Against Neonatal Circumcision. *BMJ.* 1979-09: 554.
52 Shulman, et al., p. 150.

11.17 Undetected Hypospadias

Hypospadias is a congenital deformity in which a fistula (hole) naturally occurs in the underside of the penis. This sometimes is corrected by plastic surgery. The foreskin provides an easily available piece of tissue for use in skin grafting. (Thereafter, the individual is essentially circumcised, but at least the foreskin has provided a correction for the defect.) If an infant with hypospadias is routinely circumcised, this potentially useful piece of skin has been destroyed and the operator must resort to more complicated types of skin grafts to reconstruct the penis.[53]

According to Gee & Ansell:

"In 5,882 live births, there were 22 patients with a hypospadias ... In 13 patients, the hypospadias was recognized and circumcision was not done; in 6 the hypospadias was not recognized and circumcision was done; in 2 the hypospadias was noted but circumcision was done anyway; and in one patient hypospadias was recognized after the dorsal slit was made, and the incision was then reapproximated with fine chromic gut." [15]

11.18 Preputial Cysts

A cyst is an abnormal, closed pocket of body tissue which contains fluid or solid material. Occasionally cysts develop along the remaining edge of foreskin at the site where the skin was severed.

Kaplan discusses this:

"These occur either by rolling in epidermis at the time of circumcision, or perhaps by implanting smegma in the circumcision wound. These inclusion cysts may grow to rather large proportions ... Even those that remain small can become infected ... Obviously the treatment is surgical excision." [54]

11.19 Complications of Anesthesia

Complications can ensue from use of any type of anesthesia for any medical procedure, including circumcision.

Kaplan states:

---

53 Hypospadias is hardly a life threatening condition. It is merely an annoyance because urine may drip out of the opening under the penis. Some individuals with hypospadias have preferred to live with the condition or have it surgically corrected without sacrificing the foreskin.
54 Kaplan, p. 26.

Circumcision – The Painful Dilemma

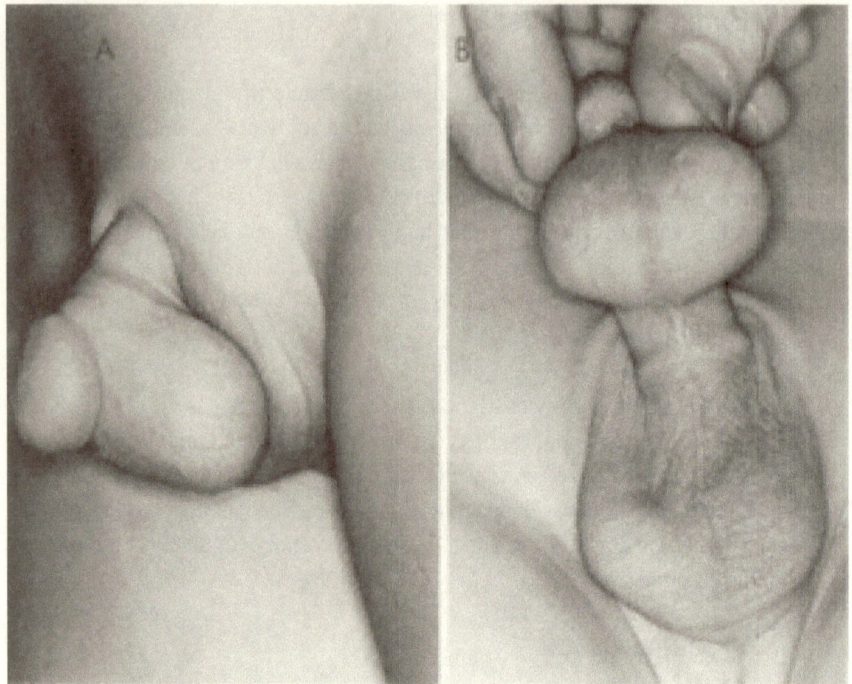

Preputial inclusion cyst following circumcision. A. lateral view. B. ventral view of the same patient.
Kaplan GW. Circumcision – An Overview. *Current Problems in Pediatrics.* 1977-03; 7(5): 25.

"Over the period 1942-1947 in England there were 16 deaths per year related to anesthetics used for circumcision. It is presumed that anesthetic techniques today have greatly reduced this incidence. This once again, however, reaffirms the observation that no general anesthetic is used lightly and without due consideration of the risks and benefits therefrom." [18]

Critics of infant circumcision frequently express outrage that newborn infants are usually given no anesthesia for an operation considered painful enough to warrant anesthesia for an older child or an adult. However, administration of such drugs to newborn infants is riskier than anesthetizing an older individual. Certainly if all newborn infants undergoing circumcision were being given general anesthesia for the operation we would see many more cases of deaths or difficulties from the anesthetic.

11.20 Tuberculosis and other Diseases from Mezizah

Mezizah is the third step of the Jewish ritual circumcision ceremony, in which the mohel applies his mouth to the fresh circumcision wound. Diseases have been spread due to this practice. Today, few ritual circumcisors practice it.

According to Bromley:

"A few years ago [1929] one of our leading medical journals published an account of an infected operator, who, during the third stage of the operation [mezizah] had infected seven children with tuberculosis and it proved fatal to all within a short time after this religious rite ..." [55]

(Please see Chapter 3 "Circumcision and Judaism", for additional discussion of this practice.)

11.21 Strangulation of the Glans by Hair

Medical reports have described cases of small boys who have, either accidentally or intentionally, had long strands of human hair tightly wrapped around the coronal sulcus (the indentation beyond the outer rim of the glans). This can be considered an indirect complication of circumcision, because the intact penis with the foreskin covering the glans has one smooth continuous surface and the glans and the coronal sulcus are not exposed.

Singh, Kim, & Wax describe three cases:

"A four year old boy presented discoloration of the glans with swelling due to an encircling hair. The hair was cut free ... the child recovered fully with no complications.

A three year old boy presented a history of dysuria [painful urination]. He had an excoriated [abraded, traumatized] glans. A hair was wrapped around the glans which was cutting into the tissue. The hair was removed and the infection was treated with antibiotics. He recovered fully with no complications.

A five year old boy was voiding through an opening on the underside of the penis. He had an infection around the urethral meatus for six months which did not clear on local antibiotic therapy. Examination revealed a urethral fistula located ventrally in the line of a deep groove which completely encircled the penis just proximal to the glans. Ten months later the fistula was repaired. Six months later he experienced a three day history of discoloration at the tip of his

---

55 Bromley RI. Circumcision. *Medical Journals and Records.* 1929-08-21: 212-3.

penis. A hair was removed from the groove proximal to the glans. His glans was black and dry. Two days later the glans sloughed off leaving a clean, dry, proximal urethra. The healing was normal." [56]

11.22 Recurrence of Pneumothorax

A pneumothorax is a collection of air or gas in the membranes that surround the lungs or pleural cavity. Auerbach & Scanlon tell of a case involving an infant who developed a pneumothorax as a result of mechanical assistance with breathing for severe respiratory distress at birth. After it was treated the infant was circumcised. His excessive crying from the pain of the operation caused the pneumothorax to recur:

> "A baby was delivered after spontaneous labor at 35 weeks' gestation. He weighed 2.51 kg. [about 4 ½ lbs.] His Apgar scores were 5 at 1 minute, and 9 at 5 minutes. He was given oxygen. The infant developed severe respiratory distress syndrome documented by chest x-ray and clinical course. Assisted ventilation was required via an endotracheal tube. At 15 hours of age a right-sided tension pneumothorax was noted, followed in three hours by a left-sided leak. Assisted ventilation was discontinued on the fifth day ... On the fifteenth day he was electively circumcised prior to anticipated discharge. Circumcision was complicated by moderate bleeding, which required several pressure dressings. After the procedure the baby had circumoral cyanosis [blueness around the mouth] and tachypnea [abnormally rapid breathing] that persisted. The infant was ... irritable and frequently crying. A right sided pneumothorax was diagnosed on the seventeenth day of life and necessitated chest tube insertion and drainage. The infant required an additional 19 days of hospitalization for this problem ... Circumcision and subsequent bleeding with frequent dressing, resulted in crying and sobbing sufficient to raise intrapulmonary pressures and rerepture a previously weakened site." [57]

11.23 Pulmonary Embolism

A pulmonary embolism is a clot of blood which travels through the circulatory system and becomes lodged in one of the blood vessels in the lungs. This causes severe

---

56 Singh B, Kim H, Wax S. Strangulation of Glans Penis by Hair. *Urology.* 1978-02; 11(2): 170-2.
57 Auerbach MR, Scanlon JW. Recurrence of Pneumothorax as a Possible Complication of Elective Circumcision. *AJOG;* 132(5): 583.

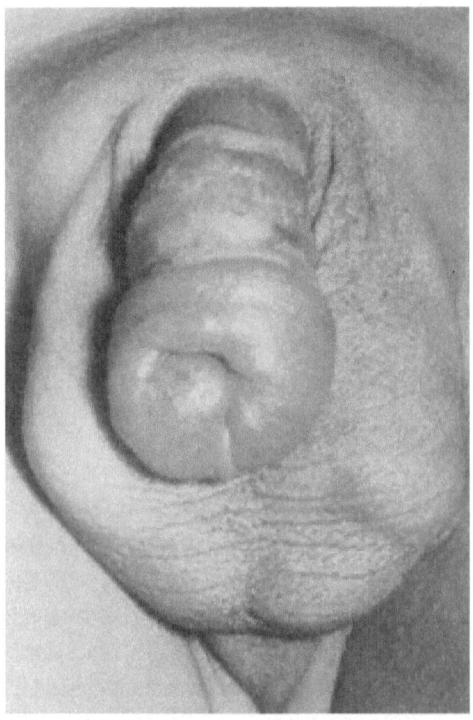

Distal lymphedema following circumcision complicated by wound separation and infection.
Kaplan GW. Circumcision – An Overview. *Current Problems in Pediatrics.* 1977-03; 7(5): 27.

breathing difficulties and can result in death. This is a small but potential risk of any surgery.

One medical report lists a case of pulmonary embolism following adult circumcision:

> "The day before his discharge he felt vaguely unwell and lost his appetite. He awoke during the night and complained of back pains which radiated to his right shoulder and were aggravated on breathing ... Two days later he experienced severe pleural pain. He had difficulty breathing and was coughing up blood. He had at least two pulmonary emboli. He became seriously ill and was operated on. The recovery was satisfactory." [58]

---

58 Curtis JE. Circumcision Complicated by Pulmonary Embolism. *Nursing Mirror.* 1971-06-18; 132(25): 28-30.

11.24 Keloid Formation

A keloid is an abnormal development consisting of a raised, firm, thickened, red piece of scar tissue. Such a formation at the site of circumcision creates a grotesque deformation of the organ, with obstruction of its function.

Ecstein describes an extensive keloid scar which developed on a small boy 6 months after he was circumcised "without any good clinical indication." The author concludes: "Fortunately this complication is unusual." [59]

11.25 Lymphedema or Elephantiasis of Skin

These terms refer to the swelling or obstruction of the lymph vessels. This can result from circumcision.

According to Shulman, et al.:

"A baby with lymphedema of the penis had been circumcised at 8 days. He was referred at age 10 months. Several days after circumcision the penis and scrotum had become swollen. On examination at 25 days it was found that a large portion of the prepuce remained and covered the glans. The penis and scrotum were edematous. Several weeks later the scrotal edema regressed but the penile skin of the ventral surface remained edematous. On admission, marked edema of the lower part of the penile skin was found ... At operation, the lymphedematous tissue was excised down to the penile fascia. The defect on the ventral surface was easily closed by the remaining dorsal flaps." [30]

11.26 Reaction of Older Sibling

Perhaps the following experience can be considered a complication of circumcision. A doctor reports:

"One Sunday afternoon I received an urgent call from a harassed mother who informed me that her two-year-old son had tried to amputate his penis and was bleeding profusely.

"He had a moderately deep laceration halfway around the base of the penis. The urethra was intact. The laceration was sutured and recovery was uneventful.

---

[59] Ecstein HB. Minor Surgery in Infancy and Childhood. *Update.* 1979-01-15: 141, 144.

"The youngster had witnessed his baby brother's ritual circumcision one week previously and had obviously been impressed by the procedure and all the attention his brother had received." [60]

11.27 Cosmetic Problems

The Gomco clamp and Plastibell devices produce an even circular cut – although if applied crookedly can still result in cosmetic problems. Older methods such as smashing the skin with a hemostat and slicing it off present greater risk that an uneven cut will result. Browne uses the quaintly British expression: "Untidy tags of skin." [37]

Removal of only a tiny bit of foreskin can cause dissatisfaction on the part of parents who are conditioned to believe that the denuded state is preferable. Sometimes such parents will take their babies back to the doctor to have more foreskin cut off because they believe that his penis does not look circumcised "enough."

Kaplan comments:

> "An inconsequential but frequent source of parental dissatisfaction with the results of circumcision is the removal of insufficient skin and inner preputial epithelium. Often in such instances one is hard pressed to determine that circumcision has been performed. Obviously this is merely a cosmetic problem, but it is amazing how much time is required to convince the parents of these children that repeat circumcision is not necessary." [61]

11.28 Loss of Penis

I have purposely saved the most dramatic and devastating complication for last. There have been cases in which the penis has been lost due to circumcision, caused by mishandling of the operation, as a result of an infection, or by a burn from electrocautery technique. In some cases enough penile shaft remained so that after extensive operations a functional penis could be reconstructed. In other cases the child has been surgically made into a "girl."

Hamm and Kanthak describe two infants who underwent penile reconstruction:

> "Two cases of gangrene of the penis in newborn infants occurred following circumcision for which a high frequency cutting current was utilized. In each instance the procedure was done by the physician in this way for the first time

---

60 Lewin P. Ritual Circumcision Sequel. *CLP*. 1971-10: 583.
61 Kaplan, pp. 21-2.

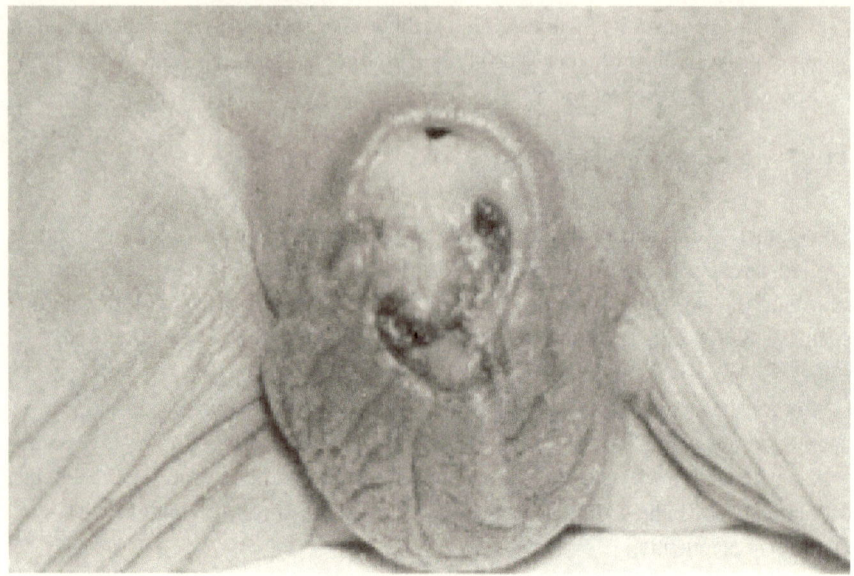

Total penile slough due to electrical burn of penis during circumcision.
Kaplan GW. Circumcision – An Overview. *Current Problems in Pediatrics*. 1977-03; 7(5): 30.

and had been utilized in the hope that a simple, hemostatic method of circumcision would result. Each of these cases was attended by more or less complete sloughing of the external portion of the penis resulting, on spontaneous healing, in a flat, smooth area of skin continuous with the scrotum on which no evidence of penile projection was present. In each of these cases a satisfactory penis was reconstructed.

... The penis has been reconstructed utilizing the remains of the corpora cavernosa penis and the corpus cavernosum urethrae with its enclosed urethra ...

Repair of the penis utilizing the remains of the penile stump by exteriorizing the deep portions of the corpora cavernosa and covering the newly formed shaft with a free skin graft provides a direct approach and a penis composed of more physiologically normal elements than is otherwise possible." [62]

There are documented cases of sex change due to total loss of the penis following circumcision. A newspaper article reports the following:

---

62 Hamm WG, Kanthak FF. Gangrene of the Penis Following Circumcision With High Frequency Current. *SMJ*. 1949-08; 42(8): 657-9.

"A boy injured so badly during a circumcision that specialists later advised a sex change operation, has been awarded $750,000 in medical malpractice damages. Circumcision was performed when the child was five months old. According to testimony in the two-day trial, the baby's genital area was burned so badly that specialists eventually recommended sex-change surgery which was performed ... the child had undergone eight operations and that several more might be necessary. The parent-child relationship is affected. In future years they will look at certain of her activities and wonder if she's beginning to revert to being male. She's suffered severe surgical scarring. How will she look at herself as she grows older? Doctors testified that lifetime treatment with hormones would develop and maintain a feminine body, but she would never be able to bear children and would have only a 50-50 chance of achieving orgasm." [63]

Money has studied a number of cases of sex reassignment of male to female in infancy. (Occasionally this is also done because of congenitally defective, abnormally small genitals, apparently what is now known as 'intersexed.') He describes a most interesting case example in which one of identical twin boys lost his penis during circumcision and was subsequently raised as a girl. Circumcision had been recommended for the twin boys at age 7 months due to "phimosis." Following the disastrous result of the first twin's surgery, the other baby was sent home intact. His "phimosis" cleared up on its own within a few days – a poignant indication of the non-necessity of the surgery.

"... The child was born a normal male and an identical twin, without genital malformation or sexual ambiguity ... at the age of 7 months ... the penis was ablated flush with the abdominal wall. The mishap occurred when a circumcision was being performed by means of electrocautery. The electrical current was too powerful and burned the entire tissue of the penis, which necrosed and sloughed off.

... [The parents] implemented their decision [for sex-change] with a change of name, clothing, and hair style when the baby was 17 months old. Four months later the surgical step of genital reconstruction as a female was undertaken, the second step, vaginoplasty, being delayed until the body is fully grown. Pubertal growth and feminization will be regulated by means of hormonal replacement therapy with estrogen." [64]

---

63 Malpractice Leads to Sex Change. *Philadelphia Inquirer.* 1975-10-31.
64 Money J. Ablatio Penis: Normal Male Infant Sex-Reassigned as a Girl. *Arch Sex Behav.* 1975; 4(1): 67.

> "Concerning the status of her organs, the girl knows that she needs to apply finger pressure above the urethral opening to insure complete downward deflection of the urinary stream, and that she can request minor surgery to correct it when she is ready. She had recovered [!] from what in infancy was a terror of white-coated doctors, but is not yet ready for a voluntary hospitalization. She knows also that some girls are born without the baby canal properly opened, for which correction is possible in teenage years. Eventually she will be told about her medical history." [65]

There is an old Freudian theory of "castration anxiety" and "penis envy" on the part of the small girl who, upon seeing a little boy's penis believes that she once had one and lost it. While I consider such theory totally ridiculous, it is incredible to learn that such an event has happened in reality!

Being female is wonderful if one is born that way. But one can only begin to speculate the anxieties and identity problems that an unwittingly converted female will experience as "she" grows up.

This individual was never able to adjust to his reassigned female status and experienced severe emotional and adjustment difficulties during childhood and adolescence. Upon being informed at age 14 of his male origin and subsequent loss of his penis, he immediately chose to re-assume his male identity. Although his original name had been Bruce, he chose the name David for himself and has been publicly known as David Reimer. He underwent surgical penile reconstruction, has married and had become an adoptive father to his wife's children. Later, as a man in his 30's he chose to come forward with his story. Sadly, David Reimer took his own life in 2004.

The entire story of this family's horrendous, lifetime tragedy is related in detail in *As Nature Made Him: The Boy Who Was Raised as a Girl*, by John Colapinto, HarperCollins Publishers, 2000.

"Just When You Think You've Heard it All!"

I've received countless phone calls about circumcision related matters. During the mid-90's I was contacted by an individual who was in the process of undergoing male to female sex-change. This person had been born a male and was routinely circumcised shortly after birth. For unstated reasons he had never accepted his male gender-status, and at age 50 had chosen to be surgically changed into a woman. He/she was requesting information from me on circumcision and informed me that because of the lack of foreskin, the vaginoplastic surgery was going to be conside-

---

65 Ibid., p. 71.

rably more complicated. If the individual has an intact foreskin, the surgeon has considerably more tissue to work with to construct an artificial vagina. This person used a pseudonym with me and wished not to be identified or contacted by anyone else.

Evidently this can be listed as yet another "complication" of circumcision. If the individual later wishes to be changed into a female, subsequent vaginoplasty is much more difficult. – R.R.

11.29 Informational Resources

- 100+ circumcision deaths each year in United States: circinfo.org/USA_deaths.html
- 41,250 Referrals, 18,562 Corrective Surgeries Annually *(doctor's quote)*:
  facebook.com/photo.php?fbid=10207619204217273&set=p.10207619204217273
- A Gallery of Circumcisions *(skin bridges – graphic pictures)*: circumstitions.com/Botched1.html
- A Kid-Friendly Approach to Meatal Stenosis:
  web.archive.org/web/20151101090730/http://www.hopkinschildrens.org/a-kid-friendly-approach-to-meatal-stenosis.aspx
- A play about Human Genital Mutilation: BOY: by AnnaZiegler:
  hooded2016.wordpress.com/2016/03/31/boy-by-anna-ziegler
- A Strange Case of Double Standards: indymedia.org.uk/en/2009/02/423057.html
- Adding Insult to Injury: Acquisition of Erectile Dysfunction from Circumcision:
  researchgate.net/publication/322056383
- Alexithymia and Circumcision Trauma: A Preliminary Investigation: researchgate.net/publication/270190401
- Amputation of Glans Penis: A Rare Circumcision Complication and Successful Management with Primary Anastomosis and Hyperbaric Oxygen Therapy: synapse.koreamed.org/articles/1093932
- Answers to Your Questions about Circumcision and MRSA *(infection)*:
  nocirc.org/publish/12-AnswersMRSA.pdf
- Answers to Your Questions about Infant Circumcision: nocirc.org/publish/3pam.pdf
- Baby Dies after Circumcision Surgery Blood Loss and Heart Failure:
  www.drmomma.org/2010/10/baby-dies-from-circumcision-surgery.html
- Baby Dies from Circumcision *(NY)*: www.drmomma.org/2009/10/new-york-baby-dies-from-circumcision.html
- Baby Dies From Circumcision during Jewish Brit:
  www.drmomma.org/2009/09/baby-dies-from-circumcision-during.html
- Baby Dies from Circumcision in South Dakota:
  www.drmomma.org/2009/09/baby-dies-from-circumcision-in-south.html
- Baby Dies Post Plastibell Circumcision:
  www.drmomma.org/2007/06/baby-dies-post-plastibell-circumcision.html
- Baby Titus from PA: circumcisioninsanity.blogspot.com/2016/01/baby-titus-from-pa.html
- Baby's penis reattached in hospital after brit goes wrong *(penile amputation)*:
  web.archive.org/web/20150905065930/http://www.israelhayom.com/site/newsletter_article.php?id=27435

- BC man's foreskin op a success *(repair of adult botched circumcision)*:
    nationalreviewofmedicine.com/issue/2006/06_30/3_patients_practice01_12.html
- Body of 9-Week-Old Infant Allegedly Found Dead; Parents Under Custody:
    web.archive.org/web/20160616174958/http://www.morningledger.com/body-of-9-week-old-infant-allegedly-found-dead-parents-under-custody/1311193
- Botched circumcision deforms man's organ:
    web.archive.org/web/20160216092659/http://www.thevoicebw.com/2016/02/15/penis-pain
- Brayden Tyler Frazier Memorial *(infant death from circumcision)*:
    facebook.com/media/set/?set=a.10152661415665331.1073741826.10150152211840331
- Brayden Tyler Frazier Obituary:
    facebook.com/photo.php?fbid=10153233664926937&set=p.10153233664926937
- Breastfeeding & Circumcision *(add breastfeeding difficulties to complications list)*[66]:
    www.drmomma.org/2009/11/breastfeeding-circumcision.html
- Brooklyn Toddler Dies After Circumcision:
    abcnews.go.com/Health/Wellness/brooklyn-toddler-dies-circumcision/story?id=13544632
- Circumcision – your rights in wrongful or botched circumcisions:
    web.archive.org/web/20151006111558/http://www.examiner.com/article/circumcision-your-rights-wrongful-or-botched-circumcisions
- Circumcision Complications Result in Disfigurations, Lawsuit, and Severe Stress for Family:
    peacefulbeginningsrosemary.wordpress.com/circ-information/complications-from
- Circumcision death posted on Craigslist:
    facebook.com/photo.php?fbid=10153233665676937&set=p.10153233665676937
- Circumcision death renews controversy:
    facebook.com/photo.php?fbid=10153910938985407&set=p.10153910938985407
- Circumcision Deaths: cirp.org/library/death
- Circumcision Harm Survey Published: doctorsopposingcircumcision.org/circumcision-harm-survey-published
- Circumcision Herpes Baby: Fourth Case Blames Baby Procedure For Herpes *(mezizah)*:
    web.archive.org/web/20160404232943/http://www.newsoxy.com/health/circumcision-herpes-baby-175029.html
- Circumcision in young boys can DOUBLE chance of developing autism:
    mirror.co.uk/news/uk-news/circumcision-young-boys-can-double-4945643
- Circumcision Kills: circumcision-kills.tumblr.com
- Circumcision Part 1: Uninformed Consent – The REAL Dangers That Doctors Don't Tell You About:
    motherwiselife.org/guest-post-circumcision-part-1-uninformed-consent-the-real-dangers-that-doctors-dont-tell-you-about
- Circumcision: dirty little secrets exposed: wisewomanwayofbirth.com/circumcision-dirty-little-secrets-exposed

---

66 More newborn baby boys die from circumcision surgery each year in the United States than from choking, from auto accidents, from suffocation, from SIDS, from sleep positioners and from (the newly banned) drop-side cribs (from *Dr. Momma*).

- Circumcision: Techniques, Results, Complications *(good source of graphic pictures of complications)*:
  coloradonocirc.org/files/handouts/Circumcision_Techniques_and_Complications.pdf
- Circumcision: Your Legal Rights *(litigation for complications)*:
  arclaw.org/publications/circumcision-your-legal-rights
- Circumcision's complications: what could go wrong?:
  web.archive.org/web/20141022104051/http://www.examiner.com/article/circumcision-s-complications-what-could-go-wrong
- Clinical presentation and pathophysiology of meatal stenosis following circumcision:
  cirp.org/library/complications/persad
- Complications of Circumcision: circumstitions.com/Complic.html
- Complications of Circumcision:
  med.stanford.edu/newborns/professional-education/circumcision/complications.html
- Complications of circumcision *(Williams & Kapila)*: cirp.org/library/complications/williams-kapila
- Contraindications to Routine Circumcision:
  med.stanford.edu/newborns/professional-education/circumcision/contraindications.html
- Death From Circumcision: www.drmomma.org/2010/05/death-from-circumcision.html
- Death from Circumcision Higher Than Suffocation and Auto Accidents:
  www.drmomma.org/2010/05/death-from-circumcision-higher-than.html
- Deaths from Circumcision: circumstitions.com/death.html
- Do you have to pee standing up to be a real man?: ihra.org.au/21870/alice-dreger-hypospadias
- Documented severe complications of circumcision *(IntactiWiki)*:
  en.intactiwiki.org/wiki/Documented_severe_complications_of_circumcision
- Does Circumcision Cause Erectile Dysfunction?:
  thewholenetwork.org/twn-news/does-circumcision-cause-erectile-dysfunction
- Estimated U.S. Incidence of Neonatal Circumcision Complications (physical only) Affecting Males Born between 1940 and 1990 *(interesting graph)*: noharmm.org/incidenceUS.htm
- Evidence on: The Vitamin K Shot in Newborns *(interesting – read all the facts)*:
  evidencebasedbirth.com/evidence-for-the-vitamin-k-shot-in-newborns
- Excessive bleeding during circumcision sign of hemophilia:
  theexpressnews.com/excessive-bleeding-during-circumcision-sign-of-haemophilia
- Extreme trauma from male circumcision causes damage to areas of brain:
  naturalnews.com/048907_male_circumcision_brain_damage_child_abuse.html
- Felice v. Valleylab, Inc. *(penile loss of 2 year old child following circumcision & infection)*:
  leagle.com/decision/19871440520so2d92011201.xml
- Forced infant circumcision harms transsexual women too:
  hooded2016.wordpress.com/2016/03/27/forced-infant-circumcision-harms-transexual-women-too
- Foreskin is normal, circumcision is not:
  web.archive.org/web/20160630060136/http://brianointacto.tumblr.com/post/132622559260/millions-of-men-walk-around-the-us-with-botched

- Genital reconstruction allows Miss. man to father child *(loss of penis through childhood circumcision):* eu.clarionledger.com/story/news/2014/04/24/genital-reconstruction-allows-miss-man-father-child/8134415
- Global Survey of Circumcision Harm: circumcisionharm.org/research.htm
- Grace Adeleye guilty of killing baby in botched circumcision *(newborn, death from hemorrhage following circumcision):* bbc.com/news/uk-england-manchester-20733674
- Haemorrhage (Bleeding): circumstitions.com/Complic.html#haemorrhage
- How 11 New York City Babies Contracted Herpes Through Circumcision *(mezizah):* healthland.time.com/2012/06/07/how-11-new-york-city-babies-contracted-herpes-through-circumcision
- How I Almost Lost My Son to Circumcision: web.archive.org/web/20161104052232/http://family-sprouts.com/almost-lost-son-circumcision
- Hypospadias in Boys: facebook.com/brotherk.bloodstainedman/posts/294920423998452
- I almost killed my baby: facebook.com/photo.php?fbid=10153233668666937&set=p.10153233668666937
- Increased Dangers of Neonatal Circumcision: web.archive.org/web/20150330012312/http://www.doctorsopposingcircumcision.org/pdf/specialstatement.pdf
- Infant circumcision causes 100 deaths each year in US: intactamerica.org/newborn-circumcision-linked-to-100-deaths-in-us-each-year
- Injury and harm: Circumcision is surgery: circinfo.org/account.html
- Intact vs. Circumcised Outcome Statistics: www.drmomma.org/2010/01/cut-vs-intact-outcome-statistics.html
- Introduction to the natural, intact penis *(photo gallery, graphic):* circumcisionharm.org/gallery%20intact.htm
- Is Hypospadias Repair Necessary? Most of the time, no, and it can be very damaging surgery!: facebook.com/notes/circumcision-resources/is-hypospadias-repair-necessary-most-of-the-time-no-and-it-can-be-very-damaging-/650149735062867
- Lack of post-surgery info angers grieving parents: facebook.com/photo.php?fbid=10153233677961937&set=p.10153233677961937
- Legal Victories *(list of 52 botched settlements circumcision cases):* arclaw.org/resources/legal-victories
- Long-Term Adverse Effects of Circumcision: i2researchhub.org/articles/ch-6-long-term-adverse-effects-of-circumcision-doc-genital-integrity-statement
- Lost Boys: An Estimate of U.S. Circumcision-Related Infant Deaths *(117 per year):* academia.edu/6394940
- Maaz our Little Angel, 20 days old: facebook.com/photo.php?fbid=10153233656451937&set=p.10153233656451937
- Massive Infection Takes Over Body After Plastibell Circumcision: www.drmomma.org/2009/11/massive-infection-takes-over-body-after.html
- Mayor de Blasio and Rabbis Near Accord on New Circumcision Rule *(infections from mezizah):* nytimes.com/2015/01/15/nyregion/mayor-de-blasio-and-rabbis-near-accord-on-new-circumcision-rule.html
- Meatal Stenosis Article Scrubbed from Website *(Johns Hopkins):* joseph4gi.com/2016/08/johns-hopkins-meatal-stenosis-article.html
- Meatal stenosis is a common result of infant circumcision: facebook.com/CircumcisionHarmsBreastfeeding/photos/a.275276959162858.75469.200048563352365/10

- 27145893975957
- Metzitzah B'Peh and Herpes: nocirc.org/publish/NOCIRC%202015%20nwsltr-17.pdf
- Mohel Cuts Off A Third of Baby's Penis During Circumcision:
  web.archive.org/web/20120420234114/http://www.algemeiner.com/2012/04/18/mohel-cuts-off-a-third-of-babys-penis-during-circumcision
- Montreal doctor sanctioned for 31 botched circumcisions: circumstitions.com/news/news72.html
- Name Shield for Mohel Who Gave Herpes to Baby:
  hooded2016.wordpress.com/2016/04/03/name-shield-for-mohel-who-gave-herpes-to-baby
- Neonatal Circumcision *(fairly neutral and blah, but does discuss complications)*:
  aafp.org/about/policies/all/neonatal-circumcision.html
- New Study Estimates Neonatal Circumcision Death Rate Higher Than Suffocation and Auto Accidents:
  web.archive.org/web/20160707201301/http://www.examiner.com/article/new-study-estimates-neonatal-circumcision-death-rate-higher-than-suffocation-and-auto-accidents
- New study: male circumcision and sexual difficulties for men and female partners:
  web.archive.org/web/20130312091702/http://www.examiner.com/article/new-study-male-circumcision-and-sexual-difficulties-for-men-and-female-partners
- Ontario newborn bleeds to death after family doctor persuades parents to get him circumcised:
  nationalpost.com/health/ontario-newborn-bleeds-to-death-after-family-doctor-persuades-parents-to-get-him-circumcised
- Orthodox Jews in talks with health officials over oral suction circumcision which has been linked to herpes in children: dailymail.co.uk/news/article-2963564
- Pittsburgh rabbi getting sued for allegedly severing newborn's penis:
  web.archive.org/web/20160711082645/http://www.nydailynews.com/news/national/rabbi-sued-allegedly-severing-newborn-penis-article-1.1561056
- Plastibell circumcision degloved her baby's penis, he will not have a normal sex life, needs more surgery:
  facebook.com/photo.php?fbid=543897989100693&set=a.105147402975756.9541.100004414898074
- Plastibell circumcision step by step: facebook.com/photo.php?
  fbid=1596862997233506&set=a.1432011917051949.1073741827.100007294630022
- Poor baby died after he had a botched circumcision, got an uti, high fever:
  facebook.com/photo.php?fbid=207162829627337&set=p.207162829627337
- Post-operative Complications of Circumcision: i2researchhub.org/articles/ch-5-post-operative-complications-of-circumcision-doc-genital-integrity-statement
- R.I.P. Baby Brayden: facebook.com/photo.php?fbid=10153910937405407&set=p.10153910937405407
- R.I.P. Little Dave *(3 days old):*
  facebook.com/photo.php?fbid=10153233669726937&set=p.10153233669726937
- Ritual circumcision and risk of autism spectrum disorder in 0- to 9-year-old boys: national cohort study in Denmark: journals.sagepub.com/doi/full/10.1177/0141076814565942
- Ritual circumcision linked to increased risk of autism in young boys, research suggests:
  sciencedaily.com/releases/2015/01/150109093725.htm

- Should surgery for hypospadias be performed before an age of consent?: academia.edu/13117940
- Stricken teen ends his life after penile amputation due to circumcision complication: dispatchlive.co.za/news/2016-03-25-stricken-teen-ends-his-life-after-penile-amputation-due-to-circumcision-complication
- The Immediate Complications of Circumcision: i2researchhub.org/articles/ch-4-immediate-complications-of-circumcision-doc-genital-integrity-statement
- The Lesser Known Complication Of Circumcision: web.archive.org/web/20201111230434/ravishly.com/lesser-known-complication-circumcision
- The Perils of Plastibell Circumcision: A Mythical "No Cutting, No Risk" Method: www.drmomma.org/2010/05/the-perils-of-plastibell-circumcision.html
- The Plastibell Lie: www.savingsons.org/2012/03/plastibell-lie.html
- Tot's shock hosp death at New York City hospital: facebook.com/photo.php?fbid=10153233666871937&set=p.10153233666871937
- Tuberculosis Acquired Through Ritual Circumcision *(mezizah)*: cirp.org/library/complications/holt1
- Two-Week Old Baby Boy Dies Of Herpes After Rabbi Performs "Holy Oral Circumcision": facebook.com/photo.php?fbid=10153233671066937&set=p.10153233671066937
- Video testimonies of harm: circumcisionharm.org/testimony.htm
- Week-old boy died after circumcision: facebook.com/photo.php?fbid=10153233679666937&set=p.10153233679666937
- When a baby dies from circumcision you find out the truth that circumcision is valued more than a baby's life: mondofown.blogspot.com/2012/01/when-baby-dies-from-circumcision.html
- Why I Chose to Circumcise My Son... *(includes video clip of infant death from hemorrhage following circumcision)*: everythingbirthblog.com/2011/12/13/why-i-chose-to-circumcise-my-son

Videos:
- Circumcision Accidents: youtu.be/jaWiBzZYG9Y
- Ethical Doctor Discusses Deaths and Complications from Circumcision: youtu.be/TPWqB4SGjgk

12   Urinary Tract Infections and Infant Circumcision

In 1989 the American Academy of Pediatrics, which had repeatedly pronounced infant circumcision unnecessary since the early 70's,[1] reviewed the subject again in light of more recent data on urinary tract infections (UTI). They released a fairly neutral statement, differing only slightly from their previous pronouncements.[2] Upon release, their verdict immediately underwent immense media distortion which has led the public to believe that the AAP is more pro-circumcision than they truly are. In 1999 the AAP restated:

> "… these data (in support of the operation) are not sufficient to recommend routine neonatal circumcision. … the procedure is not essential to the child's current well-being …" [3]

In 1985 Maj. Thomas E. Wiswell, a U.S. Army physician at Brooke Army Medical Center in San Antonio, TX., reported his observations of a significantly increased incidence of urinary tract infections among intact (non-circumcised) male infants over that among circumcised male infants. Upon reviewing the medical records of all infants born at Brooke Army Medical Center between January 1, 1982 and June 30, 1983, out of 1,919 circumcised male infants, 4 subsequently experienced infection of the urinary tract (0.21%). Out of 583 intact male infants, 24 experienced urinary tract infections during infancy (4.12%) In other words roughly 1 out of 500 circumcised male infants experienced UTIs, while approximately 1 out of 25 intact male infants experienced UTIs, a 20-fold increase in the rate of urinary tract infection among intact infant boys in this group.[4]

Prior to these observations Wiswell had opposed routine infant circumcision, but upon the publication of this and several subsequent similar articles, he has become an avid proponent of the controversial surgery.

Infection of the urinary tract is virtually always caused by contamination from fecal bacteria. A suspected contaminant is stool in the baby's diaper.

Wiswell comments:

---

1 Thompson HC, King LR, Knox E, Korones SB. Ad Hoc Task Force on Circumcision – Report. *Pediatrics*. 1975-10; 56(4).
2 Schoen EJ, Anderson G, Bohon C, Hinman F Jr., Poland RL, Wakeman Emaurice. Report of the Task Force on Circumcision. *American Academy of Pediatrics* – Reprint. 1989. (The above report pronounced the Wiswell studies inconclusive, stating: "It should be noted that these studies in army hospitals are retrospective in design and may have methodologic flaws. For example, they do not include all boys born in any single cohort or those treated as outpatients, so the study may have been influenced by selection bias.")
3 Lannon CM, Bailey AGD, Fleishman AR, Kaplan GW, Swanson JT, Doustan D. American Academy of Pediatrics Task Force on Circumcision. Circumcision Policy Statement. *Pediatrics*. 1999; 103(3): 686-93.
4 Wiswell TE. Decreased Incidence of Urinary Tract Infections in Circumcised Male Infants. *Pediatrics*. 1985-05; 75(5): 901-3.

"The male urethra is apparently more exposed to contaminating fecal bacteria than is the female urethra. The measured concentration of periurethral aerobic flora decreases with increasing age. Circumcision may reduce the extent of meatal contamination and thereby, decrease the likelihood of bacterial ascent into the bladder. With increasing age, the foreskin is more easily retracted. Penile hygiene should subsequently improve, resulting in decreased bacterial exposure and fewer urinary tract infections." [5]

Most of the infants in Wiswell's above mentioned report were less than 3 months of age. Out of a total of 5,261 infants, 41 in all experienced urinary tract infection. (13 girls out of 2,759 also were included in the report.)[6]

It would seem that the foreskin would protect the glans from simple fecal contact, as it is known that the foreskin serves as a covering for the more delicate glans. Therefore Wiswell's findings are surprising, if not arousing of suspicion. Some commentators have hypothesized that the enclosed area under the foreskin could provide a breeding ground for bacteria, while the exposed glans of the circumcised infant penis would be less likely to harbor such contaminants. However, the entirely sealed structure of a normal newborn's glans and foreskin comprises virtually no space, resembling more closely the nature of an interior organ. The only substance with which it should ever come in contact would be the baby's own urine which normally is sterile and harmless. When left alone the normally tightly sealed newborn foreskin gradually separates from the glans of the penis – a process which can take from several months to several years. Therefore it is curious that circumcision would apparently reduce the possibility of meatal contamination when the absence of the foreskin creates an exposed meatus. The rates of urinary tract infections among infants and young children decrease with age. However, toilet training with subsequent absence of soiled diaper contact is probably a more significant factor than age or foreskin retractility.

In a subsequent report Wiswell observed no urinary tract infections among 1,575 circumcised infants (0%), while 8 urinary tract infections occurred among 444 intact male infants (1.80%).[7]

In yet another, much larger study, upon reviewing 10 years worth of medical records of all infants born at Brooke Army Medical Center, Wiswell reported the

---

[5] Ibid. (Wiswell's resources: Stamey TA. Urinary Infections in Infancy and Childhood. In: *Pathogenesis and Treatment of Urinary Tract Infections.* Baltimore: Williams & Wilkins. 1980: 294-6; Lincoln K, Winberg J. Studies of Urinary Tract Infections in Infancy & Childhood. *Acta Paediatr Scand.* 1964; 53: 307-16; Bollgren I, Winberg J. The Periurethral Aerobic Bacterial Flora in Healthy Boys and Girls. *Acta Paediatr Scand.* 1976; 65: 74-80.)

[6] Ibid., p. 902.

[7] Wiswell TE. Corroborative Evidence for the Decreased Incidence of Urinary Tract Infections in Circumcised Male Infants. *Pediatrics.* 1986-07; 78(1): 96-9.

following figures: Out of 175,317 circumcised male infants, 193 (0.11%) developed urinary tract infection. Out of 46,112 intact male infants, 468 (1.12%) experienced urinary tract infections. The rate of UTIs among the intact males in this study was roughly ¼ that of his first study, and the intact to circumcised ratio of UTI occurrence is roughly half as large. In his 1987 study, roughly ten times as many infants in the intact group experienced UTIs than did the circumcised group. Urinary tract infection occurred among approximately one out of one hundred intact baby boys, and approximately one out of a thousand circumcised baby boys.[8]

Wiswell notes that the rate of infant male circumcision had significantly decreased over the previous decade. (From 1975-1979, 84.3% of baby boys were circumcised, while from 1980-1984, 74.0% were circumcised, a greater than 10% decrease.) He predicts that increasing incidences of infant UTI will occur as a result of our nation's declining rate of infant circumcision.[9]

At face value one could conclude that a valid health benefit of infant circumcision has been observed. The intact baby movement has focused upon infant pain and trauma imposed by circumcision, the invalidity of purported health claims, the protective role of the foreskin, the value of the wholeness of the body in its unaltered state, and the personal rights of the infant. But when this information was originally compiled, we knew nothing of infant urinary tract infections. In light of these findings, have we made a mistake?

12.1 Observations Reported by Others

Many doctors have questioned Wiswell's findings, including several whose letters subsequently appeared in *Pediatrics*:

Cunningham comments:

"There being no plausible explanation for such a finding, before we accept any cause and effect relationship and the possible consequence (reversal of the worldwide trend away from routine circumcision of the newborn), we should seek alternative explanations.[10]

---

8 Wiswell TE. Declining Frequency of Circumcision: Implications for Changes in the Absolute Incidence and Male to Female Sex Ratio of Urinary Tract Infections in Early Infancy. *Pediatrics*. 1987-03; 79(3): 338-42.
9 Ibid., p. 341.
10 Cunningham N (Division of General Pediatrics, Department of Pediatrics, Clinical Pediatrics and Public Health, College of Physicians and Surgeons of Columbia University, NY). Circumcision and Urinary Tract Infections (Letter to the Editor). *Pediatrics*. 1986-02; 77(2): 267.

Cunningham mentions socio-cultural differences between families of circumcised and intact infants, interventive care of the infant foreskin and the catheterization process (sometimes used for collecting urine samples) as possible variables.[10]

Cunningham also mentions a recent Swedish study which reported an incidence of only 0.56% (1/200) of UTIs among infant males. (Presumably all were intact since circumcision is rare in Sweden.)[11]

Altschul analyzed data on all infants younger than 1 year of age with urinary tract infection admitted to Northwest Region Kaiser Foundation Hospitals from 1979 to 1985. 25,000 infants were born in those hospitals over that 6 year period, during which the rate of newborn circumcision declined from 83% to 76%. 19 infants had the diagnosis of urinary tract infection. Five were boys and fourteen were girls. Presumably half of the 25,000 total infants were boys. Hence there were five cases of UTI among approximately 12,500 baby boys. The 13% to 24% of baby boys left intact over those years translates as approximately 2500 intact infant males. Of the five infant boys with UTI, one was circumcised, two had congenital defects (kidney obstruction), and two were normal intact males. Altschul cites a 3/2500 rate of infant UTI in this report (he includes one of the infants with congenital defects among the intact boys) for a rate of 0.12%, or roughly 1 out of 833 cases of UTI among intact infant males.[12] This is considerably lower than Wiswell's figures which ranged from 1.1% (1/100) to 4.1% (1/25).

But there exists no universally agreed upon standard or percentage by which endorsement or rejection of a medical practice should be based.

12.1.1 Non-Surgical Preventability

"Leave it alone" has been a virtual battle-cry in instructing people in proper care of the child's foreskin. An infant's foreskin is normally tight and unretractile. Virtually all problems known to be associated with the foreskin, such as infection, or phimosis (abnormal tightness) are caused by adults' attempts to force it loose for "cleaning."

Peaceful Beginnings, NOCIRC and most similar organizations support a "total hands off" philosophy towards care of an infant's or young child's foreskin. Although most foreskins become loose and retractile by age 3 or 4, in most little boys there is rarely anything there to clean. Not until adolescence, when penile size increases and adult body odors begin does regular simple retraction of the foreskin during bathing become advisable.[13, 14, 15]

---

11 Tullus K, Kallenius G. Epidemiological Aspects of P-fimbriated Escherichia Coli IV. Extraintestinal E. Coli Infections Before the Age of One Year and Their Relation to Fecal Colonization with P-fimbriated E. Coli. *Acta Paedr Scand.* 1987; 76: 463-9.

12 Altschul MS. Larger Numbers Needed. *Pediatrics.* 1987-11; 80(5): 763.

The area between the foreskin and glans in a normal newborn is a sealed, sterile site. Infecting bacteria do not originate under the foreskin. Urinary tract infections are normally caused by pathogens which originate in the bowel from fecal material. Therefore it can only reach the foreskin and the urethra and bladder if the infecting agent somehow becomes introduced into this area. Many have suggested that misadvised, interventive care of the infant foreskin could be a means of introducing contaminants into the urinary tract.

In Wiswell's report:

> "The parents of all male infants were advised to routinely clean the glans with a mild soap and water solution. The parents of uncircumcised male infants were additionally counseled to gently retract the foreskin to allow the easily exposed portion of the glans to be cleaned ..." [16]

In response other doctors have countered: "... the advice given to the parents, i.e., to retract the foreskin, led to trauma and thereby opened a portal of entry for pathogenic bacteria ..." [10]

> "As it is generally accepted that the prepuce is adherent to the glans penis and that retracting the foreskin in an infant may traumatize the penis and prepuce, I would wonder whether this advice may have contributed to the increased urinary tract infection rate seen in the uncircumcised male infants.[17]

> "After 40 years of pediatric practice, I am firmly convinced that the best hygiene is to keep hands off and leave the prepuce alone. I have had many infants with problems from inadequate and poorly done circumcisions; similarly, I have had many uncircumcised infants who got into trouble when a 'helpful' nurse, doctor, or grandmother forcibly retracted and cleaned a tight prepuce. ... I have never seen a problem in an uncircumcised infant when the mother just left it the way the Lord made it – no retractions, no vigorous cleansing, just left it alone. ... Historically, many 'scientific interventions' have proven to be more injurious

---

13 Øster J. Further Fate of the Foreskin – Incidence of Preputial Adhesions, Phimosis, and Smegma among Danish Schoolboys. *Arch Dis Childh.* 1986-04; 43: 200-3.
14 Gairdner D. The Fate of the Foreskin – A Study of Circumcision. *BMJ.* 1949-12-24: 1433-7.
15 Reichelderfer TE, Fraga JR. *Care of the Well Baby.* Reprint by Shepard KS (ed). Philadelphia, PA: J.B. Lippincott; 1968: 10.
16 Wiswell TE. *Pediatrics.* 1986-07: 96.
17 Malleson P (Pediatric Rheumatology, BC Children's Hospital Vancouver, British Columbia, Canada). Prepuce Care (Letter to the Editor). *Pediatrics.* 1986-02; 77(2): 265.

than helpful. Perhaps vigorous cleaning of the prepuce and glans are in that category." [18]

An even more intriguing consideration concerning infant colonization of maternal intestinal flora is reported in a recent Swedish study:
Home birth proponents emphasize that at home one is surrounded by one's "own" germs, to which most individuals have natural tolerance. Therefore, despite normally less than antiseptic conditions, a mother and her baby are usually less likely to become infected following delivery at home than in a hospital or birth center. Large numbers of people congregate in hospitals, while particularly virulent strains of bacteria abound that have become genetically resistant to antibiotics and antiseptic cleaning solutions. Hospital employees and patients, commonly develop staphylococcus infections. The fresh wound of an infant's circumcision has been observed to be a portal of entry for infection, sometimes with tragic outcome.[19]

The authors of the Swedish study under discussion consider the importance that newborn babies become colonized at birth with familiar bacteria from their own mothers' intestinal tracts rather than from foreign infectious agents in the hospital environment.

In their words:

"Retrospective studies suggest that circumcision of newborn boys will reduce the frequency of male early infantile urinary tract infection (UTI) by about 90%. If they are correct, this will be the first known instance of a common potential lethal disease being preventable by extirpation of a piece of normal tissue. To reconcile the phenomenon with existing views of evolution and biology, it is suggested that the effects of one unphysiological intervention are counterbalancing those of another – i.e., colonisation of the baby's gastrointestinal tract and genitals in maternity units by Escherichia coli strains of non-maternal origin, to which the baby has no passive immunity. As an alternative to circumcision to prevent early infantile male UTI, more natural colonisation could be promoted by strict rooming-in of mother and baby or by active colonisation of the baby with his mother's anaerobic gut flora. ...

... in biologically natural settings, when giving birth in the squatting or kneeling position, mothers often defaecate during delivery and thus colonise the baby with their own aerobic and anaerobic intestinal flora. Together with this gift

---
[18] Watson SJ. Care of Uncircumcised Penis. *Pediatrics*. 1987-11; 80(5): 765.
[19] Kravitz H, Murphy JB, Edadi K, Rosetti A, Ashraf H. Effects of Hexachlorophene-Detergent Baths in a Newborn Nursery with Emphasis on the Care of Circumcisions. *Ill Med J*. 1962-08; 122(2): 133-9.

they provide specific protection – immunoglobulins transferred before delivery through the placenta and later through breast milk. ...

If the composition of the normal flora is as important as many think it is, the colonisation of newborn babies may be too serious a matter to be left to chance in environments – the modern obstetric hospital or the neonatal intensive care unit – which from a biological point of view are unphysiological and possibly hazardous. ...

Attempts to manipulate the faecal flora might in the long run be a more physiological approach than to remove the prepuce from all newborn boys. Pending further research strict rooming-in might increase the likelihood of the baby being colonised by maternal strains." [20]

Further information on the rooming in status of the Wiswell and Altschul studies, including the extent to which each infant was kept in the central nursery (even if he "roomed in" for a portion of the hospital stay), might shed further light on Winberg's hypothesis. (Kaiser hospitals, from which the Altschul data was obtained, are known to offer rooming in.)

Proponents of breastfeeding can cite a long list of scientifically documented health advantages of breast milk over infant formula. Breast milk has now been found to contain high contents of oligosaccharides (a type of carbohydrate), which in turn are excreted in the urine of both nursing mothers and their breastfed babies. In one study oligosaccharides have been tentatively demonstrated to cause inhibition of bacterial adhesions which in turn may have a preventative effect against urinary tract infections.[21]

The breastfed/bottlefed status of the infants in the Wiswell and Altschul reports would be of interest to note. Bottlefeeding appears to be another "unphysiological intervention" which can increase the likelihood of infant uti.

The Winberg, et al. and Coppa, et al. studies suggest that the mother who keeps her baby with her from birth on and who breastfeeds can safely leave her infant son intact with scarce risk of urinary tract infection.

12.1.2 Comparative Pain and Trauma

Severe pain and trauma is inflicted upon a helpless newborn when undergoing circumcision. Our literature abounds with graphic descriptions of infants strapped to "circi" boards, screaming frantically while their genitals are clamped and cut.

---

20 Winberg J, Bollgren I, Gothefors L, Herthelius M, Tuelus K. The Prepuce: A Mistake of Nature? *Lancet.* 1989-03-18: 598-9.
21 Coppa GV, Gabrielli O, Giorgi P, Catassi C, Montanari MP, Varaldo PE, Nichols BL. Preliminary Study of Breastfeeding and Bacterial Adhesion to Uroepithelial Cells. *Lancet.* 1990-03-10; 335(8689): 569-71.

Usually no anesthesia is used. (Use of a local injection has been purported to reduce the infant's crying time by half – which still equals much trauma.[22])

Urinary tract infection is also a highly stressful, traumatic event characterized by fever and painful urination. Other symptoms can include lethargy, irritability, and lack of appetite. Wiswell describes vomiting and diarrhea occurring in a few patients, although none with jaundice or "failure to thrive" syndrome.[23]

He describes urine samples obtained by catheterization, and less frequently by suprapubic aspiration (bladder tap.) Blood samples were taken in all infants and lumbar puncture (spinal tap) was obtained in some.[23]

How the stressful, traumatic experience of UTI would compare to the obvious stress and trauma of circumcision of a healthy infant would be difficult to evaluate. The circumcised baby experiences pain and trauma and permanent body alteration/mutilation with the loss of the protective foreskin. Usually he heals normally, although many complications – infection of the circumcision wound, hemorrhage, removal of excessive skin, injury to the glans and/or surrounding tissues, meatal ulceration (urine burns on the exposed glans), and in rare cases loss of the penis and death – have all been well documented.

The baby with a urinary tract infection undergoes pain and trauma. Unlike the circumcised baby, he does not undergo permanent body alteration with loss of a normal, useful body structure. Urinary tract infection is normally readily treatable with antibiotics. Although rare cases of long term detrimental effects of urinary tract infections have been mentioned in the literature, no honest evaluation has been made to consider this alongside the known, well-documented long term complications of circumcision.

Wiswell clearly states:

> "It is unclear at this time whether the increase in incidence of urinary tract infection in uncircumcised infants has any long-term medical significance other than the immediate cost of diagnosis, treatment, and follow-up evaluation of the acute infection." [24]

Elsewhere the same author states: "In the preantibiotic era, the mortality from urinary tract infection was 20%, whereas an additional 20% may have ended up with hypertension and chronic renal failure." [25]

---

22 Stang HJ, Cunnar MR, Snellman L, et al. Local Anesthesia for Neonatal Circumcision. Effect on Distress and Cortisol Response. *JAMA*. 1988; 259: 1507-11.
23 Wiswell TE, Smith FR, Bass JW. Decreased incidence of urinary tract infections in circumcised male infants. *Pediatrics*. 1985; 75: 902.
24 Ibid., p. 903.
25 Wiswell TE. Letter to the Editor (reply to Altschul's "Larger Numbers Needed"). *Pediatrics*. 1987-11: 764.

However, today with readily available antibiotics, the above consideration cannot apply.

If the concern is towards preventing a high stress/trauma event for an infant, or balancing medical costs between that of universal circumcision versus individual costs of medical treatment for urinary tract infections, a proposal of routine circumcision for all infants to purportedly prevent a small number of urinary tract infections hardly appears to be valid medical logistics.

12.1.3 Medical "Just In Case-ism"

The proposal to destroy hundreds, if not thousands, of infant foreskins to possibly prevent one instance of urinary tract infection, is yet another example of medical "just in case-ism" with which the public has been bombarded. Soaring Cesarean rates, universal use of fetal heart monitors, hysterectomies, mastectomies, dilation and curettages, and routine episiotomies are but a few questionable, invasive procedures which frequently have failed to improve or preserve overall patient health.

As consumers we have a responsibility to ourselves and to our children to be aware and informed about all medical procedures. The orientation of the medical profession reflects an aggressive, "cut it away" approach to health care. But most surgery, particularly non-emergency surgery, has feasible noninterventive alternatives.

12.1.4 The Purpose of Surgery

Most surgery involves correcting an abnormal body condition – i.e. repair of injury, removal of diseased tissue, or correction of a deformity. Some surgery is cosmetic – which can only be considered ethical if chosen by the individual.

Birth associated surgeries such as episiotomies and Cesareans have been sources of intense debate within obstetrical circles.

But can surgery be preventative medicine? Never has the routine destruction of a normal body part been proven to be an effective health measure.

Other body structures, such as ears, toes, or fingernails could be similarly viewed as superfluous with medical data constructed around an amputative philosophy. For example, a widespread practice of routine toe amputation at birth could be demonstrated to spare the individual of a lifetime of bouts of corns, bunions, and athlete's foot, and save him from the nuisance of washing between the toes. We dismiss any similar amputative philosophy as ludicrous, hence proving that a mystical irrationality surrounds circumcision and foreskins that we apply to no other normally occurring body part.

12.1.5 "Knives Versus Washcloths" – Medical Dictatorship Versus Wholeness of the Body and Personal Autonomy

Many people have pointed out that any and all purported "health benefits" related to circumcision are merely a side issue to avoid facing the facts clearly.

John Erickson, an outspoken advocate of infants' rights has stated:

> "When you cut off a baby's foreskin, you are literally censoring his life. The vast majority of males who are not circumcised value their wholeness – even beyond price – and keep their foreskins intact, for the same reason they keep the rest of their bodies intact. When you circumcise a baby, you are cutting off a part of his penis that you *can* cut off only because the person you're cutting it off of can't protect himself because he *is* a baby. ... Many males circumcised as babies see themselves as harmed by that amputation – *regardless of the reason they were circumcised* (emphasis mine) – just as they would see themselves as harmed if any other healthy, sensitive, normally functioning part of their body had been cut off. The endlessly debated "health benefits" of infant circumcision are therefore a false issue and would not justify depriving a baby of his foreskin even if they were real." [26]

Warren F. Smith, another activist in the intact baby movement, has quipped: "Never ask the barber if you need a haircut." [27]

12.2 Conclusion

When my fourth son was born in 1985 I found the matter so absurdly simple as to warrant hardly any thought or action at all. During his infancy I was thankful to forgo subjecting him to the traumatic, violating experience that his brothers experienced. I was also thankful that he could be spared the troublesome problems with meatal ulceration that my older sons experienced as infants.

I later gave birth to another baby, a daughter in 1989. Had this baby been another boy, he too would have remained intact.

Peaceful Beginnings continues to oppose routine infant circumcision as highly traumatic to newborn infants, of dubious benefits, and violating of individual, personal rights with which an infant or small child is not afforded if his foreskin is taken away. We welcome the challenge of investigating new findings which may support or refute this stand.

---

26 Erickson J. Letter to the Editor. *The Baby News Connection Journal,* San Antonio, TX. 1990-05/06; 6(2).
27 Smith WF. (personal correspondence.)

12.3 Informational Resources

* 66 Infants with Urinary Tract Infection in First Month of Life: cirp.org/library/disease/UTI/littlewood1
* AAP Circumcision Policy Statement 1999: cirp.org/library/statements/aap1999
* Bacterial contamination rates for non-clean-catch and clean-catch midstream urine collections in uncircumcised boys: cirp.org/library/disease/UTI/llorens
* Breast feeding and biological properties of faecal E. coli strains: cirp.org/library/disease/UTI/gothefors1
* Breast-feeding and urinary tract infection *(1992)*: cirp.org/library/disease/UTI/pisacane1992
* Breastfeeding and urinary tract infection *(Pisacane)*: cirp.org/library/disease/UTI/pisacane
* Breastfeeding and urinary-tract infection *(Maarild)*: cirp.org/library/disease/UTI/marild
* Burrowing bacteria may explain recurrent urinary tract infections: bmj.com/content/317/7171/1473.1.full
* Canadian Paediatrics Society 1989 on Routine Circumcision: cirp.org/library/statements/cps3
* Care of Uncircumcised Penis: cirp.org/library/hygiene/watson1
* Circumcision and Acquisition of Human Papillomavirus Infection in Young Men: journals.lww.com/stdjournal/Fulltext/2011/11000/Circumcision_and_Acquisition_of_Human.16.aspx
* Circumcision and Lifetime Risk of Urinary Tract Infection *(by circumcision supporters Morris & Wiswell)*: auajournals.org/article/S0022-5347%2812%2905623-6/abstract
* Circumcision and newborn utis: Winberg's solution: bjui-journals.onlinelibrary.wiley.com/doi/full/10.1046/j.1464-410X.2003.04113.x
* Circumcision and urinary tract infection: cirp.org/library/disease/UTI
* Circumcision and Urinary Tract Infections *(Cunningham)*: cirp.org/library/disease/UTI/cunningham
* Circumcision causes increase in infant UTI: forum09.faithfreedom.org/viewtopic.php?p=29520#p29520
* Circumcision for the Child at Risk of UTI: yourwholebaby.org/circumcision-for-uti
* Circumcision for the prevention of urinary tract infection in boys: adc.bmj.com/content/90/8/853.full
* Circumcision is for weiners! *(cartoon at end of article)*: womanuncensored.blogspot.com/2010/01/circumcision-is-for-weiners.html
* Circumcision of the Newborn Male and the Risk of Urinary Tract Infection During the First Year: cirp.org/library/disease/UTI/amato
* Circumcision reduces lifetime risk for UTIs *(Morris, Wiswell – pro circ advocates, pushing circumcision for UTI prevention)*: contemporarypediatrics.com/view/circumcision-reduces-lifetime-risk-utis
* Circumcision: Is the Risk of Urinary Tract Infection Really the Pivotal Issue?: cirp.org/library/disease/UTI/chessare
* Circumcision: is the risk of urinary tract infection really the pivotal issue?: pubmed.ncbi.nlm.nih.gov/1544271
* Circumcision: Pros and cons: ncbi.nlm.nih.gov/pmc/articles/PMC2878423
* Circumcision: The Uniquely American Medical Enigma: cirp.org/library/general/wallerstein
* Circumcisions: Again: cirp.org/library/disease/UTI/newman1
* Circumcisions: Again: cirp.org/library/disease/UTI/robson1
* Cohort study on circumcision of newborn boys and subsequent risk of urinary-tract infection: cirp.org/library/disease/UTI/to2

- Cultural Bias in the AAP's 2012 Technical Report and Policy Statement on Male Circumcision:
  pediatrics.aappublications.org/content/131/4/796
- Decreasing the risk of urinary tract infections *(by breastfeeding)*: cirp.org/library/disease/UTI/outerbridge
- Decreasing the risk of urinary tract infections *(immunological functions of prepuce)*:
  cirp.org/library/disease/UTI/outerbridge
- Developmental factors of urethral human papillomavirus lesions:
  bjui-journals.onlinelibrary.wiley.com/doi/abs/10.1046/j.1464-410x.1999.00104.x
- Differentiation and developmental pathways of uropathogenic Escherichia coli in urinary tract pathogenesis:
  pnas.org/content/101/5/1333.full
- Doubt over Wiswell's conclusion concerning an association between the foreskin and urinary tract infections:
  cirp.org/library/disease/UTI/vanhowe
- Effect of Circumcision on Incidence of Urinary Tract Infection in Preschool Boys:
  cirp.org/library/disease/UTI/craig
- Effect of circumcision on urinary tract infection after successful antireflux surgery:
  pubmed.ncbi.nlm.nih.gov/15329127
- Effect of confounding in the association between circumcision status and urinary tract infection:
  cirp.org/library/disease/UTI/vanhowe_uti2005
- How the Foreskin Protects Against UTI *(urinary tract infection)*:
  www.drmomma.org/2009/12/how-foreskin-protects-against-uti.html
- Incidence rate of first-time symptomatic urinary tract infection in children under 6 years of age:
  cirp.org/library/disease/UTI/marild3
- Intracellular bacterial biofilm-like pods in urinary tract infections: cirp.org/library/disease/UTI/anderson1
- Is ritual circumcision a risk factor for neonatal urinary tract infections?:
  adc.bmj.com/content/94/3/191.abstract
- Male Neonatal Circumcision and the Subsequent Risk of Urinary Tract Infection:
  cirp.org/library/disease/UTI/to
- Options in antimicrobial management of urinary tract infections in infants and children:
  cirp.org/library/disease/UTI/mccracken
- Overview of urinary tract infection (UTI) in children:
  healthline.com/health/urinary-tract-infection-children#Overview1
- Postcircumcision Urinary Tract Infection: cirp.org/library/disease/UTI/cohen
- Preliminary study of breastfeeding and bacterial adhesion to uroepithelial cells:
  cirp.org/library/disease/UTI/coppa
- Protective effect of breastfeeding against urinary tract infection: cirp.org/library/disease/UTI/marild4
- Protective effects of breastfeeding against urinary tract infection: cirp.org/library/disease/UTI/hanson1
- Rebuttal of Schoen's proposal of universal child circumcision in Europe:
  cirp.org/library/disease/UTI/winberg-bollgren2
- Recent Contributions to the Study of Pyelitis in Infancy: cirp.org/library/disease/UTI/smith1916
- Risk Compensation Following Male Circumcision: Results from a Two-Year Prospective Cohort Study of Re-

cently Circumcised and Uncircumcised Men in Nyanza Province, Kenya: link.springer.com/article/10.1007/s10461-014-0846-4
- Routine Circumcision in the Newborn: An Opposing View: cirp.org/library/disease/UTI/thompson
- Routine neonatal circumcision for the prevention of urinary tract infections in infancy: cochranelibrary.com/cdsr/doi/10.1002/14651858.CD009129.pub2/full
- Study: Uncircumcised Boys Have a Higher Risk of UTI *(pro circ but good responses from intactivists)*: healthland.time.com/2012/07/09/study-uncircumcised-boys-have-a-higher-risk-of-uti
- The Circumcision Controversy: cirp.org/library/disease/UTI/altschul1990
- The Effects of Circumcision on Breastfeeding *(breastfeeding helps preventing UTIs)*: nocirc.org/statements/breastfeeding.php
- The Incidence of Genitourinary Abnormalities in Circumcised and Uncircumcised Boys Presenting With an Initial Urinary Tract Infection By 6 Months of Age: cirp.org/library/disease/UTI/mueller
- The Prepuce: A Mistake of Nature?: cirp.org/library/disease/UTI/winberg-bollgren
- Urinary Pathogens in the Male: cirp.org/library/disease/UTI/maskell/UrinPathMale.pdf
- Urinary Tract Infection Following Ritual Jewish Circumcision: cirp.org/library/disease/UTI/goldman
- Urinary tract infections and circumcision: cirp.org/library/disease/UTI/herzog2
- Urinary Tract Infections in Young Infants: cirp.org/library/disease/UTI/ginsburg
- Urinary tract infections per se do not cause end-stage kidney disease: cirp.org/library/disease/UTI/sreenarasimhaiah1
- Urologic Diseases in America Project: Trends in Resource Use For Urinary Tract Infections in Women: auajournals.org/article/S0022-5347%2805%2961083-X/abstract
- UTI Testing on Boys: DO NOT RETRACT!: www.drmomma.org/2009/09/uti-testing-on-boys-do-not-retract.html
- What is the effect of circumcision on risk of urinary tract infection in boys with posterior urethral valves? *(pro circumcision but states that more studies are needed)*: pubmed.ncbi.nlm.nih.gov/19231547

13 Penile Cancer

The supposed correlation between circumcision, especially when performed in infancy or early childhood, and lack of subsequent penile cancer, has been one of the biggest medical arguments in favor of the operation. *Is* circumcision during infancy justified as a preventive measure against this disease? Are the pain and trauma of circumcision, the risk of immediate complications, and the lifelong deprivation of one's foreskin outweighed by a *high* possibility of eventual cancer of the penis? Is amputation of the foreskin an effective means of insurance against this disease? If so, is it the *only* effective means of preventing this disease?

One of the earliest studies of penile cancer took place in 1907. Barney observed 100 cases of epithelioma (skin-cell based cancer) of the penis. These were observed over 33 years of practice. He noted that the disease is rare, equaling about 2.8 cases yearly at Massachusetts General Hospital where he conducted his research, and constituting around 1% of all cancers. He mentions that no Jews were included in his study.[1]

During the 1920s and '30s medical authorities gave considerable attention to penile cancer and attempted to link it to lack of circumcision. Because the disease is rare among Jews and Muslims, and because both of these groups practice circumcision, authorities concluded that cutting off the foreskin was an effective means of preventing penile cancer.

In 1932 Wolbarst conducted a study based on a nationwide (U.S.) questionnaire, medical literature, and personal correspondence. From this he made the following observations:

1. Cancer of the penis does not occur in Jews circumcised in infancy.[2] It has occurred in an uncircumcised Jew.
2. Penile cancer does occur in Mohammedans (Muslims), who practice ritual circumcision between the 4th and 9th year, but not in infancy. A few cases have been recorded.
3. Penile cancer occurs almost exclusively in the uncircumcised, who also suffer from phimosis, and occasionally in men circumcised in adult life.
4. There is no racial immunity[3] against penile cancer in Jews or Mohammedans. The one common factor which induces immunity is circumcision in early life.
5. Penile cancer constitutes at least 2-3% of all cancer in men.

---

1 Barney JD. Epithelioma of the Penis. An Analysis of One Hundred Cases. *Ann Surg.* 1907; 46: 890.
2 A small number of Jews who were circumcised in infancy and later developed cancer of the penis *have* been reported since Wolbarts's study was made.
3 There is some speculation today that genetic immunity may indeed be responsible for Jews' relative immunity to certain diseases, including penile cancer.

6. The annual mortality from penile cancer in the U.S. is about 225, all or at least most of which can be prevented by circumcision in early life.[4]

These findings are still being cited today as the basis for the alleged medical arguments in favor of neonatal circumcision. However, today there is growing evidence that his observations are only partially true. The wisdom of a surgical approach as a means of preventing a rare disease is highly questionable. The facts about cancer of the penis must be carefully scrutinized.

13.1   What is Cancer of the Penis? How Does it Develop? What are its Causes and Related Factors?

According to Bruhl:

"Carcinoma of the penis occurs rarely, and among our patients it takes with a frequency of 0.6%, last place among the malignant disease of the male urogenital tract after carcinoma of the kidney, prostate, bladder, and testicles. It originates mostly in the inner part of the prepuce of the penis or the inner part of the glans, and sparing the corpus spongiosum penis urethrae, spreads within the corpus cavernosum [the body of the penis]. In our department, from 1928-1974, 124 penile cancers were observed. In 69 of these the histologic diagnosis could be reviewed. In 95.7% a squamous cell carcinoma had been found." [5]

The condition is almost invariably associated with *phimosis* – the condition in which the foreskin cannot be easily retracted over the glans for washing. This fact is repeatedly stated by nearly all authors who have studied the disease.

According to Barney: "In many cases the patient said he 'was never able to retract his foreskin.' " [6]

Graham states:

"In penile cancers the prepuce is almost always tight or long and may be adherent to the underlying glans. There is retention of smegma, a peculiarly odiferous sebum, with continuous irritation. This continual irritation of the smegmatic debris results in redness, itching, a foul discharge, edema of the prepuce, and ulceration." [7]

---

4   Wolbarst AL. Circumcision and Penile Cancer. *Lancet.* 1932-01-16: 150.
5   Bruhl P. Problems of Therapeutic Surgery in Penis Carcinoma. *Cancer Res.* 1977; 60: 120-6.
6   Barney, p. 894.
7   Lenowitz H, Graham AP. Carcinoma of the Penis. *J Urol.* 1946; 56: 462.

However, in a few cases, previous circumcision appears to have been the cause or provided the originating site for the penile cancer.

Barney observed:

> "... six cases who had previous circumcision, and who said that the wound had either never healed or that the cancer had first begun in its edges. This surely is a form of trauma and in these cases it was apparently the beginning of the trouble." [8]

Cancer of the penis is nearly always a slow growing cancer which is easily curable, especially if detected in its earlier stages. However, many writers have observed that patients with this disease often delay treatment until it has reached advanced stages.

Colon, who researched the subject in 1952, comments:

> "Carcinoma of the penis is a lesion of the skin, definitely a skin carcinoma. Its very early lesions are not often seen because being relatively painless at first, the patient usually seeks medical advice at an unbelievably late stage of the disease." [9]

Cancer of the penis is frequently associated with sexually transmitted disease. In Graham's study 32% had either syphilis or gonorrhea.[10] The question arises as to whether STD is a causal factor in the development of penile cancer, or whether both diseases are associated with other factors.

Graham also comments that sometimes doctors misdiagnose the condition: "In the medical lifetime of any general practitioner few such cases are seen. The physician is not cancer conscious and generally mistakes the condition for a venereal disease. Thus valuable time is lost." [11]

Cancer of the penis is a disease that is commonly associated with *extremely poor* personal hygiene.

Wolbarst, one of the leading proponents of routine infant circumcision as a cancer preventive, states:

> "... There is a direct relationship between the lack of hygienic care of the male genitals and the occurrence of penile cancer, and that *it is most common among peoples in whom ignorance and poverty combine to maintain hygiene at its lowest standard."* [4]

---

[8] Barney, p. 896.
[9] Colon JE. Carcinoma of the Penis. *J Urol.* 1952-05; 67(5): 702-8.
[10] Lenowitz & Graham, p. 464.
[11] Ibid., p. 482.

While cancer of the penis has been virtually non-existent among Jews, it is also true that neither "ignorance" nor "poverty" have been typical characteristics of Jewish people. Jews are a remarkably intelligent people, commonly achieving financial success, attaining higher education, and are well represented among the professional classes. These people almost always have a high standard of living and are consequently clean in their personal habits *regardless* of circumcision.

Cancer of the penis is rare, but not non-existent in individuals circumcised in infancy or early childhood. There are a few documented cases of penile cancers which have developed in individuals circumcised in infancy.[12, 13, 14]

According to one recent study:

"Thirty-six biopsy specimens taken from 11 men ranging from age 21 to 36, each of whom had multiple reddish to violaceous papules, some distinctly verrucoid or velvety on either or both the shaft and glans of the penis ... histologically ... all specimens submitted showed indubitable changes of squamous cell carcinoma in situ. *Ten of the 11 men had been circumcised in infancy.* In none of the cases was there evidence of squamous cell carcinoma extending into the dermis. All were treated and resolved by either chemicals which were applied topically, or by surgical excision."[15] [Apparently this condition is not a typical penile cancer.]

Most victims of penile cancer are elderly men. According to one study: "... The average age of our patients was 65; the youngest patient was 38 years old."[16]

A curious finding is that while penile cancer is extremely rare among males circumcised in infancy or early childhood, somehow circumcision during later childhood or adulthood confers less "immunity." For example, penile cancer is extremely rare among Jews circumcised in infancy, but occasionally does occur among Moslems who practice circumcision during childhood. The reason for this is not known.

Kennaway cites Dean's speculations:

"It may be that when an infant is circumcised and the glans is no longer protected by the prepuce, a denser, thicker epidermis develops, which is resistant to the formation of cancer by chronic irritation. When circumcision is performed in later years the glans may have lost its ability to produce a resistant covering, and

---

12 Marshall VF. More on Circumcision. *Med Trib*. 1965-07-12; 83: 11.
13 Sorrells ML. Still More Criticism. *Pediatrics*. 1975-08; 56(2): 339.
14 Leiter E, Lefkovits A. Circumcision and Penile Carcinoma. *NY State J Med*. 1975; 75(9): 1520-2.
15 Wade TR, Kopf AW, Ackerman AB. Bowenoid Papulosis of the Penis. *Cancer*. 1978-10; 42(4): 1890-1903.
16 Bruhl, p. 121.

although there is no longer irritation from retained secretions, the glans remains relatively sensitive to the contacts of everyday life." [17]

Another possibility is that Moslems, as well as some medical practitioners tend to not do as "complete" of a circumcision as do the Jews. They do not cut off as much skin and often do not force the remaining skin away from the glans in the manner of the Jewish "Periah." Perhaps for a few individuals the remaining foreskin does become phimosed to the glans, collect smegma and develop infection. This can be a problem among people who believe that genital hygiene is unnecessary because circumcision is practiced. A poorly cared for penis that is partially circumcised may also predispose the individual to penile cancer in a small number of cases.

In other cases, previous circumcision has been the direct *cause* of penile cancer – the cancer developing at the site of the poorly healing circumcision scar. This would only develop as a result of an adult circumcision, since cancer of the penis does not occur in infants or children.

13.2   Laboratory Experiments That Have Tested the Alleged Carcinogenic Properties of Smegma

Smegma is simply dead epithelial (skin) cells, which if allowed to accumulate provides a medium for the growth of bacteria. It collects on the genitals of both males and females, and for most people is washed away by simple, regular bathing. Circumcised males do develop smegma, although to a lesser extent than their intact counterparts. If a male is not circumcised smegma may collect underneath the foreskin in a manner similar to wax developing in one's ears. Like earwax, smegma has a natural tendency to dissipate as fast as it is produced. If this does not happen, retracting the foreskin and cleaning out the smegma is a very simple matter. For a few intact males who have never been taught that the foreskin should be retracted and cleaned, or who are extremely negligent in their personal cleanliness habits, smegma build-up beneath the foreskin can be a troublesome problem. (Needless to say, neglect and poor habits of personal hygiene bring about problems with all parts of the body!)

Nearly all victims of penile cancer have tight foreskins and extremely poor habits of personal cleanliness. It is not certain what predisposes the penis to cancer in such cases, but the hypothesis has been presented that smegma is somehow a cancer causing agent. A few laboratory experiments with animals have attempted to answer the question.

---

[17] Kennaway EL. Cancer of the Penis and Circumcision in Relation to the Incubation Period of Cancer. *Br J Cancer.* 1947-12; 1(4): 312.

In 1947 Plaut and Kohn-Speyer applied horse smegma (collected from dead animals in rendering plants) to mice. In 190 mice the smegma was placed in an artificially created skin tunnel. 122 mice received subcutaneous injections of smegma. 88 mice had it applied to the skin surface. 150 control mice were treated with cerumen (ear wax). After 500 days 47% of those treated with smegma were alive as compared with 30% of the controls. After 600 days 26% and 6% had survived respectively. After 700 days the survival rate was 12% and 1 ½ %. (Author's note: Apparently this experiment proves that earwax is more lethal than smegma!)

No tumors grew out of any of the control mice. 7 tumors grew out of the 400 smegma-treated mice. These included 4 papillary warts, 2 hornifying squamous-cell carcinomas, 1 undifferentiated skin carcinoma, and 1 spindle-cell sarcoma.

The authors conclude: "There is nothing to indicate the possible nature of the supposed carcinogenic factor in smegma." [18]

Reddy and Baruah conducted a similar experiment with mice, but involving fewer subjects, in 1961:

Fresh human smegma was injected in mice. There were 29 males and 16 females. 10 of each were used for controls. Nearly 50% of the animals died during the first year, some of infection of the genital tract probably caused by irritation from application of smegma and bacteria.

No macroscopic (visible to the naked eye) changes were observed in the male test animals. Microscopic examinations failed to show neoplastic changes.

No macroscopic growths were observed among the females. Microscopic examinations showed varying degrees of irritation, and hyperplasia (an excessive amount of normal cells).

Their conclusion: "Definite proof of the carcinogenic potentialities of smegma in its fresh state or in its altered form due to bacterial decomposition is lacking." [19]

13.3 Socioeconomic Factors Related to the Incidence of Penile Cancer

Many authorities have noted that nearly all victims of penile cancer come from lower socioeconomic groups for whom health care and information about disease symptoms are less available than for the middle class.[20]

For a myriad of unfortunate reasons a large proportion of Black people have been relegated to the lower classes.

---

18 Plaut A, Kohn-Speyer AC. The Carcinogenic Action of Smegma. *Science*. 1947; 105: 391.
19 Reddy DG, Baruah IK. Carcinogenic Action of Human Smegma. *Arch Pathol*. 1963-04; 75: 414-20.
20 Paige KE. The Ritual of Circumcision. *Hum Nat*. 1978-05: 44.

In 1944 Schrek noted a significantly high percentage of Black[21, 22] patients with penile cancer. He observed 120 cases of cancer of the penis (out of 11,790 patients at that hospital) and found 27.5% of these men were Black, compared to 8.45% Black people among the control group.[23]

In 1946 Schrek and Lenowitz conducted a study. Out of a group of 139 men with carcinoma of the penis, 28.1% were Black, compared to 7% of the control group. They hypothesized that the higher incidence of this disease among Black males was related to: (a) lower incidence of circumcision, (b) greater incidence of STD, or (c) racial susceptibility.

The authors found that the Black people observed in their study had a *higher* incidence of early circumcisions than did the men of other ethnicities. This was explained as a result of interns and residents in hospitals, particularly in the South, practicing circumcision on Black infants. Apparently the parents were poor, on welfare and/or in clinic-like settings, and parental consent for circumcision was not obtained.

The authors concluded that lack of circumcision is not the factor which is responsible for the high incidence of carcinoma of the penis among Black men.

Black men had approximately twice the incidence of syphilis as men of other ethnicities (17.5% and 7.6%) and twice the incidence of gonorrhea (42.1% and 22.0%). Half of the Black men and three-fourths of men of other ethnicities were free of STD.

Schrek and Lenowitz concluded:

"... White and [black] men who do not develop venereal disease are equally susceptible to carcinoma of the penis. There is then no evidence of any unusual susceptibility of [blacks] to carcinoma of the penis or of any immunity of white men to this lesion ... It has been shown that patients with carcinoma of the penis have a very high incidence of venereal disease. Evidently there is a correlation between the tumor and the infection ... The findings suggest that environmental, not racial, factors determine the incidence of carcinoma of the penis." [23]

---

21 Several articles such as this one, written several decades ago, use the outdated terms "Negroes" or "colored people." I have chosen to use the more modern term "African American."
22 Editor's note: R.R. didn't adjust the usage of 'African American' consequently but kept some passages unchanged, using the term 'Black' which she used before. Because many Black people in the USA don't want to be linked to Africa where there haven't been born, I have reset all occurances of the term 'African American' to 'Black', also in tribute to the current human rights movement BLM (Black Lives Matter).
23 Schrek R, Lenowitz H. Etiologic Factors in Carcinoma of the Penis. *Cancer Res.* 1964-11-12: 185-6.

13.4 Worldwide Distribution of Penile Cancer

It is true that cancer of the penis is rare among males who have been circumcised. However, it is also true that disease is *equally rare* in many parts of the world where males keep their foreskins.

Rates of penile cancer in various countries throughout the world have been reported as follows:

Number of Cases of Penile Cancer per 100,000 Males:[24]

Country	Years	#	Country	Years	#
United States		0.8 to 1.2	Italy & Bulgaria	1969	0.5
Canada	1971	0.7	Poland	1970	0.7
	1960-1962	0.9	Yugoslavia	1956-1960	0.7
Norway	1959-1961	1.0	Hungary	1971	0.7
Denmark		1.3		1969	0.8
Sweden		1.3		1966	0.9
Finland	1970	0.8	Israel	1960-1963	0.1
	1967	0.5	Puerto Rico	1950s & 1960s	4.5
	1966 & 1963	0.4	Columbia	1962-1964	2.3
	1959-1961	0.7	Mozambique	1959-1960	1.9
Iceland	1955-1963	1.0	Nigeria	1960-1965	0.2
Netherlands	1969	0.8	South Africa		4.6
	1960-1961	0.8	Uganda		3.3

Statistics were reported differently for the following countries:

---

24 Persky L. Epidemiology of Cancer of the Penis. *Recent Results of Cancer Res.* (Berlin) 1977: 97-9, 101-2.

Percentage of Incidence of Penile Cancer Out of All Cancers in Males:[24]

Mexico	10.0%	Thailand	6.6%
Brazil	4.5%	Kenya	1.9%
Burma	15.0%		

Percentage of Incidence of Penile Cancer Out of All Cancers:[24]

Paraguay & Venezuela	3.0%	China (1919)	22.0%
Ceylon	13.7%	(1919-1939)	12.6%

Percentage of Incidence of Penile Cancer Out of All Neoplasms (Abnormal Growths) in Males:[24]

India	2.8% to 22.0%

It is most important to note that the rates of penile cancer, while low in Israel which has an exclusively circumcised male population, and low in the U.S. with a largely circumcised male population, are *equally low* in Canada and all of the European countries listed which have a standard of living similar to ours. Circumcision is practiced only sporadically in Canada and *rarely* among non-Jews in all European countries. The rates of penile cancer are somewhat higher in "underdeveloped" countries which have hotter climates and significantly lower standards of living – *although the disease is still relatively rare.*

As the standards of living in underdeveloped countries improve the rates of penile cancer will diminish. (Note that in China the rate of penile cancer after 1919 diminished to almost half that country's previous rate even though Chinese men are not circumcised.) Therefore, if we wish to help poorer countries, we should do so by improving their living conditions and teaching them better hygienic practices rather than by bringing our clamps and scalpels to cut off the foreskins of their infants. For many countries, such as China and India, are *culturally resistant* to adopting circumcision. *Cutting off the foreskin is a foreign and repugnant concept to many people throughout the world, just as female circumcision is to us.* It is ironic that a country such as ours, where virtually all homes have bathrooms and modern plumbing, has adopted circumcision as a supposed "cleanliness" measure, while other countries in which many people lack such "luxuries" are loathe to amputate foreskins.

Persky notes that circumcision is not the only, or the most significant variable in the rates of penile cancer. He comments:

> "Great variation in incidence among noncircumcising tribes in Uganda suggest social and hygienic factors. The Lugbara, who do not circumcise but have high standards of cleanliness, have lower rates than the nearby Nyoro ... High rates in East Africa have been attributed to poor hygienic practices." [25]

According to Shabad, the rates of penile cancer in the U.S.S.R. (now Russia), a population that does not commonly practice male circumcision, is approximately the same as that of the United States, Canada, and other European countries.

> "In the U.S.S.R., the incidence of penile cancer has varied in recent years from 0.5% to 1% of dangerous disease in male subjects. The morbidity of penile cancer in the Russian Soviet Federative Socialistic Republic in 1960 was 0.3 per 100,000." [26]

From the available statistics it can be concluded that cancer of the penis is an extremely rare disease. Personal hygiene is an important variable in the development of penile cancer. An intact penis is *not* a significant factor in the development of the disease in countries with modern standards of living and adequate personal hygiene.

13.5 Methods of Treatment of Cancer of the Penis

Why has the medical profession been so eager to amputate foreskins in the hopes of preventing a disease which is quite rare and is equally preventable with adequate washing? The answer apparently is that the cure for more advanced cases of penile cancer is particularly horrible. The prognosis for cancer of the penis is relatively favorable. The cure rate is high. A smaller percentage of patients die of penile cancer than from many other types of cancer. However, the cure for the more advanced cases of penile cancer is amputation of the penis – a "fate worse than death" in the minds of most men. This fact has been avoided by all of the other opponents of routine circumcision – but it must be dealt with squarely. For doctors' *perception* of human health tends to become distorted because they see so much illness and this is the reason that the medical profession has been unusually concerned with this rare disease.

The less advanced cases of penile cancer are remedied by simpler measures.

---

25 Ibid., p. 104.
26 Shabad AL. Some Aspects of Etiology and Prevention of Penile Cancer. *J Urol.* 1964-12; 92(6): 697.

According to Bruhl: "A small lesion, confined to the prepuce, is mostly managed by circumcision alone. Local radiation is added to circumcision when the lesion is in the glans and biopsy shows it to be limited to the superficial surface of the epithelium." [5]

Bleich adds: "Carcinoma of the penis may be treated ... radiologically. If the tumor is superficial and no larger than 2.5 cm. in diameter, it is treated with X-rays. Sterility is inevitable.[27]

(Fortunately most men who contract penile cancer are past the age of desiring to father children.)

Young reports on the "Radical Operation for Cancer of the Penis." However devastating, it is reassuring to learn that total amputation and emasculation are not necessary. The scrotum, testicles, and a stump of the penis remain. The author describes this:

"... We have had no recurrence at the penile stump and no evidence of extension to the scrotum or contents to show that the most radical operation of total emasculation is not necessary nor is the more radical removal of the entire penis necessary ... The patients upon whom [this] radical operation for cancer of the penis has been carried out are not incapacitated in any way. Their wounds have healed within a reasonable time and they are able to void with a well directed stream. Satisfactory intercourse has been reported ... and firm erections of the remaining portions of the penis. Patients appear satisfied with the result." [28]

During the 1920s and '30s when many doctors came out strongly in favor of infant circumcision as a prophylaxis against penile cancer, radical amputation of the penis was more commonly done as a cure for this disease than it is today. Today more sophisticated types of X-ray treatments have enabled cases of penile cancer to be cured by radiation that in years past would have been treated by amputation.

According to Bruhl:

"When the tumor involves both the prepuce and the glans and also extends into the shaft of the penis for a short distance, partial amputation is recommended. But it should be noted that today possibilities of applying supervoltage rays in this stage of carcinoma of the penis apparently show at least the same results as surgery, thus avoiding mutilation." [16]

---

27 Bleich AR. Prophylaxis of Penile Carcinoma. *JAMA. 1950-07-22;* 143(12): 1057.
28 Young HH. A Radical Operation for the Cure of Cancer of the Penis. *J Urol.* 1931-08; 26(2): 285-316.

In addition, today more sophisticated methods of restorative plastic surgery have been developed which can reconstruct a functional phallus and restore sexual function when the penis has been lost either from accidents or by an operation.

Bruhl discusses this:

> "With the nerves intact in the stump and with testicles present, both sensory and hormonal factors remain and titillation of the remnant cavernous bodies can result in a sexual impetus to the extent of ... ejaculation. The patient is not necessarily sterile although the modus apparandi [sic] for the transmission of sperm through the pendulous urethra is missing.
>
> The repair of this deficiency by plastic reconstruction of the amputated penis can be satisfactorily accomplished. The new organ can assume the normal physiological functions not only of urination but also can afford connubial gratification to both participants during coitus ...
>
> Restoration [is] accomplished by utilizing tube skin grafts into which rib cartilage was implanted." [16]

There are additional considerations. The man with cancer of the penis is almost always elderly. If he is having sexual relations it is almost invariably with a wife to whom he has been married for many years. She is certainly going to be understanding and accepting of his healing and limitations as well as thankful to have him alive. He is not in the same position as a younger man who is out to impress new girlfriends.

Also, in the complications chapter many documented cases of serious damage to and amputation of the penis resulting from circumcision were covered. *An infant runs a considerably greater risk of experiencing a serious complication of circumcision than he does of ever contracting penile cancer.* If an infant is circumcised he faces a risk of approximately one in 500-1,000 of suffering from a *serious* complication of circumcision. Penile cancer occurs at a rate of approximately 1 in 100,000 per year in most "developed" countries, and 1 in 20,000 to 30,000 per year in most "underdeveloped" countries – thus constituting a much smaller individual risk. Since only a few victims of penile cancer ever undergo partial penile amputation, and even fewer die of the disease, the individual risk of disfiguration or death is even smaller.

When weighing the possibility of serious complications of circumcision against the risk of penile cancer, we must also remember that the infant is at the *beginning* of his life, while the penile cancer victim has already lived most of his life. Therefore, serious damage to the penis resulting from infant circumcision is ultimately more devastating than serious damage to the penis as a cure for penile cancer in an elderly person.

Circumcision – The Painful Dilemma

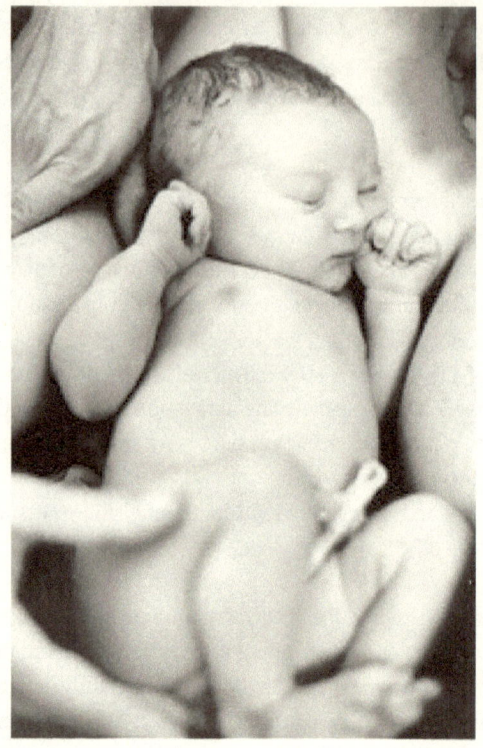

© *Suzanne Arms*

Apparently a "sacrificial" psychology has been in effect for the rationale of infant circumcision as a prophylaxis against penile cancer. Most men would prefer to go through life without their foreskins and choose the same for their sons *if* this were the *only* insurance against a *strong* possibility of losing one's entire penis to cancer. However, the facts all indicate beyond any doubt that *penile cancer is extremely rare, penile amputation is even rarer, total amputation is not necessary, and circumcision is not the only prevention.*

13.6 Conclusions

The choice of prevention of penile cancer is *either* to cut the foreskin off, *or* wash it. Many, many authors have made this point. Even Wolbarst, one of the first advocates of infant circumcision as a cancer preventive, clearly states: "The common denominator ... appears to be poor sex hygiene. The incidence of carcinoma of the penis could be reduced *either* by early circumcision *or* by good hygiene".[29]

The 1975 Ad Hoc Task Force of the American Academy of Pediatrics on Circumcision concluded the following:

> "There is evidence that carcinoma of the penis can be prevented by neonatal circumcision. There is also evidence that optimal hygiene confers as much, or nearly as much, protection. Although circumcision is an effective method of preventing penile carcinoma, a great deal of unnecessary surgery, with attendant complications, would have to be done if circumcision were to be used as prophylaxis against this disease. Promulgation of the principles of adequate penile hygiene is an alternative prophylactic measure." [30]

Many authors have emphasized that it is not merely the foreskin, but phimosis and poor hygiene that is the significant factor in the etiology of penile cancer. Preston emphasizes this fact by stating that *"if a man has a foreskin which he can retract and which he keeps clean, the risk of cancer of the penis is removed."* [31]

(In Chapter 19 "The Intact Penis" the condition of phimosis, and its remedies, is thoroughly discussed. A tight foreskin is *normal* for an infant or young boy, and should be left alone. For an older person, phimosis can usually be remedied by very simple measures.)

In emphasizing the rarity of the disease and the *inefficiency* of routine surgery as prevention, Morgan quotes Marshall's statement that:

> " 'If a surgeon would perform one circumcision every ten minutes, eight hours a day, and five days a week, he would seem able to prevent one penile cancer by working steadily for between 6 and 29 years. Since a significant number of penile cancers are curable, still more time and labor might be required to prevent a fatality from this disease.' " [32]

Gellis adds: "It is an incontestable fact ... that there are more deaths each year from circumcision than from cancer of the penis." [33]

Ritter, a strong opponent of neonatal circumcision, points out that there is no other part of the body that we routinely cut off simply because it has the *potential* of

---

29 Wolbarst, p. 187. [emphasis mine]
30 Thompson HC, King LR, Knox E, Korones SB. Report of the Ad Hoc Task Force on Circumcision. *Pediatrics.* 1975-10; 56(4): 610.
31 Preston EN. Whither the Foreskin? A Consideration of Routine Neonatal Circumcision. *JAMA.* 1970-09-14; 213(11): 1856.
32 Morgan WKC. Reply to Dr. Greenblatt. *Am J Dis Childh.* 1966-04; 3: 448-9.
33 Gellis SS. Circumcision. Am J Dis Childh. 1978-12; 132: 1168.

becoming cancerous. He states that penile cancer is so rare that many physicians never see a case of it in their entire practice, or may see only a few cases during their entire professional lives. Many other parts of the body are considerably more cancer-prone than the foreskin and many other things that we encounter in life are significantly more carcinogenic. According to Ritter:

> "If one wishes to practice an amputative type of preventive medicine, one could find many more rewarding structures to cut off rather than the foreskin.
>
> The *ear.* Cancer of the skin of the top of the ear is common. We could hear without the protruding aural appendage.
>
> The *female breast* ... Removing the minute breasts of all female infants in the immediate postnatal period would ultimately save tens of thousands of lives each year ... [A] new flat chest contour could ... be accepted as the norm, just as the multitude of surgically pruned penises are now accepted as normal.
>
> The *testis.* Cancer of the prostate, and benign prostatic hypertrophy ... could be greatly reduced in incidence or possibly eliminated, if every male had his testes removed at about the age of 35 or 40.
>
> The *cervix.* Cancer of the cervix is common ... therefore we could amputate all cervixes of women past childbearing age.
>
> *Cigarettes.* The scientific evidence tying the inhalation of the carcinogens in cigarette smoke to cancer of the lung is substantial. It would be interesting to compile statistics on how many of the routine circumcision advocates have amputated themselves from smoking cigarettes. Cancer of the lung is very common in both men and women." [34]

The two choices of prevention of penile cancer – *cutting* the foreskin off versus *washing* it – represent two different approaches to health care: the traditional, surgical approach versus the wholistic approach. Unfortunately the established medical profession has tended to prefer the surgical approach. Many doctors have preferred to routinely cut foreskins off of infants rather than *teach* new parents and later the individuals to wash this area.

Both *politics* and *economics* are strongly involved in this issue. For too often many choices in human health care have *not* centered on what is most beneficial for the individual. Instead they have centered on who is in *control* and who is getting *paid*. A doctor is the person in *control* when he performs a circumcision. He cannot *control* whether or not that person is going to wash himself. Similarly, doctors get *paid* for doing circumcisions, but they do not get *paid* for telling people to wash.

---

34   Ritter TJ. Personal Research and Conclusions on Circumcision and Cancer of the Penis (unpublished).

> "As representatives of the American Cancer Society, we would like to discourage the American Academy of Pediatrics from promoting routine circumcision as a preventative measure for penile or cervical cancer. The American Cancer Society does not consider routine circumcision to be a valid or effective measure to prevent such cancers..."
>
> Hugh Shingleton, M.D.
> National Vice President Detection & Treatment ACS
> Clark W. Heath, Jr., M.D.
> Vice President Epidemiology & Surveillance Research ACS

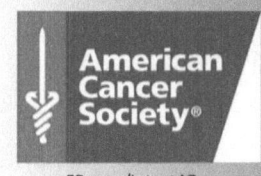

FB.com/IntactAZ

13.7 Informational Resources

- ACS (American Cancer Society) mime: no circumcision recommendation:
  dropbox.com/s/zz23nzayyrmih0t/ACScirc.jpg
- ACS letter (1996) discouraging the AAP from promoting routine circumcision as cancer prevention:
  cirp.org/library/statements/letters/1996-02_ACS
- Can Penile Cancer Be Prevented?: cancer.org/cancer/penile-cancer/causes-risks-prevention/prevention.html
- Cancer of the penis at Kenyatta National Hospital: pubmed.ncbi.nlm.nih.gov/12862118
- Carcinoma in Situ of the Penis in a 76-Year-Old Circumcised Man: cirp.org/library/disease/cancer/vanhowe
- Circumcision and Cancer: circumstitions.com/Cancer.html
- Cultural Bias in the AAP's 2012 Technical Report and Policy Statement on Male Circumcision:
  pediatrics.aappublications.org/content/131/4/796
- Dispelling Miscommunications: cirp.org/library/statements/letters/1996-02_ACS/commentary.html
- History of Circumcision, Medical Conditions, and Sexual Activity and Risk of Penile Cancer:
  cirp.org/library/disease/cancer/maden
- Human papillomavirus and circumcision: cirp.org/library/disease/cancer/vanhowe2006b
- Key Statistics for Penile Cancer: cancer.org/cancer/penile-cancer/about/key-statistics.html
- Male Circumcision *(CDC report):* stacks.cdc.gov/view/cdc/13546

- Male Circumcision and Serologically Determined Human Papillomavirus Infection in a Birth Cohort: cebp.aacrjournals.org/content/18/1/177.long
- Outcome of penile cancer in circumcised men: pubmed.ncbi.nlm.nih.gov/16406995
- Penile cancer in elderly circumcised man: pubmed.ncbi.nlm.nih.gov/9374971
- Penile cancer, cervical cancer, and circumcision: cirp.org/library/disease/cancer
- Penile cancer: epidemiology, pathogenesis and prevention: rd.springer.com/article/10.1007/s00345-008-0302-z
- Penile verrucous carcinoma in a 37-year-old circumcised man: pubmed.ncbi.nlm.nih.gov/9270540
- Risk Factors for Penile Cancer: cancer.org/cancer/penile-cancer/causes-risks-prevention/risk-factors.html
- Squamous cell carcinoma of the penis in a circumcised man: a case for dermatology and urology: pubmed.ncbi.nlm.nih.gov/9466082
- What Is Penile Cancer?: cancer.org/cancer/penile-cancer/about/what-is-penile-cancer.html
- You circumcised your son to prevent penile cancer?: dropbox.com/s/tnmmxqdl1batucf/penilecancer.jpg

14   Sexually Transmitted Infection

Prevention of sexually transmitted infection (STI) is frequently listed as one of the supposed advantages of circumcision. *Is* the foreskin a likely site to harbor such infections? *Does* its absence confer immunity to these infections?

Few studies have attempted to answer these questions. The American Academy of Pediatrics' Ad Hoc Task Force on Circumcision concluded in 1975: "Adequate studies to determine the relationship between circumcision and the incidence of venereal disease have not been performed." [1]

STI has become epidemic within the United States. Our primarily circumcised male population has done little to abate this. One could hardly blame our widespread rates of these infections on the small proportion of intact males within our population. *Obviously* circumcised males are not immune to sexually transmitted infection. Other countries which practice male circumcision frequently report similarly high rates of STI. According to Morgan: "The Middle East, where the men are circumcised, has a venereal disease rate second to none." [2]

The rates of syphilis have dropped dramatically since the 1940s – from 352,000 reported cases in 1945 to 20,000 reported cases in 1977. This has been primarily due to more widespread identification techniques and effective antibiotics.[3] However, the rates of gonorrhea and Herpes II have been rapidly increasing. Some strains of gonorrhea have become resistant to antibiotics. There is no known cure for Herpes II.[4] According to Wallerstein, Dr. Stanley Falkin wrote in 1977 that: "... gonorrhea is the most common bacterial infection in humans and that there are probably as many as 2 million cases in the United States." [5]

Some observations have revealed *no* differences in rates of STI among intact and circumcised men. Other observations have suggested that males with foreskins do contract the infections more frequently.

Taylor and Rodin investigated the rates of Herpes II virus and circumcision status and found the infection to be somewhat less common among males without foreskins. 214 male patients with genital herpes were compared with a randomly selected group of 410 male patients without the infection. They found that 24.5% of the men in the control group were circumcised, and 12.1% of those in the herpes group were

---

1   Thompson HC, King LR, Knox E, Korones SB. Report of the Ad Hoc Task Force on Circumcision. *Pediatrics.* 1975-10; 56(4): 611.
2   Topp S. Why Not to Circumcise Your Baby Boy. *Mothering.* 1978-01; 6: 76.
3   Wallerstein E. *Circumcision: An American Health Fallacy.* NY: Springer; 1980: 83-4. (Syphilis statistics source: U.S. Department of the Census, Statistical Abstract of the United States, Washington D.C., 88th ed., 1967, p. 86 for the years 1945-1965: the 97th ed., 1976, p. 91 for the years 1970-1974; for 1975, 1976, 1977 see *Sexually Transmitted Diseases,* Statistical Letter, U.S.D.H.E.W., issue no. 127, May 1978, p. 9.)
4   Ibid., p. 84.
5   Ibid., p. 83.

circumcised.[6] However, *other factors* besides whether or not the individual has his foreskin may be responsible for the difference. Knowledge of the rates of *exposure* to Herpes II among the unaffected men would reveal more definite answers.

According to Shepard:

"Venereal disease is no respecter of the host. Schrek and Lenowitz found that the incidence of venereal disease in hospitalized patients was no different in circumcised and uncircumcised. Studies in the Canadian Army (1947) showed that venereal disease was more common among uncircumcised soldiers. However, it is believed that most of the uncircumcised soldiers came from the lower socioeconomic group, and that this may have accounted for the higher rate." [7]

Socioeconomic factors, lifestyle, values, sexual practices, personal cleanliness, awareness of disease symptoms, and access to and willingness to seek medical treatment have considerably greater effect on whether or not one will contract a sexually transmitted infection than does the presence or absence of one's foreskin. In past decades the middle and upper classes have been more likely to choose circumcision for their sons, while the lower classes were more likely to leave the penis intact. Members of the lower classes have also tended to be more sexually active, less attentive to personal hygiene, and less likely to seek medical treatment.

The foreskin is a site where STI infections can be harbored. A break in the skin can be a point of entry for infection germs. However, the same can be said for many other parts of the body. Wallerstein points out that sexually transmitted infection germs enter the body via the mouth, rectum, eyes, and that the urinary meatus is the main point of entry for males.[8] They can harbor in the labia, anus, mouth, underarms, and between the toes. He concludes:

"The major problem of venereal disease is to prevent it and, failing that, to treat it promptly. The surgical removal of a possible infection site is not a solution." [9]

Contraceptive use has a dramatic effect on the prevalence of STI: Obstructive contraceptives, particularly condoms, help prevent the spread of infection.[10] Some spermicidal preparations, foams, creams, and jellies tend to inhibit the growth of infection

---

6   Taylor PK, Rodin P. Herpes Genitalis and Circumcision. *Br J Ven Dis.* 1975; 51: 274-7.
7   Shepard KS. *Care of the Well Baby.* Philadelphia, PA: J.P. Lippincott; 1968: 304-5.
8   Wallerstein, p. 85.
9   Ibid., p. 87.
10 *Our Bodies, Ourselves.* 2nd ed. NY: Simon and Schuster. 1976: 170. (Their reference: Cautley R, Beebe GW, Dickinson R. Rubber Sheaths as Venereal Disease Prophylactics. *Am J Med Sci.* 1950[1938]: 155-63.)

causing agents.[11] Use of birth control pills not only causes people to forego usage of obstructive contraceptives and spermicides, but changes the chemistry of the vagina, making women more susceptible to the infection.

According to the authors of *Our Bodies, Ourselves:*

> "For women it is estimated that for one exposure to gonorrhea you have a 40-50 percent chance of catching it if you use no protection and are not taking the Pill. If you use the Pill you have a nearly 100-percent chance of catching gonorrhea during any exposure to it. The Pill makes the vagina more alkaline than normal and stimulates carbohydrate production in the vagina. This is an extremely favorable environment for the bacteria. The Pill also seems to help the spread of gonorrhea into the fallopian tubes, even as soon as two or three weeks after infection.[12]

14.1 Yeast Infections

Yeast infection is not solely an STI. It can be spread by a variety of methods including sexual contact. However it can be a troublesome, nuisance infection. Circumcision status appears to have little or no effect on the prevalence of yeast infections among males according to two different studies.

Davidson studied 66 circumcised men and 69 intact men. He found the yeast isolation rate to be nearly the same in both groups. 14% of the circumcised men and 17% of the intact men had yeast infections.[13]

In Rodin and Kolater's study 175 men were tested for yeast infections. Of these 32 had yeast infections. Six of these 32 men were circumcised (19%). Of the remaining 145 unaffected subjects, 35 (24%) were circumcised. Therefore, a slightly higher percentage of circumcised males were found in the group without yeast infections. However, this study involved relatively small numbers.[14]

14.2 Benign Transient Lymphagiectasis

A relatively rare condition that is sometimes STI related, "Benign Transient Lymphagiectasis" may be complicated by the fact that the individual has been circumcised. Benign means not cancerous or permanently harmful. Transient means lasting for

---

11 Ibid., p. 170 (Their reference: Singh B, Cutler JC, Utidjian HMD. Studies on the development of a vaginal preparation providing both prophylaxis against venereal disease and other genital infections and contraception. II – Effect *in vitro* of vaginal contraceptive and non-contraceptive preparation on treponema pallidum and neisseria gonnorrhoeae. *Br J Ven Dis. 1972;* 48: 57-64.)
12 Ibid., pp. 168-9, 191.
13 Wallerstein, p. 86.
14 Rodin P, Kolater B. Carriage of Yeasts on the Penis. *BMJ.* 1976-05-08: 1123-4.

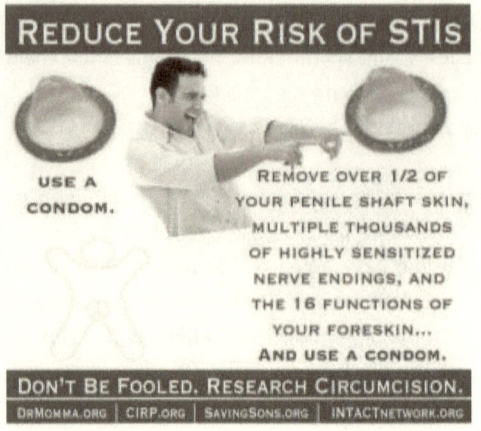

Intactivism Meme: Reduce Your Risk of STIs

only a short time. Lymphagiectasis is a dilation of the lymphatic vessels. The authors describe the condition as follows:

> "The presence of a painless, hard nodular, translucent cord that suddenly appears in the penis and is usually confined to the coronal sulcus ... not caused by infection, [apparently caused by] trauma during recent vigorous sexual activity ... It is possible that circumcision may disturb the normal lymphatic drainage of the glans and prepuce, making the trauma of coitus more likely to provoke this condition. 41.2% of their patients [in Britain with an expected rate of 25%] were circumcised." [15]

The lack of ease afforded by the gliding mechanism of the foreskin may also have contributed to the "trauma" of coitus.

14.3   Conclusion

Insufficient studies have been carried out to indicate whether or not the presence of a foreskin predisposes one to developing STI. Present studies indicate little or no relationship. Socioeconomic factors related to sexual activity, personal hygiene and access to medical treatment are apparently responsible for some instances of more sexually transmitted infections among intact males. Circumcised males are certainly

---

15   Hutchins P, Dunlop EMC, Rodin P. Benign Transient Lymphangiectasis (Sclerosing Lymphangitis) of the Penis. *Br J Ven Dis.* 1977; 53: 379-87.

not immune to sexually transmitted infections. Even *if* the foreskin were proven to predispose the individual to a greater chance of contracting a sexually transmitted infection, it is reasonable to conclude that regular washing, especially washing immediately after coitus, would inhibit its development. The problems that can result from the neglected, unwashed foreskins of a *few* individuals do not indicate any need for routine amputation of *all* infant foreskins!

Wallerstein adds: "Venereal disease complications result from neglect of the infection, whether the man is circumcised or not. On the other hand, prompt treatment usually mitigates complications, regardless of the presence or absence of a foreskin." [16]

There are only two ways that a person can be assured of not contracting STI. One is abstinence from sexual contact. The other is long-term fidelity of both partners of a marriage or relationship. STI is so prevalent that virtually anyone who has a number of sexual partners will inevitably get an infection of some sort. It is also not uncommon for one faithful partner of a marriage or relationship to contract an STI from the other partner who has had sexual contact elsewhere.

Parents who are concerned about their children contracting STI are best advised to teach them a sense of responsibility about sexual matters. Although most parents hope that their children will marry or at least form loving, committed relationships, rather than have numerous casual sexual encounters, this responsibility should also include advising any sexual partner(s) if an STI is discovered, and seeking prompt medical attention. Teaching one's children important values along with the facts about these infections is vastly preferable to subjecting them to unnecessary surgical procedures.

14.4 Informational Resources

- A CDC-requested, Evidence-based Critique of the Centers for Disease Control and Prevention 2014 Draft on Male Circumcision: How Ideology and Selective Science Lead to Superficial, Culturally-biased Recommendations by the CDC: academia.edu/10553782
- A fatal irony: Why the "circumcision solution" to the AIDS epidemic in Africa may increase transmission of HIV: blog.practicalethics.ox.ac.uk/2012/05/when-bad-science-kills-or-how-to-spread-aids
- ABC, not circumcision *(questioning of AIDS prevention)*: web.archive.org/web/20120203140317/http://www.medicalnewstoday.com/opinions/83902
- African Mass Circumcision Programs: A Dangerous Leap!: web.archive.org/web/20120818214646/http://www.pediatricsdigest.mobi/content/130/1/e175/reply
- After Condom Remarks, Vatican Confirms Shift *(Catholic ok for condom use for aids prevention)*: nytimes.com/2010/11/24/world/europe/24pope.html

---

16 Wallerstein, p. 86.

- Americans are 'more likely to have an STD than Europeans': New research reveals Iceland is the chlamydia capital of Europe while Washington D.C. tops the HIV league: dailymail.co.uk/health/article-2989697
- Background, Methods, and Synthesis of Scientific Information Used to Inform the "Recommendations for Providers Counseling Male Patients and Parents Regarding Male Circumcision and the Prevention of HIV infection, STIs, and other Health Outcomes." *(leans toward pro-circ)*: regulations.gov/document?D=CDC-2014-0012-0002
- Believing Circumcision Prevents HIV, Malawi Men Go on 'Sex Spree': web.archive.org/web/20160424013937 /http://www.aidscirc.org/2012/11/believing-circumcision-prevents-hiv.html
- Boys' HPV vax going well: insightplus.mja.com.au/2013/20/boys-hpv-vax-going-well
- Can Circumcision Cut HIV in Gay Men?: webmd.com/hiv-aids/news/20081007/can-circumcision-cut-hiv-in-gay-men
- Cancer-causing HPV plummeted in teens since vaccine, study finds: edition.cnn.com/2016/02/22/health/hpv-vaccine-teen-girls-effective
- Catholic Church and HIV/AIDS *(Wikipedia)*: en.wikipedia.org/wiki/Catholic_Church_and_HIV/AIDS
- CDC Ignores Boys' Rights: nocirc.org/publish/NOCIRC%202015%20nwsltr-17.pdf
- CDC, circumcision and misleading headlines: circwatch.org/cdc-circumcision-and-misleading-headlines
- Cervical mucus monitoring prevalence and associated fecundability in women trying to conceive: fertstert.org/article/s0015-0282%252813%252900696-1/fulltext
- Circumcision & HIVAIDS: A Life-Saving Cut?: intaction.org/circumcision-hiv-aids-an-unprecedented-disaster
- Circumcision against AIDS, between lie, sexism, and apartheid: academia.edu/2098232
- Circumcision and Acquisition of Human Papillomavirus Infection in Young Men: journals.lww.com/stdjournal/Fulltext/2011/11000/Circumcision_and_Acquisition_of_Human.16.aspx
- Circumcision and HIV – the Randomised Controlled Trials: circumstitions.com/HIV-SA.html
- Circumcision and HIV *(good charts)*: circumstitions.com/HIV.html
- Circumcision and HIV infection: cirp.org/library/disease/HIV/vanhowe4
- Circumcision and HIV: Harm Outweighs "Benefit": circumcision.org/circumcision-and-hiv-harm-outweighs-benefit
- Circumcision and HIV: It's a Dangerous Mistake for Prevention: intaction.org/circumcision-hiv-a-dangerous-mistake
- Circumcision and Its Potential Impact on the Spread of HIV Among Gay and Bisexual Men: thebodypro.com/article/circumcision-potential-impact-spread-hiv-among-gay-bisexual-men
- Circumcision and Risk of Sexually Transmitted Infections in a Birth Cohort: jpeds.com/article/S0022-3476%2807%2900707-X/abstract
- Circumcision and risk of sexually transmitted infections in a birth cohort: pubmed.ncbi.nlm.nih.gov/18280846
- Circumcision and Sexually Transmitted Infections: cirp.org/library/disease/STD
- Circumcision disaster: Malawi HIV infection rate doubles: web.archive.org/web/20200806104024/ malawi24.com/2015/08/04/circumcision-disaster-malawi-hiv-infection-rate-doubles
- Circumcision does not affect HIV in U.S. men: study: reuters.com/article/us-aids-circumcision-idUSN0345545120071204

- Circumcision DOES NOT prevent AIDS or other Sexually Transmitted Diseases. Circumcision is NOT a vaccine: facebook.com/notes/nairobi-circumcision-resources/circumcision-does-not-prevent-aids-or-other-sexually-transmitted-diseases-circum/526870410664822
- Circumcision does not stop HIV infections:
  web.archive.org/web/20111231193715/http://www.timeslive.co.za/ilive/2011/11/28/circumcision-does-not-stop-hiv-infections-hiv
- Circumcision gives men an excuse not to use condoms:
  thenewhumanitarian.org/news/2008/07/31/circumcision-gives-men-excuse-not-use-condoms
- Circumcision in HIV-infected men and its effect on HIV transmission to female partners in Rakai, Uganda: a randomised controlled trial *(promotion of circumcision for AIDS prevention)*:
  thelancet.com/journals/lancet/article/PIIS0140-6736(09)60998-3/fulltext
- Circumcision in the United States: Prevalence, Prophylactic Effects, and Sexual Practice:
  cirp.org/library/general/laumann
- Circumcision is for weiners!: womanuncensored.blogspot.com/2010/01/circumcision-is-for-weiners.html
- Circumcision is not enough to fight HIV:
  timeslive.co.za/ideas/2013-11-27-circumcision-is-not-enough-to-fight-hiv-ilive
- Circumcision is reducing HIV incidence in Uganda, Rakai community study shows (pro circumcision):
  aidsmap.com/news/feb-2015/circumcision-reducing-hiv-incidence-uganda-rakai-community-study-shows
- Circumcision makes no difference to HIV infection in UK gay men:
  aidsmap.com/news/feb-2013/circumcision-makes-no-difference-hiv-infection-uk-gay-men
- Circumcision may not cut HIV spread among gay men:
  reuters.com/article/us-circumcision-gay-idUSTRE6283Z820100309
- Circumcision May Not Protect White U.K. Gay Men From HIV:
  web.archive.org/web/20150922003257/http://www.aidsmeds.com/articles/circumcision_tops_1667_23630.shtml
- Circumcision not "significant" in HIV rates among men who have gay sex:
  pinknews.co.uk/2008/10/08/circumcision-not-significant-in-hiv-rates-among-men-who-have-gay-sex
- Clinical presentation of genital warts among circumcised and uncircumcised heterosexual men attending an urban STD clinic *(no relation found between circumcision & STIs)*:
  ncbi.nlm.nih.gov/pmc/articles/PMC1195083
- Could Circumcision Really Prevent AIDS?:
  nocircofmi.org/Portals/0/Documents/Pamphlets/AIDSPamphlet.pdf
- Cultural Bias in the AAP's 2012 Technical Report and Policy Statement on Male Circumcision:
  pediatrics.aappublications.org/content/131/4/796
- Culture Shock: Declining Ebola, Rising STDs:
  medpagetoday.com/InfectiousDisease/GeneralInfectiousDisease/54919
- Developmental factors of urethral human papillomavirus lesions:
  bjui-journals.onlinelibrary.wiley.com/doi/abs/10.1046/j.1464-410x.1999.00104.x
- does circumcision prevent hiv transmission among msm?:

- vtcares.org/does-circumcision-prevent-hiv-transmission-among-msm
- Findings about circumcision and HIV from visit to Western and Nyanza provinces in Kenya: facebook.com/owino.qane/posts/442249975810540
- Flawed African Circumcision Trials Cannot Be Used to Inform U.S. Circumcision Debate: web.archive.org/web/20170703083027/https://www.intactamerica.org/sites/default/files/IASummaryAtlanta.pdf
- Flawed Studies Used to Claim Circumcision Reduces HIV Infection: salem-news.com/articles/december112011/circumcision-hiv-rg.php
- Gay community + HIV + Circumcision *(Google Scholar link to hundreds of articles on these keywords)*: scholar.google.com/scholar?q=gay+community+%2B+HIV+%2B+circumcision&hl=en&oi=scholart
- Genital Warts Among 18- to 59-Year-Olds in the United States: journals.lww.com/stdjournal/Fulltext/2008/04000/Seroepidemiology_of_Human_Papillomavirus_Type_11.8.aspx
- Genital warts in young Australians five years into national human papillomavirus vaccination programme: bmj.com/content/346/bmj.f2032
- Global HIV rates in decline: pbs.org/newshour/nation/global-hiv-rates-in-decline
- High HIV Prevalence Among Men Who have Sex with Men in Soweto, South Africa: link.springer.com/article/10.1007/s10461-009-9598-y
- HIV & male circumcision fact sheet *(some untruths)*: avert.org/learn-share/hiv-fact-sheets/circumcision
- HIV Prevalence by Male Circumcision: facebook.com/photo.php?fbid=1470787216572875&set=a.1398441323807465.1073741828.100009248324970
- HIV Prevention Tops the News at AIDS 2014: web.archive.org/web/20181202062755/http://betablog.org/hiv-prevention-news-at-aids-2014
- HIV risk reduction behaviours in gay men: ncbi.nlm.nih.gov/pmc/articles/PMC2768371
- HIV-AIDS: The new bogeyman: circinfo.org/hiv.html
- HIV, AIDS & Circumcision: web.archive.org/web/20150928055847/http://www.aidscirc.org
- HIV/AIDS: What's behind the decline in new infections: csmonitor.com/World/Progress-Watch/2015/0112/HIV-AIDS-What-s-behind-the-decline-in-new-infections
- How the circumcision solution in Africa will increase HIV infections: publichealthinafrica.org/index.php/jphia/article/view/44
- Human papillomavirus and circumcision: cirp.org/library/disease/cancer/vanhowe2006b
- Humiliation for Circumcision Industry: Junk Science Behind HIV/Circ Exposed: facebook.com/photo.php?fbid=1020771657986172&set=p.1020771657986172
- Impact of Male Circumcision on HIV Doubted: salem-news.com/articles/february292012/circumcision-hiv.php
- In case you missed it: Two Video Interviews from CROI 2015: hiv.gov/blog/in-case-you-missed-it-two-video-interviews-from-croi-2015
- Infant Circumcision – A giant leap towards an HIV-free generation *(pushing infant circ in Africa as a supposed aids prevention)*: bw.usembassy.gov/embassy/government-agencies/cdc/infant-circumcision-giant-leap-towards-hiv-free-generation
- Is male circumcision substituting condom use and abstinence in Malawi: web.archive.org/web/20170424141332/http://malawinewsnow.com/2015/08/is-male-circumcision-

- substituting-condom-use-and-abstinence-in-malawi
- Langerhans cells and more: langerin-expressing dendritic cell subsets in the skin: pubmed.ncbi.nlm.nih.gov/20193016
- Langerhans cells limit HIV invasion: ncbi.nlm.nih.gov/pmc/articles/PMC2064110
- Langerin is a natural barrier to HIV-1 transmission by Langerhans cells: pubmed.ncbi.nlm.nih.gov/17334373
- Levels and Spread of HIV Seroprevalence and Associated Factors: Evidence from National Household Surveys: dhsprogram.com/pubs/pdf/CR22/CR22.pdf
- List of countries by HIV/AIDS adult prevalence rate *(Wikipedia)*: en.wikipedia.org/wiki/List_of_countries_by_HIV/AIDS_adult_prevalence_rate
- Malawi to conduct HIV impact survey: web.archive.org/web/20200927104930/malawi24.com/2015/10/12/malawi-to-conduct-hiv-impact-survey
- Malawian circumcised men most likely to be infected by HIV, research shows: web.archive.org/web/20200809150249/http://malawi24.com/2015/07/25/malawian-circumcised-men-most-likely-to-be-infected-by-hiv-research-shows
- Malawians blasts the US: 'We don't need aid for circumcision': web.archive.org/web/20201025022525/malawi24.com/2015/10/25/malawians-blasts-the-us-we-dont-need-aid-for-circumcision
- Male Circumcision – A Dangerous Mistake in the HIV Battle: web.archive.org/web/20171006011728/http://www.intactamerica.org/dangerousmistake
- Male Circumcision *(CDC report)*: stacks.cdc.gov/view/cdc/13546
- Male circumcision and HIV prevention insufficient evidence and neglected external validity: pubmed.ncbi.nlm.nih.gov/20965388
- Male Circumcision and HIV Prevention: Is There Really Enough of the Right Kind of Evidence?: sciencedirect.com/science/article/abs/pii/S0968808007293024
- Male Circumcision and Serologically Determined Human Papillomavirus Infection in a Birth Cohort: cebp.aacrjournals.org/content/18/1/177.long
- Male circumcision for HIV prevention in men in Rakai, Uganda: a randomised trial: thelancet.com/journals/lancet/article/PIIS0140-6736(07)60313-4/fulltext
- Male circumcision may not make much difference to overall male HIV incidence in Caribbean context: aidsmap.com/news/aug-2012/male-circumcision-may-not-make-much-difference-overall-male-hiv-incidence-caribbean
- Male circumcision to reduce the risk of HIV and sexually transmitted infections among men who have sex with men: journals.lww.com/co-infectiousdiseases/Abstract/2010/02000/Male_circumcision_to_reduce_the_risk_of_HIV_and.9.aspx
- Many Doctors Unaware of Truvada, Drug for Preventing H.I.V.: nytimes.com/2015/11/26/health/many-doctors-unaware-of-truvada-drug-for-preventing-hiv.html
- Metzitzah B'Peh and Herpes: nocirc.org/publish/NOCIRC%202015%20nwsltr-17.pdf
- Might circumcision benefit gay men?: web.archive.org/web/20181211071207/http://www.aidsmap.com/Might-circumcision-benefit-gay-men/page/1746342
- More Circumcision Myths You May Believe: Hygiene and STDs: psychologytoday.com/intl/blog/moral-

- landscapes/201109/more-circumcision-myths-you-may-believe-hygiene-and-stds
- More than foreskin: circumcision status, history of HIV/STI, and sexual risk in a clinic-based sample of men in Puerto Rico: pubmed.ncbi.nlm.nih.gov/22897699
- Neonatal circumcision does not reduce HIV/AIDS infection rates: cirp.org/library/disease/HIV/sidler2008
- New Foreskin Is Really a Stretch: pool.intactiwiki.org/images/Fs2102.pdf
- Penile circumcision to reduce the risk of HIV infection: web.archive.org/web/20161208193251/http://www.catie.ca/en/fact-sheets/prevention/penile-circumcision-reduce-risk-hiv-infection
- Per-contact probability of HIV transmission in homosexual men in Sydney in the era of HAART: ncbi.nlm.nih.gov/pmc/articles/PMC2852627
- Prevalence and risk determinants of human immunodeficiency virus type 2 (HIV-2) and human immunodeficiency virus type 1 (HIV-1) in west African female prostitutes: pubmed.ncbi.nlm.nih.gov/1442755
- Prevalence of Circumcision and Its Association with HIV and Sexually Transmitted Infections in a Male U.S. Navy Population: apps.dtic.mil/sti/citations/ADA458066
- Public Comments on Proposed CDC Circumcision Guidelines: web.archive.org/web/20190407233525/http://cdc.intactivist.net
- Randomized, Controlled Intervention Trial of Male Circumcision for Reduction of HIV Infection Risk: The ANRS 1265 Trial: journals.plos.org/plosmedicine/article?id=10.1371/journal.pmed.0020298
- Recommendations for Providers Counseling Male Patients and Parents Regarding Male Circumcision and the Prevention of HIV Infection, STIs, and other Health Outcomes *(CDC's pro-circ stance)*: regulations.gov/document?D=CDC-2014-0012-0001
- Recommendations for Providers Counseling Male Patients and Parents Regarding Male Circumcision and the Prevention of HIV Infection, STIs, and other Health Outcomes *(full text PDF)*: regulations.gov/document?D=CDC-2014-0012-0003
- Risk Compensation Following Male Circumcision: Results from a Two-Year Prospective Cohort Study of Recently Circumcised and Uncircumcised Men in Nyanza Province, Kenya: link.springer.com/article/10.1007/s10461-014-0846-4
- Risk Factors Associated with Prevalent HIV-1 Infection among Pregnant Women in Rwanda: academic.oup.com/ije/article-abstract/23/2/371/680720
- Risk factors for HIV-1 infection in adults in a rural Ugandan community: cirp.org/library/disease/HIV/malamba
- Scarification and Male Circumcision Associated with HIV Infection in Mozambican Children and Youth: webmedcentral.com/article_view/2206
- Scientists announce anti-HIV agent so powerful it can work in a vaccine: medicalxpress.com/news/2015-02-scientists-anti-hiv-agent-powerful-vaccine.html
- Seroepidemiology of Human Papillomavirus Type 11 in the United States: journals.lww.com/stdjournal/fulltext/2008/03000/seroepidemiology_of_human_papillomavirus_type_11.16.aspx
- Sexually Transmitted Infections and Male Circumcision: hindawi.com/journals/isrn/2013/109846
- Solving the "Negro rape problem": Yet another advantage of circumcision: web.archive.org/web/20151123232847/http://www.historyofcircumcision.net/index.php?option=content&task=view&id=63
- South Africa passes law to restrict circumcision: circinfo.org/South_Africa_Childrens_Act.html

- Study of potential HIV 'cure' wins FDA nod:
  bizjournals.com/sanfrancisco/blog/biotech/2015/03/hiv-aids-cirm-stem-cells-sangamo-sgmo-usc.html
- Sub-Saharan African randomised clinical trialsintomale circumcision and HIV transmission: Methodological, ethical and legal concerns: salem-news.com/fms/pdf/2011-12_JLM-Boyle-Hill.pdf
- The association between circumcision status and human immunodeficiency virus infection among homosexual men: cirp.org/library/disease/HIV/kreiss
- The CDC Dives Into the Great American Circumcision Debate:
  poz.com/article/CDC-circumcision-proposal-26661-6016
- The Cost to Circumcise Africa: researchgate.net/publication/244941272_The_Cost_to_Circumcise_Africa
- The Man Who Had HIV and Now Does Not: nymag.com/health/features/aids-cure-2011-6
- The Reemerging HIV/AIDS Epidemic in Men Who Have Sex With Men:
  jamanetwork.com/journals/jama/article-abstract/209555
- The relationship between HIV seroprevalence and the proportion of uncircumcised males in African countries:
  journals.lww.com/aidsonline/Abstract/1989/06000/The_relationship_between_male_circumcision_and_HIV.6.aspx
- [The role of Langerhans cells in the skin immune system]: pubmed.ncbi.nlm.nih.gov/19388527
- U.S. has highest STD rates among developed countries:
  web.archive.org/web/20130122163048/https://www.stdtestexpress.com/std-news/us-has-highest-std-rates-among-developed-countries-800943204
- U.S. Navy Finds That Circumcision Does Not Prevent HIV or STIs:
  thewholenetwork.org/twn-news/us-navy-finds-that-circumcision-does-not-prevent-hiv-or-stis
- Update on male circumcision: Prevention success and challenges ahead (pro; abstract):
  rd.springer.com/article/10.1007/s11908-008-0040-9
- Vaccine Blocks Herpes in Some Women (HPC vaccine): abcnews.go.com/Health/story?id=117961
- Vaginal ring to prevent HIV on the cards:
  mpumalanganews.co.za/265134/vaginal-ring-to-prevent-hiv-on-the-cards
- Voluntary medical male circumcision for HIV prevention *(WHO, pro)*:
  who.int/hiv/topics/malecircumcision/fact_sheet/en
- When Bad Science Kills: intactamerica.wordpress.com/2012/05/26/when-bad-science-kills
- Why Circumcision Does NOT Slow The Spread of HIV: web.archive.org/web/20130309083246/
  http://www.4eric.org/why-circumcision-does-not-slow-the-spread-of-hiv
- 'Why don't you just use a condom?': Understanding the motivational tensions in the minds of South African women *(condom use, cultural factors, etc.)*: phcfm.org/index.php/phcfm/article/view/79/101
- Why Men Don't Use Condoms in a HIV Epidemic: Understanding Condom Neglect through Condom Symbology: warwick.ac.uk/fac/cross_fac/iatl/reinvention/archive/bcur2013specialissue/farrar
- Why The Benefits of Circumcision Are Based On False Assumptions, Erroneous Conclusions and Misleading Medical Information: preventdisease.com/news/14/072114_Benefits-Circumcision-Based-On-False-Assumptions-Erroneous-Conclusions-Misleading-Medical-Information.shtml
- Zimbabwe Demographic and Health Survey 2010-11: measuredhs.com/pubs/pdf/FR254/FR254.pdf

15 Circumcision and HIV/AIDS

Circumcision has been dubbed "a solution in search of a problem". As soon as one supposed "benefit" is thoroughly discounted another seems to crop up in its place. Never in history has any other body part been put on trial like this, its fate to be condemned to mass annihilation upon suspicion of any supposed transgression.

15.1 Research to Find a Reason for Circumcision

Since my book was first published in 1985, a huge influx of speculation and action has arisen as to whether or not foreskins or lack of same are related to HIV. A thorough examination of every published article would result in a book ten times the size of this one, so my hope here is to present a valid synopsis with resources for those who wish to delve more deeply.

According to the observations reported by Bongaarts, et al.:

"The existence of an ecological correlation between lack of male circumcision and HIV prevalence suggests that circumcision could potentially be an important determinant in the prevention of the spread of HIV, but individual-level data are needed to demonstrate such a relationship. A review of the epidemiological studies that have evaluated the association between male circumcision status and risk of HIV infection included 21 cross-sectional and two prospective studies in sub Saharan Africa. Of these studies, 14 were conducted among patients recruited at clinics for sexually transmitted diseases (STDs). Most of these studies of male STD patients showed a protective effect of circumcision against HIV infection, with odds ratios (OR)[1] between 0.12 to 0.77. It has been noted that most of the studies were conducted in urban populations and that several had methodological limitations." [2]

"Data from men in the Mwanza region suggest that there is a modest protective effect of male circumcision on the risk of HIV infection among men, with an adjusted OR of 0.62. A stronger protective effect was observed in urban Mwanza (adjusted OR 0.46) and to a lesser extent in roadside villages (OR 0.65) while in rural areas and islands there was no significant reduction in HIV prevalence among circumcised men. The overall results from the urban areas and roadside

---

[1] **OR** stands for "odds ratio" – a measure of association between an exposure and an outcome.
[2] Bongaarts J, Reining P, Way P, Conant F. The relationship between male circumcision and HIV infection in African populations. *AIDS*. 1989-06; 3(6): 373-7.

villages are in agreement with findings from other studies in Africa, although the protective effect is smaller than reported in most studies of STD patients." [2]

"Male circumcision may have a direct effect on the risk of HIV infection, perhaps because it reduces the risk of preputial lesions and renders the glans penis less vulnerable [6]. It may also have an indirect effect on HIV risk by reducing the risk of STDs, particularly as self-reported STD is an unreliable indicator of STD occurrence. Anecdotal reports suggest that some men may be circumcised as a traditional remedy for STD, especially genital ulcers, and this may further the association." [2]

"In summary, our analysis between male circumcision and risk of HIV and STD has shown a modest protective effect of circumcision against HIV infection." [2]

According to a study by Gray, Kigozi, et al., 4,996 uncircumcised, HIV negative men aged 15-49 years who agreed to HIV testing and counseling were enrolled in this randomized trial in rural Rakai district, Uganda. Men were randomly assigned to receive immediate circumcision (2,474) or have circumcision delayed for 24 months (2,552.) HIV testing, physical exam and interviews were repeated at 6, 12, & 24 months of follow up visits. 90-92% of the participants stayed in both groups. 0.66 cases of HIV per 100 person-years occurred in the group that had been immediately circumcised, while 1.33 cases of HIV per 100 person-years occurred in the control (non-circumcised) group. Adverse effects of circumcision occurred in 84 men (3.6%).[3]

In the authors' words:

"Observational findings do not consistently show protective associations in all studies, and to exclude the possibility of confounding due to differences in sexual risk behaviors and cultural or religious practices associated with circumcision is difficult. Thus the potential efficacy of circumcision for HIV prevention can be determined only by randomized trials. One randomized trial done in South Africa was ended early after an interim analysis showed that circumcision reduced HIV by 60%. Two other randomized trials, one in Kisumu, Kenya and the other in Rakai, Uganda were also stopped early after interim analyses showed significant efficacy." [3]

---

3   Gray RH, Kigozi G, Serwadda D, Makumbi F, Watya S, Nalugoda F, et al. Male Circumcision for HIV Prevention in Rakai, Uganda: A Randomised Trial. *Lancet.* 2007-02-24; 369(9562): 657-66.

Because the trial was ended early, the analysis for the 0-24 month interval was weighted by the preponderance of person-time accrued during the first twelve months. (Some men did not return, got circumcised elsewhere or changed their minds.) Socio-demographic characteristics that were noted during the study included age, marital status, religion, education and sexual risk behavior including number of partners, condom use, alcohol consumption with sex and sex for money or gifts.[4]

The authors further state: "Further circumcision programs must emphasize that circumcision provides only partial protection and that there is a critical need to practice safer sex after circumcision (i.e. partner limitation and consistent condom use.)"[4]

Circumcision also reduced the rate of self-reported symptoms of genital ulcer disease with efficacy of 48%.[4] It is not known if circumcision reduces rates of ulcerative infections due to syphilis, herpes simplex virus 2 and hemophilus ducreyi. Genital ulcer disease is a risk factor for acquisition of HIV.[5, 6, 7]

No effects of circumcision were observed on symptoms of discharge or dysuria (painful urination) which is consistent with data from observational studies that indicate a lack of an effect of circumcision on gonorrhea or chlamydia prevalence.[8, 9] Circumcision was also not observed to be protective against urethral infections which are apparently unaffected by the removal of the foreskin.[10]

The 24-month transmission risks were 2.6% in the control group and 1.11% in the intervention group, giving a difference of 1.49% Therefore these authors estimate that about 67 circumcisions are needed to prevent one HIV infection. Any long term effectiveness of circumcision or possible need for secondary reductions is not known. (In the authors' words:) "Is this appropriate or cost-effective?"[3]

Adult male circumcision is not without risk. In this study moderate to severe adverse events related to surgery were almost 4% and follow up management was needed.

Auvert, Taljaard, et al. have reported the following information on their study in Uganda. 3,274 uncircumcised men, ages 18-24 were randomized to a control or an

---

[4] Auvert B, Taljaard D, Lagarde E, Sobngwi-Tambekou J, Sitta R, Puren A. Randomized, Controlled Intervention Trial of Male Circumcision for Reduction of HIV Infection Risk: the ANRS 1265 Trial. *PLoS Med.* 2005-11; 2(11): e298.

[5] Weiss HA, Thomas SL, Munabi SK, Hayes RJ. Male Circumcision and Risk of Syphilis, Chancroid and Genital Herpes: A Systematic Review and Meta-Analysis. *Sex Transm Infect.* 2006-04; 82(2): 101-9.

[6] Freeman ED, Weiss HA, et al. Recent Herpes Simplex Virus Type 2 Infection in Men and Women: Systematic Review and Meta-analysis of Longitudinal Studies. *AIDS.* 2006; 20: 73-83.

[7] Reynolds SJ, Risbud AR, et al. Recent Herpes Simplex Virus Type 2 Infection and the Risk of Human Immunodeficiency Virus Type 1 Acquisition in India. *J Infecti Dis.* 2003; 187: 1513-21.

[8] Rottingen JS, Cameron DW, Garnett GP. A Systematic Review of the Epidemiologic Interactions Between Classic Sexually Transmitted Diseases and HIV. *Sex Transm Dis.* 2001; 28: 579-97.

[9] Reynolds SJ, Shepherd ME, Risbud AR, et al. Male Circumcision and Risk of HIV-1 and Other Sexually Transmitted Infections in India. *Lancet.* 2004; 363: 1039-40.

[10] Gray RH, Azire J, Serwadda D, et al. Male Circumcision and the Risk of Sexually Transmitted Infections and HIV in Rakai, Uganda. *AIDS.* 2004; 18: 2428-30.

intervention group. The intervention group was immediately circumcised while the control group was offered circumcision at end of the follow up.

20 HIV infections occurred in the circumcised group while 49 infections occurred in the control group. Condom use, sexual behavior and health seeking behavior can be factors. The studies were based on observational rather than experimental data. A causal relationship between male circumcision and protection against HIV infection could not be determined.[4] Direct experimental evidence is needed to establish this relationship.[11, 12, 13]

In 2002 a randomized, controlled, blindly evaluated intervention trial was carried out in Orange Farm (near Johannesburg, South Africa). Men were paid 200 South African Rand after participating in the study. Voluntary counseling and testing was offered. Blood samples were taken. Men who were already HIV+ were not included in the statistical analysis.[4]

The background characteristics of the participants was recorded as follows: age (less than 21, or over 21), religion (Catholic, Protestant, African traditional, or other,) ethnic group (Zulu, Sotho, or other), alcohol consumption, at-risk behavior (lack of condom use), spousal partner, number of non-spousal sexual partners, number of sexual contacts, and health seeking behavior.[4]

The impact of the intervention itself was assessed, including the recommended six week period of abstinence (post-circumcision). 42 days was the median interval of abstinence. The median age was twenty one years. Very few of the men were married or living as married and about half were at high-risk behavior.[4]

The authors acknowledge that the study has limitations. It was conducted in one area in sub-Saharan Africa and therefore may not be generalizable to other places. Some participants were lost during the follow up (due to moving away or otherwise being unreachable, not to HIV), thus leading to a smaller cohort.[4]

Participants were followed up for a short period of time. The study did not explore the long term protective effect of circumcision. Some believe the keratinization of the glans when not protected by the foreskin, allows for a short drying after sexual contact, reducing the life expectancy of HIV on the penis and reduction of target cells on the foreskin. The study does not allow for identification of the mechanisms of the protective effect of circumcision on HIV acquisition. Partial, spurious protection emphasizes the need for a true and effective vaccine for HIV, and effective retroviral treatments.[4]

---

11 Gray RH, Kiwanuka N, Sewankambo NK, Serwadda D, et al. Male Circumcision and HIV Acquisition and Transmission: Cohort Studies in Rakai, Uganda. Rakai Project Team. *AIDS*. 2000; 14: 2371-81.
12 Siegfried N, Muller M, Volmink J, Egger M, et al. HIV and Male Circumcision – A Systematic Review with Assessment of the Quality of Studies. *Lancet:* Infectious Diseases; 5: 165-73.
13 Halperin DT, Bailey RC. Male Circumcision and HIV Infection: 10 Years and Counting. *Lancet*. 1999-11; 354: 1813-5.

There are potential risks in promoting circumcision as a way of reducing the risk of HIV infection. Circumcision can be performed under poor hygienic conditions leading to infection, bleeding and permanent injury or death especially if appropriate treatment during healing is not provided. During the healing period, sexually active men are likely to be at a higher risk of HIV infection. Circumcision does not provide full protection. If misunderstood this could lead to reduction of protection for men who decrease condom use or otherwise engage in riskier behavior. The authors observed that the intervention group had significantly more sexual contacts due to a perceived effectiveness or belief in immunity due to circumcision. Circumcision is not a universal cultural practice and culture can be a barrier in policy considerations.[4]

Infections were 60% fewer in the treatment group which seems to indicate that circumcised men are less likely to be infected with HIV when having sex with infected women. More research is needed. There have been flaws in the methodology used. Circumcised men can still become infected, even though the risk might be lower. They should still take other steps to prevent themselves from getting HIV.[4]

The researchers Halperin and Bailey, whose works have largely pushed for advancement of male circumcision in Africa have observed the following:

"A decade has passed since publication of Cameron and colleagues study that showed a greater than eight fold increased risk of HIV1 infection for uncircumcised men. Today, many observers of the AIDS pandemic are puzzled by the glaring discrepancies in HIV seroprevalence between different countries and regions, despite the presence of what seem to be similar regions and risk factors. For example, the November, 1998 UNAIDS/WHO Report on the AIDS Epidemic concludes, 'It is not fully understood why HIV infection rates take off in some countries while remaining stable in neighboring countries over many years.' " [13]

"Four studies reported significant relative risks that ranged from 2.3 to 4.5 after multivariate analyses, and in the other two prospective studies, multivariate risk rates were 3.0 or greater, but were not significant. Of 38 cross-sectional studies, 27 from eight countries found a significant association between lack of male circumcision and HIV infection, five found a trend towards an association, five found no association, and one reported an increased risk of infection in men who had been circumcised. In 1994 Moses and colleagues established that on the basis of the information available at the time the association between lack of male circumcision and HIV infections met all but three of Hill's criteria for making causal inferences: an additional 17 studies from eight countries have since been published. That circumcision is partially protective has been documented even in settings in which circumcised men have higher risk profiles for HIV transmission (i.e. more sexual partners, alcohol use and some sexually transmitted infections.) [13]

"A wider public discussion has occurred as to why, 20 years into the pandemic, some countries continue to retain fairly low HIV seroprevalence whereas in other places sometimes even neighboring regions rates of infection are many times higher." [13]

"The varying rates of HIV-1 infection: Philippines – 0.6%, Bangladesh – 0.03%, Indonesia, – 0.05%, Thailand – 2.2%, Cambodia – 2.4% (have yielded) dramatic discrepancies with 10 to 20 fold differences (which are) not easily explained." [13]

15.2 Refuting Biased Research

In response to the observations reported by Halperin and Bailey the following appeared: "Why does Europe, where the men are largely uncircumcised, enjoy one of the lowest HIV rates in the world, while North America, where men are usually circumcised, suffers one of the highest?" [14]

> "Until such questions are answered [medical publications] should refrain from promoting the controversial public policy outlined in [the viewpoint that all of Africa should embrace routine male circumcision as a potential AIDS preventative.]
>
> The popular press, famously unable to distinguish between sensational editorials and solid research, has dangerously distorted these reviews.
>
> Halperin and Bailey rightly warn that a public misunderstanding of their position might have disastrous effects on HIV containment. [Publicity and propaganda promoting circumcision as a 'vaccine' to prevent AIDS has given people the false assumption that being circumcised gives full protection against AIDS.]" [14]

Halperin and Bailey have acknowledged that five cross-sectional studies found no association between male circumcision and HIV infection and one reported an increased risk of infection in men who have been circumcised.

> "Whenever there is some evidence that surgery may reduce the risk of developing a particular disease, but there is also evidence the surgery may have no prophylactic effect whatsoever, or even increase the risk of developing that disease, then

---

14 Pittas-Giroux JA. Infection: Letters to Editor. *Lancet*. 2000-03-11; 355.

the surgery should still be done on every person in whom the disease could develop??

Clearly a great many body parts would be candidates for such surgery. What would the total cost come to and what would be the overall impact on public health?? Condoms & safe sex practices are preventative measures, but do not involve amputation of healthy erogenous tissue." [15]

"Medecins Sans Frontieres (MSF) (Doctors Without Borders), one of the world's renowned NGOs working on public health has released statistics showing that HIV infection rate in Malawi has doubled in recent years despite a range of interventions put in place to tackle the spread of the virus have included relentless campaigns on condom use and circumcision.[16]

"According to the statistics by MSF, HIV rates have doubled in Malawi moving from 10% to 20% in 1 year. Strangely, this has been the same period that Malawians have been manipulated and forced to go through circumcision in masses with the promise that it reduced the contraction of HIV. The results which were published on BBC revealed that of every five people, one person is HIV positive making Malawi the country worst hit by the HIV pandemic of all countries in the world.[16]

Kangwele (a researcher from Malawi) has observed:

"The research which was conducted long before the championing of the circumcision campaign dispelled the assumptions that circumcision reduces the chances of contracting HIV, the virus that causes AIDS." [17]

"A document which Malawi24 has seen and throws back to a 2010 research on the prevalence rate of HIV among Malawian men established that over 10% of Malawian men who had undergone circumcision were HIV+ compared to only 7% of uncircumcised men." [17]

"The report dubbed 'The Malawi Health and Demographic Survey' states on page 207 that the prevalence rate of HIV was higher among circumcised men than the uncircumcised in Malawi." [17]

---

15 Harrison DC. Infection: Letters to Editor. *Lancet.* 2000-03-11; 355.
16 Malawi: Circumcision Disaster – Malawi HIV Infection Rate Doubles. *Malawi24.* 2015-07-25.
17 Kangwele MJ. Malawian Circumcised Men Most Likely to be Infected by HIV, Research Shows. *Malawi24.* 2015-07-25.

"However, regardless of these statistics the World Bank went ahead to pump $15,000,000 into the circumcision campaign for Malawian men when research had proved to them that circumcision did not reduce the chances of Malawian men contracting HIV. Recently medical male circumcision has been embroiled in controversy as it has emerged that most men had contracted HIV after being circumcised because they had been told that it would reduce their chances of contracting the virus." [17]

According to study researcher Mickey Daugherty, MD, (a urology resident at the State University of New York Upstate Medical University presentation at The Annual Meeting of the American Urological Association in 2017), "Circumcised participants in a study presented at the annual meeting [...] were twice as likely as their uncircumcised counterparts to have either of two HPV strains associated with penile cancer, researchers said." [18]

Daugherty told Infectious Disease News: "Classically, circumcision has been shown to be protective against HPV infection. We're not completely sure why, but there was a higher rate of these higher-risk HPV infections in men who are circumcised." [18]

Daugherty said the high proportion of men in the United States who are circumcised could account for the prevalence of HPV in that population. Nonetheless, he said, "The results show that circumcision alone is not a preventive measure." [18]

The men provided penile swabs which were tested for 37 HPV strains. The researchers stratified two strains of low-risk HPV linked to genital warts, HPV-6 and HPV-11. They also stratified two strains of high-risk HPV linked to penile cancer, HPV-16 and HPV-18. Most participants (77.8%) were circumcised. Results showed a higher risk for high-risk HPV among circumcised but no significant increase in risk for low-risk HPV in circumcised men.[18]

The information presented by Daugherty was subsequently published in *JAMA Oncology* by J.J. Han, et al.,[19] in *The Journal of Infectious Diseases* by B.Y. Hernandez, et al.[20] and in *Meeting News Perspective*.[21]

Rodriguez-Diaz reports on a study in Puerto Rico which found "Male circumcision may not make much difference to overall male HIV incidence in Caribbean

---

18 Daugherty M, et al. Abstract MP 11-03. Presented at: *The Annual Meeting of the American Urological Association, 2017-05-14/16, Boston, MA.*
19 Han JJ, et al. Prevalence of HPV in Adults Aged 18–69: United States, 2011–2014. *NCHS Data Brief.* 2017-04; 280. URL: cdc.gov/nchs/data/databriefs/db280.pdf
20 Hernandez BY, et al. Circumcision and Human Papillomavirus Infection in Men: A Site-Specific Comparison. *J Infecti Dis.* 2008-03; 197(6): 787-94.
21 Green J. Circumcised men at twice the risk for cancer-causing HPV, study shows. *Infectious Disease News.* 2017-05-22.

context." [22] Researchers concluded, "A blanket roll-out of an MMC (Medical Male Circumcision) program in the context of a Caribbean country such as Puerto Rico would not necessarily make much difference to HIV prevalence in men as a whole." [22]

Doerner has observed: "An analysis of an online and gay-venue survey of white, British-born gay and bisexual men in the UK has found no association between whether they were circumcised and whether they had HIV." [23]

Intaction[24] reports:

"A study in Israel showed that the HIV rate skyrocketed 55% between 2005-2012. Between 1981 through the end of 2011 there were 6,579 [Israeli] men diagnosed as having HIV or full-blown AIDS. Of this total, only 1,265 in Israel were homosexual men. That means there were 5,314 heterosexual circumcised men who contracted HIV leading to this stunning increase. Authorities attribute the increase to more people having unprotected sex and lack of fear of the disease. Since Israeli men are all circumcised, it would be logical to assume their willingness to engage in unprotected sex was in part due to the widely publicized belief that circumcision offers protection. Furthermore, Israel has a much higher HIV infection rate than Japan where most men are intact." [25]

"The HIV virus can attack the mucosa at the meatus (urethral opening) or inside the urethra just as easily as the foreskin. Most men of sexually active age in the United States are already circumcised, but the infection rates are higher in the USA than in other developed countries where circumcision is rare. Common sense tells us that circumcision is unreliable in protecting against HIV." [25]

Intaction has also shared a list of comments questioning the validity of attempts to support lack of foreskin as an HIV/AIDS preventative:

"In only three highly controversial, short-term clinical trials circumcision was purportedly shown to reduce risk of HIV by 50-60% in heterosexual males engaging in male/female intercourse. The results did not show that females had any

---

22 Rodriguez-Diaz CE, Clatts MC, Jovet-Toledo GG, Vargas-Molina RL, Goldsamt LA, García H. More than Foreskin: Circumcision Status, History of HIV/STI, and Sexual Risk in a Clinic-Based Sample of Men in Puerto Rico. *JSM.* 2012-11; 9(11): 2933-7.
23 Doerner R, et al. Circumcision and HIV Infection Among Men who Have Sex With Men in Britain: The Insertive Sex Role. *Arch Sex Behav.* 2013-10; 42(7): 1319-26.
24 **Intaction** is a well-known on-line source of information questioning and opposing genital cutting of all non-consenting infants and children.
25 "Circumcision and HIV – It's a Dangerous Mistake for Prevention" | URL: intaction.org/circumcision-hiv-a-dangerous-mistake/

protection from HIV as a result of their partners being circumcised, nor was transmission prevented in same sex partners. Drug use and other non-sexual vectors of HIV infection are not prevented by circumcision. The vast majority of other studies on the relationship between circumcision and HIV have shown either that circumcision offers no protection or that the results are inconclusive." [26]

"Some say clinical research is fraught with fraud as researchers and academics chase grant money. Others have suggested that touting phony benefits of circumcision will increase unwanted pregnancies and promiscuity." [26]

"The ability to have unrestricted sex is the subtle message behind the African circumcision marketing campaigns. Meanwhile the drastic reduction in sensitivity caused by circumcision due to the loss of 20,000 nerve endings will make African men engage in riskier behavior to achieve sexual gratification. Pro-circumcision propaganda will decrease use of contraception (i.e. condoms.)" [26]

A 2008 study examined data from 13 sub-Saharan countries found no association.[27]

Another 2008 study found that circumcision made no difference in HIV rates in South Africa.[28]

A 2007 study concluded that once commercial sex-worker patterns are factored in, male circumcision is not significantly associated with lower rates of HIV.[29]

A recently released report from the Zimbabwe Health Demographic Survey found that circumcised Africans had a higher HIV infection rate (14%) than Africans left intact (12%).[30]

"Researchers in Uganda say circumcision only reduces HIV transmission by 1.3%, not 60% as claimed in previous clinical trials. Based on a recent male-to-female transmission of HIV study in Uganda, researchers Gregory Boyle and George Hill in a study published by Australia's Thomson Reuters showed that more women contracted the virus after unprotected intercourse with infected circumcised male partners." [26]

"The New York Times reports that the infection rates in Uganda from 2005-2012 have increased while the United States, through its AIDS prevention strategy known as PEPFAR (The President's Emergency Plan for AIDS Relief) spent

---

26 "Researchers: Circumcision Doesn't Reduce HIV Spread" | URL: intaction.org/417/
27 Garenne M. Long-term Population Effect of Male Circumcision in Generalized HIV Epidemics in sub-Saharan Africa. AJAR. 2008, 7(1): 1-8.
28 Connolly C, Simbayi LC, Shanmugam R, Nqeketo A. Male circumcision and its Relationship to HIV Infection in South Africa: Results of a National Survey in 2002. SAMJ. 2008; 98(10): 789-94.
29 Talbot Jr. Size Matters: The Number of Prostitutes and the Global HIV/AIDS Pandemic. PloS One. 2007; 2(6): e543.
30 "African HIV infection rate higher on circumcised men". URL: intaction.org/african-hiv-infection-rate-higher-on-circumcised-men-2/

$1.7 billion in Uganda to fight AIDS. The results raise questions about the efficacy of a U.S. strategy largely based on circumcision." [26]

The following are the findings of yet another report by Intaction:

"The World Health Organization (WHO) wants to have 20 million men in Southern and Eastern Africa circumcised. WHO officials claim that circumcision will prevent HIV infections. To convince them to undergo the operation, men are assured that without a foreskin they will be 'vaccinated against AIDS.' It is an unprecedented undertaking: never before have aid organizations attempted to surgically alter so many people. It could end up being an unprecedented disaster." [26]

"Should the campaign be successful, 3.4 million new HIV infections would be prevented between now and 2025, but critics warn that the mass circumcisions are based on disputed studies and could end up having the opposite of the hoped-for effect: more HIV infections." [26]

"The first sign of a connection between foreskin and HIV were in the mid 1980's. Scientists noticed that fewer circumcised men were infected and construed that the foreskin was a possible point of attack for the virus. The inner foreskin is an area of concentration of lymphocytes and specialized cells called Langerhans cells. These specialized immune cells actually serve to protect against infection, so while Langerhans cells normally intercept and destroy HIV, under other conditions, for example in the presence of parallel infections, they can relay the virus on the HIV target cells and raise the infection rate." [26]

"For Doctor Bertran Auvert's study in South Africa, 1,339 men in the Johannesburg township of Orange Farm were voluntarily circumcised. After the procedure, Auvert compared their infection rate with a control group of 1309 non-circumcised men in the same region. His hypothesis was that the HIV target cells and thereby the risk of infection could be eliminated along with the foreskin." [26]

" 'TOTAL NONSENSE', says the German circumcision expert Wolfgang Buhmann, 'To help people in areas with high HIV rates, you have to make it clear to them that sex without a condom is life threatening. Sex with a condom however is safe, regardless of whether the foreskin is still there or not. Shades of grey, in-between just create confusion.' " [26]

"Nearly all forms of circumcision are accompanied by significant health risks, particularly when the operation takes place in often unhygienic, traditional settings. In South Africa between 2008 and 2014, approximately half a million boys were treated in hospitals for botched circumcisions, and more than 400 of them died. Even in very good hygienic conditions, medical problems are often noted, including deformed scarring, hemorrhage, wound infection, diminished sensation and other consequences. The effort to circumcise the majority of men in Southern Africa may, even by a conservative estimate, lead to hundreds of thousands of complications, some of them lifelong." [26]

"The effect of circumcision alone is something we can't calculate in isolation. HIV tests and condoms are crucial." [26]

"In Southern Africa the pressure to get circumcised is enormous. Posters in the streets depict a horrified African woman tearing at her hair and shouting, 'What?! You're not circumcised?!' Men with intact penises are branded as disease-causing pathogens. Non-circumcised men in Lusaka now have hardly any chance of finding a female partner." [26]

"An investigation in Uganda shows how fatal this development is. For women with circumcised husbands the HIV rate in the six months after the circumcision has drastically increased by 61%." [26]

"Confusing, false, missing information? More HIV due to riskier behaviors by circumcised men? 'We have no indications that would substantiate such hypotheses,' says George Sinyangwe of USAID[31] in Lusaka, but how can that be? The health report from Malawi has indicated that circumcised men are already showing higher HIV rates than non-circumcised men. Some have contracted the HIV virus not sexually but from contaminated needles, blood transfusions and surgical instruments. Many participants have disappeared and could not be tested or questioned." [26]

Dr. Robert Van Howe, MD, MS, FAAP, professor at Michigan State University, who has been researching this issue for years is convinced: "The circumcision campaign will ultimately increase the number of HIV infections." [26]

After returning to Germany, the author of this article, Michael Obert, tried for weeks to obtain an official statement from the WHO. He received no response. [32]

Van Howe's thorough investigation has revealed the following:

Three randomized, controlled trials (RCTs) done in sub-Saharan Africa appeared to show during the study period a 38-66% relative reduction for the circumcised subjects in the risk of heterosexual, female to male only, transmission of HIV. [4, 33, 3] All three studies were terminated early due to their apparently clear results. However Dowsett and Couch examined the results of the three RCTs but found insufficient

---

31 **USAID** is the world's premier international development agency and a catalytic actor driving development results. USAID's work advances U.S. national security. The initials stand for "United States Agency for International Development."
32 Obert M. Circumcision & HIVAIDS – A Life-Saving Cut?. URL: intaction.org/circumcision-hiv-aids-an-unprecedented-disaster/ (Original: *GEO Magazin* (German). 2015-07. Translated by Curtis Murphy.)
33 Bailey RC, Moses S, Parker CB, Agot K, Maclean I, Krieger JN, et al. Male Circumcision for HIV Prevention in Young Men in Kisumu, Kenya: a Randomised Controlled Trial. *Lancet*. 2007; 369: 643-56.

evidence to recommend circumcision to prevent HIV infection.[34] Green, et al. reviewed the evidence and also found "insufficient data" as well as contrary evidence.[35, 36]

Factors influencing these studies have included:
- Participant expectation bias – participants believed that circumcision would reduce the risk of HIV.
- Lead time bias – Men randomized to the intervention arm of the trials (group that was circumcised) were considered to be at risk for becoming infected from the time of the surgery, even though they were told to avoid sexual activity during the period of wound healing. Men in the control arm (who were not circumcised) were able to be sexually active from the beginning of the study.
- Selection bias – only men who were interested in a free circumcision were eligible to participate and may not have been representative of the general population.
- Attrition bias – for every man who became infected with HIV during the trials, 3.5 – 7.4 men were lost to follow up. This is a serious methodological problem that could alter the statistical significance of the findings.[37]
- Early termination bias – studies that are terminated early are more likely to overestimate any treatment effect.[38, 39]
- Duration bias – because men who were not initially circumcised were circumcised at the end of the study, long-term comparison of the effects cannot be accurately extrapolated as some modelers have proposed.[40]
- Source of infection unknown. If the studies were designed to determine whether circumcision reduced the risk of heterosexually-transmitted HIV, the investigators should have confirmed that the infections were indeed transmitted through heterosexual contact. They did not. Using the data reported, it is estimated that about half of the infections of the men in these studies were not sexually transmitted.[41]

---

34 Dowsett GW, Couch M. Male circumcision and HIV prevention: Is There Really Enough of the Right Kind of Evidence? *SRHM*. 2007; 15(29): 33-44.
35 Green LW, McAllister RG, Peterson KW, Travis JW. Male Circumcision is not the HIV 'Vaccine' We Have Been Waiting For! *Future HIV Therapy*. 2008; 2(3): 193-9.
36 Green LW, Travis JW, McAllister RG, Peterson KW, Vardanyan AN, Craig A. Male Circumcision and HIV Prevention: insufficient Evidence and Neglected External Validity. *Am J Prev Med*. 2010; 39(5): 479-82.
37 Akl EA, Briel M, You JJ, Sun X, Johnston BC, Busse JW, et al. Potential Impact on Estimated Treatment Effects of Information Lost to Follow-up in Randomised Controlled Trials (LOST-IT): Systematic Review. *BMJ*. 2012; 344: e2809.
38 Pocock S, White I. Trials Stopped Early: Too Good to be True? *Lancet*. 1999; 353: 943-4.
39 Bassler D, Briel M, Montori VM, Lane M, Glasziou P, Zhou Q, et al. Stopping Randomized Trials Early for Benefit and Estimation of Treatment Effects: Systematic Review and Meta-Regression Analysis. *JAMA*. 2010; 303: 1180-7.
40 Williams BG, Lloyd-Smith JO, Gouws E, Hankins C, Getz WM, Hargrove J, et al. The Potential Impact of Male Circumcision on HIV in Sub-Saharan Africa. *PLoS Med*. 2006; 3: e262.
41 Van Howe RS, Storms MR. How the Circumcision Solution in Africa Will Increase HIV Infections. *JPHiA*. 2011; 2: e4.

The cumulative treatment claimed a 38-66% relative risk reduction[42] which is an absolute risk reduction of 1.3%. This is a small effect which could have resulted from the various forms of bias. Data released before the trials began found a number of African countries where the prevalence of HIV infection was greater in circumcised men than in intact men.[43, 27] "Since the mass circumcision campaigns began in Uganda and Kenya, the incidence of new cases of HIV in both countries has increased." [44, 45, 46]

As with other STIs there is no evidence that circumcision has had any impact on lowering the incidence of HIV infection in the United States. Of the eight HIV studies in North American heterosexual men,[43, 47, 48, 49, 50, 51, 52] only one has found a significant association between circumcision and HIV infection risk. It actually found that circumcised men were at greater risk of HIV infection.[22]

The HIV epidemic in the U.S. is concentrated among men who have sex with men (MSM) and injection drug users. A meta-analysis of the studies published on

---

42 Siegfried N, Muller M, Deeks JJ, Volmink J. Male Circumcision for Prevention of Heterosexual Acquisition of HIV in Men. *Cochrane Database Syst Rev.* 2009; 2: CD003362, 23a.
43 Mishra V, Medley A, Hong R, Yuan Gu Y, Robey B. Levels and Spread of HIV Seroprevalence and Associated Factors: Evidence from National Household Surveys. *DHS Comparative Reports*, Calverton (MD): Macro International Inc. 2009; 22.
44 Ministry of Health, ICF International, Centers for Disease Control and Prevention, U.S. Agency for International Development, WHO Uganda, Uganda AIDS Indicator Survey 2011, Kampala (Uganda): Ministry of Health; 2012.
45 National AIDS Control Council, National AIDS and STD Control Programme – "The Kenya AIDS Epidemic: Update 2011" Nairobi (Kenya): National AIDS Control Council; 2012.
46 Orido G. Push for Male Circumcision in Nyanza Fails to Reduce Infections. *Standard (Kenya) website.* 2013-09-11. | URL: standardmedia.co.ke/nyanza/article/2000093293/push-for-male-circumcision-in-nyanza-fails-to-reduce-infections
47 Chiasson MA, Stoneburner RL, Hildebrandt DS, Ewing WE, Telzak EE, Jaffe HW. Heterosexual Transmission of HIV-1 Associated with the use of Smokable Freebase Cocaine (Crack). *AIDS.* 1991; 5: 1121-6.
48 Telzak EE, Chiasson MA, Bevier PJ, Stoneburner RL, Castro KG, Jaffe HW. HIV-1 Seroconversion in Patients With and Without Genital Ulcer Disease. *Ann Intern Med.* 1993; 119: 1181-6.
49 Laumann EO, Masi CM, Zuckerman EW. Circumcision in the United States: Prevalence, Prophylactic Effects, and Sexual Practice. *JAMA.* 1997; 277: 1052-7.
50 Thomas AG, Bakhireva LN, Brodline SK, Shaffer RA. Prevalence of Circumcision and its Association with HIV and Sexually Transmitted Infections in a Male US Navy Population. *Naval Health Research Center, San Diego (CA).* Report No. 04-10.
51 Mor Z, Kent CK, Kohn RP, Klausner JD. Declining Rates in Male Circumcision Amidst Increasing Evidence of its Public Health Benefit. *PLoS ONE.* 2007; 2(9): e861.
52 Warner L, Ghanem KG, Newman DR, Macaluso M, Sullivan PS, Erbelding EJ. Male Circumcision and Risk of HIV Infection Among Heterosexual African American Men Attending Baltimore Sexually Transmitted Disease Clinics. *J Infecti Dis.* 2009; 199: 59-65.

this topic by the CDC found that the risk for HIV infection in MSM is the same in intact and circumcised men.[53, 54, 55, 56]

In another study by Van Howe: "The notion that circumcision significantly reduces the risk of STIs is a piece of medical folklore dating back to Victorian-era medicine, before a modern understanding of the causes of disease and before the advent of evidence-based medicine.[57]

"When the results of STI studies are considered in aggregate using meta-analysis, circumcision has been shown to have no significant impact on the risk of gonorrhea, chlamydia,[57, 58] genital herpes simplex virus infections, human papilloma virus (HPV),[58] or chancroid.[57, 58] Being circumcised is associated with an increased risk of non-specific urethritis,[56, 57] genital discharge syndrome (which includes gonorrhea, chlamydia, and non-specific urethritis).[57] Being circumcised is associated with a slightly lowered risk of genital ulcerative disease (which includes chancroid, syphilis, and genital herpes infection)[57, 58, 5] and syphilis (primarily in Africa).[58, 5] However, prospective studies have found a slight increase in the incidence of syphilis in circumcised males.[59, 60]

"In the case of HPV, sampling bias can occur if only the glans of the penis is tested. Several studies have shown that circumcised men are more likely than intact men to harbor the HPV virus on the shaft of the penis instead of the glans.[60, 61, 62, 63, 64, 65, 20]

---

53 Millett GA, Flores SA, Marks G, Reed JB, Herbst JH. Circumcision Status and Risk of HIV and Sexually Transmitted Infections Among Men who Have Sex with Men. *JAMA.* 2008;300:1674-84. Errata: *JAMA.* 2009; 301: 1126-9.
54 Crosby RA, Graham CA, Mena L, Yarber WL, Sanders SA, Milhausen RR, et al. Circumcision Status is not Associated with Condom use and Prevalence of Sexually Transmitted Infections Among Young Black MSM. *AIDS Behavior.* 2015-10-07, Epub ahead of print.
55 Van Howe RS. Alleged Medical Benefits. *Doctors Opposing Circumcision* website. URL: doctorsopposingcircumcision.org/for-professionals/alleged-medical-benefits/
56 Darby R. A Surgical Temptation: the Demonization of the Foreskin and the Rise of Circumcision in Britain. University of Chicago Press. 2005.
57 Van Howe RS. Genital Ulcerative Disease and Sexually Transmitted Urethritis and Circumcision: a Meta-Analysis. *Int J STD AIDS.* 2007; 18(12): 799-809.
58 Van Howe RS. Sexually transmitted infections and male circumcision: a systematic review and meta-analysis. *ISRN Urology.* 2013: 109846.
59 Tobian AAR, Serwadda D, Quinn TC, Kigozi G, Gravitt PE, Laeyendecker O, et al. Male Circumcision for the Prevention of HSV-2 and HPV Infections and Syphilis. *N Engl J Med.* 2009; 360(13): 1298-309.
60 Mehta SD, Moses S, Parker CB, Agot K, Maclean I, Bailey RC. Circumcision Status and Incident HSV-2 Infection, Genital Ulcer Disease, and HIV Infection. *AIDS.* 2012; 26: 1141-9.
61 Weaver BA, Feng Q, Holmes KK, Kiviat N, Lee SK, Meyer C, et al. Evaluation of Genital Sites and Sampling Techniques for Detection of Human Papillomavirus DNA in Men. *J Infecti Dis.* 2004; 189: 677-85.
62 VanBuskirk K, Winer RL, Hughes JP, Geng Q, Arima Y, Lee SK, et al. Circumcision and the Acquisition of Human Papillomavirus Infection in Young Men. *Sexually Transmitted Diseases.* 2011; 38: 1074-81.
63 Aynaud O, Piron D, Bijaoui G, Casanova JM. Developmental Factors of Urethral Human Papillomavirus Lesions: Correlation with Circumcision. *Br J Urol International.* 1999; 84: 57-60.

"There is no evidence that circumcision has reduced the incidence of STIs in the U.S, while the prevalence of chlamydia, gonorrhea and syphilis has declined steadily in Europe since 1980 (where circumcision is rare.) In the U.S. (with a primarily circumcised adult male population) the incidence of syphilis has increased and the incidence of chlamydia has soared.[66] The incidence of gonorrhea in the U.S. is 20 times higher than in Europe while the incidence of chlamydia in the U.S. is 45 times higher than in Europe.[67] A recent study of men visiting public STI clinics found that circumcised men were less likely than intact men to use condoms which may in part explain these STI trends.[58]

"Even if circumcision did reduce the risk of STIs, pre-emptive amputation is not a preferred approach to diseases that can readily be cured with a short course of antibiotics or prevented by simple safe-sex behaviors." [68]

Darby and Van Howe have observed and reported on the following, their objective being to conduct a critical review of recent proposals that widespread circumcision of male infants be introduced in Australia as a means of combating heterosexually transmitted HIV infection. Logic, coherence and fidelity must be applied to the principles of evidence-based medicine. Such proposals ignore doubts about the robustness of the evidence from the African random-controlled trials as to the protective effect of circumcision as a means of HIV control, but they misrepresent the nature of Australia's HIV epidemic and exaggerate the relevance of the African random-controlled trials findings. They also underestimate the risks and harm of circumcision and ignore questions of medical ethics and human rights. The notion of circumcision as a 'surgical vaccine' is criticized as polemical and unscientific.[68]

Darby and Van Howe continue to express doubts about the African random controlled trials which claim that circumcision prevents heterosexual HIV transmission from women to men. The trial was based on three non-double-blinded, non-placebo-controlled, random controlled trials in Africa in which 5,000 men were circumcised. After 20 months, 64 of the men in the circumcised group had HIV compared to 137 in the non-circumcised group. The trial contained several forms of bias. Only

---

64 Aynaud O, Ionesco M, Barrasso R. Penile Intraepithelial Neoplasia. Specific Clinical Features Correlate with Histologic and Virologic Findings. *Cancer.* 1994-09-15; 74(6): 1762-7.
65 Oriel JD. Natural History of Genital Warts. *Br J Ven Dis.* 1971; 47(1): 1-13.
66 Sexually Transmitted Diseases Across Space and Time. *OnlineDoctor (UK)* website | URL: onlinedoctor.superdrug.com/std-us-eu/
67 Crosby R, Charnigo RJ. A Comparison of Condom use Perceptions and Behaviours Between Circumcised and Intact Men Attending Sexually Transmitted Disease Clinics in the United States. *Int J STD AIDS.* 2013; 24(3): 175-8.
68 Darby R, Van Howe R. Not a Surgical Vaccine: There is No Case for Boosting Infant Male Circumcision to Combat Heterosexual Transmission of HIV in Australia. *Australian and New Zealand Journal of Public Health.* 2011-10; 35(5): 459-65.

men interested in a free circumcision were eligible. It would have been impossible to blind researchers or subject (as to who received immediate circumcision).[67, 58]

Garenne found that in 8 countries (Burkina Faso, Cote d'Ivoire, Ethiopia, Ghana, Niger, Rwanda, Tanzania and Zimbabwe) there was no significant difference in HIV seroprevalence between circumcised and uncircumcised men. In two countries (Kenya and Uganda) HIV seroprevalence was higher among uncircumcised men, and in three countries (Cameroon, Lesotho and Malawi), HIV seroprevalence was higher among circumcised men. In Lesotho the difference was striking: HIV seroprevalence was 22.8% among the circumcised men but only 15.2% among the uncircumcised population.[27]

In South Africa where one-third of the male population is circumcised and HIV prevalence is among the highest on record, both Garenne, and Connolly, et al. found no difference in HIV status between circumcised and uncircumcised samples.[27, 28]

"Both the U.S. and Indonesia with predominantly circumcised male populations have a significantly higher incidence of HIV than Australia, Canada, Britain and New Zealand where circumcision is in decline or extremely rare."[27]

No convincing biological explanation of circumcision's protective effect has been proven. Pro-circumcision speculation has suggested that the interior mucosa of the prepuce is thinner and more prone to tearing.[27] The mucosa of the inner and outer prepuce have been shown to be of the same thickness in some studies but not in others.[69]

Langerhans cells[70] have been believed to be the entry point for the virus. Actually Langerhans cells repel HIV. The transmission rate of HIV is low – about 1 per 1,000 unprotected coital acts.[71] Inner foreskin secretes langerin[72] which kills numerous pathogens.[68]

> "Until we understand how circumcision works biologically, we cannot be certain whether the observed reduction in risk of infection in the random-controlled trials is the result of changed anatomy resulting from surgery, changed behavior resulting from counseling and provision of condoms, or various forms of bias." [73]

---

69 Ganor Y, Bomsel M. HIV-1 Transmission in the Male Genital Tract. *American Journal of Reproductive Immunology.* 2011; 65: 284-91.
70 **Langerhans cells** are dendritic (branching) **cells** of the skin which stimulate an immune response to foreign substances.
71 Dinh MH, McRaven MD, Kelley L, Penugonda S, Hope TJ. Keratinization of the Adult Male Foreskin and Implications for Male Circumcision. *AIDS.* 2010; 24(6): 899-906.
72 **Langerin** is a microscopic structure within a Langerhans which becomes a specific organelle called the Birbeck granule, which is specific for producing an immune response to invasive pathogens (i.e. diseases.).
73 Chin J. The AIDS Pandemic: The Collision of Epidemiology with Political Correctness. Oxford (UK): *Radcliffe Publishing.* 2007.

"It is now firmly established that circumcision provides no protection to men who have sex with men and there is evidence from Britain that circumcised gay men may be at greater risk. The annual number of new HIV diagnoses has remained relatively stable at around 1,000 over the past 4 years. HIV continues to be transmitted primarily through sexual contact between men and of 1,185 cases of heterosexually acquired infection newly diagnosed in 2005-2009, 58% were in people (or their partners) from high prevalence countries." [74, 75]

According to Darby and Van Howe (based on figures of new HIV exposures (during the early 2000's) via heterosexual contact:

"It would be necessary to circumcise several thousand babies now to prevent one case of HIV from 2030 onward, a proposal that would be ruled out on cost-benefit considerations alone." [68]

This would be inconsistent with principles of evidence-based medicine: Infants are not at risk of infection by sexual contact and will not be at risk until they become sexually active in 16-20 years, by which time treatment and prevention options and the virus itself may have altered beyond recognition. Assuming that the African evidence is reliable and applicable, logically – sexually active adult men who have regular intercourse with numerous female partners and do not always use condoms should consider circumcision for themselves. Instead some researchers have proposed circumcision of baby boys as a precaution against a risk they will not face until adulthood and against a disease that is very rare among heterosexually active adult men anyway. If it is still necessary to wear a condom, there seems little point in getting circumcised.[68]

Research has confirmed that the WHO recommendations arising from the African random-controlled trials cannot be applied to developed nations.[68, 76] "Behavioral factors appear to play a far more important role than whether or not one has a foreskin." [77, 78]

---

74 de Witte L, Nabatov A, Pion M, Fluitsma D, de Jong MAWP, de Gruijl T, et al. Langerin is a Natural Barrier to HIV-1 Transmission by Langerhans Cells. *Nat Med.* 2007; 13(3): 367-71.
75 Reid D, Weatherburn P, Hickson F, Stephens M. *Know the Score: Findings from the National Gay Men's Sex Survey 2001.* London (UK): Sigma Research, Faculty of Humanities & Social Sciences, University of Portsmouth. 2002.
76 McDaid LM, Weiss HA, Hart GJ. Circumcision Among Men who have Sex with Men in Scotland: Limited Potential for HIV Prevention. *Sex Transm Infect.* 2010; 86: 404-6.
77 Wei C, Raymond H, McFarland W, Buchbinder S, Fuchs J. What is the Potential Impact of Adult Male Circumcision on the HIV Epidemic Among men who have Sex with Men (MSM) in San Francisco? *J Sex Transm Dis.* 2010; 37: 1-3.
78 Royal Dutch Medical Association. Non-therapeutic circumcision of male minors. | PDF available at URL: knmg.nl/actualiteit-opinie/nieuws/nieuwsbericht/international-physicians-protest-against-american-academy-of-

A study by Perera, et al. found the benefits of neonatal or childhood circumcision to be negligible and the possibility of reduced vulnerability to HIV irrelevant to children. If uncircumcised boys are more subject to "adverse medical conditions" we should expect this to show up in child health reviews, but the Australian Institute of Health and Welfare found no decline in child health as the incidence of circumcision in Australia has fallen, and indeed that child health has improved over the same period. The RACP[79] concluded that there was no medical justification for prophylactic circumcision of minors in Australia.[80]

The harm and risks of circumcision and the ethics of performing amputative surgery on minors, which includes the loss of both sexual satisfaction and psychological well-being, has been ignored by many researchers. "Any consideration of the costs of circumcision will be woefully inadequate if it fails to factor in the value of the foreskin to the individual and the cost of surgical complications and other adverse sequelae, both physical and psychological." [80]

According to the Australian Institute of Health and Welfare:

"There is no evidence for the assertion that neonatal circumcision presents a lower incidence of complications than circumcision in adulthood. The risk of harm is likely to be greater if the operation is performed before the natural separation of foreskin from the glans, and lower in adulthood when the mature size of the penis and final foreskin length can be observed and taken into account. Males differ so much in these variables that one cut does not fit all. Also safe anesthesia is normally provided for adults." [81]

The results of these findings pose the issues of medical ethics and human rights. Does the proposed procedure provide a net therapeutic benefit to the patient, considering the risk, pain and loss of normal function? Also, does the procedure avoid permanently diminishing the patient in any way that could be avoided? Will the final result provide a significant net benefit to the patient in proportion to the risk undertaken and the losses sustained? Will the patient be treated as fairly as we would all wish to be treated? Lacking life-threatening urgency, will the procedure honor the patient's right to his or her own likely choice.) Could it wait for the patient's assent?[81]

Darby & Van Howe also criticize the use of unscientific language.

---

pediatrics-policy-on-infant-male-circumcision.htm
79 **RACP** stands for "Royal Australasian College of Physicians."
80 Royal Australasian College of Physicians. *Circumcision – RACP Position Statement.* Sydney, Australia: RACP. 2010-09: 13.
81 Australian Institute of Health and Welfare. *A Picture of Australia's Children Canberra (Australia).* AGPS. 2005.

"Circumcision as a 'surgical vaccine' is regrettable and misleading, with no basis in science and is irresponsible in that it may encourage high risk behavior. Circumcision advocates seem unwilling to acknowledge the difference between amputating body parts to provide limited protection against a rare disease to which the individual is unlikely to be exposed, and giving a person an injection that confers a high level of immunity to common or highly contagious diseases." [68]

"The rapid spread of HIV in Africa was associated with a high level of sexual activity involving numerous concurrent, but often transient sexual partnerships, widespread prostitution, both formal and informal, various forms of polygamy and reluctance to practice safe sex including use of condoms. It is also probably that a significant proportion of HIV infections are the result of non-sexual transmission such as non-sterile medical procedures." [82]

"Much of Africa has poorly developed health services with the co-presence of numerous other epidemic diseases such as malaria, tuberculosis and other STIs." [83]

"Safe sex education, needle and syringe programs and provision of condoms appear to be the most successful strategy against AIDS." [84]

Darby & Van Howe have also observed: "Langerin is a protein based substance which is said to have disease preventative properties. Langerhans cells which produce Langerins are present in the epithelium (human skin) and are abundant in foreskins." [68] This is important knowledge since some writers have believed that the foreskin only harbors disease pathogens. [85, 86]

According to the study by de Witte, et al.:

"Human immunodeficiency virus-1 (HIV-1) is primarily transmitted sexually. Dendritic cells (DCs) in the subepithelium (inner layer of skin) transmit HIV-1 to T cells through the C-type lectin DC-specific intercellular adhesion molecule ICAM-3-grabbing nonintegrin (DC-SIGN). However the epithelial Langerhans

---

82 Cold CJ, Taylor JR. The prepuce. *Br J Urol International.* 1999; 83(Suppl 1): 34-44.
83 Darby R, Svoboda JS. A Rose by any Other Name: Rethinking the Similarities and Differences Between Male and Female Genital Cutting. *Medical Anthropology Quarterly.* 2007; 21: 301-23.
84 Beauchamp TL, Childress JF. *Principles of Biomedical Ethics* – Part II. 6th ed. NY: Oxford University Press. 2009.
85 Gisselquist D. *Points to Consider: Responses to HIV/AIDS in Africa, Asia, and the Caribbean.* London (UK): Adonis & Abbey. 2008.
86 Bowtell WD. World AIDS Day. *Medical Journal of Australia.* 2010;193(11/12):653-4.

cells (LOCs) are the first DC subset to encounter HIV-1. It has generally been assumed that LCs mediate the transmission of HIV-1 to T cells through the C-type lectin Langerin, similarly to transmission by DC-SIGN, Langerin prevents HIV-1 to T cells through the C-type lectin Langerin, similarly to transmission by DC-SIGN on dendritic cells (DCs). Here we show that in stark contrast to DC-SIGN, Langerin prevents HIV-1 transmission by LCs. HIV-1 captured by Langerin was internalized into Birbeck granules and degraded. Langerin inhibited LC infection and this mechanism kept LCs refractory to HIV-1 transmission; inhibition of Langerin allowed LC infection and subsequent HIV-1 transmission. Notably, LCs also inhibited T-cell infection by viral clearance through Langerin. Thus Langerin is a natural barrier to HIV-1 infection, and strategies to combat infection must enhance, preserve or, at the very least, not interfere with Langerin expression and function." [74]

Van Howe has also reported the following:

"Meta-analyses (have been carried out) on studies of genital discharge syndrome versus genital ulcerative disease, genital discharge syndrome, nonspecific urethritis, gonorrhea, chlamydia, genital ulcerative disease, chancroid, syphilis, herpes simplex virus, human papillomavirus and contracting a sexually transmitted infection of any type. Chlamydia, gonorrhea, genital herpes and human papillomavirus are not significantly impacted by circumcision. Syphilis showed mixed results. Intact men were at greater risk for genital ulcerative disease & lower risk for genital discharge syndrome, nonspecific urethritis, genital warts and the overall risk of any sexually transmitted infection (STI). In general populations there is no clear or consistent positive impact of circumcision on the risk of individual STIs." [68]

Prevention of STIs cannot rationally be interpreted as a benefit of circumcision, and any policy of circumcision for the general population to prevent STIs is not supported by the evidence in the medical literature. Van Howe has continued to state: "The AAP 1999 Task Force on Circumcision concluded 'evidence regarding the relationship of circumcision to STD in general is complex and conflicting.' " [58]

In 2012 the AAP concluded that "evaluation of current evidence indicates that the health benefits of newborn male circumcision outweigh the risks; furthermore, the benefits of newborn male circumcision justify access to this procedure for families who choose it. Specific benefits from male circumcision were identified for the prevention of UTIs, acquisition of HIV, transmission of some STIs and penile cancer." [87]

Within the body of the statement the committee admitted that they were unable to precisely measure the benefits of infant circumcision and unable to quantify the risks.

> "While a number of review articles and systematic reviews of the association between male circumcision and individual types of STIs have been published, many of these need updating while others have methodological shortcomings." [5, 88, 89, 90]

> "Three randomized clinical trials of adult male circumcision in Africa failed to adjust for lead-time bias. Men who were assigned to immediate circumcision were instructed to either not engage in sexual activity or use condoms with all sexual contacts until the circumcision healed (approximately 4-6 weeks) Analyses that included these trials were conducted with the reported data and with the data adjusted for a 6 week lead time bias.[86]

> "Sampling bias (was not considered.) Circumcised men are more likely to have genital warts or have positive lesions or positive swabs on the penile shaft than intact men.[57, 65, 91, 92, 93, 94, 95] Studies that sampled only the glans or urethra would underestimate the incidence and prevalence of HPV infection in circumcised males." [74]

A study published by VanBuskirk, et al. reveals that if only the glans is sampled, only 66.1% of the intact men with genital HPV would be identified, while only 45.2% of the circumcised men with genital HPV would be identified.[96] Additionally, patient report of circumcision status can be inaccurate.[67]

---

87 American Academy of Pediatrics, Task Force on Circumcision. Circumcision Policy Statement. *Pediatrics.* 1999; 103: 686-93.
88 AAP 2012 Task Force on Circumcision. Male Circumcision. *Pediatrics.* 2012; 130: e756-e785.
89 Van Howe RS. Does Circumcision Influence Sexually Transmitted Diseases?: A Literature Review. *BJU Int.* 1999; 83(suppl. 1): 52-62.
90 Van Howe RS. Human Papillomavirus and Circumcision: A Meta-Analysis. *J Infect.* 2007; 54(5): 490-6.
91 Rehmeyer CJ. Male Circumcision and Human Papillomavirus Studies Reviewed by Infection Stage and Virus Type. *J Am Osteopath Assoc.* 2011; 111(suppl. 3): S11-S18.
92 Chelimo TA, Wouldes LDC, Elmwood JM. Risk Factors for Prevention of Human Papillomaviruses (HPV), Genital Warts and Cervical Cancer. *J Infec.* 2012; 66(3): 207-17.
93 Albero X, Castellsague AR, Bosch FX. Male Circumcision and Genital Human Papillomavirus: a systematic Review and Meta-Analysis. *J Sex Transm Dis.* 2012; 39: 104-13.
94 Larke N. Male Circumcision, HIV and Sexually Transmitted Infections: A Review. *Br J Nurs.* 2010/05-06; 19(10): 629-34.
95 Cook LS, Koutsky LA, Holmes KK. Circumcision and Sexually Transmitted Diseases. *Am J Public Health.* 1994; 84(2): 197-201.
96 VanBuskirk K, Winer RL, Hughes JP, et al. Circumcision and the Acquisition of Human Papillomavirus Infection in Young Men. *Sex Transm Dis.* 2011; 38: 1074-81.

As to genital ulcerative disease (GUD) and genital discharge syndrome (GDS): intact men are more prone to GUD and circumcised men are more prone to GDS. Non-specific (nongonococcal) urethritis (NSU) is significantly lower in intact males. With chlamydia and gonorrhea, no significant difference in prevalence has been noted between circumcised and intact males.[96]

Genital ulcerative disease is more common in developing countries and is more likely to grow in mucosal surfaces, hence more likely in intact males.

Syphilis has shown a positive association for intact men primarily in populations at high risk for acquiring STIs, while in general populations, there is no significant difference.

Genital Herpes/Herpes Simplex virus type 2 shows no statistically significant association for circumcised versus intact males. Chancroid is uncommon in developing nations and is extremely rare in developed nations. No statistically significant relationship has been found in regard to circumcised or intact status. Genital warts have shown a strong trend of being lower in intact males in general population.[63, 64, 67, 97, 98]

Prevalence of human papillomavirus has shown conflicting results.[67, 89] Many types may be related to penile cancer with some sampling bias. There have been barely statistically significant results based on circumcision status (i.e. some men are unsure of their circumcision status and sometimes only the glans was sampled but not the shaft.)[99, 100] Studies have indicated that the clearance of HPV takes longer from the intact penis.[59, 94, 101, 102] If this is true, it would be more likely to be detected in intact men.

Among all STIs the prevalence of acquiring any STI is lower in intact men.[67] STIs with genital discharges are more common than genital ulcers, which may explain why the prevalence of any STI is lower in intact males. It is clear that despite these methodological concerns, the impact of circumcision on the overall risk of contracting any STI is to increase the overall risk of infection. Because of the highly conflicting amount of data included in this analysis and disparate results on the incidence of infection, more studies are needed.[67]

---

97 Hernandez BY, Shvetsov YB, Goodman MT, et al. Reduced Clearance of Penile Human Papillomavirus Infection in Uncircumcised Men. *J Infecti Dis.* 2010; 201(9): 1340-3.
98 Barile MF, Blumberg JM, Kraul CW, Yaguchi R. Penile Lesions Among U.S. Armed Forces Personnel in Japan. *Dermatology.* 1962; 86: 273-81.
99 Cameron DW, D'Costa LJ, Maitha GM, et al. Female to Male Transmission of Human Immunodeficiency Virus Type 1: Risk Factors for Seroconversion in Men. *Lancet.* 1989; 2(8660): 403-7.
100 Nasio JM, Nagelkerke NJD, Mwatha A, Moses S, Ndinya-Achola JO, Plummer FA. Genital Ulcer Disease Among STD Clinic Attenders in Nairobi: Association With HIV-1 and Circumcision Status. *Int J STD AIDS.* 2009; 7(6): 1251-7.
101 Van Howe RS. Errors in Meta-Analysis by Van Howe. *Int J STD AIDS.* 2009; 20(3): 218-20.
102 Auvert B, Sobngwi-Tambekou J, Cutler E, et al. Effect of Male Circumcision on the Prevalence of High Risk Human Papillomavirus in Young Men: Results of a Randomized Controlled Trial Conducted in Orange Farm, South Africa. *J Infecti Dis.* 2009; 199(1): 14-9.

"The summary effect for the prevalence of every disease was greater in studies of high-risk populations than in general populations." [67] Calls for population-wide implementation of male circumcision on the grounds that it prevents sti's are not supported by the findings of these analyses. A major problem with infant circumcision is the lack of an accurate method of identifying which infants will find themselves in high risk population when they become sexually active.[103]

Sexual partners are usually not found randomly but within ones cultural or ethnic group.[104] Circumcision is associated with religious, tribal and cultural factors. Men with a particular circumcision status will likely have sexual partners from within a group that has a predominance of men with the same circumcision status. The smaller the group, the more quickly the rise and the higher the peak prevalence for a particular STI.[105] When circumcision rates are high, intact men would be more likely to be in a smaller ethnic, religious or cultural group and thus have a higher peak prevalence of a disease. As circumcision prevalence drops, circumcised men would find themselves in the smaller groups that would be more likely to have a higher peak prevalence of infections.[67]

The lack of any significant association between high risk HPV infections and circumcision status undermines the argument made by the few who believe that circumcision reduces cancer risk.[106, 107] Lack of association between HPV, HSV & other STIs also undermines the analysis published by the same researchers at Johns Hopkins that selectively reported their HPV findings in Africa.[67]

The results of these analyses also further undermine the argument of how the increased risk of HIV infection in intact men is biologically plausible. The plausibility has been based on several assumptions which are purely speculative, that the inner mucosa of the foreskin is thin and more prone to abrasions, the subpreputial space is a breeding ground for sexually transmitted viruses, and that Langerhans cells on the mucosal surface act like HIV virus magnets pulling the virus into the body.[105]

The preputial mucosa is not unusually thin.[106, 107] Circumcised men have a trend toward more penile abrasions (presumably from lack of adequate lubrication).[108] Langerhans cells are quite efficient in killing HIV cells, hence the low rate of trans-

---

103 Tobian AAR, Kigozi G, Gravitt PE, et al. Human Papillomavirus Incidence and Clearance Among HIV-positive and HIV-negative men in Rakai, Uganda. *AIDS.* 2012; 26: 1555-65.
104 Gray RH, Serwadda D, Kong X, et al. Male Circumcision Decreases Acquisition and Increases Clearance of High-risk Human Papillomavirus in HIV-negative men: A Randomized Trial in Rakai, Uganda. *J Infecti Dis.* 2010; 201: 1455-62.
105 Lu B, Wu C, Nielson M, et al. Factors Associated with Acquisition and Clearance of Human Papillomavirus Infection in a Cohort of U.S. Men: A Prospective Study. *J Infecti Dis.* 2009; 199(3): 362-71.
106 Van Howe RS. AAP: 'Spurious but Entertaining'. 12th International Symposium on Law, Genital Autonomy and Human Rights Helsinki, Finland, September 2012.
107 Laumann EO, Gagnon JH, Michael RT, Michaels S. *The Social Organization of Sexuality: Sexual Practices in the United States.* Chicago, IL: University of Chicago Press. 1994.
108 Morris BJ, Gray RH, Castellsague X, et al. The Strong Protective Effect of Circumcision Against Cancer of the Penis. *Advances in Urology. 2011;* Article ID 812368.

mission through sexual contact (approximately 1 in 1,000 unprotected acts of coitus) and require activated T cells.[108, 109] Langerhans cells are the first line of mucosal defense. There is no difference in the incidence and prevalence of HSV or HPV based on circumcision status. Research has found that the higher viral replication rates and viral load of HPV is on the penile skin rather than in the subpreputial space.[110]

Twenty percent or more genital infections in Africa are not spread through sexual contact.[71, 73, 74, 111, 112, 113, 114, 115] Data from three African randomized clinical trials in adult males looking for association between circumcision and any incidence of HIV infection[116, 117] found that apparently half of the infections documented were transmitted through nonsexual means.[118] Also, they observed a relatively small number of patients which would effect the validity of results.[67]

The control group (which were men without any STIs) may introduce bias due to differing behavioral patterns. Most forms of bias are insidious and difficult to measure. Circumcision status is linked to socioeconomic status, which may impact healthcare-seeking behaviors.[85]

In addition the men who were randomized to immediate circumcision were not exposed to STIs for 4-6 weeks following their procedures. Therefore, their exposure to disease was not the same as men who were assigned to later circumcision. When the reduced exposure time is accounted for, several of the associations found that these trials were no longer statistically significant.[67]

Sadly, the promotion of circumcision in Africa has had some tragic consequences. Circumcision has led many men to believe that they no longer need to use condoms, be faithful to one partner or use any other means of caution in their sexual lives, therefore in many instances it has increased the risk of aids and other STIs.

---

109 Zetola N, Klausner JD. Male Circumcision Reduces Human Papillomavirus Incidence and Prevalence: Clarifying the Evidence. *Sex Transm Dis.* 2012; 39: 114-5.
110 Morris BJ, Mindel A, Tobian AAR, et al. Should Male Circumcision be Advocated for Genital Cancer Prevention? *Asian Pac J Canc P.* 2012; 13: 4839-42.
111 Morris BJ, Wamai RG. Biological Basis for the Protective Effect Conferred by Male Circumcision Against HIV Infection. *Int J STD AIDS.* 2012; 23: 153-9.
112 Dinh MH, Hirbod T, Kigosi G, et al. No Difference in Keratin Thickness Between Inner and Outer Foreskins from Elective Male Circumcisions in Rakai, Uganda. *PLoS One.* 2012; 7(7): e41271.
113 Bailey RC, Neema S, Othieno R. Sexual Behaviors and Other HIV Risk Factors in Circumcised and Uncircumcised Men in Uganda. *J Acquir Immune Defic.* 1999; 22(3): 294-301.
114 Iores R, Beibei L, et al. Correlates of Human Papillomavirus Viral Load with Infection Site in Asymptomatic Men. *Cancer Epidemiol Biomarkers Prev.* 2008; 17(12): 3573-6.
115 Gisselquist D, Rothenberg R, Potterat JJ, Drucker E. Non-Sexual Transmission of HIV Has Been overlooked in Developing Countries. *BMJ.* 2002; 324(7331): article 235.
116 Gisselquist D, Potterat JJ. Heterosexual Transmission of HIV in Africa: An Empiric Estimate. *Int J STD AIDS.* 2003; 14(3): 162-73.
117 Gisselquist D, Potterat JJ, Brody S, Vachon S. Let it Be Sexual: How Health Care Transmission of AIDS in Africa was Ignored. *Int J STD AIDS.* 2003; 14(3): 148-61.
118 Gisselquist D, Potterat JJ, Brody S. Running on Empty: Sexual Co-Factors are Insufficient to Fuel Africa's Turbocharged HIV Epidemic. *Int J STD AIDS.* 2004; 15(7): 442-52.

"In 2005 came the report, 'Male circumcision protects against HIV like a vaccination.' A sensation! Hope bubbled up everywhere. The catalyst for the euphoria was the French Doctor Bertan Auvert. For his study in South Africa 1,339 men in the Johannesburg township of Orange Farm were voluntarily circumcised. After the procedure Auvert compared their infection rate with a control group of 1,309 non-circumcised men in the same region. His hypothesis was that the HIV target cells, and thereby the risk of infection could be eliminated along with the foreskin." [119]

"After one and a half years he appeared to prove his theory correct. Among the non-circumcised men in the control group, Auvert assessed 49 cases of HIV while he found only 20 among the circumcised men. From this the Frenchman inferred an up to 60 percent reduced HIV risk which was soon to become the mantra of the WHO campaign in Africa." [120]

However the WHO has also stated: "They are emphatically aware that condoms still need to be used after a circumcision. This is stressed in the training for local partners run by USAID, the authority which is coordinating the development partnership project for the U.S. government." [121]

"We're not just cutting off foreskins" says George Sinyangwe, the primary health advisor for USAID in Lusaka. "All men receive information which totally clears up mistaken ideas about the use of the procedure before, during and after their circumcision." [3]

"But is that message about safe sex getting through? When you have unprotected sex your penis gets tiny cracks into which the virus can penetrate, but circumcision makes your glans hard and tough." explains Margaret Nkunika. [33]

A 28-year-old man commented "I know the protection (via circumcision) amounts to 60 percent, which is better than nothing. But condoms offer a much higher level of protection, up to 95 percent." But the men laugh. "Using condoms in vaginal intercourse would be like eating candy in its plastic wrapper." [41]

A great many of recent studies warn of "mixed messages." Because of the unclear information of the campaign, scientists at the Makere University in Uganda have determined that circumcised men are more likely to take risks sexually than non-circumcised men.[122]

---

119 Gisselquist D. Denialism Undermines AIDS Prevention in sub-Saharan Africa. *Int J STD AIDS*. 2008; 19(10): 649-55.
120 Gisselquist D, Potterat JJ, St. Lawrence S, et al. How to Contain Generalized HIV Epidemics? A Plea for Better Evidence to Displace Speculation. *Int J STD AIDS*. 2009; 20(7): 443-6.
121 Gisselquist D, Potterat JJ, St. Lawrence S, et al. Repeating a Plea for Better Research and Evidence. *Int J STD AIDS*. 2011; 22(7): 416-7.
122 de Vincenzi I, Mertens T. Male Circumcision: A Role in HIV Prevention? *AIDS*. 1994; 8(2): 153-60.

The WHO has stated that while circumcision is supposed to reduce the risk of HIV transmission from women to men, it does not work the same in the other direction. Male circumcision offers no protection to women.[58]

In Uganda, for women with circumcised husbands the HIV rate in the six months after the circumcision has drastically increased, by 61 percent. Bertan Auvert ("the father of the circumcision solution") has stated, "I am absolutely convinced that some women will become HIV positive because of the circumcision of their partners because the men fall into a false sense of security." [32]

"Circumcision likewise offers hardly any protection to homosexual men who are among the high risk groups around the world. Yet one gay man in Zambia has stated: 'Most gays in Zambia think that circumcision protects them from HIV too. We are swearing off condoms and dying like flies.' " [123]

15.3 CDC's Misleading Headlines

The Center for Disease Control (CDC) has published misleading headlines such as "Benefits of Circumcision Outweigh the Risks" and "CDC Endorses Circumcision for Health Reasons." [124]

There is growing opposition by Africans to the current circumcision campaign. A 2017 on-line press release has stated: "Is it that the media is hungry to present benefits and call for a universal endorsement for something that really hasn't happened? Is this a feeble attempt to manipulate the public opinion, under the assumption that everybody is too lazy to go to the source materials? The CDC refers people to counseling rather than immediate and universal endorsement. Their aim is to aid a person through a decision making process. Sexual orientation and lifestyle choices are factors to be considered. When parents are asked to decide about circumcision for a newborn, this raises concerns about personal body autonomy, since a man with a foreskin can elect to be circumcised, but if circumcised as a newborn, cannot easily reverse the decision. The CDC has recognized that there are advantages and disadvantages to performing male circumcision at various stages of life, but the newborn has no ability to participate in the decision." [124]

The CDC's stance is based on the African trials on circumcision and HIV. They recognize that circumcision does not replace the need for condoms and safe sex, nor does it reduce the risk of male-to-female or male-to-male transmission. Circumcision also does not reduce the transmission through anal or oral sex or for intravenous drug

---

[123] See ref. 32 (Obert's sources not stated.)
[124] CDC, circumcision and misleading headlines. *CircWatch* (website). 2014-12-03. URL: circwatch.org/cdc-circumcision-and-misleading-headlines/

users. Circumcision will only curb the transmission of HIV from females to males during vaginal penetration.[124] Therefore the person's HIV risk behavior, HIV status, sexual preferences and gender of partner must be assessed.[124]

The CDC also states: "The prevalence of HIV infection in the U.S. is not as high as in sub-Saharan Africa and most men do not acquire HIV through penile-vaginal sex. Targeting recommendations for adult male circumcision to men at elevated risk for heterosexuality acquired HIV infection would be more cost effective than offering routine adult male circumcision. Men may be targeted according to sexual practices or an elevated prevalence of HIV within a geographic region or race/ethnicity group." [124]

The CDC continues by stating: "All sexually active adolescent and adult males should continue to use other proven HIV and sti risk reduction strategies such as reducing the number of partners and correct and consistent use of male latex condoms, and HIV preexposure or postexposure prophylaxis among others."[124]

Finally, according to the CDC: "The foreskin is a highly innervated structure and some authors have expressed concern that its removal may compromise sexual sensation or function. However, in one survey of 123 men following medical circumcision in the U.S., men reported no change in sexual activity and improved sexual satisfaction, despite decreased erectile function and penile sensation. A small survey conducted among 15 men before and after circumcision found no statistically significant difference in sexual function or sexual satisfaction. Other studies conducted among men after adult circumcision have found that relatively few men report that there is a decline in sexual functioning after circumcision. Most report either improvement or no change." [124] (Of course what a person can report that he feels or does not feel is highly subjective, and difficult to measure or assess. Men will be understandably reluctant to report reduced sexual sensation or satisfaction. – R.R.)

> "The VMMC Experience Project is a non-for-profit organization to empower Africans to raise their voices on the issue of mass circumcision as provided by Western health organizations. Its investigation into the 'voluntary medical male circumcision' (VMMC) campaign in rural East Africa revealed less than voluntary recruitment methods for circumcision, including $3 vouchers to impoverished men and the targeting of schoolboys without their parents' consent. Vulnerable populations such as orphaned children and prison inmates become frequent targets, as the recruiters (called 'mobilizers') are compensated per head. Some of these boys and men later regret undergoing the procedure. Others report they never consented at all." [124]

VMMC representatives have stated: "The mass circumcision campaign also results in confusion about HIV immunity. At least 7 respondents attributed their own infections to misinformation derived from the campaign. Others have mourned the loss of loved ones to HIV/AIDS following circumcision which they underwent for HIV/AIDS prevention." [125]

Prince Hillary Maloba, a native of Kenya and Uganda, is the Director of the Project. His uncles are members of the Bagisu, a circumcising tribe with one of the highest HIV rates in Uganda. "Millions of circumcised men are living with HIV," he reports. "Millions of children with circumcised parents are left AIDS orphans. Now traditionally non-circumcising tribes are being forced to accept circumcision based on blatant lies." He concludes, "We demand the banning of mass circumcision in Africa!" [125]

In other parts of the world there has been widespread condemnation of the practice of infant circumcision. Norway, Sweden, Finland, Denmark, Iceland and Greenland have all called for a ban on medically unnecessary circumcisions performed on underage boys. The Danish Medical Association's 2016 policy on male infant circumcision describes the practice as "ethically unacceptable," while the Royal Dutch Medical Society urges a "powerful policy of deterrence." [125]

"In 2013 the Council of Europe adopted a resolution which classifies medically unnecessary circumcisions as a violation of children's right to physical integrity. UNICEF'S African infant circumcision initiative is backed by the American agencies USAID and PEPFAR. To some Africans this conjures up images of American colonialism and even a cultural assault. 'Circumcision' says Maloba. 'We totally reject this.' " [125]

A letter has been written to UNICEF by the VMMC Experience Project by Dr. Piotr Czauderna (former president of the Polish Association of Pediatric Surgeons), and Dr. Dean Edell (Well-known American physician-broadcaster.) (There has been no response from UNICEF as of Aug. 2017.)[125]

15.4 Conclusion

Behavioral factors obviously play the most important role in preventing all types of STIs including HIV. Having multiple sexual partners, especially with prostitutes and lack of condom use are the most significant factors in acquiring STIs. However, human behavior cannot truly be controlled in laboratory experiments. It would be

---

[125] Fisch M. African Opposition to UNICEF's Mass Infant Circumcision Campaign: UNICEF Responds. So do Africans. *The VMMC Experience Project* (website). 2017-08-01. URL: www.digitaljournal.com/pr/3434194.

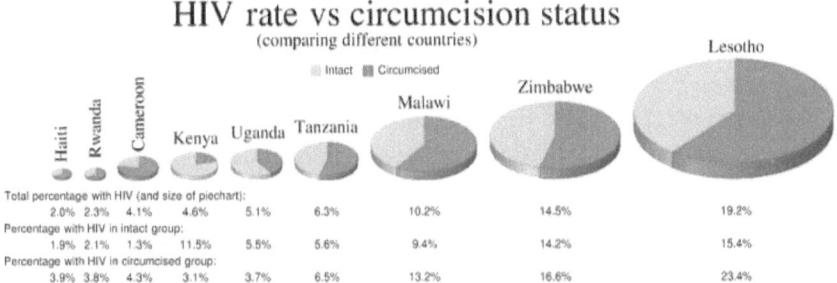

neither ethical nor feasible to isolate people and observe their every action. Following the surgery of circumcision, or being interviewed and left intact, patients are released to lead their own lives. Scientists cannot observe, much less control the behavior of their subjects. Upon follow-up the men are asked about their sexual contacts, frequency of sex, condom use, etc., but subjects may lie or fail to remember their specific actions. Also, some participants get lost to follow up. Therefore any study of human behavior is bound to be flawed. In the studies listed here, men who are sore and recovering from painful genital surgery are almost certainly going to abstain from sex or do it less frequently.

They may also be more likely to use condoms (due to their soreness.)

Part of the aim in the ongoing attempt to amputate as many African foreskins as possible is one of doctor control. Medical professionals are trained to be active in their approach to human health conditions. Therefore, their aim is to tackle any injury or illness with chemicals and/or surgery. (Of course in many situations these are the preferred treatments.) By cutting off foreskins a doctor is in control. Doctors cannot control (or get paid) for telling people to be responsible for themselves, be it telling them to bathe, eat healthfully, confine their sexual contacts to one healthy and faithful partner, or to use condoms.

Billions of dollars have been spent on the "Circumcise Africa" campaign. Africa is a country where millions of people lack the basic necessities of life which most of us in the western world take for granted. A significant portion of the African populations could have been supplied with food, safe drinking water, housing and access to education with the billions of dollars that have been spent to cut off foreskins. Since the supposed HIV preventative possibility offered by amputating foreskins is speculative at best, this is especially a tragic and wasteful use of these funds.

Finally, an important consideration for those who refer to the Bible as a source for endorsing circumcision (despite the many passages in the New Testament which clearly define its irrelevance and wrongness for Christians): Judaeo/Christian values include fidelity within marriage and clearly denounce all types of random, non-committal sexual behavior. Most STIs do result from sex with multiple partners, frequenting prostitutes, etc. Whatever spiritual significance may have been attached to circumcision by the ancient Hebrews, one can hardly interpret this as having been some "medical prescription" from God as a license for any rampant sexual risk taking.

15.5   Informational Resources

- Are circumcised men safer sex partners? Findings from the HAALSI cohort in rural South Africa:
  journals.plos.org/plosone/article?id=10.1371%2Fjournal.pone.0201445
- Circumcision doesn't and won't prevent HIV. This is why?:
  web.archive.org/web/20170521230951/newsghana.com.gh/circumcision-doesnt-and-wont-prevent-hiv-this-is-why
- More than foreskin: circumcision status, history of HIV/STI, and sexual risk in a clinic-based sample of men in Puerto Rico: pubmed.ncbi.nlm.nih.gov/22897699

16 Prostate Cancer

A tight, unretractable foreskin, associated with extremely poor hygiene, can in rare instances be an implicating factor in cancer of the penis. Does the presence of the foreskin have any similar effect on the prostate gland? This gland is located at the base of the penis and surrounds the neck of the bladder. Although it is nowhere near the foreskin, lack of circumcision has been suggested to be a factor in the development of prostate cancer.

While cancer of the penis is extremely rare, prostatic cancer is relatively common. It has been cited as the third leading cause of American male cancer deaths.[1]

In 1942 Ravich observed 840 cases of obstruction of the prostate, and found that among 768 Jewish patients, only 1.7% had prostate cancer, while among 75 non Jewish patients, 20% had cancer of the prostate. From this Ravich concluded that circumcision among the Jews was responsible for their low rate of this disease.[2]

In 1965 Apt observed that prostate cancer was the most common form of cancer among males in Sweden. Virtually none of the males in Sweden are circumcised. Apt noted that: "... The occurrence of prostatitis (which can develop into prostatic carcinoma) ... seems to be favoured by phimosis and balanitis." [3]

He compared the statistics for mortality of Sweden and Israel, and for Scandinavian Jews, and found that the cancer mortality for all types of cancer was roughly the same among Jews and non-Jews but the prostatic cancer mortality was considerably lower among Jews.[3]

Apt observed:

"The annual rate [of prostatic cancer] in Sweden is 414 [cases] per million males, in Israel 88. This suggests a very great difference between the two countries. But as prostatic cancer occurs typically within certain age groups, one must look at the relative age distribution ... Prostatic cancer is thus 4.7 times more frequent in Sweden than in Israel, but in the ages in which it is most common only 2.3 times." [3]

From this he inferred that universal circumcision in countries such as Sweden would greatly reduce that country's future rate of prostate cancer.

Other authorities have challenged and discounted such claims:

Preston interpreted Apt's statistics differently and challenged his findings. There are seven times as many men over age 60 in Sweden than in Israel. Since prostate

---
1 Wallerstein E. *Circumcision; An American Health Fallacy.* NY: Springer; 1980: 100. (His reference: American Cancer Society. *Cancer Facts and Figures.* 1978: 10.)
2 Ravich A. The Relationship of Circumcision to Cancer of the Prostate. *J Urol.* 1942; 48: 298-9.
3 Apt A. Circumcision and Prostatic Cancer. *Acta Med Scand.* 1965-04; 178: 493-504.

cancer rarely occurs in men younger than 60, one would expect that Sweden would have a rate of prostate cancer at least seven times greater than that of Israel. However prostatic cancer is only 4.7 more frequent in Sweden than in Israel. "Would this mean that non-circumcision protects against prostatic cancer?" [4]

Wallerstein challenges Apt's study by pointing out that he chose a country with an unusually high rate of prostatic cancer for his study:

"He selected Sweden – a country with one of the highest rates of prostatic cancer – as a basis for comparison with Israel, which was bound to bias the results. Had another noncircumcising country with a very low rate been chosen, completely opposite results would have been obtained." [5]

Wallerstein cites the statistics of the American Cancer Society in which the United States (with a high percentage of circumcised males), and Israel (with virtually all males circumcised), fall in the *middle* when the death rates per 100,000 population of various countries in 1972-1973 are listed. The Netherlands, Sweden, and Switzerland rank highest with rates of 22.9, 21.1, and 19.3 respectively. The males in these countries are intact. The United States has a rate of 14.4. Israel's rate is 7.5. However, El Salvador, Honduras, and Thailand, all countries which do not practice circumcision, report extremely low rates of 1.2, 0.8, and 0.2 respectively.[6]

Age is not accounted for in these figures. It may be that the countries with lower rates of prostatic cancer have fewer elderly men. However, it is still significant to note that the United States and Israel do not have unusually low rates of prostatic cancer despite their adoption of circumcision.

Heredity may be a factor in the lower rates of prostatic cancer among Jews compared to some other peoples.

Kaplan and O'Conor observed 886 patients with prostate hyperplasia (excessive growth of normal tissues). 184 of these showed carcinoma. 182 were Jewish, 16 of whom had carcinoma. 23.9% of the non-Jewish patients and 8.8% of the Jewish patients had carcinoma. *However,* 40.2% of the Gentile patients were circumcised, and 35.9% of the Gentiles with prostatic carcinoma were circumcised.

They state: "There seems to be a general agreement in the literature that the incidence of carcinoma of the prostate is lower in Jews than in Gentiles." [7]

---

4 Preston EN. Whither the Foreskin? A Consideration of Routine Neonatal Circumcision. JAMA. 1970-09-14; 213(11): 1853-8.
5 Wallerstein, p. 101
6 Ibid., p. 100. (His reference: American Cancer Society. *Cancer Facts and Figures 1978.* 1978: 15.)
7 Kaplan GW, O'Conor VJ Jr. The Incidence of Carcinoma of the Prostate in Jews and Gentiles. JAMA. 1966-05-30; 196(9): 803.

This appears to be independent of lack of foreskin, for according to their statistics, *among the non-Jewish patients there is no appreciable difference in the percentage of circumcised males who did and did not develop prostatic carcinoma.*

Kaplan and O'Conor add:

"Ravich postulated that a carcinogen present in smegma migrates up the urethra and is a factor in the development of carcinoma of the prostate. Since carcinoma usually arises in the posterior lobe of the prostate, this hypothesis seems untenable ... More likely [there is a] genetic predilection for the development of carcinoma of the prostate among Gentiles as compared to Jews ...

Despite other arguments mustered for or against the practice of circumcision, the relation of this operation to the subsequent development of prostatic carcinoma does not seem evident. If one supports circumcision as a routine procedure, the prevention of prostate cancer should not be used as a reason to countenance such action." [7]

Wallerstein points out that regional differences of the rates of prostatic cancer vary widely throughout different parts of the United States, Canada, and other parts of the world, irrespective of circumcision status.[8]

He also adds that according to the American Cancer Society, the incidence of prostatic cancer has increased in the United States "by more than 20% in the past 25 years" despite our country's increasing circumcision rate.[9]

The cause of prostatic cancer is not known. Many factors have been implicated. Sexually Transmitted Diseases may be a significant factor. According to Stagg: "One investigator found that 67 percent of his patients with cancer of the prostate had a prior history of venereal disease." [10]

The 1975 Ad Hoc Task Force of the American Academy of Pediatrics has concluded: "There is presently no convincing scientific evidence to substantiate the assertion that circumcision reduces the eventual incidence of cancer of the prostate." [11]

It appears that the lower incidence of prostate cancer among Jewish males is related to heredity, lifestyle, personal health and cleanliness. The presence or absence of the foreskin appears to have nothing to do with the development of this disease.

---

8   Wallerstein, p. 102. (His ref.: Franks LM. Etiology, Epidemiology and Pathology of Prostatic Cancer. In: *Proceedings of the National Conference on Urologic Cancer.* NY: American Cancer Society. 1973: 1092-5.)
9   Ibid., p. 102. (His reference: American Cancer Society. *Cancer Facts and Figures 1978.* 1978: 7.)
10 Stagg D. A Basis for Decision on Circumcision (ch. 63). In: *Compulsory Hospitalization or Freedom of Choice in Childbirth?* Transcripts of the 1978 NAPSAC Convention, vol. III. Stewart & Stewart; 1978: 833.
11 Thompson HC, King LR, Knox E, Korones SB. Ad Hoc Task Force on Circumcision – Report. *Pediatrics.* 1975-10; 56(4): 610-1.

16.1 Informational Resources

- A Conscientious Objector in the War on Cancer:
  medpagetoday.com/HematologyOncology/ProstateCancer/56091
- Circumcision and Prostate Cancer: circumstitions.com/cancer-pros.html
- Does circumcision prevent prostate cancer?: 15square.org.uk/does-circumcision-prevent-prostate-cancer-2/
- Prostate cancer *(see note about diet role)*: prostatecancerprevention.net/index.php?p=prostate-cancer
- Prostate cancer incidence statistics: cancerresearchuk.org/health-professional/cancer-statistics/statistics-by-cancer-type/prostate-cancer/incidence

17 Cervical Cancer

Does the foreskin, or smegma, cause or contribute to cancer of the female uterine cervix? Cancer of the cervix (the lower, rounded part of the uterus which opens into the vagina) is second in frequency only to breast cancer among cancers that affect women.

According to Wynder and his associates:

> "The uterine cervix is the second most frequent site of cancer in American women, accounting for approximately 10% of all newly diagnosed cases and for about the same percentage of total cancer deaths. In different American cities, its annual incidence varies from 30 to 60 per 100,000 females. The incidence rates are about the same in Western Europe. Scattered reports from Asia suggest that in these countries the uterine cervix is the most important site and may account for 40 or more percent of all newly diagnosed cases of cancer. Cancer of the cervix is infrequent among Jewish and Moslem women." [1]

The presence or absence of the foreskin of a woman's sexual partner has been one of *many* factors suggested as a variable in cancer of the cervix. The fact that the rates of this disease occur with approximately the same frequency in Europe (with a largely intact male population) as in the United States (with a largely circumcised male population) suggests that circumcision has little or no effect on the incidence of cervical cancer. However, because Jewish and Moslem women have relatively low rates of this disease, and because both of these peoples practice male circumcision, some authorities have concluded that the circumcision of Jewish and Moslem males is responsible for their women's relative immunity to this disease.

Unfortunately, observations such as this often reach lay people in garbled bits and pieces. As a result, some women believe that "You can get cancer of the cervix if you have sex with a man who is not circumcised!" They have the idea that one could have sex once with an intact male and a few days later show up at a doctor's office with an active case of cervical cancer – in a manner similar to catching a sexually transmitted infection. I know of one man who had himself circumcised shortly before getting married out of fear that he would give cervical cancer to his wife.

Should all males sacrifice their foreskins to protect womankind from cancer of the cervix? Numerous studies must be analyzed carefully before an answer can be reached.

---

[1] Wynder EL, Cornfield J, Schroff PD, Doraiswami KR. A Study of Environmental Factors in Carcinoma of the Cervix. *AJOG.* 1954-10; 68(4): 1016.

17.1 Factors Related to Cancer of the Cervix

A large number of variables have been mentioned in the literature as possible contributory factors to cervical cancer. Although in this review, each of these will be discussed separately, it can be seen that a cluster of interrelated variables tend to be associated with the disease. For example, cervical cancer has been purported to be related to non-use of contraceptives. It has also been suggested that the disease is related to repeated childbearing. Obviously lack of contraceptive use and frequent childbearing are also interrelated. Similarly, cancer of the cervix appears more frequently in patients with a history of sexually transmitted infection. It also appears to be associated with frequent intercourse and numerous sexual partners. However, sexually transmitted infection and frequent intercourse with numerous sexual partners also tend to be interrelated.

While many factors appear with significantly greater frequency among cervical cancer patients than they do among other women with similar backgrounds, but without the disease, thus suggesting a causal relationship, it is interesting to note that *there is no factor that is invariably present in all cases of cervical cancer.* For example, although cervical cancer occurs more frequently among women who have had numerous sexual partners, it does occur in women who have had only one sexual partner and even in virgins.

17.1.1 Ethnicity

In the United States, Black women have a significantly higher incidence of cervical cancer than do *white* women. The incidence ranges from 28 to 59 cases per 100,000 among *white* women and 54 to 73 cases per 100,000 among Black women, throughout various American cities.[2]

Heins, et al. report a study of 1,000 Pap smears of 98% Black women, 3.1% of whom had cervical carcinoma, among clinical patients, compared to a rate of 0.9% cervical cancer cases among 1,000 Pap smears of primarily *white* private patients.[3]

Terris, Wilson, & Nelson studied 1,148 cases of cervical cancer in various stages. 454 of these women had invasive carcinoma of the cervix (spreading to other healthy tissue). 411 had carcinoma in situ (cancer confined to one area). 283 patients had cervical dysplasia (abnormal, precancerous changes in the tissue). 65% of the patients with invasive carcinoma, 72% of those with carcinoma in situ, and 82% of those with dysplasia were Black. Puerto Ricans accounted for 15% of the patients with invasive

---

[2] Ibid., p. 1017.
[3] Heins HC Jr, Dennis EJ, Pratt-Thomas HR. The Possible Role of Smegma in Carcinoma of the Cervix. *AJOG.* 1958-10; 76(4): 726-7.

carcinoma, 19% of those with carcinoma in situ, and 12% of those with dysplasia. 18% of those with invasive carcinoma, 9% of those with carcinoma in situ, and 12% of those with dysplasia were *white*.[4] The authors do not state, however, the normal distribution of these three racial/ethnic groups in the population group from which these patients came.

The question arises as to whether a genetic factor among Black people, Puerto Ricans, or other minority groups predisposes them to a greater frequency of the disease, or whether cultural factors such as early marriage, frequent childbearing, hygiene, or sexually transmitted infection are related.

Similarly, cultural factors may be involved irrespective of Jewish women's husbands' circumcision status.

17.1.2 Socioeconomic Status

Apt mentions: "In England the incidence of cervical carcinoma among doctor's wives, lawyer's wives, and clergymen's wives is barely one fifth that in the remainder of the population." [5]

The significant variables are not the husband's occupation or income level per se, but other factors which are interrelated with socioeconomic status.

Wynder, et al. mention studies which link low economic status with other factors such as: "Poor obstetrical care and postpartum care, improper housing and poor nutrition ... neglect of symptoms of the lacerated and ulcerated cervix ... [which] account for the greater frequency of cervical cancer among the poorer classes." [6]

Elsewhere in the article, the same authors suggest: "The social-class difference derives from the difficulty that men in unavoidably dirty occupations have in keeping clean, and from the different patterns of intercourse and marriage in the less favored classes." [6]

17.1.3 Personal Hygiene

Personal cleanliness, on the part of both men and women, appears to be a crucial factor in the development of cervical cancer.

Wynder, Mantel, and Licklider (who advocate neonatal circumcision as a supposed cancer preventative), claim that they have found a relationship between lack of circumcision *and* poor penile hygiene in connection with the development of cancer of the cervix. They concede that:

---
4 Terris M, Wilson F, Nelson JH Jr. Relation of Circumcision to Cancer of the Cervix. *AJOG*. 1973-12-15; 117(8): 1056-66.
5 Apt A. Circumcision and Prostatic Cancer. *Acta Med Scand*. 1965; 178: 496.
6 Wynder, Cornfield, et al, p. 1024-52.

"... only one of three retrospective studies in the U.S. has obtained results suggestive of a positive association between cervical cancer and circumcision status ... it is clear that the [supposed] protective effect of circumcision would be less pronounced in the U.S than in many other countries. The higher level of personal hygiene would tend to provide many of the [supposed] protective benefits otherwise afforded by circumcision." [7]

Heins, et al. mention poor vaginal hygiene among their previously mentioned clinic patients who had a significantly higher rate of cervical cancer than the private patients.[3]

Rates of cervical cancer have been observed among three different groups of people in Macedonia, Yugoslavia. These are Eastern Orthodox Christians (who do not practice circumcision), and two Moslem groups – Shqyptars and Turks (both of which practice circumcision). While the Christian group had the highest rate of cervical cancer, the Turks had higher rates of the disease than the Shqyptars although both groups were circumcised. The author cites major differences in social life, sexual practices, and hygienic practices as accounting for the differences. The Shqyptars practiced a much stricter lifestyle, including shaving of the genital region and regular washing after intercourse.[8]

17.1.4   Age of First Coitus

Many studies mention that early marriage, or more specifically intercourse before the age of 20 years, is associated with increased risk of cervical cancer.

In Terris and Oalmann's study they found that 53% of the patients with cervical cancer and 26% of the controls had experienced their first coitus before age 17. 39% of those who were diagnosed after age 50 had their first coitus before age 17.[9]

Rotkin conducted an in-depth study of adolescent coitus in relation to cervical cancer. He poses the following:

"Speculation suggests a male contribution that becomes established in adolescent girls because they are then most susceptive. This agent may be a substance, organism or particle not related to the ejaculate, perhaps borne on the unsanitary male

---

[7] Wynder EL, Mantel N, Licklider SD. Statistical Considerations on Circumcision and Cervical Cancer. *AJOG.* 1960-05; 79(5): 1027-9.
[8] Damjanovski L, Marcekic V, Miletic M. Circumcision and Carcinoma Colli Uteri in Macedonia, Yugoslavia – Results from a Field Study. *Br J Cancer.* 1963; 17: 406-9.
[9] Terris M, Oalmann M. Carcinoma of the Cervix; An Epidemiologic Study. *JAMA.* 1960-12-03; 174(14): 1848-9.

organ or contraceptive, and remaining dormant during the mean latent period of 30 years before developing into carcinoma ..." [10]

(In other words, a girl could have her first coitus at age 13 and ultimately get cervical cancer at age 43.)

Rotkin notes that adolescent coitus tends to be interrelated with other factors. He quotes Jones' suggestion:

> "... [The] importance of the socioeconomic complex of relative poverty (at least in early life) with rapid maturation sexually and a haste to begin early, and early to terminate, the reproductive phase of biologic destiny – marriage, intercourse, first and last pregnancies, separation, divorce – all of these events occur significantly earlier in the life of the woman destined to develop cervical carcinoma than the woman without this disease ..." [10]

(Rotkin's studies and observations were published in 1962. In the years since, social mores have changed and more middle class teenagers are having intercourse. Adolescent coitus today is certainly not confined to the lower socioeconomic groups. Some authorities have noted that the rates of cervical cancer in the United States are increasing, and will continue to increase, possibly because of this.)

Rotkin conducted a study involving interviews and questionnaires, with the following results: 9 patients and 8 controls experienced first coitus before age 15. 32 patients and 20 controls experienced first coitus between ages 15 and 17. 33 patients and 27 controls experienced first coitus between ages 18 and 20. 15 patients and 24 controls experienced first coitus between ages 21 and 23. 9 patients and 9 controls experienced first coitus between ages 24 and 26. 1 patient and 8 controls experienced first coitus after age 26. 1 patient and 4 controls had never experienced coitus.

Rotkin speculates that hormonal factors based on the rapid maturation, body changes, and emotional stresses of adolescence may somehow predispose the cervical tissue to eventual carcinoma if coitus is begun at this time.[10]

17.1.5 Marriage

Cancer of the cervix is more prevalent in women who are or have been married than it is in women who have never married. However, factors other than simply being married are involved.

---

10 Rotkin ID. Relation of Adolescent Coitus to Cervical Cancer Risk. *JAMA*. 1962-02-17; 179(7): 486-9.

Stern and Neely investigated a number of possible variables associated with cervical cancer and found the number of "marital events", i.e., marriages, divorces, widowhoods, and remarriages, to be the most significant factor in their study.[11]

Terris and Oalmann compared 122 patients with cervical carcinoma with 122 matched (by ethnicity and age) controls and found that 47% of the patients and 16% of the controls had been married more than once. 1 patient and 5 controls had never married. 34% of the patients and 14% of the controls were married before age 17.[9]

The woman's age at the time of her first marriage has been mentioned as a factor in cervical carcinoma. This usually interrelates with her age at the time of first coitus.

17.1.6 Childbearing

Studies have revealed conflicting results over whether or not pregnancy or childbearing have any effect on eventual cervical cancer. It is not certain whether the disease is associated with early or repeated pregnancies, or method of delivery.

An article in the CMA Journal states that: "... the risk of cervical cancer is twice as high in married infertile women as in single women ..." [12]

Therefore, sexual intercourse, rather than childbearing alone appears more likely to be the important factor.

Wynder and his associates quote Hofbauer who speculates that: "... excessive ovarian stimulation in multiparous women might be of etiologic significance." [13]

Towne noted that cervical carcinoma is approximately eight times more frequent in parous (having given birth) women than in non-parous women. She poses that pregnancy and labor with their attendant cervical trauma bear a causal relationship to cervical carcinoma. Towne reviewed the date collected between 1933 and 1953 and noted that among 574 patients with cervical cancer, 83.4% had borne children.[14]

The obvious discrepancy in her findings, however, is that she failed to account for age. Cervical cancer is most common in women past childbearing age. It occurs most frequently in women in their 40s and 50s. The older a woman is, the greater is the likelihood that she has ever been pregnant or borne a child. An age-controlled study would yield more conclusive results.

It is plausible that damage to the cervix during birth, especially from forceps, other obstetrical interventions, or precipitous delivery, especially if the damage was never repaired, could contribute to cervical cancer. A more detailed study investigating types of birth complications involving cervical damage would shed further

---

11 Stern E, Neely PM. Cancer of the Cervix in Reference to Circumcision and Marital History. *J Am Med Womens Assoc.* 1962-09; 17(9): 739-40.
12 Cleanliness, Continence, Constancy, and Cervical Carcinoma. *CMAJ.* 1964-05-09; 90: 1132.
13 Wynder, Cornfield, et al, pp. 1019-20.
14 Towne JE. Carcinoma of the Cervix in Nulliparous and Celibate Women. *AJOG.* 1955-03;69(3):606-613.

light on the subject. Would women who have given birth only by Caesarian delivery be less susceptible to cervical cancer than women who have given birth vaginally? Is there a relationship between cervical cancer and induced abortion which forces the cervix open prematurely?

Wynder, Cornfield, et al. conducted an extensive, detailed study of cervical cancer. Their findings in regards to the correlation between pregnancies and cervical cancer revealed that among the *white* women in their study, 9% of the patients with cervical cancer and 12% of the controls had never been pregnant. Among Black women, 11% of the patients and 17% of the controls had never been pregnant. However, they found that the event of pregnancy and early marriage were strongly associated.[6]

The age of a woman's first pregnancy may be a factor in eventual cancer of the cervix. More likely, the significant factor is the age of first coitus, the pregnancy simply being the outcome of the coitus.

17.1.7 Use of Contraceptives

Different authors have posed the possibility that cervical cancer may be related to non-use of contraceptives. Some have speculated that use of obstructive type contraceptives such as condoms and diaphragms could decrease a woman's susceptibility to the disease.

In Terris and Oalmann's study of 122 cervical cancer patients and 122 matched controls the authors noted that: "... few of the women had ever used contraceptives, but the proportion doing so was significantly lower in the patients than in controls." [9]

In Aitken-Swan and Baird's study, they found that 13% of the patients and 43% of the controls had used a sheath (condom) or cap (diaphragm) type of contraceptive.[15]

Wynder, Cornfield, and associates found no significant differences between their cervical cancer and control groups in regards to contraceptive practice.[6]

If smegma were an implicating factor in cervical carcinoma, use of obstructive contraceptives would presumably result in lower rates of cervical cancer since they would prevent smegma from reaching the cervix. However, the findings on contraceptive use fail to support this. Non-use of contraceptives would also, for most women, be related to numerous pregnancies, thus tying this in with the possible correlation between repeated childbearing and cervical cancer. A study relating use of different types of contraceptives, investigating rates of cervical cancer among those using non-obstructive contraceptives such as birth control pills, would shed further light on the subject.

---

15 Aitken-Swan J, Baird D. Circumcision and Cancer of the Cervix. *Br J Cancer.* 1965-06;19(2):217-227.

17.1.8 Sperm Contact

Sandler mentions studies that have suggested that sperm may contribute to factors in the development of cervical carcinoma. He cites: "Dr. Reid and colleagues correlate the protein chemistry of sperm with the socioeconomic status as an important etiological factor in carcinoma of the cervix uteri." [16]

If sperm were indeed an implicating factor in cervical carcinoma, it would follow that use of obstructive contraceptives would protect the cervix from sperm contact therefore diminishing one's susceptibility to this disease. Aitken-Swan and Baird acknowledge this possibility in their study. They suggest:

> "This method (obstructive contraceptives), like circumcision, would protect the cervix from contact with smegma. Unlike circumcision, it would also prevent contact with spermatozoa, if epithelial penetration by spermatozoa could initiate the process leading to cancer." [15]

However, since other studies have found no differences between patients and controls in regards to contraceptive use, and since cervical cancer has been noted in women who regularly use obstructive contraceptives and even in women who have never experienced coitus, it is questionable whether either smegma contact or sperm contact are implicating factors. Since sperm contact unquestionably leads to pregnancy, it may be that repeated pregnancies are the significant factor in cervical cancer. However, data on the relationship between cervical cancer and childbearing are also inconclusive. It may simply be that non-use of contraceptives is related to a number of other factors associated with lower socioeconomic status, poorer hygiene and general health.

17.1.9 Diet

Some authors have suggested that differences in diet may cause some women to be more predisposed to cervical cancer than others. It is plausible that nutritional deficiencies may contribute to the development of this disease.

Wynder and associates cite Khanolkar's theory that: "... women in the lower income groups with resulting inadequacy of diets might develop liver dysfunction and subsequently might have a higher hormonal blood level because the damaged liver is unable to detoxify the estrogens."

They add:

---

16 Sandler B. Sperm Basic Proteins in Cervical Carcinogenesis. *Lancet.* 1978-07-22.

"Khanolkar feels that cancer of the cervix is most common in Hindu women who have a badly balanced and deficient diet, especially during the childbearing stage ... Horwitz considers ritual dietary laws among Orthodox Jewish women to be of possible etiological significance. Ayre proposes that deficiencies of thiamine and riboflavin might lead to a greater susceptibility of cervical tissues to cancer formation." [13]

Clearly further investigation is needed in this area before a conclusion can be reached.

17.1.10 Coal Tar Douches

It seems incredible that women would douche with coal-tar based products such as Lysol. However, this has been a practice among some groups. Some authors have suggested that this practice may be a factor in cancer of the cervix. However, studies have failed to find a correlation.

Wynder and associates state: "Lombard and Potter suggest that this may be of etiological significance. Smith notes no significant difference in the type of douches used by Italians and Jews in his study." [13]

Terris and Oalmann found no differences between patients and controls in the duration and frequency of douching.[9]

Similarly, Wynder, Cornfield, et al. found no differences between patients and controls in the type or frequency of douching.[6]

17.1.11 Nidah – Jewish Ritual Abstinence Following Menstruation

Traditionally Jewish women have observed a practice called "Nidah." This involves ritual abstinence from intercourse during menstruation and for several days thereafter, followed by a ritual "Mikvah" bath. Some have suggested that this practice may be responsible for Jewish women's lower rates of cervical cancer. However, Heins, et al. mention that the possibility is unlikely since today only about 5% of Jewish women observe the laws of Nidah.[3]

Wynder and associates quote Kennaway who mentions the possible correlation between ritual abstinence and relative immunity to cervical cancer. They add that Parsis (a group in India) who have a relatively low frequency of cervical cancer also have a period of abstinence after menses. Weiner suggests that the apparent greater frequency of cervical cancer in Jewish women today, as compared to the beginning of this century, might possibly be explained by a greater laxity of Jewish women in following the law of abstinence." [17]

17.1.12 Menstrual Disorders

Menstrual difficulties, as well as age of onset of menstruation have been suggested as possible factors in cervical cancer.

Wynder, Cornfield and associates found no differences between patients and controls in regards to the age of the onset of menses, the length of menstrual flow, or abstinence during or after menstruation.[6]

Other reports mention menstrual factors briefly, but apparently little has been studied about this.

17.1.13 Sexually Transmitted Disease

Higher rates of sexually transmitted disease appear to be associated with cervical cancer. It is not clear whether STD is a direct cause of cervical cancer, or if the two simply tend to appear together and are interrelated to other causal factors such as frequency of intercourse and number of sexual partners.

In 1942 Levin, Kress, and Goldstein noted that:

> "… it appears that in women with cancer of the uterine cervix, syphilis is found approximately three times as frequently as in women with cancer of the other sites … Out of 930 patients with cervical cancer, 36, 3.9% had syphilis. Out of 3,680 female patients with other types of cancer, 41, 1.1% had syphilis. In a previous study, Belote, in 1931, found a percentage of 15.1% syphilis out of 232 patients with cervical cancer, and 3.8% syphilis among 393 females with other types of cancer, yielding a ratio of 4 to 1." [18]

In Terris and Oalmann's study, comparing 122 cervical cancer patients with an equal number of controls, 13 patients and only 6 controls had positive tests for syphilis.[10]

In Wynder, Cornfield, and associates' study, they found twice as many syphilitic patients among women with cervical cancer as in controls among the non-Jewish *white* group. No difference was found, however, between the Black patients and controls. They comment:

---

17 Wynder, Cornfield, et al, p. 1018-9.
18 Levin ML, Kress LC, Goldstein H. Syphilis and Cancer. *NY State J Med.* 1942-09-15: 42, 46.

"Of interest, however, is the fact that those reporting a past history of syphilis also reported, as one might expect, earlier age at first coitus. These could operate together, or be related to more frequent coitus among this group." [6]

In the same study the authors found no differences between patients and controls in regards to history of gonorrhea.[6]

One study suggests that Herpes Type 2 appears to be more prevalent in the history of women with cervical cancer. Taylor and Rodin state that antibodies to HSV Type 2 have been found more frequently in patients with cervical atypia and carcinoma than in controls.[19]

Use of obstructive contraceptives has been listed as a possible preventive factor in decreasing one's susceptibility to cervical cancer. Obstructive contraceptives also help prevent sexually transmitted infections. Therefore, these two factors may interrelate.

17.1.14 Chronic Cervicitis and Lacerations to the Tissues

Cervical cancer appears to be preceded, in most cases for many years, by irritation or damage to the tissues.

Rieser quotes Besseson who states: "Cancer of the cervix is rarely seen without chronic endocervicitis, unhealed lacerations, erosions, scarring or chronic infections of types undetermined." [20]

Wynder and associates mention Gagnon's suggestion: "The eradication of cervicitis equals the suppression of cancer of the cervix." [13]

They also add: "Lombard and Potter found a rate of 26% of unrepaired lacerations (presumably from childbirth or abortion) among patients with cancer of the cervix and 13.2% among matched controls." [13]

This obviously interrelates with other factors such as childbearing, obstetrical help, type of delivery, sexually transmitted infections, and personal hygiene.

17.1.15 Vaginal Discharge

Wynder and associates mention: "Hausdorff suggests vaginal discharge as a causative factor in the production of cervical cancer." [13]

More plausibly it would seem that the vaginal discharge is related to sexually transmitted infection or cervicitis, or may be a result of cervical cancer itself.

---

19 Taylor PK, Rodin P. Herpes Genitalis and Circumcision. *Br J Ven Dis*. 1975; 51: 274.
20 Rieser C. Circumcision and Cancer. *SMJ*. 1961-10; 54: 1133-4.

17.1.16 Hormones

Some have speculated that hormonal factors may have an effect on whether or not women develop cervical cancer.

Wynder and associates quote Clemmesen's suggestion of a "special hormonal status in these [Jewish] women," that may be responsible for this group's relative immunity to the disease." [17]

Elsewhere the same authors mention:

"... Ayre believes estrogen to be a growth-stimulating factor to cervical cancer. 90% of 50 patients with cervical cancer had evidence of excessive tissue estrogens on the basis of vaginal and cervical cornification ... Niebergs advances the contrasting idea that low estrogen levels might be of etiologic significance. Lombard and Potter propose that hormonal factors may account for earlier marriage and high divorce rates among patients with cervical cancer." [!][13]

Hormonal levels would in turn be interrelated with diet, pregnancy, and sexual stimulation.

17.1.17 Number of Sexual Partners

A most significant factor in cervical cancer relates to lifestyle, number of marriages, and number of sexual partners. Women who have had many sexual partners throughout their lifetimes appear to be more likely to develop cervical cancer. This is *not* to say that *every* woman who develops cervical cancer has had a number of sexual partners. However, the *likelihood* of developing the disease is greater among women who have had numerous sexual partners.

Wynder and associates note that prostitutes are four times as numerous among women with cancer of the cervix as are other women of comparable socioeconomic groups. Conversely, there is a very low incidence of cervical cancer among nuns.[17]

Wynder, Cornfield, and associates found that:

"There is a consistently larger proportion of women who have been married two or more times in the cervical cancer group. 29% of the white, non-Jewish patients, and 12% of the controls had been married twice or more. Among blacks, 35% of the cancer patients and 22% of the controls had been married more than once." [6]

The same authors found significantly low rates of cervical cancer among women who had had intercourse only with their husbands who also happened to be circumcised: "Among the white, non-Jewish groups, 3% of the patients and 9% of the controls had intercourse with only their circumcised husbands. For the blacks, the rates were 0% and 9% respectively." [6]

They note, however, that 10% of the *white* and 20% of the Black subjects were unable to report on the circumcision status of their partners.[6]

Data about any woman's number of sexual partners is understandably difficult to obtain. She may not wish to disclose this information, and there is no way of verifying what she reports. Therefore, studies about this facet of the cervical cancer question have been limited.

It may be, however, that marital fidelity is a crucial variable in the development of this disease. Certain peoples who have practiced male circumcision, such as the Jews, have *also* practiced a more conservative lifestyle in which marital fidelity is especially important.

Information about the cervical cancer rates among women who have had intercourse only with their *intact* husbands would help to answer the question. (Such data was not reported in Wynder, Cornfield, and associates' study.)

Jeffrey R. Wood has posed the possibility that the absence of foreskin with resultant difficulty in sexual penetration and accompanying frustration leads to considerable sexual dissatisfaction. This would mean less satisfactory relationships. Consequently people would seek more sexual partners. *If* the above is indeed true, and *if* having numerous sexual partners does relate to cervical cancer, then *theoretically* circumcision could be a *causative* factor in cancer of the cervix.[21]

17.1.18 Circumcision Status of Sexual Partner

Because Jewish and Moslem women have relatively low rates of cervical cancer, and Jewish and Moslem males are circumcised, it has been hypothesized that the presence of the foreskin is a factor which can contribute to cancer of the cervix.

Most of the studies that have investigated this possibility have found that when Jewish women are omitted from the group under investigation, circumcision is no longer a significant factor. Among American non-Jewish women, there appear to be no differences in the rates of cervical cancer between those married to circumcised husbands and those married to intact husbands.[22]

---

21 Wood JR, (personal correspondence).
22 Dunn JE Jr, Buell P. Association of Cervical Cancer with Circumcision of Sexual Partner. *JNCI*. 1959-04; 22(4): 751-2.

During the years 1951-1955, Dunn and Buell interviewed 429 patients with cervical cancer. The same number of controls were selected by matching age, ethnicity, ever married, and ever parous (having given birth). Five Jewish patients and 21 Jewish controls were omitted from the study.

Among the 334 cervix cases, 114 had circumcised husbands. Among the 364 controls, 126 had circumcised husbands. 220 patients and 238 controls had intact husbands.

Interestingly, instead of simply concluding that circumcision of the husband obviously has no effect upon cervical cancer, they attempt the hypothesis that intermittent exposure to other uncircumcised partners not accounted for in the study (which Jewish women supposedly would be less likely to encounter), or the remaining fragment of foreskin left by medical circumcision (which is sometimes less "complete" than Jewish circumcision) may be the culprits. (Some authors have even hypothesized that the higher rates of cervical cancer among American Jewish women, compared to those in Israel, are caused by extra-marital affairs with intact American men.) The foreskin or smegma would have to be *extremely* carcinogenic to cause cervical cancer by brief extramarital contacts, or from a small fragment of foreskin!

In 1961 Stern and Dixon published a report comparing 403 women with atypical hyperplasia (excessive growth of normal cells) and pre- and invasive cancer of the cervix, with 4,738 controls. Age of first marriage, present marital status, number of marriages, divorces, widowhoods (termed "marital events"), religious affiliation, circumcision of husband, and contraception, were the variables studied. They found "marital events" and "Jewish" to be of primary importance. As in Dunn and Buell's study, they found that omission of Jewish women from the study had an appreciable effect on the relationship of the other variables to the cancer status. In particular, the status of circumcision as a predictor of cancer remains of secondary importance.[23]

In Terris and Oalmann's study of matched groups of cervical cancer patients and controls, the husbands of 44% of the patients were intact as were 25% of the controls. *However,* in *one-half* of the patients and controls the circumcision status was unknown.[9]

In a study by Terris, Wilson, and Nelson, involving more subjects, *no significant differences* were found: Among the patients with invasive carcinoma and their matched controls (89 of each) 18.7% of the patients and 19.6% of the controls had intact husbands.

---

23 Stern E, Dixon WJ. Cancer of the Cervix – A Biometric Approach to Etiology. *Cancer.* 1961/Jan-Feb; 14(1): 154, 158-160.

Among those with carcinoma in situ and their controls (133 of each) 18.0% of the patients and 22.4% of the controls had circumcised husbands, and 41.6% of the patients and 39.2% of the controls had intact husbands.

Among those with dysplasia and their controls, (74 of each) 20.8% of the patients and 21.6% of the controls had circumcised husbands, and 39.9% of the patients and 35.5% of the controls had intact husbands.[4]

Aitken-Swan and Baird's study suggests that perhaps use of an obstructive contraceptive *combined with* the husband being circumcised may be a factor in preventing cervical cancer. However, only a small number of subjects were involved. Most other studies have revealed no relationship between cervical cancer and either of these factors. Socioeconomic factors may simply be related to contraceptive use, circumcision, *and* cervical cancer.

Among the couples in which the husband was circumcised *and* a sheath or cap was used, there were no cancer patients and 7 controls. Among those in which the husband was circumcised and no sheath or cap used, there were 12 patients and 7 controls. Of those in which the husband was not circumcised, and a sheath or cap was used, there were 6 patients and 13 controls. Of those in which the husband was not circumcised and no sheath or cap was used, there were 26 patients and 15 controls.[15]

It appears from these findings that if either of these factors is valid, then use of an obstructive contraceptive seems to be a more important protective factor than lack of foreskin. Among the group in which the husband was intact and an obstructive contraceptive was used, there were more than twice as many controls as patients.

Interestingly, Aitken-Swan and Baird cite the rates of 2.2 cases of cervical cancer per 100,000 among Jewish women in Israel; 17 per 100,000 among women in Sweden, and 44 per 100,000 among American women. The second and third statistics are especially worth noting for Sweden has a nearly exclusively intact male population and yet a lower rate of cervical cancer than does the United States which has a largely circumcised male population.[15]

Similarly, the World Health Organization reports statistics on the mortality rates from cancer of the cervix during the years 1958 to 1967. Among every 1,000,000 females, the percentage of deaths from cervical cancer was 7.3 to 9.8 in the United States; 6.2 to 6.9 in the Netherlands; 6.0 to 7.3 in Finland; and 6.5 to 8.3 in Sweden. Obviously the death rates from this disease are higher in our country with its largely circumcised male population, than they are in the Netherlands, Finland, or Sweden, all of which have a primarily intact male population.[24]

The low rates of cervical cancer among Jewish women may be determined by lifestyle, sexual practices, personal hygiene, or genetic factors, instead of circum-

---
24 World Health Statistics Annual World Health Organization, Geneva.

cision. The higher rates of cervical cancer among American Jewish women compared to Israeli Jewish women may be due to more intermarrying and conversion to Judaism of different types of peoples among the American Jewish population, thusly affecting their genetic makeup.

17.2   Controlled Experiments with Smegma

A number of experiments have been conducted with laboratory animals in an attempt to investigate the alleged carcinogenicity of smegma. Some of these have already been discussed in the chapter on penile cancer. Four other such studies, most of which have involved the direct application of smegma to the cervixes of mice, are discussed here.

Fishman, Shear, Friedman, and Stewart injected human smegma subcutaneously into 12 mice. There was abscess formation and ulceration at the sites of injections, but no tumors grew.

Smegma was applied intravaginally in 20 mice repeatedly over 15 to 17 months. A trauma control group of mice was regularly penetrated with a metal plunger with no substance applied. No tumors were found in either group.

20 other mice had smegma applied intravaginally with a plunger into the cervix, 203 times weekly for 12 months, receiving between 72 and 140 applications. Postmortem examinations revealed no tumors.

As a control, 10 mice had benzapyrene (a known carcinogen) applied to the cervix and vaginal canal, 2-3 times weekly. By the end of 14 months all 10 mice had cancerous tumors.[25]

Pratt-Thomas and associates injected whole human smegma into the vaginas of mice by various methods. Ovarian dermoid cyst contents were used as a control. Other mice were treated with methylcholanthrene in lard and in coconut oil, and insertion of speculum without substance applied.

Out of 12 of 15 mice that were given biweekly vaginal injections of smegma, 4 had overt invasive carcinomas, 1 had an early carcinoma, another had a "possible" carcinoma, and 6 had marked epithelial hyperplasia.

Of the mice receiving weekly vaginal injections of smegma, 11 out of 26 had marked hyperplasia, but none had definite invasive malignant tumors.

Of 21 mice that were injected with a vaginal ligation (smegma was injected and a suture was made to keep it in), 1 had a carcinoma, 1 had a questionable malignant papilloma, and 2 had sarcomas (cancer arising from underlying tissue).

---

25   Fishman M, Shear MJ, Friedman HF, Stewart HL. Studies in Carcinogenesis. XVII. Local Effect of Repeated Application of 3,4-Benzpyrene and of Human Smegma to the Vagina and Cervix of Mice. *JNCI.* 1942-02: 361-367.

Of 10 mice given estrogen injections with smegma (in an attempt to investigate a relationship between cervical cancer and hormones) 1 carcinoma developed.

Among the mice given estrogen injection, vaginal ligation and smegma, no neoplastic changes were found. Nor were any changes found among the mice given a simple vaginal ligation.

Among the mice injected with *sterile* smegma (autoclaved to kill bacteria) and vaginal ligation, no neoplastic changes or hyperplasia were found. (This suggests that the *bacteria*, not smegma itself, may be what stimulates tumors – at least for this particular group of mice. If this is so, it follows that personal hygiene, not the mere presence or absence of one's foreskin, would be the significant factor in preventing cervical cancer.)

Methylcholanthrene, a known carcinogen, was inserted in 26 mice. This produced marked to profound hyperplasia in 16 mice and moderate in 5. One had an active papilloma and one had a squamous cell carcinoma.

Insertion of dermoid cyst material with a vaginal ligation produced 2 squamous cell carcinomas, one papilloma, and one marked hyperplasia.[26]

All scientists who work with laboratory animals know that some genetic strains of animals are more prone to tumors than are others. Since a considerably larger number of tumors grew among Pratt-Thomas and associates' mice than did among the mice involved in Fishman and associates' study, Pratt-Thomas' group may have had a selection of mice that were more tumor and cancer prone than others. It should also be remembered that lab animals are often given proportionately huge doses of whatever substance is involved in the test. An injection of smegma in a tiny mouse vagina is probably the equivalent of a cup full of smegma in a human vagina.

Heins and associates applied whole raw human smegma to the cervixes and upper vaginas of mice. Female genital tract bacteria and ovarian dermoid cyst contents were applied to control mice.

In one of their studies, 50 mice were repeatedly injected with smegma. 25 of these survived the study. Of these there was no change in 7, mild to marked hyperplasia in 17, and one cancer of the cervix. This tumor developed in a mouse that received 118 injections of smegma over 13.75 months.

In several other types of smegma application experiments conducted by the same authors, no tumors grew.[27]

Reddy and Baruah inserted fresh human smegma into the vaginas of 16 female mice. 19 male mice had human smegma applied to the penis beneath the prepuce. This was done to both groups 3 times a week for 16 months. At the end of this period

---

26 Pratt-Thomas HR, Heins HC, Latham E, Dennis EJ, McIver FA. The Carcinogenic Effect of Human Smegma: An Experimental Study. *Cancer.* 1956/Jul-Aug; 9(4): 671-80.
27 Heins, et al, pp. 726-32.

4 male mice and 6 female mice were still alive. Some had died from infection of the genital tract.

Of their small experiment, no macroscopic growths were observed. Some had hyperplasia and infections, but no abnormal or metastatic growth appeared.[28]

Laboratory experiments with animals are conducted under extremely abnormal conditions. It is highly doubtful that female mice living under *normal* conditions, having intercourse with uncircumcised male mice, with exposure to the smegma produced from a mouse penis, will develop cervical cancer.

17.3 Conclusions

Cancer of the cervix is associated with a number of related factors, none of which have been proven to be a cause of the disease. No one factor is universally present in all cases of cervical carcinoma. Many of these factors tend to be based on socio-economic conditions relating to poverty, poor personal hygiene and general health, multiple sex partners, and beginning sexual relations at an early age.

When Jewish women are omitted from study groups, it is clear that there are no differences in the rates of cervical cancer between women married to circumcised husbands and those married to intact husbands.

Laboratory experiments with smegma applied to the cervixes of mice show questionable and inconclusive results in regards to the carcinogenicity of this substance.

Most studies involving the effect of obstructive contraceptives on cervical cancer rates show no differences in the rates of this disease among users and non-users of the devices, yet these would protect the cervix from smegma contact.

If smegma were to be proven to be carcinogenic, certainly regular washing of the genitals would be effective in eliminating the problem. The same "washing versus surgery" argument that has been posed regarding other supposed "health benefits" of circumcision applies here.

For the present, the most effective means of controlling cervical cancer is widespread screening by detection with regular examinations and Pap smears for all women.

Most authorities agree that routine circumcision of males is *not* justified as a means of preventing cancer of the cervix in women. Neither the presence of the male foreskin nor smegma have been proven to be associated with the disease.

Dr. King of the Ad Hoc Task Force on Circumcision for the American Academy of Pediatrics concludes:

---

28 Reddy DG, Baruah IKSM. Carcinogenic Action of Human Smegma. *Arch Pathol.* 1963-04; 75: 414-20.

"... Neonatal circumcision is unproven as a means of reducing ... carcinoma of the cervix in marital partners. The indication for neonatal circumcision most often invoked is seen as impractical. The greater question, relating to carcinoma, is the protective effect that circumcision may confer vis-a-vis carcinoma of the cervix in spouses. Here the data is less compelling [than for penile cancer] but good penile hygiene – retracting and washing under the foreskin – or genetic resistance to carcinoma of the cervix are equally plausible explanations for the relatively low incidence of carcinoma of the cervix found in Israeli or Scandinavian wives ... Compelling epidemiological data that would mandate circumcision as a means of preventing carcinoma of the cervix are presently lacking." [29]

---

29 King LR. The Pros and Cons of Neonatal Circumcision. *Surg Rounds.* 1979; 2: 29-34.

18   Is Circumcision Traumatic For a Newborn Baby?

Circumcision was often deliberately intended to be a means of torture during primitive initiation rites. Today circumcision is always performed under anesthesia if the patient is an adult or child past early infancy. Yet when the same operation is performed on a newborn infant it is almost always done without anesthesia. *Why ?!*

Does the newborn baby feel any fear or discomfort as he is strapped into the plastic circumcision board? Does he register pain when his genitals are pinched, cut, clamped, or sliced? Does he feel soreness during the following days as his freshly-cut penis heals? Or is he not sufficiently developed enough to be aware of anything?

In many of the personal accounts in this book it was *obvious* to those involved that the infant underwent a severe amount of pain. It would seem that simple common sense and basic knowledge of the feelings and responses of infants in other respects would plainly indicate that the newborn infant is sensitive and aware and is just as capable of feeling pain as any other person at any other age.

However, many people, both lay and medical professionals, insist that the infant feels little or nothing when he undergoes this operation. There are people who have dismissed me as a neurotic, overly-sensitive mother for my heartfelt concern about this matter.

One father, after watching his infant son being circumcised, assured me that the operation could not possibly have been traumatic for the baby because all he heard was "one tiny little cry!" One doctor has tried to tell me that he is able to circumcise a baby "so gently that the baby just goes to sleep during the operation." An acquaintance who is a child psychiatrist has labeled my efforts as "struggling with minutiae."

The textbook for a class on "Marriage and Parenthood" that my husband and I took during college, tells future parents the following about the newborn:

> "For the most part, the neonate is blankly unemotional, although he may smile when contented, whether he is awake or asleep. There is no indication that the neonate feels affection toward anybody or anything, although such affection develops quickly in the first few months.
>
> The neonate is also relatively insensitive to pain, but his sensitivity picks up rapidly in the first few days. Circumcision can be performed a few days after birth with no anesthetic and with apparently very little discomfort." [1]

While some people insist that the infant feels nothing, others attempt to justify neonatal circumcision by claiming that perhaps the baby feels some pain, but it is much more traumatic for an older child or an adult. For example Katz states:

---

[1] Saxton L. *The Individual, Marriage, and the Family*. Belmont, CA: Wadsworth Publishing; 1968: 426.

"Circumcision can be done at any time, but the amount of post-operative pain and irritability is proportional to the age. Up to three weeks of age, pain and irritability virtually occur only at the time of the operation. From four weeks to three months of age the baby is irritable for a night or two and an analgesic is recommended. From three months to a year the pain and irritability last three or four days, and from a year onwards the response varies with the individual. The average adult experiences pain and discomfort for seven to ten days.

While functional development does not necessarily parallel the progress of nerve myelination, it is certain [?] that not all tracts and pathways in the nervous system are fully functional at birth. No anesthetic is necessary during the first 2 ½ to 3 months after birth." [2]

It is curious that Katz is "certain" of what he states, because absolutely no studies have been conducted that support the belief that infants feel little or no pain.

Statements informing people that babies feel nothing while undergoing circumcision arouse anger and disgust among those of us who are opposed to infant circumcision. However, my own experiences when my first two sons were circumcised *seemed* to bear this out. Neither experience left *me* with any impression that the baby had undergone anything traumatic.

Eric's foreskin was cut off the morning after he was born. He was brought to me several times that day for feedings. During those feedings he was never crying, fussing, or showing any outward indication that he was in pain.

Jason underwent the same operation the morning after his birth. We had "rooming-in" and I knew exactly when it was done. I recall the doctor taking Jason in his bassinet to another room about 30 feet away and bringing him back to me about 15 minutes later. Although I was within earshot I did not hear any crying. After he was back with me the day continued as usual with Jason sleeping and nursing as before. It did not appear to me that circumcision had traumatized the baby.

Why then did Ryan's circumcision seem to be such a horrible, traumatic experience? The answer will be made clear further on in this chapter.

Others who have witnessed infant circumcision describe the event in terms of extreme trauma and incredible cruelty, For example, according to Foley:

"The circumcision of a newborn is a spectacle so appalling and revolting in its cruelty that, on their first encounter with the ordeal, many robust medical students faint. The infant is tied down securely to a circumcision board, with his genitals exposed. Next, the entire foreskin and much of the penile skin is pulled through a clamp, and as the clamp's screw is tightened the skin is crushed off. As

---

2 Katz J. The Question of Circumcision. *Int J Surg*. 1977-09; 62(9): 491.

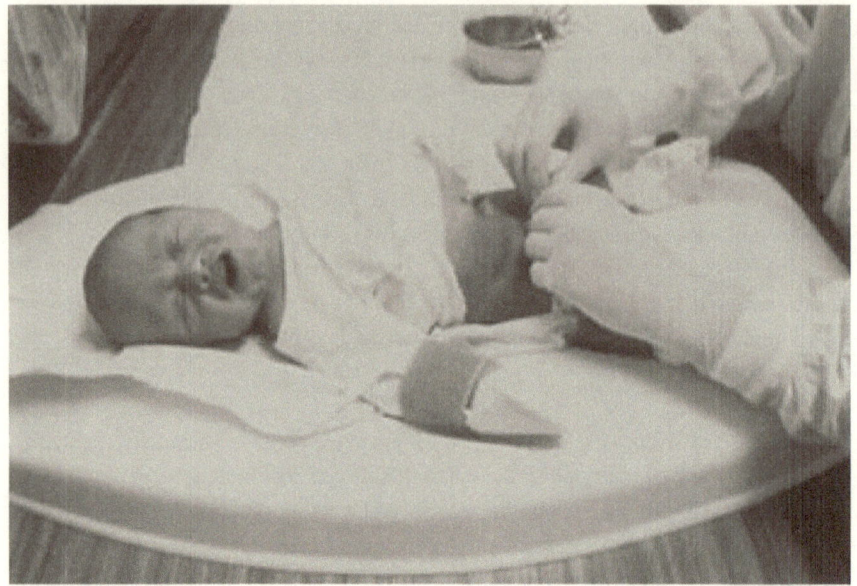

Reprinted with permission from the Saturday Evening Post Company © 1981.

much as 80% of the total penile skin is removed. In this country anesthetics are rarely used. The infant struggles and screams, and often vomits and defecates, before lapsing into unconsciousness." [3]

The psychiatrist Dr. Rene Spitz has been quoted as saying:

"I find it difficult to believe that circumcision, as practiced in our hospitals ... would not represent stress and shock of some kind. Nobody who has witnessed the way these infants are operated on without anesthesia ... the infant screaming ... in manifest pain, can reasonably deny that such treatment is likely to leave traces of some kind on the personality ... This is one of the cruelties the medical profession thoughtlessly inflicts on infants, just because these cannot tell what they suffer ..." [4]

Why do some people perceive infant circumcision as a trifling, momentary event of which the baby is scarcely aware, while others describe it as severe torture? Can people really be talking about the *same* occurrence?

---

3   Foley JM. The Unkindest Cut of All. *Fact.* 1966-07: 309.
4   Weiss C. Circumcision in Infancy. *CLP.* 1964-09; 3(9): 561-2.

18 – Is Circumcision Traumatic For a Newborn Baby?

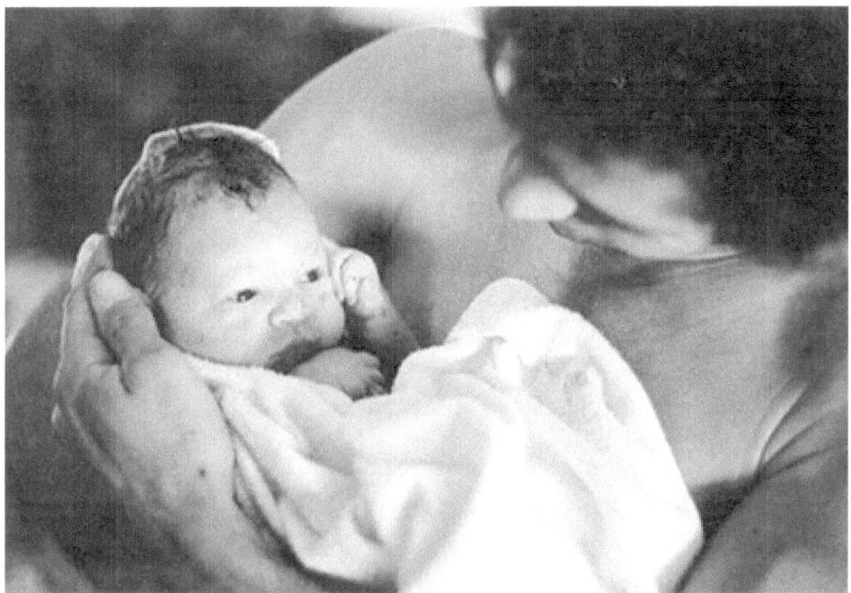

© *Suzanne Arms*

Witnessing and describing what one believes another person feels in any given situation is a highly subjective endeavor. One's own personality and involvement in the situation influence one's perception. Almost all parents who have ever had a son circumcised, or medical professionals who have ever performed or assisted with the operation – if presented with the idea that circumcision hurts babies – react with a certain amount of defensiveness. For circumcision is not done out of *deliberate* intent to harm the infant. No one *wants* to believe that what he or she is doing or advocating inflicts a great deal of pain on helpless babies! If one is to accept such a belief, then he/she would either have to recognize in himself or herself an element of cruelty and sadism, *or* he/she would have to admit that he/she was wrong in the past and quit performing or authorizing circumcisions. It is difficult for most people to admit that they have been wrong. It is difficult for many doctors to learn from lay people.

Circumcision of infants is a culturally accepted event in our society. The *context* has somehow made people fail to question this act. In most situations if someone were to forcibly restrain a child and do something to hurt his genitals, people would consider that child abuse. But we have accepted the same action within hospital nurseries! If some doctor were to cut off the little fingers of all the newborns in a hospital or to slash the vaginas of all the infant girls he would quickly be thrown in jail! Everyone would be horrified! But somehow we are inconsistent and do not give infant boys the same consideration. A few years ago a sexual psychopath was tried and convicted for the rape and murder of a two-year-old girl. People were especially aghast when they learned that he had applied vise grips to the child's tiny nipples! Yet we believe that it is okay to apply clamps to infant foreskins! Of course *we* as adults know that the *intention* is different. We assume that a doctor who circumcises babies is not a sexual psychopath or sadist. *But, his motive makes no difference to the baby!*

It is also true that for medical professionals a certain amount of callousness develops as a result of working in an environment where they deal with so many people and see an unusual amount of suffering. Compared to the serious surgery, horrible injuries and life-threatening diseases that they constantly witness, infant circumcision to them may appear trivial.

Some people are simply not particularly attuned or sensitive to the feelings of others. Some consider any sentiment about babies as maudlin or silly. Even some anti-circumcision activists are primarily concerned about unnecessary surgery and the rights of males to keep their foreskins and consider trauma to infants an extremely minor matter.

Much of the focus of the medical profession is on objective, "scientific" emotionless facts. This perspective is certainly expedient and necessary for conducting much research. It is also true that any medical professional has to maintain some level of emotional detachment in order to effectively carry out his or her responsibilities, particularly because they witness an incredible amount of injury, trauma, and tragedy. Unfortunately many medical professionals have become geared to think *only* along those lines. It is sad indeed that the people whose role is to cure the sick and attend birth in our society have so frequently fallen into the trap of being detached instead of caring about the feelings of others.

However, there are certain characteristics of the newborn and his response to the operation that have even led some basically sensitive and caring adults to believe that circumcision is not traumatic for him.

With rare exceptions no one can *consciously remember* being an infant. In a sense, infancy is a "natural amnesiac." Therefore, some people believe that since events in infancy can only rarely be recalled, nothing that happens in infancy is truly important. Sometimes men who have been circumcised as infants will say "It was done to me and I don't remember it, so it must not have hurt." The concept that events during birth, infancy, or early childhood *are* perceived, *are* remembered, *can* be recalled through therapy, and *can* have an effect on the rest of that individual's life is too "out in left field" for many people to accept. It is plausible that for some people their *own* traumas during birth and infancy, and the subsequent repression of feelings, causes them in turn to reject this concept and to fail to sympathize with the feelings of others.

It is true that newborn infants do heal rapidly from any type of injury. Usually, a circumcised infant's penis is healed within about a week. Also, stitches are not normally required following infant circumcision, but are necessary when an older child or adult undergoes the same operation. Yet another factor is that infant circumcision takes very little time. Unless complications occur, the operation should take only about 5-10 minutes. The short amount of time involved, the absence of stitches, and rapid healing process have all led some people to believe that infant circumcision is less traumatic than for someone older.

However, time as perceived by infants is undoubtedly different than what adults perceive. Most adults could stand a five minute painful procedure without being traumatized. But for an infant five minutes under a circumcision clamp must seem tremendously long! Also, a week's worth of healing undoubtedly is a tremendous amount of suffering for someone who has only been in this world for a few days. To further the contrast between infant and adult circumcision: Many lay people are unaware that the newborn's foreskin is sealed to the glans. Therefore, when the foreskin is cut off, one layer of skin has literally been torn away from another. The freshly exposed infant's glans is raw, extremely sensitive skin like new skin beneath a blister. When an adult is circumcised, in most cases his foreskin has long since freed itself from the glans. Also, the freshly-circumcised adult penis is not in constant contact with feces or urine-soaked diapers! But most importantly, the older individual is able to *understand* what is being done to his body!

As has been stated elsewhere, for many parents their babies' circumcision has been such a "behind the scenes" procedure that they are simply not aware of it. Perhaps bonding has not been allowed to take place, or perhaps the mother is still too sore, exhausted, or drugged from giving birth to be concerned over what is happening to her baby. If she does not change diapers in the hospital, she will not even see her son's penis until they both go home. By this time his circumcision is nearly healed and she simply never realizes that he underwent a traumatic operation.

How trauma and pain affect a person is a highly individual matter. Some people are not particularly bothered by pain. Two individuals, each given the same stimuli, may respond to it differently, one perceiving it as extremely unpleasant, the other hardly noticing it. Witness the incredible gamut of women's reactions to labor and birth – ranging from "there was nothing to it" to "it was the most horrible torture I have ever imagined!" While it is true that earlier traumas influence our perceptions during later experiences, some differences in pain perception may be inborn. It is reasonable to assume that such differences also exist in newborns. (Although I doubt that there has ever been any infant who felt *no* pain as his foreskin was severed.) This could be yet another explanation as to why witnesses of circumcision report such conflicting views.

A final, important consideration is that adults expect a *vocal* response to be the appropriate indicator of pain. Some infants do actively scream as they undergo circumcision. But other babies cry only a little or not at all during the procedure. If a baby does not make much noise in response to the operation, frequently adult observers conclude "It must not have hurt him because he did not cry." Also, babies, characteristically fall into a deep sleep following circumcision. This has caused some people to conclude "Look! It didn't hurt him! He just went to sleep!" The significance of both absence of crying and deep sleep manifested by babies in response to circumcision will be explored in greater depth.

It is clear that the wide range of opinions about the infant's response to circumcision reflects *selective perception* on the part of observers. Simple common sense would support the fact that the infant does indeed feel pain. Recent scientifically conducted studies also indicate that the infant feels more pain from circumcision than most people would like to believe. *There is no documented evidence or scientific study that supports the belief that infants do not feel pain.* Therefore it is curious that medical professionals have so frequently clung to this belief. Usually doctors are quick to dismiss lay people's ideas as being "not valid," "unscientific," or "unproven." Yet the idea that circumcision is not painful for babies is equally "unproven" and "unscientific."

Interestingly, the earlier medical writings about infant circumcision unquestioningly state that the operation is indeed extremely painful for an infant.

In 1904, DeLee wrote: "It is cruel to subject the helpless tiny patient to unnecessary pain. Mild anesthetics are used ..." [5]

According to Valentine in 1901:

"Ordinary humanitarian sentiment prevents consideration of circumcision without anesthesia. I do not believe ... that any physician would rend a mother's heart by so torturing her babe. It is specious to hold that an infant's sensibilities are not sufficiently developed to permit it to perceive pain. If so, why does the infant cry when a maladjusted pin pricks it, or when its delicate skin is irritated by a badly folded or moistened diaper? Is it logical to assume that its shrieks of agony, when a foreskin is cut or torn off, are but reflex?" [6]

---

5   DeLee JB. *Obstetrics for Nurses*. Philadelphia: W.B. Saunders; 1924: 437.
6   Valentine FC. Surgical Circumcision. *JAMA*. 1901-03-16: 712.

18.1 Scientific Investigations in Regard to the Infant's Reaction to Circumcision

Relatively few scientific studies have been conducted in regard to this matter. The only studies that I found worth noting during the original writing of this book all took place during the 1970's. In some of these studies the researchers' primary concern was not circumcision. They simply wanted to study infant response to a stressful procedure. In one study the intent was to observe gender differences among newborns and it was found that circumcision distorted the results.

Emde and his associates investigated the sleep patterns of newborns. People experience two types of sleep. Sleep cycles usually begin with a period of active, rapid eye movement called "REM" sleep. Dreams take place during this phase of sleep. Later in the sleep cycle people usually experience a deeper, inactive type of sleep without rapid eye movements called "non-REM" sleep.

They investigated how stressful stimulation (provided by circumcision) would affect the sleep cycles of newborns. One theory predicted that the stress of circumcision would result in an increased amount of active, restless sleep. The second theory predicted that infants would exhibit "conservation-withdrawal" behavior. In their technical language: "… a reduction of incoming stimuli by alteration of sensory thresholds with a decline of activity." In plain English, babies would withdraw into an abnormally deep sleep in response to pain and trauma.

Six normal, full-term newborn male infants were observed continuously over a 24-hour period. Midway through the observation period they all underwent circumcision with a Plastibell device. Four of the six infants evinced increased amounts of non-REM sleep of 28%, 72%, 76%, and 80% during the 12 hours following the operation. One infant was kept awake by his father and the other was clearly an exception. Three other infants of the same age who did not undergo circumcision were also observed for 24 hours. They showed no increase in non-REM sleep during the second 12 hours.

They then studied 20 normal, full-term male infants, 10 of whom were circumcised and 10 who were not circumcised. They used an electro-encephalograph polygraph machine to record sleep patterns and other behavior in more detail. They were studied on two successive nights beginning at 24 hours of age. Eight of the ten circumcised infants showed an increase in non-REM sleep, with increases ranging from 41%-121%. The amount of non-REM sleep varied little from the first night to the second among the infants who were not circumcised.[7]

---

[7] Emde RN, Harmon RJ, Metcalf D, Koenig KL, Wagonfeld S. Stress and Neonatal Sleep. *Psychosom Med.* 1971/Nov-Dec; 33(6): 491-3.

It is reasonable to conclude that this abnormal sleeping pattern on the part of the infant is a withdrawal, a self-protective reaction to the trauma.

Anders and Chalemian attempted to repeat Emde's study, but theirs differed in a number of ways and produced different results.

They observed 11 normal, 3-day-old, full-term male infants for 3 separate 1-hour periods, 1 hour prior to circumcision immediately following a feeding, a stress-circumcision hour immediately following the operation, and a recovery hour after the next feeding following circumcision. They classed the state of the infants in four categories of wakefulness and two types of sleep: Fussy Cry; Wakeful Activity; Alert Inactivity; and Drowsy; and Active REM Sleep and Quiet non-REM Sleep.

They found that total wakefulness increased during the stress-circumcision period characterized by fussy crying. The recovery hour was characterized by drowsiness. No significant changes in active REM or quiet non-REM sleep were noted in any period.

However, they do point out that Emde's study observed the infants over longer periods of time. This may account for the differences in their observations. Additionally the infants in Emde's study were circumcised with the Plastibell, while the infants in Anders and Chalemian's study had it done by a clamp device. The plastic ring and ligature is probably more painful for the infant because the device remains in place. The difference in methods may also account for the differences in behavior.[8]

Talbert, Kraybill, and Potter investigated infants' internal chemical responses to the stress of circumcision. Serum cortisol and cortisone are secreted by the hypothalamic, pituitary, and adrenal glands, and are generally produced in greater amounts following stressful situations.

Five normal newborn male infants were studied. Before 6 hours of age, heel stick and then circumcision with a Gomco clamp took place. Blood was again obtained at 20 minutes and 40 minutes after circumcision. Cortisol and cortisone levels were measured in all three samples. The average levels prior to circumcision were 5.8 µg/100 ml of cortisol and 7.3 µg/100 ml for cortisone. 20 minutes after the operation the respective mean levels rose to 14.7 and 8.5 for the infants. 40 minutes afterwards the levels remained significantly higher.

They conclude that neonates respond to stress with increased output of adrenal corticoids.[9]

Heel sticks are also painful for babies. Therefore one is led to question how might three heel sticks create additional trauma for the infant or affect the results of their study. Also, while I question the ethics of neonatal circumcision, I also question the

---

8   Anders TF, Chalemian RJ. The Effects of Circumcision on Sleep-Wake States in Human Neonates. *Psychosom Med.* 1974/Mar-Apr; 36(2): 174-5.
9   Talbert LM, Kraybill EN, Potter HD. Adrenal Cortical Response to Circumcision in the Neonate. *Obstet Gynecol.* 1976-08; 48(2): 208-10.

ethics of using infants as "guinea pigs" in studies like this even if parental consent is obtained.

Richards, Bernal and Brackbill set out to investigate possible gender differences between male and female babies. Such studies when conducted in the United States found newborn boys to be more active and restless, while similar investigations conducted in Europe found no such sex differences. Since infant circumcision is widespread in the U.S. but is rarely done in Europe, they postulated that circumcision, not gender, was responsible for the differences in behavior.

They state:

> "... circumcision requires more study in its own right and that it requires description if not control in all neonatal and infancy studies. Our purpose here is to examine the possibility that ... physical insult in the form of male circumcision, has both behavioral and physiological consequences that may have been uniformly misinterpreted by developmental scientists." [10]

More recently Brackbill and Schroder conducted a follow-up investigation of the correlation between neonatal circumcision and gender differences. They researched 38 other studies which were concerned with gender differences among newborns and included circumcision as a variable. Interestingly the data revealed few significant differences among newborns in *any* of a large number of categories. Some of the different studies yielded conflicting results.

Brackbill and Schroder do not state what methods of circumcision were employed in these different studies, nor when the operation was performed in relation to birth or to the study itself, nor what other potentially traumatic variables had been recently performed on both male and female infants (such as heel sticks) which could similarly alter their behavior.

A single, more controlled study (if such studies on newborn infants are indeed ethical) accounting for many variables such as the above listed, would reveal more conclusive answers.[11]

If Richard's, Bernal's and Brackbill's first hypothesis is valid this raises yet another question. Could another "complication" of circumcision be less affection, attention, or positive feelings on the part of parents toward their infant? Some have suggested that injury to the infant can stimulate an instinctive rejection reaction by the mother, similar to the way a mother animal is likely to kill or reject her infant if it has

---

10 Richards MPM, Bernal JF, Brackbill Y. Early Behavioral differences: Gender or Circumcision? *Dev Psychobiol.* 1976; 9(1): 89-95.

11 Brackbill Y, Schroder K. Circumcision, Gender Differences, and Neonatal Behavior: An Update. *Dev Psychobiol.* 1980-11; 13(6): 607-14.

been injured. More plausibly and less directly, circumcision may produce a fussier, crankier, less appealing baby who will in turn inspire less parental affection.

18.2 The Awareness and Consciousness of the Newborn

Books and publications about infants frequently expound on the sensitivity and awareness of newborns. Ironically these are often the same books that ignore the subject of circumcision or state that the infant feels little or nothing while this part of his body is cut off. Circumcision has truly been a "blind spot" in our thinking.

According to an *American Baby Magazine* publication:

"The newborn can also avoid pain. If you hurt any part of him, he will withdraw from you if he can. Stroking one leg will make the other cross and push your hand away. If you poke the upper part of his body, his hand comes over to grasp yours. Then he will try to push you away.

These reflexes are not just immediately useful. Your baby's brain stores and learns from all these reflex experiences, building for the future ...

Even more exciting, your baby is a thinking, feeling, being ...

They are also very sensitive to touch and pressure. Touch is almost a language for infants. Skin contact and warmth, especially from mother's body are probably the most potent stimulation for infants in the first few months of life. Like a radar screen picking up vibrations, your baby soaks in your feelings about him from your handling. He can sense rough, inappropriate, or insufficient handling, and he appreciates touch suited to his style." [12]

During the 1970's Dr. Frederick Leboyer's book and film about "Birth Without Violence" have revolutionized our understanding about the feelings and perceptions of infants at the time of birth. Until his ideas became popular people rarely considered the baby's perspective.

Babies were expected to cry and scream when they were born. Lusty, vigorous crying meant a healthy baby and made everyone happy! Although spanking the baby or holding him upside down is less common today than in the past, that has been the standard "Hollywood" image of birth.

With the advent of natural childbirth and husband participation, birth has become a time of celebration. Doctors and delivery room nurses have frequently joined in the festive mood. People would shout out the sex of the baby as soon as it was apparent. The delivery room, which is somewhat of an "echo chamber" to begin with, became full of people cheering and talking noisily. Meanwhile, people are unwrapping equip-

---

12 The First 12 Months of Life. *Am Baby Mag.* 1979: 23-24.

ment and clanging metal things around. It never occurred to anyone that all this racket was frightening or assaulting to the baby.

Delivery rooms have always been filled with bright lights! (After all, the doctor has to see what he is doing!) No one questioned silver nitrate, the caustic burning substance that is placed in baby's eyes in case the mother has gonorrhea. And babies "had" to be washed up, weighed, and roughly jostled around by the nursery personnel!

Leboyer has raised our consciousness by telling us:

"Aren't cries always an expression of pain? Isn't it conceivable that the baby is in anguish? What makes us assume that birth is less painful for the child than it is for the mother? And if it is, does anyone care?

That tragic expression, those tight-shut eyes, those twitching eyebrows ... That howling mouth, that squirming head trying desperately to find refuge ... Those hands stretching out to us, imploring, begging, then retreating to shield the face – that gesture of dread.

Those furiously kicking feet, those arms that suddenly pull downward to protect the stomach. The flesh that is one great shudder ...

Has there ever been a more heartrending appeal?

And yet this appeal – as old as birth itself – has been misunderstood, has been ignored, has simply gone unheard ...

What makes being born so frightful is the intensity, the boundless scope and variety of the experience, its suffocating richness.

People say – and believe – that a newborn baby feels nothing. He feels *everything*. Everything – utterly, without choice or filter or discrimination.

Birth is a tidal wave of sensation, surpassing anything we can imagine. A sensory experience so vast we can barely conceive of it ... The baby's senses are at work. Totally.

They are sharp and open – new ... These sensations are not yet organized into integrated, coherent perceptions. Which makes them all the stronger, all the more violent, unbearable – literally maddening ...

What about its sense of touch?

Its skin – thin, fine, almost without a protective surface layer – is as exposed and raw as tissue that has suffered a burn. The slightest touch makes it quiver ... Newborn babies arrive in our world as if on a carpet of thorns. They'll adapt to it. By withdrawing into themselves, by deadening their senses. But when they first land on these thorns, they howl. Naturally. And idiots that we are, we laugh ...

Unhappiness is so ingrained in most babies by this time that they can hope for nothing else. If someone approaches, they tremble even more.

And then we see an extraordinary thing: when the tears and the gasping and the pain become too much, *the infant flees ... The baby disappears into itself.* Doubles up again ... symbolically, it has taken itself back into the womb ... When it is no longer able to cry, it collapses. Sinks into sleep. Its only refuge. Its only friend." [13]

Leboyer has essentially made the same observation that was made by Emde and his associates, but in a different manner.

Leboyer advocates treating the infant with a great deal of gentleness and respect immediately following birth. He replaces the harsh glaring light with dim lighting, and the typical loud noises during birth are replaced with soft voices and as little sound as possible. Following birth the infant is placed on its mother's abdomen and gently massaged.

Prior to Leboyer's philosophy no one had ever given any thought to when the cord was cut. But Leboyer advocates delaying cutting of the cord:

"If the cord is severed as soon as the baby is born, this brutally deprives the brain of oxygen. The alarm system thus alerted, the baby's entire organism reacts. Respiration is thrown into high gear as a response to aggression. Everything in the body-language of the infant – the immensity of its panic and its efforts to escape ... the act of breathing for a newborn baby, is a desperate last resort." [14]

He explains his philosophy behind massaging the infant as follows:

"It is through our hands that we speak to the child, that we communicate. Touching is the primary language ...

Immediately we sense how important such contact is, just how important is the way we hold a child. It is a language of skin-to-skin – the skin from which emerge all our sensory organs. And these organs in turn are like window-openings in the wall of skin that both contains and holds us separate from the world. The newborn baby's skin has an intelligence, a sensitivity that we can only begin to imagine." [15]

Finally he eloquently describes the differences between the baby born to harsh conventional birthing techniques and the baby born non-violently.

---

13 Leboyer F. *Birth Without Violence.* Alfred A. Knopf; 1975: 5-6, 8, 15-6, 19, 29.
14 Ibid., p. 51.
15 Ibid., p. 59.

"... Our adventurer is free of fear. He or she has gone from change to change, from one discovery to the next, so slowly, so surrounded and enveloped in love and attention, that everything that happens is accepted with confidence and happiness ..." [16]

"We are touching on mysteries now. This is a grace which radiates in silence that crowns with a halo every child who arrives among us ..." [17]

"Curiously, during the final moments, all newborn babies are alike. For a brief period, it is still as if they had no identity at all ... It is simply that they all wear the same mask. The depersonalizing mask of terror. And it is only when this mask falls away that we discover the individual beneath ... there are no ugly babies. Only those deformed by fear ..." [18]

"The baby has a miraculous sureness in understanding us. The baby knows everything. *Feels* everything." [19]

"The baby sees into the bottom of our hearts, knows the color of our thoughts. All without language." [20]

"The newborn baby is a mirror reflecting our image. It is for us to make its entrance into the world a joy." [21]

Leboyer's book has sold widely. During the 1970's and 80's many parents have attempted to use his techniques when giving birth. Unfortunately many parents have been interested in Leboyer techniques only to find their doctors and local hospitals indifferent about it and unwilling to change.

Leboyer presents his ideas as a poet and not as a scientist. Because what he says is not presented as cold, hard statistics, documented "facts," and research involving thousands, many medical professionals have not been able to relate to it. Also, doctors have not been able to observe any concrete, measurable, long-term health or developmental differences among babies born by the Leboyer method. (At least among those born to hospital "token" Leboyer techniques.) Therefore many consider it of no

---

16 Ibid., p. 94.
17 Ibid., p. 95.
18 Ibid., p. 97.
19 Ibid., p. 107.
20 Ibid., p. 108.
21 Ibid., p. 112.

value. Why can't the practice of treating babies with gentleness and respect be of value *in and of itself?!*

What has been even more disturbing is that a number of doctors and hospitals have tried to "do" the Leboyer "method," without approaching it out of true consciousness and caring for the feelings of the infant. When "The Leboyer Method" was still a novel idea it proved to be a great source of publicity for a hospital. Newspapers did features on it. Hospital staff did public presentations on it for their clientele. For many it became a fad. In some hospitals the people involved would dim the lights, massage the baby, perhaps immerse the infant in a warm bath, and follow this peaceful routine for about 15 minutes. It made a great show – the latest "in" thing to do. But after that, the baby was whisked off to the nursery where he/she was jostled around, weighed, measured, exposed to bright lights, silver nitrate placed in his/her eyes, and if male his foreskin was cut off. Many doctors who have gained a lot of public recognition for offering "the Leboyer method" were regularly circumcising the same babies that they had helped into the world by "non-violent techniques!" Many parents were requesting the Leboyer method and signing circumcision papers at the same time! Where is our consciousness and awareness? We have not learned anything about the nature and well being of the infant. We have merely adopted another fad! Leboyer techniques are *worthless* if they are done without sensitivity, caring, and genuine concern for the baby's feelings. We must apply that same consciousness and caring for choosing to leave our sons intact. For as modern day intactivism progresses, for many parents, not having one's son circumcised sometimes has also become the next "fad," the next "in thing to do." Although as intactivists we consider each infant boy with an intact penis a "victory" in our cause, it must be seen that as advantageous as a foreskin may be, the choice will be worth little if it is not chosen out of love and genuine concern for the infant's well being.

Joseph Chilton Pearce in his magnificent, eye-opening book *Magical Child*, presents more ideas which complement Leboyer's message, giving us further insight into what the infant experiences following conventional birth:

> "The semi-drugged, overstressed, and exhausted infant is, of course, generally unable to get his/her breath, even if given ample time to do so. The many new, unused coordinates of muscles are confused and malfunctioning. His/her body is reacting only; all synchronous interactions have long since been destroyed. In addition to his/her prolonged body fear of oxygen deprivation, when s/he is finally sucked or clawed out of the mother, his/her entry is into a noisy, brilliantly lit arena of masked creatures and humming machines. (The hum of fluorescent lighting alone is an overload, much less fluorescence itself, which, as the world's greatest authority on lighting, John Ott, makes perfectly clear, is disastrous to

infants.) Suction devices are rammed into the mouth and nose, the eyelids peeled back to that blinding, painful light and far more painful chemicals dropped into the open eyes. S/he is held by the heels and beaten on the back or subjected to a mechanical respirator; at this critical oxygen-short period, the umbilical cord has been cut. S/he is cleaned up a bit from the blood of the episiotomy ... placed on cold, hard scales to be weighed like any other piece of meat in a factory; wrapped up ...; bundled off to a nursery crib, screaming in pain and terror if s/he is lucky; or rushed semiconscious and half dead to an incubator, far worse fate than a crib, if s/he is less lucky.

What the infant actually learns at birth is what the process of learning is like. S/he has moved from a soft, warm, dark, quiet and totally nourishing place into a harsh sensory overload. S/he is physically abused, violated in a variety of ways, subjected to specific pain and insult, all of which could still be overcome, but s/he is then isolated from his/her mother ... The failure to return to the known matrix sets into process a chain reaction from which that organism never fully recovers. All future learning is affected. The infant body goes into shock. The absorbant mind shuts down. There will be little absorption again because there is only trauma and pain to be absorbed. The infant then surely exhibits only two states ..., 'quiescence,' which means semi- to full unconsciousness, and 'unpleasure.' If awakened from his/her survival retreat from consciousness, s/he is propelled back into a state of unresolved high stress. S/he cries him/herself to sleep again ... Pleasure and smiling will surely be much later in appearing, just about two and a half months later, because it will take that long for this unstimulated and isolated body to compensate if it is to survive at all. The infant's body must manage slowly to bring its own sensory system to life, get that reticular formation functioning, and come fully alive through whatever occasional physical nurturing it gets. Stage-specific processes, once missed, must be laboriously rebuilt.

... In nearly all cases, the doctors circumcise the male infant on the second or third day of life. They cut off the foreskin of his penis, nearly always without anesthetic. After all, the infant – suffering excessive stress, in a state of shock, and all too often with a crippled reticular formation – seems to be a vegetable, so why not treat him as one? ... If the infant is not already in a complete state of shock before the operation, he certainly will be afterward, as parents would be if they were to observe and comprehend what is happening ... Ask your doctor, though, and he will scathingly dismiss criticisms, reassure you that it's perfectly all right, and make you feel rather stupid for even asking." [22]

---

22   Pearce JC. *Magical Child*. NY: E.P. Dutton; 1977: 57-9.

Much of this is, of course, speculative. No one has any way of *definitely* knowing what an infant truly feels. But much of what is now being learned about the infant's perception during birth has been based on people's own recollections that surface during regressive sessions such as primal therapy. Others who refute its validity claim that one may not be re-experiencing events the way they actually happened, or that people are simply fabricating what they tell. However, critics of such findings are probably defensive about their *own* involvement in birth or infant circumcision.

Anyone who has *only* experienced or observed conventional birth within a hospital might readily dismiss these ideas presented by Leboyer or Pierce as too "fantastic" or "strange" to be considered. "But this is a perfectly nice, cute little baby! There's nothing wrong with him!" Following the births of my first two sons in hospitals I didn't go out the door thinking "Wow! This baby is really traumatized!"

But, after having given birth at home using dim lighting, soft voices, immediate body contact, and treating the baby with only gentleness and love, I can verify that there is a *profound* and *dramatic* difference in the nature of the baby born in this manner, compared to the baby born by conventional techniques. The baby is more peaceful and contented and will smile blissfully during his first few days of life when he has been welcomed into the world knowing only warmth and gentleness. His eyes will open and look around immediately after birth when they are not assaulted with glaring lights or burning chemicals.

This explains why in my experience, my first two sons circumcisions shortly after their births in hospitals did not impress me as being traumatic, while the same operation performed on my third son following his peaceful home birth was so horrible! *The baby born to conventional birthing procedures is in a state of trauma anyway – whether he is circumcised or not!*

This explains why some babies do not cry or appear to react when their foreskins are clamped and sliced off. The baby is *already* in a state of withdrawal, simply from other common traumatic procedures associated with conventional birth. (An analogy can be drawn by the experience of having one's blood drawn – generally an unpleasant sensation for most people. If one is to have one's blood drawn when one is healthy, such as during a routine check-up, the experience usually stands out as extremely painful. The same person, while recovering from surgery or following a severe injury, may only be scarcely aware of someone drawing his blood.) Also, in some cases infants have still been under sedation from drugs given to the mother during labor, and therefore have been partially anesthetized for circumcision.

Another explanation for the absence of crying during circumcision is that for some babies the shock of the assault is so intense that they *cannot* cry! (A personal experience supporting this is based on my husband's past experience as a lab technologist. One of his most unpleasant tasks was to do routine PKU heel sticks on new-

18 – Is Circumcision Traumatic For a Newborn Baby?

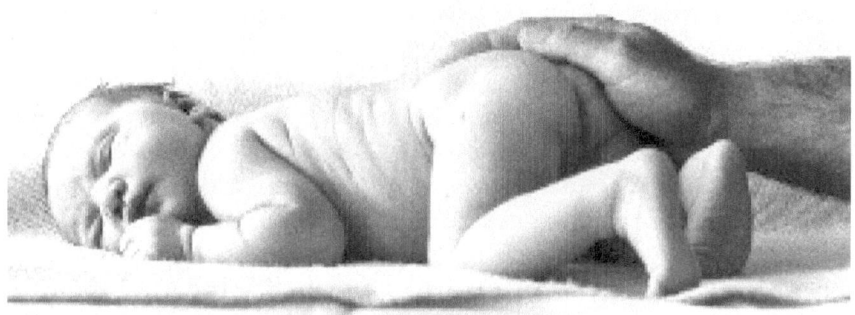

© Suzanne Arms

borns. A heel stick is painful although less intense than circumcision. He has done hundreds of heel sticks on newborns and has never seen a case in which the infant did not cry!)

Medical professionals have simply not been "tuned in" to the feelings of newborns. They work day in and day out, seeing hundreds of parents and babies every year, and forgetting about most of them. Most births are "routine" (if birth should ever be "routine!") and the mothers and babies go home healthy. The constant turnover of patients quickly fades into a blur.

I have repeatedly tried to direct the concept of the consciousness and awareness of newborn babies and the significance of trauma to medical professionals and to other parents only to receive looks of uncomprehension. *For most people have never seen an untraumatized newborn and have no understanding of what this means.* They fail to *perceive* their babies in the hospital nursery, under the glaring lights with eyes burned by silver nitrate and recently cut genitals as traumatized because this is the *only* type of baby that they have ever seen. They have no basis for comparison. For the truly untraumatized newborn infant is something truly precious and rare.

18.3 Is There a Relationship Between Circumcision and Sudden infant Death Syndrome?

Every year thousands of apparently healthy infants are put to bed and never wake up. This tragedy is called Sudden Infant Death Syndrome (SIDS), and commonly called "Crib Death." The parents are wrought with severe grief and guilt. The cause of SIDS is still uncertain. A plethora of theories have been proposed.

More male infants than female infants succumb to SIDS. For this reason, some anti-circumcision activists have suggested that perhaps circumcision leads to SIDS. Could the trauma of circumcision as remembered in the infant brain, be *the* reason, or a contributing factor, that would make a small percentage of babies give up and stop living? *If* this theory were to be proven true, dramatic results would follow. Few parents would choose circumcision for their infants if there was a strong possibility that the operation would endanger his life. Potential victims would be spared by virtue of not having experienced circumcision. However, considerable research is necessary before the answers will be known. Although numerous detailed studies have attempted to solve the tragedy of SIDS, to the best of my knowledge none have ever considered circumcision as a variable. It is hoped that researchers will investigate this in the future.

The following information is worthy of noting:

SIDS rarely occurs during the *immediate* recovery period following circumcision. Most circumcised infants undergo the operation during the first few days of life, but SIDS rarely occurs before age 1-2 months, and is most frequent between the ages of 2 and 4 months. Perhaps what has given some people the idea that circumcision may cause SIDS is the fact that there have been infants who have bled to death or succumbed to severe infections following circumcision. These tragedies, however, are *not* SIDS.

Although more male than female infants do succumb to SIDS, many girl infants are also victims of the tragedy. According to Valdés-Dapena, approximately 58-59% of SIDS victims are male and 41-42% are female. Therefore, circumcision cannot be isolated as a *sole* cause of the tragedy.[23]

If circumcision were a significant factor in SIDS it would stand to reason that the rates of its occurrence would be dramatically higher in countries such as the United States or Israel where infant circumcision is common than in other countries where the operation is not practiced. However, the distribution of the various rates of SIDS throughout various parts of the world shows no apparent correlation.

---

23 Valdés-Dapena MA. *Sudden Unexplained Infant Death 1970 through 1975.* Rockville, MD: U.S. Dept. of Health, Education & Welfare; 1978: 7, 10.

According to Valdés-Dapena, specific studies of the occurrence of SIDS report that the lowest rates (per 1,000) have appeared in Sweden: 0.06; Israel: 0.31; Netherlands: 0.42; and Czechoslovakia: 0.8. While circumcision is not practiced in Sweden, the Netherlands, or Czechoslovakia (now Czechia and Slovakia), the operation has been nearly universal for infant males born in Israel.

The middle rates on the list ranged from 1.55 per 1,000 in California to 2.32 in King County, Washington. The areas represented include various U.S. cities (with most males circumcised), Great Britain (with very few circumcised), and Australia and New Zealand (with less than 50% circumcised).[23]

The highest rates (per 1,000) appear in Western Australia: 2.5 (less than half circumcised); Oxford Linkage Area, Great Britain: 2.78 (very few circumcised); Ireland: 2.8 (almost none circumcised); and Ontario, Canada: 3.0 (about half circumcised).[23]

The above studies can only be considered estimates. The *individual* circumcision status of the victims involved, and even the male-female ratio, are not noted. Studies making note of the above statistics are confined to specific places and times. The data was collected during the early 1970s and was usually confined to one year. Statistics revealing the continuous rates of SIDS in specific areas over a period of years would be more informative.

The breakdown of the rates of SIDS among various ethnic/racial groups within the United States appears not to indicate a correlation with circumcision, for the rates are considerably higher among our racial "minority" groups than among the *"white* middle class" although the latter tend to choose circumcision to a greater extent than the former. SIDS occurs at a rate of 5.93/1,000 among Native Americans; 2.92 among Blacks; 1.74 among Hispanics, 1.32 among *whites*, and 0.51 among Orientals.[22] Again, however, specific data for the circumcision status of the victims may reveal different findings.

Positive correlations have been noted between SIDS and many other factors. The tragedy occurs more frequently among infants of younger mothers, single mothers, and mothers seeking no prenatal care. Bottle-fed babies, babies born prematurely, and babies of mothers who smoke are all at somewhat greater risk. Prenatal nutrition and general health of the mother appear to be important factors. However, babies who have been full term, breastfed, and born to healthy, non-smoking mothers *have* also been SIDS victims. No one factor appears to be universal.

Many believe that some infants are somehow *born* susceptible to SIDS. The question is posed that the trauma of circumcision, as remembered in the infant brain, *could* be a factor that could "tip the scale" for an infant who is *already* vulnerable to SIDS. *If* this is true, perhaps leaving that infant intact could mean the difference between life and death.

Circumcision – The Painful Dilemma

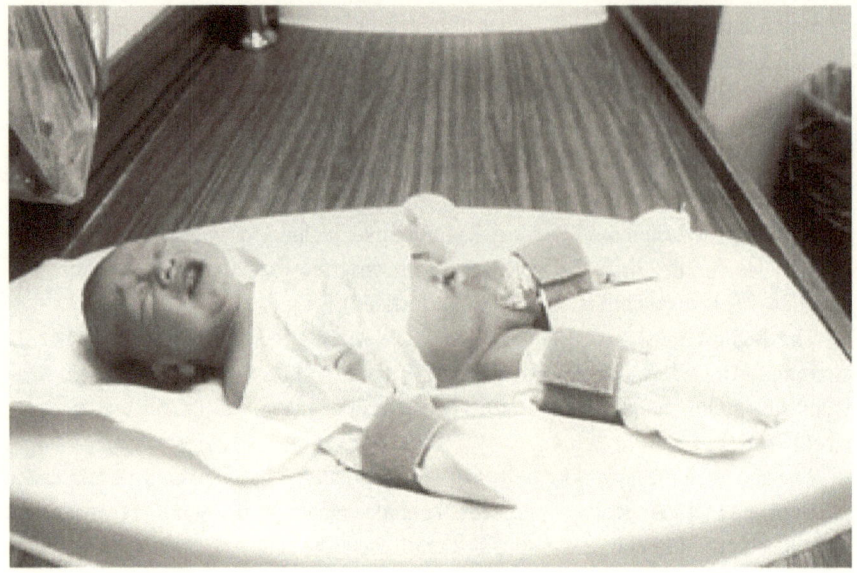

Reprinted with permission from The Saturday Evening Post Company ©1981

One intactivist (opponent of infant circumcision) has *speculated* the following on the subject:

> "During the trauma of the circumcision operation the infant often stops breathing because of the extreme pain. This lack of oxygen, though not fatal at the time, *does* damage the lowermost part of the brain that controls the semi-automatic functions such as heartbeat, breathing and swallowing. For several months after the operation the baby will often stop breathing for as long as 30 seconds while asleep. The medical term for this temporary suspension of breathing is called 'apnea' and these apnea episodes cause *further* damage to the breathing control mechanism. Finally the infant stops breathing altogether and he dies." [24]

It *must* be emphasized that these ideas are *not proven*. Further research must be done in this area. (I am in no way presenting any claim here that circumcision and SIDS are at all related. No evidence so far has proven or disproven this possibility.)

Parents who lose an infant to SIDS experience incredible grief and remorse. Frequently they torment themselves by painstakingly going over every detail of the baby's life, agonizing over what they may have done wrong. Often such parents need

---

[24] Before You Decide to Circumcise. (Informational brochure – their source of information is not stated.) Larchwood, IA: Dep. of Family and Community Welfare, div. of The Remain Intact Org.

professional therapy to recover from the tragedy. Such parents, if their child happened to be a circumcised baby boy, may, upon hearing our speculations, blame themselves for having allowed him to undergo the operation. Therefore, intactivists are admonished to be careful so as not to needlessly add to these parents' grief. It is easy to become so caught up in one cause as to ignore people's feelings in other areas. SIDS parents can, of course, consider leaving a future son intact for any of the *known* advantages of not circumcising. But if they are in the throes of grief, they must be reassured that it is *not known* whether or not circumcision contributes to SIDS.

In the years since this book was originally published, some newer studies have taken place.

In Paul D. Tinari's study at Kingston General Hospital (Kingston, Ontario, Canada in 1998), infants were strapped into Circumstraints and then placed into an MRI chamber while the lower part of the infant's body was accessible to the doctor performing the circumcision.

> "The baby was kept in the machine for several minutes to generate baseline data of the normal metabolic activity in the brain. This was used to compare the data gathered during and after the surgery. Analysis of the MRI data indicated that the surgery subjected the infant to significant trauma. The greatest changes occurred in the limbic system concentrating in amygdala and in the frontal and temporal lobes.
>
> A neurologist who saw the results postulated that the data indicated that circumcision affected most intensely the portions of the victim's brain associated with reasoning, perception and emotions. Follow up tests on the infant one day, one week and one month after the surgery indicated that the child's brain never returned to its baseline configuration. In other words, the evidence generated by this research indicated that the brain of the circumcised infant was permanently changed by the surgery." [25]

(The reactions on the part of the medical system bears witness to the conscious attempt on the part of medical hierarchy to silence all questioning of infant circumcision [aka male genital mutilation]: Upon attempts to publish their findings in the open medical literature – "All of the participants in the research ... were called before the hospital discipline committee and were severely reprimanded. We were told

---

25 Tinari PD. Circumcision Permanently Alters the Brain. Pacific Institute for Advanced Study. URL: circumcision.org/brain.htm

that while male circumcision was legal under all circumstances in Canada, according to their dubious interpretation of the ethical regulations, any attempt to study the adverse effects of circumcision was prohibited. Not only could we not publish the results of our research, but we also had to destroy all of our results. If we refused to comply we were all threatened with immediate dismissal and legal action.")

A more recent report by James McIntosh in 2015 (Oxford University, England) shows similar results and has been published in medical media.

> "The researchers examined the brains of 10 healthy infants aged 1-6 days old and 10 healthy adults aged 23-36 years. [...] the babies were placed inside an MRI scanner where the bottoms of their feet were poked with a special retracting rod. [...]
>
> The researchers observed significant brain activity in 18 of the 20 brain regions that are active in adults when experiencing pain. The babies' brains responded in the same way to a poke (force 128mN) as adults did to a stimulus that was four times stronger (512mN).
>
> Dr. Slater states that their findings stand in contrast with previous understandings of infant pain. 'In fact, some people have argued that babies' brains are not developed enough for them to really 'feel' pain, any reaction being just a reflex,' she says. 'Our study provides the first really strong evidence that this is not the case.' " [26]

> "What did the researcher's find? Eighteen out of the 20 brain regions activated in the adults when experiencing pain were also activated in the infants. This suggests that infants not only feel pain the way adults do, but also that they have a lower pain threshold." [27]

MRI scans reveal brain activity in response to a painful stimulus in infants and adults.

(These findings were published online in the journal *eLife*.)

Another study set out to find out whether neonatal circumcision (with and without Emla cream as a numbing agent) altered pain response from vaccinations given at 4 or 6 months in comparison to infants who had not undergone circumcision. Infants were videotaped during vaccination done at the primary care physician's clinic. Videotapes were scored without knowledge or circumcision or treatment status by a

---

26 McIntosh J. World-first MRI study shows babies experience pain 'like adults'. *MNT*. 2015-04.
27 Gregoire C. Surprising Study Finds That Babies Feel Pain Like Adults. *Huff Post*. 2015-23-04.

research assistant who had been trained to measure infant facial action, cry duration, and visual analogue scale pain scores. Differences between the groups were assessed in regards to facial action, crying time and assessments of pain. The boys who had been circumcised without any type of anesthesia demonstrated far greater sensitivity to injection pain. Pain reaction from boys for whom the numbing agent had been used during circumcision was somewhat less, while those who had not undergone circumcision demonstrated significantly greater tolerance to the pain of injections.[28]

Goldman summarizes this by stating:

"The authors believe that 'neonatal circumcision may induce long-lasting changes in infant pain behavior because of alterations in the infant's central neural processing of painful stimuli.' They also write that 'the long-term consequences of surgery done without anesthesia are likely to include post-traumatic stress as well as pain. It is therefore possible that the greater vaccination response in the infants circumcised without anesthesia may represent an infant analogue of a post-traumatic stress disorder triggered by a traumatic and painful event and re-experienced under similar circumstances of pain during vaccination.'" [29]

18.4   A Possible Link Between Infant Circumcision and Autism

The typical baby, by the time he or she is several months old, will giggle, grin, laugh and babble in response to interaction with those who are familiar to him/her. A normal child is learning words by his/her second year of life, knows how to express his/her needs, and readily forms friendships with others. But there are others who, from early infancy on, have great difficulty communicating with other people or responding normally to the world around them. As babies they may not respond to expected smiles, games and other interactions. As children they may have difficulty learning language, forming friendships, or developing large motor skills. They may exhibit unusual, repetitive behaviors, experience mood disorders, or have sensory processing difficulties. The symptoms listed here describe the child with autism. There is no single standard definition of autism. Each individual is different. There are varying degrees of severity along the autism spectrum. Some people eventually outgrow symptoms of autism and lead relatively normal adult lives, while others remain imprisoned, life long in their limitations. Most autistic people have normal intelligence. Some are even geniuses. Whether or not autism is truly on the rise in re-

---

28 Taddio A, et al. Effect of Neonatal Circumcision on Pain Response During Subsequent Routine Vaccination. *Lancet.* 1997-03; 349(9052): 599-603.
29 Goldman R. Infant Responses to Circumcision. In: *Circumcision: The Hidden Trauma.* Boston: Vanguard; 1997: 20-6.

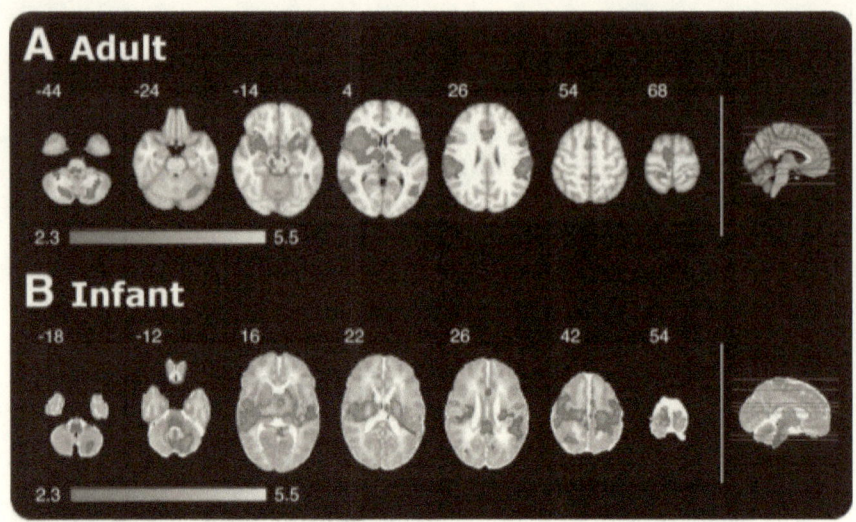

cent years is still questionable. In years past some autistic children have undoubtedly been misdiagnosed as "retarded" or "demented." Today autism is generally more recognized, treated, and better understood than in previous times.

Autism is believed to be related to early brain development, both in utero and during the early months of life. In the United States autism occurs more than 4 times as frequently in boys – 1 in 42, as it does in girls – 1 in 189. Possible causes mentioned have included genetic predisposition, prenatal exposure to environmental contaminants including pesticides and air pollution, advanced parental age, maternal illness during pregnancy (particularly diabetes), low birth weight, extreme prematurity, birth complications that have involved oxygen deprivation, and mercury poisoning from Thimerosal in vaccines.[30, 31, 32]

The results of a recent 19 year study[33] has found higher rates of autism among boys who were circumcised as infants compared to boys who were left intact. The researches have posted that the extreme pain and trauma of genital cutting in infancy impacts the brain and may hamper how the individual responds to stress. The study took place in Denmark where 342,877 boys born between 1994 and 2003 were followed until their 9th birthdays. In addition to autism spectrum disorder (ASD), the outcomes of hyperkinetic disorder and asthma was also observed. Out of the total of boys studied, 4,986 showed symptoms of ASD. The abstract reads as follows:

---

30 What are the signs of autism?: autismspeaks.org/signs-autism
31 What Is Autism?: autismspeaks.org/what-autism
32 What Is Autism?: autismallies.org/about-autism/what-is-autism
33 Frisch M, Simonsen J. Ritual circumcision and risk of autism spectrum disorder in 0- to 9-year-old boys: national cohort study in Denmark. *J R Soc Med*. 2015; 108(7): 266-79.

Objective: Based on converging observations in animal, clinical and ecological studies, we hypothesized a possible impact of ritual circumcision on the subsequent risk of autism spectrum disorder (ASD) in young boys.
Design: National, register-based cohort study.
Setting: Denmark.
Participants: A total of 342,877 boys born between 1994 and 2003 and followed in the age span 0–9 years between 1994 and 2013.
Main outcome measures: Information about cohort members' ritual circumcisions, confounders and ASD outcomes, as well as two supplementary outcomes, hyperkinetic disorder and asthma, was obtained from national registers. Hazard ratios (Hrs) with 95% confidence intervals (CIs) associated with foreskin status were obtained using Cox proportional hazards regression analyses.
Results: With a total of 4986 ASD cases, our study showed that regardless of cultural background circumcised boys were more likely than intact boys to develop ASD before age 10 years (HR=1.46; 95% CI: 1.11–1.93). Risk was particularly high for infantile autism before age five years (HR=2.06; 95% CI: 1.36–3.13). Circumcised boys in non-Muslim families were also more likely to develop hyperkinetic disorder (HR=1.81; 95% CI: 1.11-2.96). Associations with asthma were consistently inconspicuous (HR=0.96; 95% CI: 0.84–1.10).
Conclusions: We confirmed our hypothesis that boys who undergo ritual circumcision may run a greater risk of developing ASD. This finding, and the unexpected observation of an increased risk of hyperactivity disorder among circumcised boys in non-Muslim families, need attention, particularly because data limitations most likely rendered our HR estimates conservative. Considering the widespread practice of non-therapeutic circumcision in infancy and childhood around the world, confirmatory studies should be given priority.

Deciphering the above statistics into plain English, this study found that among the boys that were observed, those who had undergone circumcision displayed a 1 ½ to 2 times the development of autism spectrum disorder. I wish to add, what we now know of changes made in the infant brain due to stressful events, including painful genital cutting and recovery, it stands to reason that in some cases the trauma for some could lead to eventual difficulties in communication and interaction with others and the surrounding environment.

18.5 Primal Pain – Interview With The Primal Institute

Patricia Leis Nicholas, M.A., Assistant Director
E. Michael Holden, M.D., Medical Director
Leslie A. Pam, Ph.D., Associate Director

The Primal Institute began operation as an outpatient clinic in 1968. It was co-founded by Dr. Arthur Janov and Vivian Janov.

Dr. Arthur Janov had felt dissatisfied with the ability of most therapeutic methods to effect real and lasting change. In collaboration with Vivian Janov, a process of re-experiencing repressed psychological trauma was discovered. The Janovs observed many of their patients making an important breakthrough as they relived the pains of childhood. These deeply felt feelings became known as "Primal Pain." Further observation led to the refinement of both theory and practice, culminating in 1970 with the publication of The Primal Scream by Dr. Janov.

Rosemary: Would you recommend that parents choose not to have their infant sons circumcised specifically because it causes psychological damage?

Ms. Nicholas: Yes, and also it's going to hurt the baby!

R: But isn't pain inevitable in life? Even if the child is born by the Leboyer method and never circumcised, there's no way he can live in this world and not get hurt. He's going to fall down and skin his knee or clunk his head.

Dr. Holden: It makes a difference whether a person is going to have trauma a few days after he's born, compared to having trauma when he's a little older. The younger a child is, the closer he is to conception, the more open and vulnerable that child is to hurt. So the goal of the parent should be to minimize hurt during infancy. It is correct, of course, that in later childhood, some bumps and bruises are inevitable. But it is not inevitable for an infant.

R: This is part of why infant circumcision is such a scandal! If you were going to circumcise a three-year-old, nobody would strap him down and let him scream and do it to him without anesthesia. Yet, that's the way it is done to newborns! People have thought that newborn babies have no feelings!

H: Actually the opposite is true. Newborn babies have that much *more* feeling, *more* sensitivity, and are *more* vulnerable to pain than older children.

N: Most parents are not aware of what actually goes on during the circumcision procedure.

R: Can you explain what primal therapy is in a few words? What does it do, or prove, or solve?

H: There's a premise for primal therapy which is that neurosis and psychosomatic illnesses in adults are based on pain in childhood.

R: Physical pain *and* psychological pain?

H: We don't make a distinction between the two because suffering is suffering. Psychological pain is a representation of emotional and physical pain from childhood. Primal therapy is a system devised by Dr. Janov for reversing neurosis. It allows people to complete their total biological healing responses to traumas that happened when they were little, and too vulnerable to finish these healing responses. For example, if a child was very badly hurt and needs to cry for 40 hours, an infant may only be strong enough to cry for an hour. After that he will shut down to that pain. So there's 39 more hours of crying still to go. Primal therapy is the completion of the response to early traumas. It is the completion of the healing sequence.

R: So sometimes you get people that cry for 40 hours?

H: Yes, about a single feeling. It is desperately hard, agonized crying.

Dr. Pam: But it's not 40 hours of crying in one sitting!

H: Whether one is a baby or an adult, there is just so much pain that one can tolerate in a given unit of time. Primal therapy is a sequential re-experiencing of hurts to complete these healing sequences in response to early traumas.

P: That's not only in infancy.

H: That's right. It can be a trauma from childhood and even teenage years and early adulthood. It can be anything that you have repressed.

R: It's fascinating that a person can go back and find these things when only rarely can one consciously remember one's birth, infancy or prenatal days.

H: There's a reason why the typical person does not remember before age 3 or 4. It's because there's so much pain during that time that it's part of repression.

R: Then if someone had a particularly comfortable birth and infancy they would remember it?

H: That is basically true. If a person had an extremely good birth and a great infancy, they'd tend to remember from about age one or one-and-a-half, rather than from age 4 on. We see patients who will say that they remember nothing before age 12. So the amount of repression varies with the amount of pain.

R: I've had therapy myself, but it was more conventional. Much of it was based on *A Guide to Rational Living* by Ellis and *Your Erroneous Zones* by Dyer. I've also had assertiveness training. The basic message of my therapy was "Don't wallow around blaming your parents or blaming the past for your problems. Deal with your life in the present and future." What you do would contradict that?

P: It's just another approach.

N: The key word that you used was "wallow." We don't have people "wallow" in their pain. We have them relive their experiences so that we can resolve the past trauma and continue living as they want to live their lives. Making those changes that make their lives better is only possible if they resolve the pain that drives them to act in a certain way.

R: Then according to primal therapy a person can't just forget past traumas. One has to go back and resolve it.

N: That's right. It's a "resolving" experience rather than a "wallowing" experience.

H: Dr. Janov often makes the point that primal therapy is not for everyone. It is for people who are suffering a great deal. Perhaps other types of therapy have not worked for them. Some people will benefit greatly from other types of therapy. But if a person is really open to their pain of childhood, then primal therapy will be good for them.

P: Primal therapy deals with the causes of neurosis. If you don't have the kind of pain that requires you to go back to the cause, you can patch yourself up.

N: I think anyone *can* benefit from primal therapy. We get average neurotic people who feel that something's wrong with their life. They have families and successful jobs. They find that our therapy fulfills them. They find something that they lost along the way and then they can experience life more fully.

R: The way I understand it, usually one cannot derive ones neurosis from one isolated instance of trauma.

N: There is prototypic pain. People will have a certain type of pain and it's compounded by many different experiences that reinforce a particular trauma. When they get the other traumas out of the way, they can focus on the original trauma.

R: It's like something way back that they can't quite reach? That "forgotten" trauma is what causes a certain type of behavior.

H: It can be reached ultimately through primal therapy. There is a sequence of laying down the pain which starts with severe prototypic pain in an individual who is very open. This is continually added to throughout childhood. Primal therapy is that whole process in reverse.

R: What is the difference between a child born by the Leboyer method and one born to bright lights and typical traumatizing hospital procedures? It's a neat type of birth experience to have. But what is the ultimate difference?

H: Have you seen children that were born by the Leboyer method?

R: I gave birth to my own baby that way. He was circumcised 8 days later. I don't know if that "undid" the whole thing. He's a sweet, happy, loving child. So are my other two sons and they were born in typical hospital settings.

N: If you give birth by the Leboyer method, you are eliminating at least some of the trauma that the child would have experienced with bright lights and other circumstances.

R: Have any differences in Leboyer-born children been objectively observed?

H: There is one study that followed 104 children born by the Leboyer method for 9 years. Of those 104, 100 of them were truly ambidextrous. Also, they were not afraid to try new things. That [fear of new experiences] is something quite characteristic of children born conventionally. Thus the transition from in utero to outside appears to have some long-lasting learning value for the child. If that first transition was easy to take, then later transitions are apparently easier to take. Also, one gets the subjective impression that Leboyer-born children are more serene and tranquil than children born by the conventional method. I can see it by the relaxation muscles. They have a placid, almost beatific look to their faces.

P: Being ambidextrous is important because it has to do with brain functions.

H: The left hemisphere for 92% of people becomes the hemisphere in which one is dominant for speech and handedness. But the left hemisphere is also recruited as part of the defense against pain. Thus verbal cognitive defenses against pain are very common. That is related to the prominent right-handedness in people. In primal therapy people become more bidextrous. They don't become truly ambidextrous because it is many years later. The implication of true ambidexterity *[in Leboyer-born children]* is that the left hemisphere did not need to be recruited as a specialized, repressing portion of the brain, in the service of neurosis ... in the service of keeping one unaware of pain.

R: I can't say that I fully understand that!

N: The first time he explained it to me, I had no idea what he meant!

H: A three-year-old born by the conventional method would be predominantly right-handed, would be extremely verbal, and would be using words to defend against pain. Whereas a Leboyer-born child would be using both hands and would be speaking in a much more feeling way, not to repress pain but to express need. The brain is utilized differently in a person who has been hurt a lot in infancy.

P: You understand that the left side of the brain controls the right side of the body, and vice versa. So when a person is right-handed, the left side of the brain has a lot of power, energy, and strength, and it's used to repress feelings. Neurologically that's a known fact. That's why people who stutter don't stutter when they sing. Singing and feeling come from the right side of the brain. If someone is ambidextrous there's an equal power on both sides of the brain. Then the person could use his or her left hand equally well.

H: Which is related to feelings, emotions and expressions.

R: What would cause someone to be left-handed?

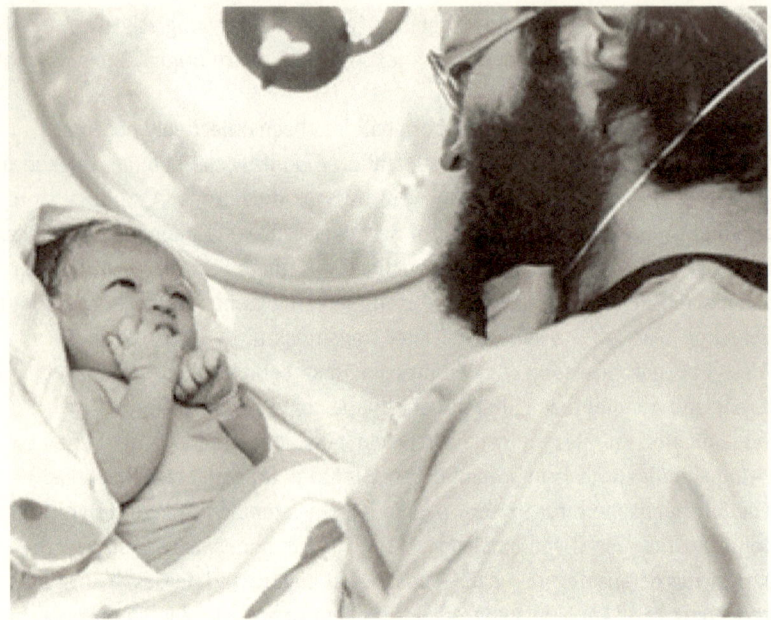

© *Suzanne Arms*

H: That's not well understood. 85% of people are left-hemisphere dominant for speech and right-handed. 7 ½% of people are left-hemisphere dominant for speech and left-handed. That means 92 ½% of people are left-hemisphere dominant for speech. Another 7 ½% of people are left-handed and right-hemisphere dominant for speech. There are anatomical differences between the left and right hemispheres. Embryologically the left hemisphere has many more neurons in it than the right hemisphere. Left-handedness can be genetic. It can also evolve in an individual who had impairment early in development, so that the right hemisphere becomes the dominant one.

R: My oldest son is left-handed. My youngest[34] who was born with Leboyer techniques appears to be solely right-handed. Maybe the circumcision took the other side away from him?

H: It is an important neurological finding that Leboyer-born children tend to be ambidextrous. But I'm not sure that because a person is right-handed or left-handed that they necessarily had a certain kind of pain in childhood. There are other factors which determine handedness.

---

34 This interview took place in 1978 after my third child was born. I later gave birth to three more children, two daughters and another son. Interestingly, my fourth son, born in 1985 and left intact happens to be left handed. Of additional interest, one of my right handed children is left foot dominant. Another one is left eye dominant. Apparently this is a genetic trait from my husband's side of the family. – R.R.

R: There is a feeling, especially among those of us who espouse such things as natural births, bonding, breastfeeding and such ... kind of a prevailing attitude of "You do it exactly this way or you don't quite measure up!" Sometimes pursuing a certain method takes priority over the actual needs of the infant. What is resulting is feelings of guilt and failure. Some parents feel "I didn't do right by my child. I have an inferior child because something went wrong." This can result from a Caesarian birth, or medication during birth, or a baby that needed surgery, or the decision to circumcise.

H: Our point of view is not that the child is "inferior" but that a child who has had trauma is *different* than he or she would have been without the trauma.

N: I'm a parent too. It's important for parents to realize that the *intent* is not to hurt the child. Sometimes people don't know the information because nothing has been published. It's like when nobody knew that smoking was harmful.

R: 20 to 30 years ago parents were led to believe that the baby wouldn't breathe right away unless the doctor spanked him!

N: Circumcision is the same kind of thing.

H: You can't change what has already happened. But you can allow them to react to pains in the present by letting them express their feelings. Parents can allow their children to express their concern, their upset, their frustration, their anger.

N: It's important that parents not allow themselves to get too hung up with guilt feelings because that will affect how they relate to that child.

R: What about the baby that has to have necessary traumatic medical procedures? I have spoken to mothers who have had badly jaundiced babies who have had to have several heel sticks. The mothers are worried about the trauma that the baby went through. Should parents seek to avoid procedures such as vitamin K shots, PKU heel sticks, or silver nitrate in the eyes in order to spare the baby the trauma?

H: Some things are medically necessary. In the case of a very jaundiced child, it's important to know the bilirubin count. But circumcision is elective.

N: Severe jaundice can result in permanent brain damage and so can PKU. Circumcision certainly does not fall into the same category.

R: What if parents have a Leboyer birth and have a boy and later have him circumcised? Some people just aren't thinking. Leboyer births have become the latest fad. People are asking for Leboyer births and signing circumcision papers at the same time. Does the latter "undo" the former?

H: If the birth is benevolent it is a great favor to the child. This has helped the child for a lifetime. But any subsequent trauma is traumatic whether it happens at 8 days, 8 years, or 18 years. It is better to have a Leboyer birth followed by circum-

cision than to have a conventional birth followed by circumcision. You don't "undo" a good experience.
R: What are the long-range detrimental effects of circumcision during infancy?
H: In general there has been an increase in the total burden of pain.
P: It has a completely different meaning and outcome for each person. I'm Jewish and I had the Bris at 8 days. Someone who had it done in the hospital by a doctor shortly after birth would experience it differently.
R: What can you tell me about your recollection of circumcision through primal therapy?
P: I remember being strapped down. I remember the Mohel. I remember several men. They're wearing dark clothes and some of the guys had beards. I see it as a bunch of evil leering monsters who are going to devour me. The feeling was that they were taking something from me. I had something they wanted and they took it from me, and I was totally helpless!!
R: Did you feel pain during the memory?
P: Oh sure! It really wasn't as much physical pain as it was pure abject terror! I mean ... you're this big, you're being strapped down!! The physical sensation isn't as bad as the psychological effect. The mental image I have is a lot more painful than the actual cutting. They sort of converge on me and the terror is so great that I almost ... I can't feel the physical pain because the mental pain is so great!!
H: The *meaning* of the trauma is the most painful thing, not the trauma per se.
R: So if you had gotten stuck on your diaper pin, that would have hurt, but it wouldn't have been the same.
P: I think human beings are capable of tolerating a certain amount of physical pain. Like you said, the kid falls down and scrapes his knee. I don't think those things are traumas. It's the meaning that's attached to it that's important. If your father deliberately stuck you with a pin that would be different than if you accidentally got stuck by a pin.
N: However, so many people think that babies don't experience pain when they're circumcised. When I watch people having the re-experience of circumcision, there *is* physical pain.
P: The pain that I experienced was afterwards. Initially I was petrified. When they did it to me I could feel the moment and I was completely numb with fear. But as my fear subsided the feeling went right back down here. It just hurt for days until it healed. During the time I was constantly aware that I was hurting, but my feeling is that it has to do with them hurting me and taking something from me. Every time I was aware of that pain, the throbbing and the healing process, I kept seeing this scene, and my body kept going into it! I was just terrified until the

pain went away. As long as it took to heal I was in absolute terror and agony ... for days.

There are two different parts to the feeling for me. One is the scene of having it happen and one is the aftermath. And the aftermath is just as bad! I could feel something trying to *turn me off*. Since the pain is there I cannot tolerate the terror in the same intensity that it was first initiated upon me. If it's 100% terror when it's happening, the body cannot tolerate that amount of pain. The only thing I could do was to turn off and shut down because the healing process is so painful.

N: But, Leslie, after you experienced and relived this by having the primal, how did you find that insight that what had happened affected your life?

P: Basically I understood why. I had a very strange birth. Then I had the Bris. Later I had my tonsils out. Then I had a hernia operation when I was three. So most of my life I was numb to feelings. I didn't know what the word "feelings" meant. I felt like I went into shock. I've also relived the hernia operation. I can relive the incision but that's not really the pain of it. The part that freaked me out is that my mother took me to the hospital and told me that she wouldn't leave me and that everything would be all right. Then when they went to put me under with the gas, I thought "she sent me here to be killed!"

H: I had a similar experience at age 10. Even for a ten-year-old your mind is not developed enough to realize that this is a service of a medical operation. The child feels that he's being assaulted. A child does not make sense out of a surgical procedure the way an adult would. One of the most important things that the parent can do is to stay with the child during the procedure if he is to remain conscious, or until the anesthesia has taken effect, if he is being put under.

R: I'm glad to hear you say this. When my second son Jason was two he had to have some stitches taken in his forehead. The doctor made me leave during the stitching. He said if I stayed there Jason would associate the trauma with me and get mad at me since he wouldn't know why I wasn't rescuing him.

H: That's just bullshit!!

R: Does an isolated physically painful experience really cause psychological maladjustment? Is a circumcision during infancy really going to screw somebody up for life?

H: What is relevant is whether a person was able to fully experience and respond to that trauma at any age. If there's some part of the healing reaction left over, it contributes to neurosis. What's relevant is whether a person could react to it fully and integrate it.

R: We have raised goats and we have their horn buds removed by disbudding them. The procedure is horrible. They're encased in this little box with just their heads sticking out. You take this hot electric iron and you burn into the animal's skull to kill the horn bud. Our friends who do this have observed that if the animal has been a pet and has had a lot of stroking then they almost always scream during the procedure. But if the animal has not been made into a pet, then they just stand there and take it.

H: That's closely related to a human counterpart which is that if a child goes to a hospital himself for an operation, he's likely not to cry during the whole hospitalization. But if the mother is there, the child will cry incessantly. Until about 1952 this was interpreted as meaning that parents should not be with children in hospitals. Finally people became more enlightened and realized that the children were crying because it was safe to cry in the presence of their parents.

R: To the doctors and nurses I'm sure it is a lot easier if the child isn't making any noise.

H: It's at the expense of the child. The child has to hold on to pain in a neurotic way which means pushing pain back which is later expressed in other ways.

R: Sometimes when babies are being circumcised they don't appear to respond to it. They don't cry. They shrink within themselves and don't react to it openly.

H: It's like the example of the baby goats. Is it safe for that child to cry? I would guess that if a mother is holding the child during circumcision the child would cry in agony ... but why circumcise? When a kid is eight days old and he's strapped to a board, it's not safe to utter a peep! The whole body has to draw within and clamp down on that experience.

R: Is this what you see people do when they're reliving circumcision?

N: When they relive it they cry and express their feelings ... the fear, the agony.

R: So evidently if a person is circumcised as a newborn he undergoes a severe trauma and as a result he is "not what he could have been" had he not had that experience. Some of our greatest spiritual leaders in ancient times ... Jesus and the prophets and the apostles ... all would have been circumcised as infants. Are you saying that these men would have all been better people had they never been circumcised?!!

H: It doesn't make a value judgment about whether a person is good, bad, or indifferent. It just means that they still have some pain to express from their childhood. In the absence of that expression it will tend to come out in other ways ... insomnia, psychosomatic symptoms. If a child has been circumcised, that child has been traumatized. The child is a different sort of person than he would have been had he never had that pain.

R: But Jesus was circumcised as an infant, and He's supposed to be the most perfect person that there ever was.

H: I don't want to get into a ...

P: No comment!

N: You are placing a value judgment on Jesus and ... we really can't answer that!!

R: In some hospitals they do immediate circumcision right there in the delivery room. In other hospitals they wait a day or two. Do you find a difference in the person who was circumcised immediately compared to the individual who was circumcised a few days later, as to what he would re-experience?

H: In general the earlier the trauma, the more vulnerable the child.

R: My basic feeling is that if you have to have it done, you should wait a few days. I think the worst thing would be to have it be his very first sensation in life.

P: At birth you are in so much shock and agony, you're shut down already. Maybe that s the time to have it.

H: I think it just should not be done. It's an avoidable trauma.

R: I agree. But do you find a difference?

N: No. It's totally individual. Both seem to be equally as bad.

P: What's worse, a crack on the hand with a hammer today or tomorrow? When you're that little those kinds of things are about 20 times more painful than you could tolerate to begin with. Whether it's done on the same day that you're born, or two days later, or eight days later ... if it's traumatic, it's traumatic. If we could absorb all the pain ... and the meaning that it has, that you're taking something from me ... that I feel unloved ... that I'm not getting what I need ... if we had tolerance for the entire amount of pain, the trauma would be resolved. Unfortunately we can't do that.

H: What I said about the timing of pain should be considered more in relation to months. If the child were circumcised at six months of age, it would be quite different than if it happened within the first month.

P: In terms of the development of the brain and the way that it can handle pain, that makes perfect sense.

H: The older the child the greater his ability to defend against pain.

R: Yet at six months parents and doctors would pay more attention to the child's reaction. At this age the child would *look* more like he's afraid and scream louder. They have more of a "personality" by then.

P: Right. They get them while they're helpless. They think they're not feeling anything right after birth and when they're six months old they can.

H: One newborn baby is extremely similar in behavior patterns to another newborn baby. When individual personal past experience begins to be reflected in a child's behavior you see the development of "personality." "Personality" in the individual characteristics derives almost entirely from maturation of the cerebral cortex which is virtually non-functional in the newborn. So that euphemism about the child's developing personality is just talking about a neural schedule, a maturation of the cortex. But the baby can feel pain at any age.

R: We just haven't thought of newborn babies as being people.

P: The way they protest is meaningless. If your mother called us now and said Michael, you're going to be circumcised.

H: Well, I certainly would react differently than I would have at that age!!!

P: In those days they could just pick you up and do it to you. Today they'd have to work to convince you. They'd have to bribe you ...

H: Extort me!! Kill me!!

R: There are different types of circumcision devices. There are clamps. The Plastibell is a ring of plastic that stays in place for about a week. If a person relives his circumcision, is he aware of which device was used?

N: No. It hurts regardless.

R: My gut feeling is to tell my sons not to ever go through primal therapy because they would have to relieve that pain of having been circumcised.

P: Well, I'm glad I did because of the meaning that it had for me. There's always been a certain kind of person that has terrified me during my whole life, based on that experience. There's a certain smell that I associate with that time. There's a certain look that I associate with the people involved. Before I had the therapy those kind of experiences used to bring up that same feeling. I had absolutely no idea why I disliked certain kinds of people. There was a certain religious overtone to this thing that I've always disliked.

R: Did you perceive it as a spiritual or religious experience?

P: No. But later on going to temple, there was always a certain uneasy feeling about meeting the Rabbi and the other men. They all had black hats and beards and they had a certain smell. Those were the guys that did it to me and I always shied away from them.

H: One has irrational fears until you know where the fear came from.

P: That memory remained with me my whole life. In some way I was responding to people in a certain way based on that experience. Whenever anybody tried to take something away from me it made me feel utterly helpless, and panicked and tense. Anybody who wanted to do something similar to that ... it would bring up that feeling. It's not very pleasant going through life being afraid of people.

R: How do your parents feel about that? Do they know? Do they feel guilty?

H: He went through primal therapy because he wanted to. It had nothing to do with his parents.

P: I haven't ever discussed that particular issue with my parents. My mother is pretty open about how she wiped me out when I was a kid. But she was a child herself when I was born. At that time people didn't know any better.

N: When people go through primal therapy and relive their infancy, they don't blame and judge their parents.

R: The books about primal therapy gave me that impression. I felt "This is fascinating, but these parents are real villains!"

H: No. That's not true. Parents do painful things to their children by accident or out of ignorance. But when you go through primal therapy you don't call your mother or father on the telephone and bawl them out.

N: Often it's just the reverse. Many people come into this therapy feeling hostile toward their parents. After understanding the isolated experiences that caused their traumas, sometimes they can have a relationship with their parents in the present that they didn't have previously.

H: Whether your children ultimately want primal therapy should be their decision, not yours or your husband's.

R: I agree. That was just my "gut" reaction! Finally, is primal therapy the same thing as rebirthing or natal therapy?

N: There's an enormous difference.

H: Rebirthing is age-regressing back to the ideas or visual impressions of one's birth. It's not a complete re-experience. It is mock primal therapy. It is dangerous because if a person had an extremely painful birth and they start to re-experience that in a swimming pool in the presence of someone who knows nothing about primal pain, then they're on the verge of psychosis! Primal pain comes up very hard for people. It produces incredible anxiety. Part of the goal of primal therapy is opening a person up to just so much pain, to give them time, and integrate it in a sequential, systematic way.

P: If they understood the way the brain was constructed they would realize that people could not connect birth experience consciousness and have its full meaning without second-line access which we call reliving other experiences that are less painful.

H: One has to go down to those painful experiences in a sequence over a long period of time. To go from the present to birth is like walking into a volcano. It's too much. It's impossible to integrate it.

18.6 Reports About Circumcisions

18.6.1 Shawn's Circumcision

Shawn was born in August of 1972 in Santa Fe, New Mexico. I had a short labor and a fairly un-traumatic birth – as much as can be expected in a hospital. I had natural childbirth and an unnecessary 3rd degree episiotomy. Shawn weighed 8 lbs. 6 oz. and was 21 inches long. I remember looking at his penis and thinking how strange it looked. (I'd never seen an uncircumcised baby before.) It took me two days to get up the courage to ask the nurse if my baby was "OK" and if his penis was "normal." She laughed and assured me they all looked that way and that he'd look "normal" after he was circumcised. I repeatedly asked the doctor if it would hurt Shawn and he repeatedly said "no," and that "it was better to do it now when it will heal quickly." So I signed the paper to have it done.

On the third day after his birth I decided to take a look at Shawn in the nursery. As I walked down the hall I heard him screaming. I rushed to the nursery and knocked on the window. The nurse came to the door and I asked where he was. She said "He's across the hall being circumcised." The next few minutes were a living hell, an eternity of torture as I listened to him scream as I have never heard anyone scream before or since. I wanted to burst through the door and say "Stop! Stop!" But I didn't know what they were doing or how long it would take. Finally the doctor came out. "Is he all right?!" I asked in panic. "You have a very strong little boy there," he said. "It took three nurses to hold him down. He did *not* like what we did to him *at all*, but he'll be fine."

A nurse brought him to me and I took him to my room. I told him I was sorry and that I didn't know it would hurt him so badly. He nursed and fell asleep. We went home from the hospital the next day. He healed and I didn't think much about it again.

Then a year and a half later, when Shawn was 19 months old, the real problems began. Shawn awakened screaming in his bed!! He flung himself and thrashed and screamed and repeatedly was brought to a position of a crucifix as if someone was holding him down. I could not wake or comfort him. He screamed for 45 minutes and then fell back to sleep. I was horrified. I had never experienced anything like this before. The next morning he did not remember anything.

He went through this same thing about once a week for two years. Times varied from 30 minutes to 1 ½ hours, but always the same high-pitched screaming, thrashing, and as he became older and more verbal he began saying, "No, no, no!!", holding his genitals, and then as if someone was holding him down, he would fling himself into the circumcision position and struggle there. Then he'd break loose of the imaginary hold, grab his penis, and scream "No, no, no!!" again. Back and forth he would go until he'd finally give up and go to sleep. He wouldn't let us comfort him. After a while we found that if he needed to urinate the screaming would last longer and if we could get him to go to the bathroom he'd usually fall asleep after that.

He started doing it about once a month when he was 3 ½. Since he was 5 he has only done it about two times a year. He still does not consciously know he has ever done this. We have told him about it in detail and he cannot remember having these experiences. He does have nightmares occasionally and he will remember these the next day. We can awaken him after a bad dream and comfort him. This other thing that he does is not dreaming.

When Shawn was 2 ½ I spoke with Arthur Janov at a Birth/Rebirth Conference in Santa Cruz, Calif. I described Shawn's behavior to him. He agreed that it was a typical circumcision trauma. He said to let him scream it out, to comfort him as much as one could, but not to worry, he would outgrow it.

When our second son, Peter, was born in 1979, my husband Jim and I had a hearty discussion about whether or not to have him circumcised. Jim felt concern that Peter wouldn't "match" him and Shawn. I couldn't believe that after all we'd been through, he'd even consider it! So I got out articles pro and con – O.B. texts, pediatric books, Mothering Magazine articles – for him to read. I told him that after he knew as much about it as I did I would then discuss it and if he still wanted to get it done I would agree. He never mentioned the subject again. Peter is still intact. I think men have a very difficult time dealing with this whether they admit it or not.

Vicki Campbell, Las Cruces, NM

18.6.2 One Man's Story

I was born in a hospital in Colorado and was circumcised there. Because my mother left the hospital the day after I was born, I must have been circumcised within 24 hours of being born. My mother tells me that I was an unusual baby because I slept so frequently. I fell asleep instantly whenever she changed my diaper or whenever she placed me in bath water. Believing that there was something wrong with me, my mother took me to her doctor. He gave me a clean bill of health. I believe that this was a conditioned response to circumcision trauma.

I grew up on a farm and while I was a pre-schooler we had a cow which provided milk for our family. When I was three years old, my mother purchased a cream separator from an older couple. I recall that they were very friendly and that they doted on me when we went to pick up the cream separator. The separator consisted of two pieces of machinery that I remember vividly: a black cast iron apparatus in the shape of a goose neck and a stainless steel basin. The night after we purchased it I had a nightmare. I had the same nightmare again and again for several weeks. In my dream I am strapped to a black table, unable to move. I am naked. Between my legs, the black gooseneck apparatus of the cream separator is clamped to the edge of the table. To my right is a shiny, steel basin. The old woman who sold us the cream separator looms over my face. She smiles and tweaks my cheeks. I remember her big teeth. Behind her is her husband. He has a knife in his hand. He slices off part of my penis. He is emotionless. I do not feel pain, but anger, nausea and powerlessness. I am especially angry with the woman. How can she be smiling while I am being butchered? I try to kick away the knife, but I cannot. I am simply incapable of making my muscles do what I want them to do. I wake up feeling nauseous. This is the earliest dream I can recall, and the picture remains vivid in my mind to this day.

I am told that our dreams are merely our brains' attempt to make sense of random electrical impulses. I am also told that infants cannot truly see anything because their eyes are unable to focus immediately after birth. However, I cannot get over the striking resemblance between a Gomco clamp and the black gooseneck of my mother's cream separator. And why does the stainless steel basin – ever-present at all circumcisions – fit so prominently into my dream? I believe that my circumcision produced an electrical pattern in my brain that was something less than random, a template of sorts waiting for the right environmental objects to give it shape.

I believe that if parents are present during the circumcision of their son, they should not be within his sight. I do not believe that the presence of parents would be comforting or reassuring to the baby. He might believe, instead, that his parents are responsible for the act. He cannot understand their words or accurately interpret their facial expressions or gestures. In my dream, I believe that the smiling woman who distracts me and tweaks my cheeks is responsible for my being butchered. The message is confusing and not to be trusted.

I do not blame my parents for what happened to me. I believe that they chose to have me circumcised thinking that they were doing something good for me. My father was not circumcised. Perhaps he believed he was giving me an advantage he didn't have. I believe that I did have some problems identifying with my father because we were different.

It is ironic that today one of the arguments for circumcision is that the boys, if left intact, might have trouble identifying with their circumcised fathers. Why didn't physicians think of that in the 'fifties, 'forties and 'thirties (when most fathers were not circumcised)? With the practice originating so recently, the identification problem must have occurred in every family at one time or another.

(Name and address withheld by request)

18.7 Interview With a Pediatrician About Pain

Dr. Justin Call, M.D., Psychoanalyst, Pediatrician, Child Psychiatrist, Professor in Chief of Child and Adolescent Psychiatry, School of Medicine, University of California, Irvine

Dr. Call: As a pediatrician and as an intern in a hospital I used to do circumcisions. I was taught that the best time to do a circumcision was right at birth in the delivery room. It was a matter of convenience.

Rosemary: Why has neonatal circumcision become a routine procedure in U.S. hospitals?

C: Nobody can tell you what the scientific indications are for circumcision. With armies traveling in a desert, if the males are circumcised, they have fewer infections and swellings of the foreskin than individuals who have not been circumcised. This is under unhygienic, hot conditions. The other reason is the religious ritual.

R: What do you think about pain and trauma experienced by the infant during circumcision?

C: If you ask the question "Does the baby feel pain?" You *bet* he feels pain!! The helpless, panicky cry of an infant when circumcised is an abnormal kind of cry. It is a breathless, high-pitched cry that is never heard in other normally occurring circumstances. Then sometimes babies who are being circumcised do exactly the opposite. They lapse into a semi-coma. Both of these states, helpless crying and semi-coma are abnormal states in the newborn.

R: The semi-coma state must explain why some babies don't cry while being circumcised. This makes people assume that it didn't hurt the baby.

C: That's right. Also people don't distinguish between that high-pitched, panicky, breathless cry and a normal loud cry. And people don't make the distinction between sleep and semi-coma. A very interesting study was done by Dr. Robert Emde and Dr. David Metcalf, et al.[35] at the University of Colorado Medical Center. They studied the sleep-wakefulness cycles of infants in relation to circumcision. They found that in the 24 hours following circumcision, a great deal more time was spent by the infant in a state of subdued sleep ... withdrawal. This is the opposite of what people would expect.

R: What about using anesthesia for circumcising babies?

C: Administering anesthesia to a child is a risky procedure. Doctors would love not to use it if they could get away with it. Also they prefer not to use a local anesthetic because it swells the tissues. They can get a better closure of the tissues if they're not swollen.

The rationale for circumcision that some doctors give is phimosis. This means that the foreskin cannot be drawn back beyond the edge of the glans. This is uncommon in the naturally occurring event when one does nothing about the fore-

---

35 Emde RN, Harmon RJ, Metcalf D, Koenig KL, Wagonfeld S. Stress and Neonatal Sleep. *Psychosom Med.* 1971/Nov-Dec; 33(6): 491-7.

skin. Phimosis[36] is normal in the newborn. The foreskin will naturally loosen and become easily drawn back by the time the child is a few years old. The operation of clipping the skin under the tongue to correct "tongue tie" used to be a popular procedure. Many doctors thought that the tongue should be able to protrude fully beyond the mouth. It has now been shown that the tongue lies in the mouth cavity and does not protrude in the newborn, but normally as the child grows older it will come out. That operation is rarely done any more.

R: I have interviewed a mother whose son was circumcised at age three. She said that his foreskin had started to grow back over the head of his penis so that he was having difficulty urinating. I wonder if his case could have been treated differently.

C: Usually phimosis can be treated successfully without circumcision or surgery of any kind. I don't know the child's circumstances.

I don't recommend that any attention be paid to the foreskin until it loosens easily. After that the mother should draw it back occasionally to clean it. I have known that some mothers develop an obsession ... a highly exciting sexual ritual around the drawing back of the baby's foreskin several times a day. So it can definitely be overdone!

R: Apart from the immediate painful effects, how do you think the trauma of circumcision affects the individual throughout his life?

C: Some people have thought that circumcision is the first real castration and subsequent castration anxiety borrows some of its power from the earlier experience with circumcision. I don't know if that theory has any validity.

But in the immediate newborn period, I believe that circumcision has a disruptive effect on the development of the mother-infant bond, because of the changes in the state of the infant. This interferes with the mother-infant bond just as medication would. The bond has been disrupted.

18.8 Interview With the Founder of the Association for Childbirth At Home

Tonya Brooks

(Tonya is the president and founder of the Association for Childbirth at Home, International, Los Angeles, CA. She worked on her Ph.D. in psychology with research done in early developmental psychology and development of infants. She is a lay

---

[36] "Phimosis" is actually an incorrect term for the normally tight, adherent foreskin of the newborn. "Phimosis" should only be applied to the abnormally tight or adherent foreskin of an older individual.

midwife, and the mother of six children, five of whom were born at home. Four of her children are intact sons.)

Tonya: I have assisted with nine circumcisions of infant sons of parents whose births I had attended. The doctor believed that babies did better if someone was holding them. I had to lean over them and hold their legs prone. It took my whole body to hold down a newborn for circumcision.

Rosemary: It must have been hard for you to watch.

T: Yes. I hated to watch the babies cry. But the hardest thing for me was to watch parents who did not seem to want it done. Twice I've watched the mothers cry. In one case the mother did not want her baby circumcised, but her husband did. It was extremely unfortunate that she who was taking the responsibility for it questioned the decision, and he, who wanted it done, wasn't even there. I have rarely seen a mother who wanted circumcision.

My feeling against circumcision is that it is the child's body and you have to grant every person a "beingness."

R: Would you say that your experiences with circumcisions have been quite traumatic?

T: I was bothered intellectually by it. But I've watched parents become traumatized. My concern is that babies have undifferentiated pain responses. They feel pain all over their bodies. I think it is more traumatic for babies to be circumcised within a few hours after birth. If you watch babies who have had easy births, their faces don't look like they're pained. Babies who have had difficult births ... you can tell by looking at them that they have been in pain. If you take a traumatized baby and subject him to circumcision, you're more likely to get a problem. You should at least wait until the baby has had a chance to be loved and calmed down before having a circumcision. Just because a baby has less differentiated pain response does not mean that it is less traumatic for him than it would be for someone older. It just seems less traumatic to adults because they don't cry as long.

R: Sometimes when babies are circumcised they really scream. Other times they don't make much noise. I wonder now if they retreat into themselves following a traumatic birth and are unable to cry out when they are circumcised.

T: When a person is injured, he can react in one of two ways. He can yell! This is a more pro-survival response than the kind of injury in which the person is so traumatized that he can't cry out. Have you ever closed your hand in a car door and it hurt so badly that you couldn't yell?! In four of the nine circumcisions that I have seen, the baby didn't cry. He just seemed to be suddenly in a state of shock! That's always easier on the parents because we expect crying to be a measure of pain.

R: We have had baby goats disbudded with the cauterizing iron burning the horn bud out of the animal's skull. Our friends who do this have observed that if the animal is a pet, if it has gotten a lot of loving from humans, then it will scream when it is being disbudded. But if it has not been a pet, it will just stand there and take it. I find that intriguing.

T: To be able to cry out is better. What you describe doesn't mean that it's less traumatic for the goats who haven't been loved, it's more. The pet goats are more able to communicate pain. So that may explain why some babies don't cry in response to being circumcised. I have seen babies so socked into it that they've been almost unconscious. I would feel more comfortable about a baby that cried than one who didn't. It's harder on the parents because screaming drives home the fact that the child has been injured, but the response is healthier for the child.

R: Some babies start to scream as soon as they are strapped to the circumcision board. Some babies scream when they're just being examined. So sometimes trauma is not connected to pain at all, but being held down and invaded and "messed with."

T: A baby that has just been born has gone from a warm, enclosed environment out into the cold, with bright lights, and they're put on a table and stretched out. That's traumatic. It's an assault on his person. That's one of the reasons I want parents to control births, so they can pick that baby up in their arms and not have anyone else mess with their baby.

R: What do you believe about the lasting effect of circumcision trauma?

T: I believe that trauma has a cumulative effect. I would like to keep my children from having as many injuries as possible. I guess it is very individualistic. Trauma during infancy may cause a child to be less responsive and more introspective. Things can be done about that. An extreme example would be a child who has been abused. I suppose that if a child was simply circumcised as an infant, he would grow up without any problems ... but there are later traumas. Possibly if a child was circumcised as an infant and the injury was so traumatic that he buried it in his subconscious, and then the first time he wanted to make love he'd have difficulty. I doubt that would happen.

R: I have wondered about the way my first son Eric screamed every time his diaper was changed when he was a newborn. This kept up for three weeks. I wonder if it was like operant conditioning. He was circumcised the first time his diaper was ever taken off, so he imprinted on the idea of "pants taken off, this part of me uncovered ... pain!!" It took several diaper changes, long after the wound itself had healed, for that behavior to be unlearned.

T: You have a conscious, analytical mind, and a reactive or subconscious mind that controls memory banks. The subconscious is the conditioned response part of the mind, where your habits are. This is where you react without reasoning. If you have been in a car accident, the first time you drive again you react with fear every time somebody comes at you.

R: Circumcision is a form of body alteration. What do you think? Do parents really have the right to alter their children's bodies in this manner?

T: I wouldn't assume to alter someone else's body unless it were needed physiologically. If a baby had a birth defect that could be corrected by cosmetic surgery, I would not hesitate. I suppose if I or my husband had been Jewish we would have had our sons circumcised. I would supersede if my child would be ostracized culturally.

R: It is very hard to question your own culture.

T: I have become increasingly less tolerant of cultural influences. One's culture has to be a consideration, but parents should give more consideration to this child in present time and what his life is going to be like. If the family is deeply involved in Judaism, went to Temple faithfully, their son would later have a Bar Mitzvah, then I suppose they should have the Bris. But otherwise people should really think about it. I know of one family whose little boy asked to be circumcised at age 6.

R: It was his decision.

T: Yes. If it hurts, it's not going to affect him traumatically because it was his decision. If any of my boys asks to be circumcised when he gets older, I'll let him get circumcised.

R: What would you say to parents if it's after the fact ... whether they had a traumatic birth, or a Caesarian, or a prolonged separation from the baby, or a circumcision? With all the ideals we've been striving for, some parents can feel that they've failed.

T: The parents should think in present time. They should give that child a lot of emotional support and love ... not anything other than good mothering. If the child has a problem I would encourage him to communicate.

R: With our involvement in home birth and our concern about babies having non-traumatic birth – what are our goals? It is impossible to live in this world without ever feeling pain.

T: The reasons are individualistic, but we should get the baby into this world with as little trauma as possible. Doctors may claim "Well, it's not that big of a deal. All of us have been born and we're all just fine!" But there is evidence that how we're born very definitely affects our emotional and psychological well-being. I have no doubt that severe birth trauma does cause long-term effect. The home birth movement is a commitment to this. Doctors have attacked the home birth movement on medical issues, but they have got to realize that the psychological aspects of birth are every bit as important as the medical ones!!

18.9   Conclusions

Most parents try to do everything that they believe will be beneficial to their infants and children. As parents we constantly experience guilt, frustration and exasperation as new idea after new idea comes along telling us to do things yet another way. As I write this I can envision other parents in kindred spirit crying "Just when I thought I was doing everything right, somebody comes along telling us that we've done something terribly wrong!!"

In 1972 when I was expecting my first child I was full of ideals and philosophies of how I would do everything right when raising my children. Today I have six children. (Now they are all adults.) I recall days when I felt that I was doing my best if I could get everybody into shoes that matched! I have seen many of my ideals "go down the drain," yet in total perspective, raising children has been a positive experience.

How important is a child's circumcised or intact penis in perspective of all that will be important in his life? I frequently have found myself caught up in a dilemma of perspective as I have worked on this manuscript, concentrating on traumas inflicted on infants, while meanwhile one or more of my children is crying or needing my immediate attention. What began in part out of personal need to resolve my own remorse over the trauma that my babies suffered has, over the years, grown into an expression of my need for intellectual fulfillment.

The trauma of the circumcision operation and lifelong deprivation of one's foreskin cannot be denied or dismissed as insignificant. We cannot afford to ignore the importance of events that surround the beginning of life. However, those of us who specialize in birth often tend to become so caught up in the importance of birth related events that we forget that the rest of our children's lives are equally important. In perspective, I do believe that many other things are more important in a child's life. I undertook this research in part because I saw a dire need for information on circumcision. Other concerns such as nutrition, breastfeeding, early childhood education, etc. are already being given attention by many other people.

So many factors contribute to the ultimate psychological makeup of an individual, that it is extremely difficult to know how any one isolated event has affected him or her. Despite all of my knowledge, I have no way of knowing how my own sons are affected today by the painful operation that they underwent during infancy. As children they were healthy, usually happy, and seemingly oblivious to their lack of foreskins. Their younger brother, who has been left intact, came along in 1985. Although

18 – Is Circumcision Traumatic For a Newborn Baby?

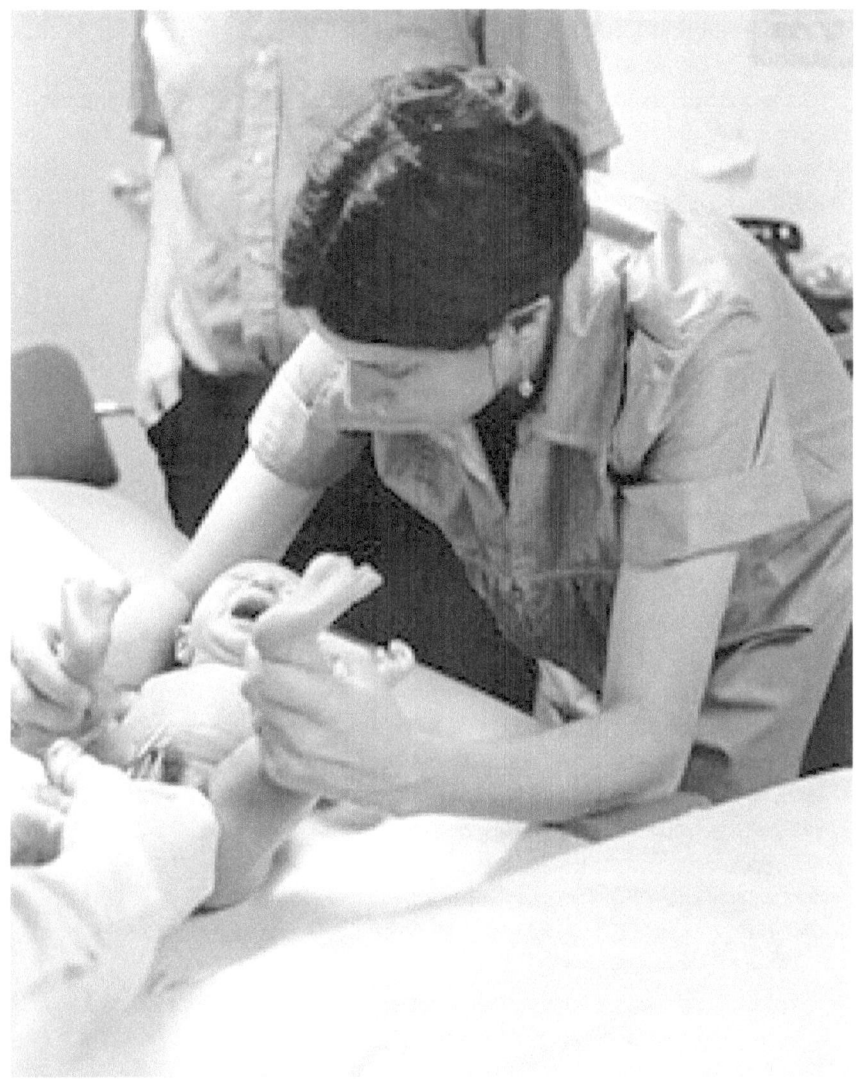

© *Suzanne Arms*

they all would tease and pester each other as much as any normal siblings, I have never heard the subject of foreskins or lack of same mentioned. Now that my three older sons are adult men, the issue is too painful and personal for me, as their mother, to bring up to them directly, even thought they are well aware of my life work in this field. I have maintained a close, loving and communicative relationship with all of my children in practically all respects, but this issue lies too close to my heart to touch.

Being wanted, and provided the opportunity to grow up in a happy, loving family are of primary importance in the life of a child. Undoubtedly many little boys who have been abandoned and unwanted have also happened to have intact penises. Therefore, the choice against circumcision will only be relevant if considered within the context of love, acceptance and of wanting what is best for the child in his life.

18.10 Informational Resources

- 12 Tips for Gently Parenting Your Adult Children (Hint: It starts when they're newborns!):
  littleheartsbooks.com/2012/07/20/12-tips-for-gently-parenting-your-adult-children-hint-it-starts-when-theyre-newborns-2/
- 19 Year Study Finds Autism Higher Among Boys Who Were Circumcised as Infants:
  www.drmomma.org/2015/01/19-year-study-finds-autism-higher-among.html
- A "Wear and Tear" Hypothesis to Explain Sudden Infant Death Syndrome:
  frontiersin.org/articles/10.3389/fneur.2016.00180/full
- A Nursing Student is Introduced to Circumcision:
  thewholenetwork.org/twn-news/a-nursing-student-is-introduced-to-circumcision
- Adverse Effects of Pain on the Nervous Systems of Newborns and Young Children: A Review of the Literature: journals.lww.com/jnnonline/Abstract/2002/10000/
  Adverse_Effects_of_Pain_on_the_Nervous_Systems_of.2.aspx
- Alexithymia and Circumcision Trauma: A Preliminary Investigation: researchgate.net/publication/270190401
- Are There Long-Term Consequences of Pain in Newborn or Very Young Infants?:
  ncbi.nlm.nih.gov/pmc/articles/PMC1595204
- ASD And Circumcision Linked, With Thoughts Of Brain Development As A Factor:
  medicaldaily.com/asd-and-circumcision-linked-thoughts-brain-development-factor-318144
- Autism and Trauma: Calming Anxious Brains:
  aldridgepalay.com/resources/Currently-unused/Autism-and-Trauma--Calming-Anxious-Brains.pdf
- Babies feel pain 'like adults': https://www.ox.ac.uk/news/2015-04-21-babies-feel-pain-adults
- Babies Form Memories In Utero, Study Finds:
  bellybelly.com.au/pregnancy/babies-form-memories-in-utero-study-finds
- Babies Remember Pain: kindredmedia.org/2016/01/babies-remember-pain
- Bipolar Christianity: How Torturing "Sinful" Children Produced Holy Wars:
  psychohistory.com/books/the-origins-of-war-in-child-abuse/chapter-9-bipolar-%20christianity-how-torturing-sinful-children-produced-holy-wars
- Blender Swirl Nightmare – One Man's Story of Circumcision Pain and Healing:
  peacefulbeginningsrosemary.wordpress.com/circ-information/blender-swirl-nightmare
- Body Pleasure and the Origins of Violence: violence.de/prescott/bulletin/article.html

18 – Is Circumcision Traumatic For a Newborn Baby?

- Brain Visualization Research during Male Infant Circumcision:
  stopinfantcircumcision.org/BrainVisualizationArticle.htm
- Breastfeeding is natural ...: facebook.com/photo.php?fbid=1008204325868390&set=p.1008204325868390
- Breastfeeding must be given priority over circumcision: cirp.org/library/birth/hill1
- Breastfeeding/Chestfeeding & Your Baby: yourwholebaby.org/breastfeeding
- Can adverse neonatal experiences alter brain development and subsequent behavior?:
  pubmed.ncbi.nlm.nih.gov/10657682
- Can mental trauma be passed on through sperm?:
  nhs.uk/news/genetics-and-stem-cells/can-mental-trauma-be-passed-on-through-sperm
- CDC estimates 1 in 68 children has been identified with autism spectrum disorder:
  cdc.gov/media/releases/2014/p0327-autism-spectrum-disorder.html
- Children Who Experience Early Childhood Trauma Do Not 'Just Get Over It':
  swhelper.org/2014/10/08/children-experience-early-childhood-trauma-just-get
- CIA Mind Control Project Financed Circumcision Psychological Research:
  thoughtcrimeradio.net/2014/06/cia-mind-control-project-financed-circumcision-psychological-research
- Circumcised boys may be more likely to develop autism and ADHD by the age of 10, study claims:
  dailymail.co.uk/health/article-2902214
- Circumcising newborn boys increases their risk of cot death due to the stress of the procedure – and could explain why it is more common in boys than girls, study finds: dailymail.co.uk/health/article-5998771
- Circumcision and Breastfeeding (Resources): kellymom.com/ages/newborn/newborn-concerns/circumcision
- Circumcision and Pain: circumstitions.com/Pain.html
- Circumcision as Attenuated Homicides:
  salem-news.com/articles/november122011/circumcision-homicide-rm.php
- Circumcision doubls autism risk, study claims:
  telegraph.co.uk/men/active/mens-health/11334800/Circumcision-doubles-autism-risk-study-claims.html
- Circumcision Harms Breastfeeding:
  sisterhoodlc.wordpress.com/2015/11/03/circumcision-harms-breastfeeding/
- Circumcision in young boys can DOUBLE chance of developing autism:
  mirror.co.uk/news/uk-news/circumcision-young-boys-can-double-4945643
- Circumcision Increases Breastfeeding Complications:
  www.drmomma.org/2009/11/circumcision-leads-to-breastfeeding.html
- Circumcision is Torture and Child Abuse: returntonow.net/2016/03/02/circumcision-is-child-abuse-and-torture
- Circumcision Made Him Sick:
  web.archive.org/web/20150216001333/http://wholewoman.hubgarden.com/circumcision-made-him-sick
- Circumcision of Males / Females:
  canadiancrc.com/Circumcision_Genital_Mutilation_Male-Female_Children.aspx
- Circumcision Permanently Alters the Brain: circumcision.org/circumcision-permanently-alters-the-brain
- Circumcision policy: A psychosocial perspective: ncbi.nlm.nih.gov/pmc/articles/PMC2724127
- Circumcision Study Ends Early Due to Infant Trauma:

- facebook.com/photo.php?fbid=10153235670205407&set=p.10153235670205407
- Circumcision study halted due to trauma: edition.cnn.com/HEALTH/9712/23/circumcision.anesthetic
- Circumcision Trauma and Brain Damage:
    facebook.com/photo.php?fbid=10204737584823738&set=p.10204737584823738
- Circumcision vs. Child Health, Breastfeeding and Maternal Bonding: cirp.org/library/birth
- Circumcision, Pain, and the Risk of Autism Spectrum Disorders:
    evolutionaryparenting.com/circumcision-risk-of-autism
- Circumcision, Serial Killing, Criminal Behavior and American Medical Violence:
    salem-news.com/articles/august312012/circumcision-violence-rm.php
- Circumcision: Medicine Practicing Below the Usual and Customary Standards of Care in Ritual:
    salem-news.com/articles/september092011/circ-rituals-rm.php
- Circumcision: The doctor told me he wouldn't feel a thing:
    everythingbirthblog.com/2013/04/27/circumcision-the-doctor-told-me-he-wouldnt-feel-a-thing
- Circumcision's Psychological Damage:
    psychologytoday.com/intl/blog/moral-landscapes/201501/circumcision-s-psychological-damage
- Did You Know [...] NO pediatric health organization in the world recommends circumcision:
    facebook.com/photo.php?fbid=1008204302535059&set=p.1008204302535059
- Dracula's Circumcision: salem-news.com/articles/august152012/dracula-circumcision-rm.php
- Early Circumcision May Be A Major Cause Of Sudden Infant Death Syndrome: iflscience.com/health-and-medicine/early-circumcision-may-be-a-major-cause-of-sudden-infant-death-syndrome
- Effect of circumcision on urinary tract infection after successful antireflux surgery:
    pubmed.ncbi.nlm.nih.gov/15329127
- Effect of Neonatal Circumcision on Pain Response During Subsequent Routine Vaccination:
    cirp.org/library/pain/taddio2
- Emotional Care of Hospitalized Children: An Environmental Approach: amazon.com/dp/0397543433
- Ending Child Abuse, Wars and Terrorism: psychohistory.com/books/the-origins-of-war-in-child-abuse/chapter-12-ending-child-abuse-wars-and-terrorism
- Examining the Mental Effects of Paedocircumcision: Fundamentals: circumcisioncomplex.com/fundamentals
- Expecting and new mothers understand circumcision is absolutely detrimental to breastfeeding relationships, and in many cases it will terminate breastfeeding completely:
    facebook.com/AshleyKaidel/posts/1073710649308501
- Extreme trauma from male circumcision causes damage to areas of brain:
    naturalnews.com/048907_male_circumcision_brain_damage_child_abuse.html
- Fine-touch pressure thresholds in the adult penis: pubmed.ncbi.nlm.nih.gov/17378847
- Global Survey of Circumcision Harm: circumcisionharm.org/research.htm
- Global Wars to Restore U.S. Masculinity: psychohistory.com/books/the-origins-of-war-in-child-abuse/chapter-11-global-wars-to-restore-u-s-masculinity
- "He won't even remember being circumcised…":
    www.savingsons.org/2015/06/he-wont-even-remember-being-circumcised.html

- "Hey LLL Circumcision Affects Breastfeeding! Tell moms the truth!":
  facebook.com/CircumcisionHarmsBreastfeeding
- How the trauma of life is passed down in SPERM, affecting the mental health of future generations:
  dailymail.co.uk/health/article-2611317
- Impact of Birthing Practices on Breastfeeding: Protecting the Mother and Baby Continuum:
  cirp.org/library/birth/kroeger1
- Infant Circumcision Increases Rates of: facebook.com/photo.php?fbid=10156350566755440&set=p.10156350566755440
- Infant Circumcision: More Painful Than We Thought:
  mom.com/toddler/19802-infant-circumcision-more-painful-we-thought
- Infant Responses to Circumcision: circumcision.org/infant-responses-to-circumcision
- Infantile amnesia reflects a developmental critical period for hippocampal learning:
  facebook.com/photo.php?fbid=650759441747880&set=a.105147402975756.9541.100004414898074
- Infants Deeply Traumatized by Common Medical Procedures, New Study Suggests:
  wakeup-world.com/2016/08/20/infants-deeply-traumatized-by-common-medical-procedures-new-study-suggests
- Information on circumcision: to cut or not to cut, that is the question:
  existere.wordpress.com/2012/02/10/information-on-circumcision-to-cut-or-not-to-cut-that-is-the-question
- Is the Pain of Circumcision Truly 'Brief'?: www.drmomma.org/2011/04/is-pain-of-circumcision-truly-brief.html
- Long-Term Adverse Effects of Circumcision:
  i2researchhub.org/articles/ch-6-long-term-adverse-effects-of-circumcision-doc-genital-integrity-statement
- Male circumcision decreases penile sensitivity as measured in a large cohort:
  pubmed.ncbi.nlm.nih.gov/23374102
- Male circumcision: pain, trauma and psychosexual sequelae: pubmed.ncbi.nlm.nih.gov/22114254
- Mental Illness Strikes Babies, Too:
  members.tranquility.net/~rwinkel/MGM/oldrefs/www.drkoop.com/newsdetail/93/512690.html
- MRI Studies: The Brain Permanently Altered From Infant Circumcision:
  www.drmomma.org/2009/10/mri-studies-brain-permanently-altered.html
- Neonatal Cortisol Response to Circumcision with Anesthesia:
  journals.sagepub.com/doi/abs/10.1177/000992288602500807
- Newborn babies should not be given sugar as pain relief, says study:
  theguardian.com/science/2010/sep/02/babies-sugar-pain-relief-warning
- Newborns experience 'too much pain' during procedures, pediatrics group says:
  ctvnews.ca/health/newborns-experience-too-much-pain-during-procedures-pediatrics-group-says-1.2750960
- Newborns, Especially Preemies, Experience Too Much Pain During Routine Procedures:
  web.archive.org/web/20170711023711/https://www.aap.org/en-us/about-the-aap/aap-press-room/Pages/AAP-Newborns-Especially-Preemies-Experience-Too-Much-Pain-During-Routine-Procedures.aspx
- One Baby's Experience: peacefulbeginningsrosemary.wordpress.com/home/babys-experience

- Pain in babies *(Wikipedia):* en.wikipedia.org/wiki/Pain_in_babies
- Pain in Infants: facebook.com/photo.php?
    fbid=532054570285035&set=a.105147402975756.9541.100004414898074
- Pain of circumcision and pain control: cirp.org/library/pain
- Pain relief for neonatal circumcision: cochrane.org/CD004217
- Peaceful Beginnings *(the author's website):* peacefulbeginningsrosemary.wordpress.com
- Predictive Factors of Postoperative Pain and Postoperative Anxiety in Children Undergoing Elective Circumcision: A Prospective Cohort Study: ncbi.nlm.nih.gov/pmc/articles/PMC4610938
- Prevention and Management of Pain and Stress in the Neonate: cirp.org/library/statements/re9945
- Protect (All) Your Boys from Early Trauma:
    psychologytoday.com/intl/blog/moral-landscapes/201501/protect-all-your-boys-early-trauma
- Ritual circumcision and risk of autism spectrum disorder in 0- to 9-year-old boys: national cohort study in Denmark: journals.sagepub.com/doi/full/10.1177/0141076814565942
- Ritual circumcision linked to increased risk of autism in young boys, research suggests:
    sciencedaily.com/releases/2015/01/150109093725.htm
- Scarred For Life: theatlantic.com/daily-dish/archive/2007/06/scarred-for-life/227429
- Scars That Won't Heal: The Neurobiology of Child Abuse:
    drive.google.com/file/d/0B6-xMDW_KilRWjhWMGF0V2hBaUE/view
- Sexual and Emotional Abuse Scar the Brain in Specific Ways:
    healthland.time.com/2013/06/05/sexual-and-emotional-abuse-scar-the-brain-in-specific-ways
- Socialization of Violence and Abuse in Child Abuse and Child Molestation:
    salem-news.com/articles/august282012/circumcision-facts-rm.php
- Sperm RNA carries marks of trauma: nature.com/news/sperm-rna-carries-marks-of-trauma-1.15049
- Stressed Newborns May Experience More Pain Than They Show:
    mothering.com/threads/study-stressed-newborns-may-experience-more-pain-than-they-show.1625887
- Studies on Circumcision: circumcision.org/studies-on-circumcision
- Study finds that babies feel pain just like adults do (and we're wondering why that wasn't obvious):
    web.archive.org/web/20170515220624/http://www.inhabitots.com/study-finds-that-babies-feel-pain-just-like-adults-do-and-were-wondering-why-that-wasnt-obvious
- Study shows that infants feel and remember circumcision pain:
    web.archive.org/web/20170803192215/http://www.sickkids.ca/AboutSickKids/Newsroom/Past-News/1997/Study-shows-that-infants-feel-and-remember-circumcision-pain.html
- Surprising Study Finds That Babies Feel Pain Like Adults: huffpost.com/entry/7117812
- "The baby was kept in the machine for several minutes ...":
    facebook.com/photo.php?fbid=10153251302941469&set=p.10153251302941469
- The Bioethics of the Circumcision of Male Children: cirp.org/library/ethics
- The Childhood Origins of Terrorism:
    psychohistory.com/books/the-emotional-life-of-nations/chapter-3-the-childhood-origins-of-terrorism
- The Circumcision Decision: facebook.com/groups/CircumcisionDecision/814161088669297

- The Effectiveness of Anesthesia for Circumcision Pain:
  www.drmomma.org/2008/11/the-effectiveness-of-anesthesia-for.html
- The Effects of Circumcision on Breastfeeding *(breastfeeding helps preventing UTIs)*:
  nocirc.org/statements/breastfeeding.php
- The Global Survey of Circumcision Harm is a groundbreaking exploration into the effects of infant circumcision on adult men: web.archive.org/web/20170716063735/http://www.intactamerica.org/sites/default/files/Circumcision%20Harm%20Survey.pdf
- The GoMo study: a randomized clinical trial assessing neonatal pain with Gomco vs Mogen clamp circumcision: ajog.org/article/S0002-9378%2815%2900249-5/abstract
- The Impact of Neonatal Circumcision: Implications for Doctors of Men's Experiences In Regressive Therapy:
  primal-page.com/neonatal.htm
- The Origins of Peace and Violence: violence.de
- The Origins of War in Child Abuse: psychohistory.com/books/the-origins-of-war-in-child-abuse
- The psychological impact of circumcision: cirp.org/library/psych/goldman1
- The Screams of My Baby *(Goldman)*: facebook.com/brotherk.bloodstainedman/videos/547684065388752
- The Vulnerable Prenate: ludwig-janus.de/images/Downloads/english/Brekhman-original/05Emerson.pdf
- The Womanly Art of Breastfeeding: Circumcision:
  www.drmomma.org/2012/06/womanly-art-of-breastfeeding.html
- Tiffany's Story: Circumcision and its Impact on My Son:
  www.savingsons.org/2015/12/buying-lies-circumcision-and-its-impact.html
- Vainglorious: The Munchausen Complex: salem-news.com/articles/may262008/circ_richardm_5-24-08.php
- What Babies Know About Their Bodies and Themselves:
  nytimes.com/2018/07/09/well/what-babies-know-about-their-bodies-and-themselves.html
- Why does children's pain get short shrift?:
  theglobeandmail.com/opinion/why-does-childrens-pain-get-short-shrift/article20842813
- World-first MRI study shows babies experience pain 'like adults': medicalnewstoday.com/articles/292717

Videos:
- Bad Science: Circumcision Doesn't Reduce Sensitivity?: youtu.be/6f9zdWy8_JM
- History of Circumcision: youtu.be/mrQrLYH-qTo
- Infant Circumcision: Injection and Procedure:
  web.archive.org/web/20150430135225/dailymotion.com/video/xjkd30_infant-circumcision-injection-and-procedure_news
- Psychiatrist Discusses the Lasting Trauma of Circumcision: youtu.be/117vEwBtEY4

19   The Intact Penis

People who live in parts of the world where circumcision is not practiced would find our attitudes quite curious, but many American parents who have chosen to leave their infant sons intact have felt that they were doing something "brave," "daring," or "radical." Often such parents worry about whether they have made the right choice, or think that their baby's penis looks "strange." Perhaps they have never before seen an intact penis.

Parents giving birth in American hospitals have often had to be quite insistent and militant about their choice against circumcision. Sometimes they have faced criticism and lectures from doctors and nurses. Some parents who have planned to leave their sons intact have allowed their doctors to talk them into the operation.

Misinformation in books on infant care and in medical textbooks has led parents and physicians alike to believe that care of the intact infant is quite complicated and painstaking, and that the penis with its foreskin will be fraught with innumerable problems. Unfortunately this misinformation often results in excessive attention to the infant's foreskin which is what *causes* most of these problems.

The movement to do away with routine infant circumcision has followed in the footsteps of the natural childbirth movement, the growing popularity of breastfeeding, and the awakening public interest in other natural health related issues. There are many similarities especially between mothers' struggle to "relearn" breastfeeding, and new parents' endeavor to leave their infant sons intact.

Within recent years the mother who chose to breastfeed her infant has faced curiosity, criticisms, and immense misinformation in our bottle feeding-oriented society. Similarly, the parent of an intact son has encountered criticism, curious remarks and misinformation about his "natural" penis.

Opponents to routine infant circumcision, like many of those involved with other wholistic health related issues, have often seemed "vehement," "fanatical," and "angry." This anger has often resulted from the outright absurdity that people should have to work so hard, and face so much misinformation, opposition, and apathy, over something so incredibly *simple!!*

19.1   The Care of the intact Penis

Correct care of the intact penis, based on knowledge of the development of the foreskin and glans during fetal life, infancy, and childhood, *should* be an essential part of medical training, especially for doctors who will specialize in pediatrics or general practice. Unfortunately, most American doctors lack this information. They know little or nothing about the function of the foreskin, or its development or correct care. Usually they also know very little about the reasons for circumcision. When asked about the advisability of the operation they often cite non-medical arguments such as conformity or "social" reasons. Most American doctors' only "knowledge" about foreskins is how to cut them off.

The most informative and helpful sources of information concerning the development and correct care of the infant's foreskin have come from Great Britain. In 1949, Gairdner, a British physician, conducted a detailed study. According to his findings:

> "The prepuce appears in the fetus at 8 weeks as a ring of thickened epidermis which grows forwards over the base of the glans penis. It grows more rapidly on the upper surface than the lower, and so leaves the inferior aspect of the shaft of the penis and the terminal part of the urethra that has yet to be constructed ...
>
> From the inferior aspect of the glans a pair of outgrowths are pushed out and meet (the sulcus on the upper aspect of the glans marks their fusion) so enclosing a tube which becoming continuous with the existing urethra advances the meatus to its final site. These outgrowths from the glans carry with them the prepuce on each side, thus completing the prepuce inferiorly and forming the frenulum.
>
> By 16 weeks the prepuce has grown forwards to the tip of the glans. At this stage the epidermis of the deep surface of the prepuce is continuous with the epidermis covering the glans, both consisting of squamous epithelium. By a process of desquamation the preputial space is now formed in the following manner. In places the squamous cells arrange themselves in whorls, forming epithelial cell nests. The centres of these degenerate, so forming a series of spaces; these, as they increase in size, link up until finally a continuous preputial space is formed.
>
> The stage of development which has been reached by the time the child is born varies greatly ...
>
> *The prepuce is still in the course of developing at the time of birth, and the fact that its separation is usually still incomplete renders the normal prepuce of the newborn non-retractable* [emphasis mine].
>
> The age at which complete separation of the prepuce with full retractability spontaneously occurs is shown ... [in a] study of 100 newborns and 200 boys up to age 5 ... Of the newborns, 4% had a fully retractable prepuce, in 54% the glans could be uncovered enough to reveal the external meatus, and in the remaining 42% even the tip of the glans could not be uncovered ... The prepuce is *non-retractable* in four out of five normal males of 6 months and in half of normal males of 1 year. By 2 years about 20% and by 3 years about 10% of boys still have a non-retractable prepuce ... Nonretractability depends on incomplete separation of the prepuce ...

Among 200 intact boys aged 5-13 years, 6% had non-retractable prepuces; and 14% could only be partially retracted. Often this involved only a few strands of tissue between the prepuce and glans so that minimal force is required to achieve retractability." [1]

Reichelderfer and Fraga, in a chapter in a British-based textbook on infant care, relate similar findings:

"Our studies have shown that less than 1% of newly born infants could retract the prepuce. We examined 495 children up to 12 years of age. 25% could retract the prepuce at less than 6 months, 61% at 6-12 months, 63% at I year, 69% at 2 years, 76% at 3 years, 85% at 4 years, 86% at 5 years, 90% at 6-8 years and 100% at 9-12 years." [2]

They include the following important information, of which parents and doctors must be aware:

"If an attempt is made to separate the prepuce from the glans at birth by running a probe around the potential preputial space, numerous raw bleeding areas are encountered where the connecting tissues have been torn. Healing then takes place by fibrosis, leaving an adherent foreskin." [2]

This information is essential because frequently parents and doctors have believed that the infant's foreskin should be forcefully retracted, either shortly after birth or during the first few months of his life before it has separated of its own accord. Sometimes new parents of intact sons have been instructed to retract and wash under their baby's foreskin every day. In a society that is only familiar with circumcised penises, people have been led to believe that care of the intact penis is quite difficult and complicated, and therefore *have proceeded to make it so.*

Forcible retraction of the infant's or young boy's foreskin before it has loosened naturally is extremely painful to the child and can create future difficulties which would not have occurred had it been left alone. While innumerable parents of circumcised infants have expressed remorse over having allowed their babies to undergo the painful operation, parents of intact sons often express just as much anger and dismay because their child had his foreskin forcefully torn back from his glans. Since the infant's foreskin is normally adherent to his glans, artificially breaking these

---

1 Gairdner D. The Fate of the Foreskin. *BMJ.* 1949-12-24: 1433-4.
2 Reichelderfer TE, Fraga JR. Circumcision. Reprinted from Kenneth SS: *Care of the Well Baby.* 2nd ed. Philadelphia, PA: J.B. Lippincott; 1968: 297-8.

adhesions literally involves tearing one layer of skin away from another. Some observers have believed that this step of the circumcision procedure appears to be more painful to the baby than the actual clamping and cutting. Since forceful retraction of the foreskin often is done to the baby more than once, *the intact baby in our unenlightened society has frequently experienced much more pain and trauma to his penis than the circumcised baby!*

Unfortunately, although British sources have clearly described the correct development and care of the foreskin, American medical sources have been replete with misinformation. For example, Taber's *Medical Dictionary*, which is widely used in the United States by all branches of the medical profession, advises the following:

> "The foreskin is often tight after birth. It should be pulled back gently at birth to see that the meatus is clear, and then left alone for 8 days. After this, if still tight, it should be picked up in the thumb and finger and gently coaxed backwards twice a day. If it is inclined to bleed, smear it with an antiseptic ointment. Care must be taken not to strip it backwards too far or constriction of the glans (paraphimosis) may occur. If tightness still persists or there is any difficulty passing urine, a doctor should be consulted. Often the gentle [?] passage of a probe by the doctor, underneath the skin of the prepuce will obviate any need to circumcise." [3]

Even though extensive studies have shown that only 1-4% of all newborns' foreskins are retractable, a leading medical text tells doctors and nurses that the tight foreskin of the newborn is abnormal and must be forcefully loosened!! I have even known of parents who have wished to leave their infant sons intact, only to have the doctor advise them shortly after birth that circumcision must be done because the baby's foreskin does not retract! This is reminiscent of new mothers who have been advised by doctors or nurses that they should not breastfeed because they "obviously don't have any milk" – both parties unaware that a new mother only secretes colostrum for the first few days!

19.2 What About the Problems that the Intact Male May Encounter?

Expectant and new parents frequently express concern that their son may have "problems" if he keeps his foreskin. However, most parents would not be able to define what those "problems" might be. Sometimes people have known an intact male or parents with an intact son who did experience a problem with his foreskin, or has

---

[3] Thomas CL, ed. *Taber's Cyclopedic Medical Dictionary.* Philadelphia: F.A. Davis; 1977: C-75.

been circumcised during childhood or adulthood, and have understandably wondered if the easiest solution would be to have the foreskin cut off at birth.

The two major problems that intact males encounter are *phimosis* – the condition in which the foreskin is either tight or adherent to the glans and cannot be easily retracted, and infection of the foreskin. A thorough analysis of both of these conditions, how and why they occur, and how they can be prevented or remedied, is necessary. Weighed against the risks of the operation itself, and the advantages of having one's foreskin, is circumcision justified as a preventive measure against either phimosis or infection? If either condition occurs, is circumcision the only, or the most advisable cure? Or can the problem be resolved by simpler, less drastic means?

19.2.1 Phimosis

There are three categories of phimosis. The first is the frequently misunderstood, normal developmental condition in the infant or young boy in which the foreskin is not yet ready to retract. This condition is *not* true phimosis because it is *normal*.

Secondly there is "congenital phimosis." This is the condition in which a foreskin which is left alone during infancy and early childhood never does loosen or retract naturally. Some authorities, aware of the non-retractability of the prepuce at birth and during early childhood, still label the remaining small percentage of boys with non-retractable foreskins at age 4 or 5 as having "congenital phimosis." However, since other studies have revealed cases of foreskins first becoming retractable during late childhood or teenage years, the use of this term is highly questionable. "Congenital" implies that the condition is a birth defect, and therefore an abnormality. Some tight foreskins are actually not adherent to the glans, but simply have small openings making retraction difficult. True congenital phimosis appears to be extremely rare.

Thirdly, there is "acquired phimosis." This is the unfortunate, troublesome complication brought about by the forceful retraction of the normally adherent foreskin of the infant or young child. When two adjacent surfaces of skin are forced apart, this causes tearing, bleeding, and exposure of raw skin surfaces, the same as if a layer of skin were pulled off of any other body surface. Then, when the two fresh, raw, bleeding skin surfaces are placed back together, such as when the infant's foreskin is replaced over the glans, these two surfaces heal together creating scar tissue, leading to a troublesome, abnormal attachment of the prepuce to the glans. This is why it is extremely important that the foreskin NOT be retracted until it has loosened of its own accord.

Occasionally parents of intact sons have been frantic with worry that their son will develop acquired phimosis after one episode with forcible retraction by an unknowledgeable doctor. Consultation with medical authorities about this has indicated that if this happens, the foreskin should subsequently be left alone. A single incident of forceful retraction appears not to lead to significant build-up of scar tissue or adhesions. A small amount of petroleum jelly or other ointment applied between the glans and the prepuce may help prevent the two surfaces from healing together. Usually the unfortunate child is in considerable pain from this event and is quite resistant to having his foreskin retracted again.

Parents of intact sons may have to take the responsibility of educating their doctors about this matter. And since doctors have been known to forcefully retract babies' foreskins without any warning or discussion, parents should discuss the matter with their doctor prior to the baby's examination. Also, since some doctors retract the foreskins of newborn infants in hospitals, parents wishing to leave their sons intact should, during prenatal care, instruct the doctor not to retract the baby's foreskin if they have a boy.

Gairdner states the following in regard to phimosis:

> "Since in the newborn infant the prepuce is nearly always non-retractable, remaining so generally for much of the first year at least, and since this normal non-retractability is not due to tightness of the prepuce relative to the glans but to incomplete separation of these two structures, it follows that phimosis (which implies a pathological constriction of the prepuce) cannot properly be applied to the infant. Further the commonly performed manipulation known as 'stretching the foreskin' by forcibly opening sinus forceps inserted in the preputial orifice cannot be justified on anatomical grounds besides being painful and traumatizing. In spite of the fact that the preputial orifice often appears minute – the so-called pinhole meatus – its effective lumen, when tested by noting whether or not a good stream of urine is passed, is almost invariably found to be adequate." [4]

In Denmark a study was made on the eventual outcome in a population group in which intact foreskins are left alone until total retractability occurs spontaneously.

> "Øster conducted 9,545 observations on the state of the prepuce in 1,968 schoolboys aged 6-17 years. The boys were examined annually for up to 8 years between 1957 and 1965. 4% of these boys had phimosis; 2% had tight prepuces; and 5% had smegma. Incidence of phimosis decreased with age ranging from 8% among the 6-7 age group to 1% among the 14-17 age group. Smegma increased slightly, ranging from 1% among the 6-9 age group to 8% among the 14-17 age

---

4   Gairdner, p. 1435.

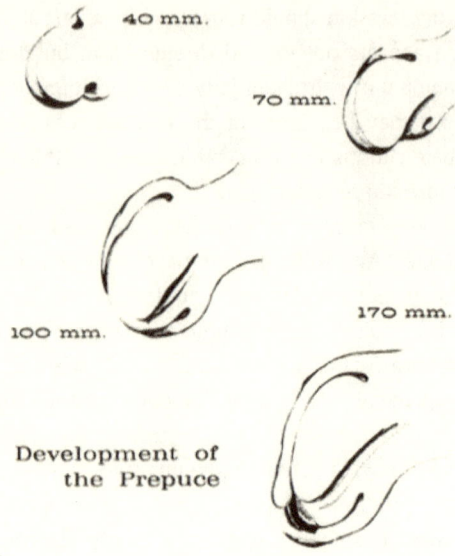

Development of the Prepuce (after Spalding, Deibert and Hunter).
From: Reicheldorfer TE, Fraga JR. Circumcision. In: Shepard, KS, ed. *Care of the Well Baby.*
J.B. Lippencott. 1968: 296.

group. Preputial adhesions which did not constitute phimosis ranged from 63% among the 6-7 age group to 3% among the 16-17 age group." [5]

The author concludes:

"Physiological (congenital) phimosis is a rare condition in schoolboys, and it has a tendency to regress spontaneously; operation is rarely indicated. Clumsy attempts at retraction probably cause secondary (acquired) phimosis, which then requires operation.

Preputial non-separation ('adhesion') occurs frequently, but separation of the epithelium takes place gradually and spontaneously as a normal biological process in the course of school life and is concluded about the age of 17.

Production of smegma increases from the age of about 12-13 years. Neither this nor the hygiene of the prepuce present any problems if the boys are regularly instructed." [5]

---

5   Øster J. Further Fate of the Foreskin. *Arch Dis Childh.* 1968; 43: 200-3.

19 – *The Intact Penis*

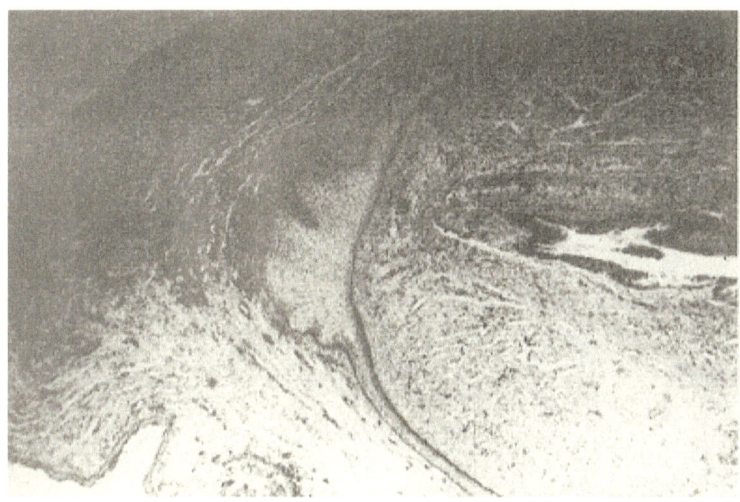

Cross section of infantile penis showing adherence of the prepuce to the glans penis. The urethra is on the right.
From: Reicheldorfer TE, Fraga JR. Circumcision. In: Shepard KS, ed. *Care of the Well Baby.* J.B. Lippencott; 1968: 297.

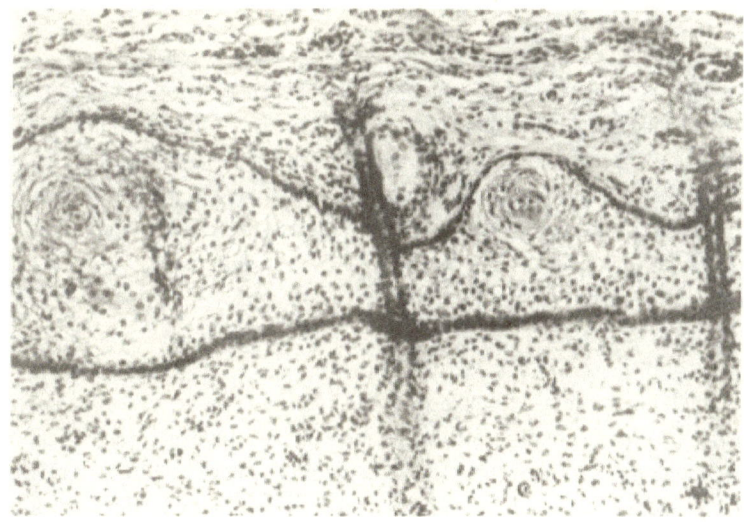

Cross section between the adherent glans and penis showing nests of epithelial cells that ultimately degenerate and bring about a separation of the two surfaces.
From: Reicheldorfer TE, Fraga JR. Circumcision. In: Shepard KS, ed. Care of the Well Baby. J.B. Lippencott; 1968: 298.

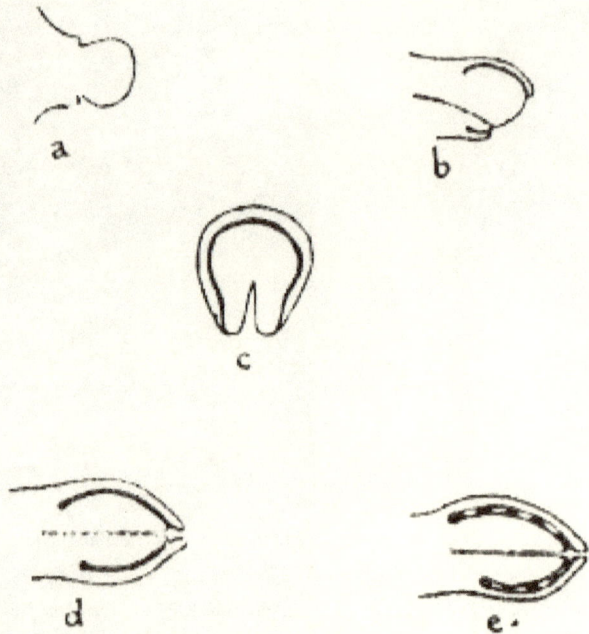

Development of prepuce. (a) Eights weeks; (b) sagittal section and (c) coronal section, 12 weeks; (d) 16 weeks; (e) at about term.

Paraphimosis is another problem which is caused by forceful, premature retraction of the infant's tight foreskin. In this condition the tight foreskin has been pushed back, exposing the glans, and then constricts so that it cannot be replaced. Swelling ensues and the helpless infant is in considerable pain. Some doctors will perform an immediate circumcision to remedy the situation, although others have found that simply soaking the penis in warm bath water will ease the swelling so that the foreskin will go back over the glans.

Gairdner discusses this:

> "Through ignorance of the anatomy of the prepuce in infancy, mothers and nurses are often instructed to draw the child's foreskin back regularly, on the supposition that stretching of the foreskin is what is required. I have on three occasions seen young boys with a paraphimosis caused by mothers or nurses who have obediently carried out such instruction: for although the size of the prepuce does allow the glans to be delivered, the fit is often a close one and slight swelling of the glans, such as may result from forceful efforts at retraction may make its reduction difficult." [4]

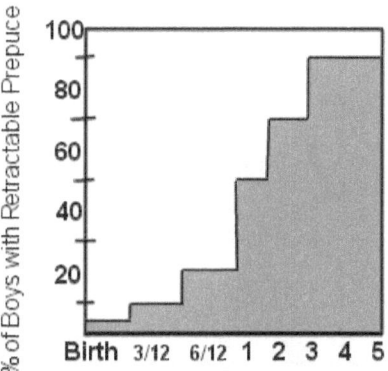

Proportion of boys of varying ages from birth to 5 years, in whom the prepuce has spontaneously become retractable. Note that it is uncommon for this to occur in the first six months.
From: Gairdner D. The Fate of the Foreskin: A Study of Circumcision. *BMJ.* 1949-12-24: 1433-4.

It is clear that the prepuce of the infant and young boy should be left alone. But what about the still-tight foreskin of the older child, teenager, or adult? Some doctors, even those who know that the infant's foreskin is normally tight, still recommend circumcision for the small percentage of boys whose foreskins do not retract after ages 4 or 5. Are there other, simpler alternatives? In the United States, any parent of an intact son, and the intact male as he grows older, is likely at one time or another to encounter a doctor who recommends circumcision. As long as our society is circumcision-oriented and regards the intact penis as an oddity, there will always be some medical authorities who think that foreskins should be cut off at the slightest indication of a problem. (This is not unlike bottle-feeding oriented doctors who recommend weaning rather than resolution for any problem with breastfeeding.) Parents of intact sons, and intact individuals *must* be knowledgeable and ready to consult other physicians or sources of information when and if cutting off the foreskin is recommended.

Many intact individuals have found that gradual stretching of one's own foreskin usually can loosen it if it is tight or adherent. Most little boys handle their own penises. During early childhood this is rarely true masturbation. It is merely curiosity about one's own body parts, similar to exploring one's toes. Many little boys have unintentionally helped their own foreskins to loosen by doing this.

Jeffrey R. Wood, Founder and President of INTACT Educational Foundation gives the following advice:

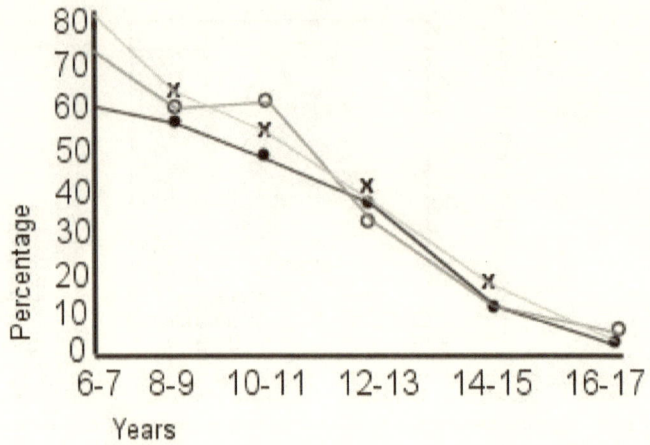

Incidence of preputial adhesions in various age-groups. – Total material (9,200 observations); 173 boys observed through 7 years (1,160 observations); ... 1,086 boys observed in 1964-65 (1,052 observations).
From: Øster J. Further Fate of the Foreskin; Incidence of Preputial Adhesions, Phimosis, and Smegma among Danish Schoolboys. *Arch. Dis. Childh (Br Med Assoc)*. 1968-04: 200.

"... Sadly, many American doctors are trained to think of circumcision as the only alternative to any problem involving the foreskin – when, in fact, there are many other choices which may be more advantageous to the patient.

... *Anyone who doesn't want to be circumcised* [or allow their son to be circumcised – R.R.] *doesn't have to be – except in the rarest cases* ..." [6]

The prescribed time for the foreskin to loosen varies greatly with the individual:

"... It may be before birth or after puberty! ... Normally it occurs before the age of four, [although] some men are not fully mature until around 25. In some cases [of late failure of the foreskin to separate into older childhood or teens], stretching exercise seems advisable to facilitate the loosening process. (Usually this can be done by the individual in private.)

... Difficulties with the foreskin can be among the many signs that one is not eating properly and an improved standard of nutrition provides benefits to the entire body not just the foreskin ... There is a theory, as yet undocumented, that continued heavy dependence on milk into early adulthood in certain individuals somehow prevents the foreskin from getting its genetic message to loosen up. Un-

---

6   Wood JR. Alternatives to Circumcision in the Treatment of Phimosis. *INTACT Educational Foundation.*

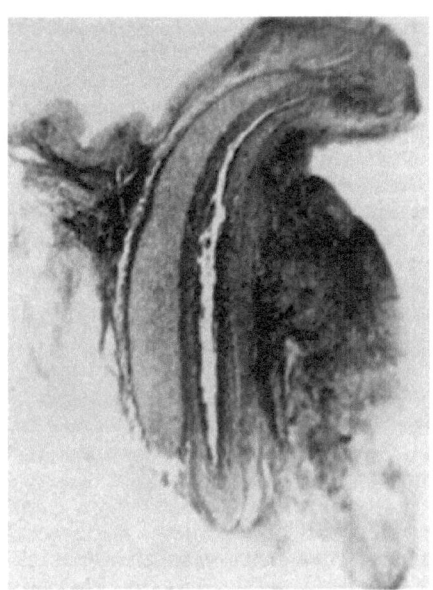

Cross section of a penis from a 120 mm fetus. Note the lack of cleavage between the prepuce and glans.
From: Kaplan GW. Circumcision – An Overview. *Current Problems in Pediatrics.* 1977-03; 7(5): 6.

fortunately, the average American diet is built around milk and dairy products as one of its key ingredients so that it is somewhat of a challenge for anyone in this country to maintain a nutritionally adequate diet that avoids these staples. But it is possible, and when refined carbohydrates and other 'junk foods' are eliminated as well, the results are incredible. One of the most notable benefits is a greater resistance to colds and all types of infections. Some uncircumcised men have even noticed that smegma has ceased to accumulate. As for the foreskin loosening up, this requires time and patience, and since it might have happened anyway, the significance of improved nutrition in this regard is difficult to establish. But it's certainly worth a try – for the other benefits alone!

In the rare cases where surgery is required, there are two alternatives to ... complete circumcision ... The simplest operation is known as the dorsal slit, in which nothing is actually removed, and the effect of which is to make the foreskin more easily retractable ... The other alternative is] partial circumcision – in which only the contractile tip of the foreskin is removed – the part which in phimosis has failed to acquire the ability to expand. What remains of the foreskin continues to protect the glans in the flaccid state ..." [6]

19.2.2 Infection of the Foreskin

When I first made plans to write this book I intended to devote an entire chapter to the problem of infected foreskins. I had so frequently heard about infection being a common, troublesome problem among males with foreskins that I expected to uncover a great deal of information about this. Surprisingly I have found very few resources that even discuss the matter.

Nonetheless, expectant and new parents are frequently told about the "danger of infections" if their baby is not circumcised. Is this argument justified when balanced against the very common problem of meatal ulceration and other problems that are exclusive to circumcised males?

If the foreskin does become infected, is immediate circumcision the best or the only appropriate remedy for the condition?

Three medical terms refer to infections of the foreskin and/or glans. *Balanitis* refers to an inflammation of the glans penis and mucous membrane beneath it. *Posthitis* refers to the inflamed condition of the foreskin. *Balanoposthitis* refers to both.

As was thoroughly discussed in the chapter covering complications, the reddened, swollen prepuce of the infant still in diapers is actually protecting the more delicate glans from the much more painful, troublesome problem of meatal ulceration.

Gairdner discusses this:

> "Inflammation of the glans is uncommon in childhood when the prepuce is performing its protective function. Posthitis – inflammation of the prepuce – is commoner, and it occurs in two forms. One form is a cellulitis of the prepuce. This responds well to chemotherapy and does not seem to have any tendency to recur. Hence it is questionable whether circumcision is indicated. More often inflammation of the prepuce is part of an ammonia dermatitis affecting the napkin (diaper) area ... The urea-splitting Bact. ammoniagenes (derived from fecal flora) acts upon the urea in the urine and liberates ammonia. This irritates the skin which becomes peculiarly thickened, while superficial desquamation produces a silvery sheen on the skin as if it were covered with a film of tissue paper. Such appearances are diagnostic of ammonia dermatitis, and inquiry will confirm that the napkins, particularly those left on through the longer night interval, smell powerfully of ammonia ...
>
> When involved in an ammonia dermatitis the prepuce shows the characteristic thickening of the skin, and this is often labeled a 'redundant prepuce' – another misnomer which may serve as a reason for circumcision. The importance of recognizing ammonia dermatitis lies in the danger that if circumcision is performed, the delicate glans, deprived of its proper protection, is particularly apt to share in

the inflammation and to develop a meatal ulcer. Once formed, a meatal ulcer is often most difficult to cure." [7]

As the individual matures and his foreskin loosens, virtually all potential problems with foreskin irritation or infection can be prevented by simple, regular washing. Some problems with foreskin infection can result from the individual's not knowing how to properly clean this part of his body. Although retracting one's foreskin while bathing is extremely simple, in our society, where the intact male has been an oddity, he may grow up never knowing that his foreskin *should* be retracted. Another factor is that circumcision has sometimes followed social class patterns in our society, so that in past decades the upper and middle classes have been more likely to choose circumcision for their sons, while the lower classes have been more likely to leave their sons intact. (Sometimes the "choice" was made for financial reasons – hence, unfortunately associating foreskins with poverty.) This has contributed to people's prejudice against foreskins. Also, sometimes people at lower income levels may have had less access to bathing facilities, general healthcare or nutritious foods, while many have worked at jobs requiring hard physical labor and/or contact with dirt, thus possibly predisposing them to infections regardless of their circumcision status.

Sylvia Topp comments:

"It seems to be true that a person who is not circumcised can develop infections of the foreskin, obviously a problem that would be unknown to a circumcised man. However, these infections are usually not serious and not one of the uncircumcised men I interviewed mentioned having such problems. A few said they had had warts which had been removed but one said he knew a circumcised man who also got warts. Now, although an infection can be annoying, is it really a good enough reason to perform an operation on every male baby? Other parts of the body get infected all the time, but this as far as I know is the only case where surgery instead of cure is preferred as treatment ...

Unfortunately, few of the (intact) men I talked to had been trained in the care of the foreskin, since this knowledge is not easily available to this minority of American boys and men. Two of the men hadn't pulled back their foreskins until they were adults because there was no one around to explain anything to them. Another had his foreskin attached in a thin line at the back of the penis head and had assumed that everyone's was since he had no one to compare himself with. He lived with the difficulty of cleaning in the corners that this attachment formed until intercourse ripped the skin loose, and of course frightened him." [8]

---

7   Gairdner, pp. 1435-6.
8   Topp S. Why Not to Circumcise Your Baby Boy. *Mothering.* 1978-01; 6: 73.

Some types of irritations can occur as a result of *too much* attention to cleaning. One doctor relates: "I have never seen any penile condition that could be attributed to smegma. Many irritations are due to excessive cleansing – especially soap." [9]

Much of the need to inform the public about the correct care of the intact penis is similar to the need to enlighten and educate the public about breastfeeding. The doctor who advises that all infant males should be circumcised because "He *might* develop an infection of the foreskin" is very much like the doctor who advises that all mothers should bottle-feed because otherwise "She *might* develop sore nipples or a breast infection." Some doctors, upon treating breastfeeding problems (which can be *much* more troublesome than foreskin problems!) conclude that "Breastfeeding is too fraught with difficulties for today's mother." Those of us who seek the benefits of more natural choices for our children prefer positive alternatives rather than such a defeatist attitude.

19.3 The Intactivism Movement

Ever since man first decided that foreskins should be cut off, other people have been objecting to the practice. Tribes that left the penis alone often criticized or sneered at other tribes who practiced circumcision. Since circumcision has only rarely been the choice of the individual, complaints and protests have often come from the victims themselves. Their laments were usually unheard. Years later they would be circumcising their own sons.

As soon as circumcision first became a medical practice during the late 1800's, the operation had its share of critics. Yet the operation's popularity grew throughout the early decades of the 20th century, as birth became "assembly line processed" in hospitals. Circumcision has always had its dissenters, but during recent decades when the rate of neonatal circumcision approached 98% in many parts of the United States, these individuals have been "voices crying in the wilderness."

Most circumcision critics have been men who have been victims of complications of the operation, or who have simply resented their lack of foreskin. Some were born during the earlier part of the 20th century and now feel dismayed to find that nearly all boys today are deprived of their foreskins. Usually their efforts have ended in burn-out and frustration. They have had few listeners and rarely did their efforts reach the people that *need* to be educated – prospective parents! Out of their frustration, or due to poor methods of dealing with people their cries were usually extremely vehement and bitter. Most were dismissed as angry fanatics. One of the most vitriolic of the anti-circumcision crusaders was Joseph Lewis, a Jewish man who in the 1950's wrote *In The Name of Humanity*, an angry tirade against infant circum-

---

9   Wood JR. General Letter. *INTACT Educational Foundation.*

cision, especially the Jewish ritual. Lewis was an atheist and wrote many treatises on atheistic causes. Therefore, his efforts were bound to alienate anyone with religious beliefs. Lewis had few listeners.

Many intactivists have condemned doctors who perform the operation as evil, money-hungry butchers, and label parents who choose circumcision as sadistic child abusers! Others rant and rave about the mutilated, sexually deficient circumcised organ. As one of the "pioneers" in modern day intactivism I understand and empathize fully with their ardor, especially since after so many years and so much effort infant circumcision continues to happen. I call their expression justifiable, righteous anger. Unfortunately, too many people fail to understand that an angry, condemning approach is only a detriment to the cause. Most people will not listen or learn from such epithets. Some may actually feel driven to have their sons circumcised so that they will not be like "those angry fanatics." For parents do not choose circumcision out of conscious intent to harm their child. Nor do most doctors perform the operation out of sadism. People have simply been *misinformed*. No one *wants* to believe that they have done something wrong. Nor does any man *want* to believe that there is something wrong with his penis. Many doctors are resistant to learning from lay people. Even when the circumcision issue is presented calmly, factually, and gently some people find the subject too difficult to handle. (So fellow intactivists, let's keep our angry rants to ourselves in our closed groups and try to be kind and understanding, although informative, when dealing with the general public. I remember how I once felt as a naive new mother.)

In order for our intactivism to have a significant impact on the American public, the message must reach expectant parents and the professionals who work with them. The childbirth education movement has had to emerge and develop as a powerful force before the two concerns could join.

During previous ages there was little need for organized childbirth education. Such knowledge was passed down and shared from woman to woman in a direct, informal way. Most babies were born at home with female friends and relatives in assistance. Families were large and girls grew up with knowledge about birth and infant care. During the 20th century families have become smaller and more fragmented. Birth was transferred to the domain of male medical professionals and became centralized within hospitals. Parents were left knowing virtually nothing about birth or infant care. Usually they placed their trust in the medical profession, but the support received therein was often woefully lacking. Organized classes in childbirth education have, in part, been an effort to fill this gap.

The childbirth education movement began as an effort to develop and introduce methods of giving birth comfortably without medication, thus providing psychological and physiological benefits to mother and baby. Psychoprophylaxis and conditioned response were first studied in Russia during the late 1800's by Pavlov. These techniques were subsequently applied to women in labor for dealing with contractions. Dr. Fernand Lamaze, a French doctor, learned these methods during the 1920's and further developed them. During the 1950's an American woman, Marjorie Karmel, gave birth in France under Dr. Lamaze's direction. She subsequently introduced the "Lamaze method" in the United States. Concurrently, during the 1920's and '30's Dr. Grantly Dick-Read developed the "Read method" which is based on relaxation, deep breathing, and spirituality. During the 1940's and 50's Dr. Robert Bradley, using Read's philosophy, plus his own observations of animals giving birth, introduced the "Bradley method." His most important contribution was the introduction of the husband as "labor-coach" and active participant during birth.

Until the late 1960's classes in childbirth education were often difficult to find. Doctors tended to be skeptical if not adamantly opposed to childbirth classes. Many resisted the idea of allowing fathers into delivery rooms. Frequently doctors and nurses did not want their patients to be informed or knowledgeable because that made them "ask too many questions." Expectant parents often had to search far and wide simply to find doctors and hospitals willing to allow the father to be present during birth or agree to let the mother deliver without medication.

The popularity of childbirth education classes has burgeoned during the past few years due to increasing interest in natural health and consumer awareness. Consumer pressure has contributed to acceptance of childbirth education by most doctors and hospitals. Today, classes in prepared childbirth are available in virtually all communities in the United States and most developed countries.

During the latter half of the 1970's some factions within childbirth education have become increasingly critical of standard procedures within hospitals, such as episiotomies, pubic shaves, enemas, heart monitors, and separation of mothers and babies. The childbirth education movement has produced a plethora of books and publications. The first books centered on basic issues such as father participation during birth and the advantages of giving birth without medication. Many books published more recently have been increasingly openly critical of dehumanizing hospital procedures and doctor control of birth. Within childbirth education the home-birth movement has emerged, as many parents, desperate for a humane and meaningful birth experience have chosen to stay home to give birth. As an alternative to both hospital and home birth, alternative birthing centers have provided a comfortable choice for many.

Throughout all of this, infant circumcision has received very little attention. There have simply been too many other important issues to bring light and question. Questioning circumcision is still just beginning to emerge as a worthy issue to be covered in childbirth education classes. Unfortunately, too many childbirth educators still provide only vague, neutral advice to prospective parents.

Dr. Frederick Leboyer's book and philosophy about *Birth Without Violence* became popular during the mid-1970's. Being French, it never occurred to Dr. Leboyer to mention circumcision. However, he introduced the concept that newborn babies have *feelings!* Never before had we thought about the baby's perception of birth! Some new parents began trying the "Leboyer method" when giving birth. But we were typical Americans who had never thought to question the cutting off of baby boys' foreskins. Those of us who gave birth to sons found ourselves shocked with the painful reality!!

During this time, in 1976, Jeffrey R. Wood established INTACT Educational Foundation in Wilbraham, Massachusetts. He promoted the adjective "intact" to define the state of the penis that has its foreskin. Whenever possible we use this term as a more positive sounding alternative to "uncircumcised."

Some of Mr. Wood's letters to his followers relate this organization's history and purpose:

"As we begin to understand something of the complex psychosexual processes that underlie this barbaric assault against masculine integrity, there is a link being established between the violence inflicted upon helpless infants, and the unrest which they may in turn manifest when older. We are discovering that emotionally as well as physically, the results of circumcision are unpredictable and often disastrous. Only in a religious context does there seem to be any less potential for lifelong psychological consequences, yet even progressive elements within the Jewish culture are calling for reform on this vital issue. What has been taken for centuries to symbolize a covenant of faith now increasingly appears to be symbolic of the same contempt for nature that has brought mankind to the very brink of self-destruction. Today's trend toward more natural living is not merely another fad, it is an expression of humanity's deepening concern for its ultimate survival." [9]

"Inspired by the work of Roger and Peggy Saquet, whose Non-Circumcision Information Center offered free material to readers of Boston's alternative newspapers, I established INTACT in the fall of 1976 to serve Western Massachusetts in much the same capacity. Both N-CIC[10] and INTACT work harmoniously together, each sharing its ideas and reprints with the other, and in recent months, each has received some degree of national publicity. The name INTACT came

---

10 Today Saquet's "Non-Circumcision Information Center" is virtually inoperative, while INTACT is working nationwide. An article written by Saquet is included among INTACT's informations sheets.

about in the following manner. The alternative newspaper here in the Pioneer Valley, the *Valley Advocate* was my initial advertising medium, and it charges by the word for classified ads. *'NonCircumcision Information Center of Western Massachusetts'* would come to seven words, running up the advertising bill considerably. Not wanting to use a mysterious, unpronounceable bunch of initials, I hit upon INTACT as a good code word. The name stuck; actually, it's our entire message condensed into just one word! Incidentally I've always thought that the letters in our name should all stand for something, as in '**I**mmediate **N**eed to **A**bolish **C**ircumcision **T**otally' – but that particular choice sounds too extreme for good public relations [He later came upon "**I**nfants **N**eed to **A**void **C**ircumcision **T**rauma."] [11]

Most books and publications about childbirth education or infant care say nothing or only give vague advice about circumcision. However, within the latter half of the 1970's and early 1980's a few books and publications have given more attention to the circumcision question. The *Home Birth Book* by Charlotte and Fred Ward includes a chapter on Primal Therapy by Patricia Nicholas which mentions circumcision trauma. (Inscape 1976.) *Labor and Delivery, An Observer's Diary* by Constance A. Bean (Doubleday 1977) includes a poignant, eye opening chapter entitled "The Circ Room" which describes infant circumcision in detail. (This chapter, entitled "The Circ Room" is now included on Peaceful Beginnings' website.) *Magical Child* by Joseph Chilton Pearce (Dutton 1977) strongly denounces circumcision. *Mothering* magazine has included a number of articles, including some written by me, opposing circumcision. In the winter of 1980, ICEA News (the newsletter of the International Childbirth Education Association) published a brief article opposing infant circumcision. Paul Zimmer, a pioneer intactivist in Pennsylvania, was listed as a resource and was deluged with requests for information. *Right From the Start* (Rodale Press 1981) by Gail Sforza Brewer and Janice Presser Greene includes a highly informative chapter about circumcision. The December 1981 issue of *The Saturday Evening Post* included two informative articles and an eye-opening picture display of a baby being circumcised. (*The Saturday Evening Post* later sold the slide series used for this article to me. I reprinted them and for several years sold them to childbirth educators and others for use in informing the public. They are now printed on *Peaceful Beginnings'* website as the feature entitled "One Baby's Experience." Some have also been reprinted and used widely in intactivist literature.)

My concern about infant circumcision dawned in 1977 following my third son's home birth and subsequent circumcision. In 1979 I began selling copies of my circumcision slides and information sheets to childbirth instructors. In 1980 Jeffrey

---

11   Wood JR. Notes from Jeff Wood. *INTACT Educational Foundation.*

Wood appointed me as Vice President of INTACT Educational Foundation. Shortly thereafter I wrote out INTACT's Philosophy and Policy and made several of our informational sheets available singly and in bulk to the public. Two sets of informational slide series' on circumcision were also made available. (Many of these information sheets now appear on my website.) Numerous ads and references in various childbirth education-related newsletters and magazines have kept the public informed of our cause.

In 1979 Nicholas Carter's book *Routine Circumcision: The Tragic Myth* was published by Noontide Press. His book was well researched, but is somewhat dated as he wrote it during the 1960s and searched 10 years for a publisher. The tone is quite angry and vehement and it has not been well received.

In 1980 Edward Wallerstein, a Jewish man, published *Circumcision: An American Health Fallacy* through Springer Publications. It is well documented and factual, with a calmer, more academic tone than many other works on the subject. It gained some respect among medical professionals.

In October of 1981 *NBC Magazine* did a feature on infant circumcision showing several infants actually undergoing the operation. I was on that program as was Edward Wallerstein and several doctors including Dr. Paul Fleiss whose interview appears in this book.

In 1983 Mr. Wood and I mutually decided to split forces due to personal, philosophical differences. Since my writings also cover a number of other baby and birth related topics in addition to circumcision I renamed my efforts Peaceful Beginnings and continued mailing out materials as before. Today Peaceful Beginnings exists as a website which is readily available to the online public.

Jeffrey Wood has retired from his efforts but his work will always be remembered as having played an essential role in the pioneering efforts of modern day intactivism. Roger Saquet's "Non-Circumcision Information Center" has been inoperative for many years.

What type of people are involved in this cause? Many, like myself, are parents of circumcised sons who regret our decision and have seen a desperate need for more information to be made available about circumcision. Others are parents of intact sons who have been uncertain or put on the defensive about their less conventional decision. Some intactivists are circumcised men who resent the fact that they lack their foreskins. Others are intact men, resentful about the absurdity of being "unusual" for having a natural penis. Many concerned individuals come from Jewish backgrounds. Some are childbirth instructors wanting to share this information with their students. Some are doctors and nurses who seem to be as frustrated with the medical establishment as the rest of us.

Like all causes, intactivism has had its critics. No matter how gently or factually we present our information, some people find our information too upsetting to accept. Some publications have been approached with articles about circumcision and have flatly turned it down. It is an absurdity that something as simple as not cutting off part of the body should be considered "radical."

One of the major goals of intactivism is that our information become an accepted, vital concern within all programs of childbirth education. We urge that our materials and information be included in childbirth preparation classes, classes in infant care, and during prenatal care.

We have experienced immense concern and participation from childbirth educators and groups throughout the United States and elsewhere. We have also experienced our share of dissension and apathy. Like most major endeavors, the field of childbirth education has many factions and conflicts. Some classes are offered through specific hospitals and merely prepare the expectant parents to accept and cooperate with all of the hospital's routines. Some instructors merely teach exercises and breathing techniques for labor and birth, and even consider such basic issues as nutrition or breastfeeding inappropriate to cover in class. Independent instructors are more likely to be true parent advocates, raising challenging questions and issues and urging parents to actively make choices and seek changes that will better their birth experiences.

Not all childbirth educators agree with intactivism's total opposition to all genital cutting of non-consenting infants and children. Some advise in favor of circumcision. Many do not cover the topic at all. Others basically agree with us but are afraid to discuss it in their classes for fear of getting others upset if they present this vital information. Some feel that it is not right for the childbirth educator to influence people's thinking on such a "personal" decision. This is just a cop-out, for virtually all parents have had so little information about circumcision that their "decision" scarcely deserves to be called such. And while the childbirth educator may not have thought the issue through, a neutral stance on infant circumcision is taking the position that only the needs and feelings of the *parents* are important, and that the *babies'* rights and well-being have no significance. This approach may be easier and "safer" from the childbirth instructor's perspective. However, growing awareness and true concern for the best interests of the helpless infants involved should hopefully inspire more and more childbirth educators to come out opposing the painful and unnecessary operation.

Making changes in society and inspiring people to think about something that they have never before considered is immensely challenging, frustrating, and rewarding. Fortunately, within childbirth education changes do take place relatively fast. Many issues that have been considered "radical" and "controversial" have become widely accepted and commonplace within a few years. During the early 1970's delivering without medication and fathers' participation in the delivery room were "hot" issues, "causes" for which we had to fight. Most childbirth educators considered other issues such as immediate contact with the baby, total rooming in, and home birth too "radical" to cover in their classes. Alternative birth centers, "birth rooms" in hospitals, or Leboyer births were unheard of. Today these practices have become commonplace in most parts of the country. In the years since, however, especially with the advent of widespread information available on the internet, our information soundly opposing infant circumcision continues to reach more expectant parents and increasing numbers of expectant parents have been leaving their baby boys intact.

Leaving ones child intact does have one major advantage. It is a far *simpler* matter than most other issues concerning infants and children. Similar causes such as alternative education for one's children, specific diets, or even natural childbirth and breastfeeding require their followers to learn and do many things. Some choices require considerable expense and sacrifice. In contrast, leaving one's son intact (as long as parents know to leave their child's foreskin entirely alone) usually requires very little commitment or action (save for fending off critical relatives – especially in the United States).

19.3.1 Intactivism Goals

Intactivism is a healing process by which humanity can grow to fruition. Our goals are threefold.

1. **Infants deserve and merit from a trauma free introduction into this world.** Surrounding them with only love and tenderness with an unbroken parent/infant bond will provide the courage and freedom to begin a positive, healthy life journey.
2. **Respect for individual autonomy.** No infant or young child has ever chosen genital or any type of unnecessary body modification.
3. **Healing of our sexuality.** Sexuality is one of life's greatest blessings, possessing the awesome power of uniting the souls of the partners and creating new lives. Sexuality is an essential part of our life essence, but sadly has become severely damaged by a myriad of cultural forces. I have likened sexuality to an exquisitely beautiful stained glass window with a rock thrown through it. Genital damaging has been one of many ways that our sexuality has become numbed, blunted, literally amputated from the totality of our life essence. If we cannot heal ourselves, we can heal the future of humanity by freeing the new generation from this destruction that has attacked our souls.

19.4 Interviews and Letters

19.4.1 Dr. Paul M. Fleiss, M.D., Los Angeles, CA (Pediatrician)

Dr. Fleiss: The basis of circumcision is not in preventive medicine, but as a ritual. But it has become common practice in the United States for about 80% of all males. We are now learning that babies ... they have eyes and they see, they have ears and they hear ... they have feelings. The findings about how important early bonding is makes you realize that an infant is more than just a lump of clay. You should treat a baby the same way that you expect to be treated yourself. *I wouldn't want to be strapped down to a board, taken away from all the security and love that I have known, and then have part of my body cut off without an anesthetic.*

I'm Jewish and I've been circumcised. I have one boy that was circumcised when he was born in 1968. I yielded to what I thought were cultural reasons for doing it. My younger boy was born in 1977. 1 didn't have him circumcised and I feel much better about it. He was born at home. He stayed next to his mother after birth. Circumcision would have been completely contradictory to all the other things we've done for the baby.

Rosemary: If anybody past infancy is circumcised it is done under anesthesia. Yet with a baby it is done without anesthesia. Why?

F: It's easy to strap him down. The newborn baby is not considered a human being. They're considered without feelings. Obviously it hurts. Once we put them back with the mother they appear to forget it.

R: You used to do circumcisions?

F: Yes. I'm not sure I ever believed in it. I did them because people asked to have them done. But I stopped when I just didn't want to do that to babies any more.

R: If you are studying to be a pediatrician, obstetrician, or general practitioner, are you automatically trained to do circumcisions in medical school?

F: It's a simple procedure to learn. Most doctors who work with newborn infants can learn the procedure if they want to. Some don't choose to learn it. It's not automatic. You just somehow learn it in your training.

R: Have you, being Jewish, found any family pressures with having your youngest son remain intact?

F: There might be. There comes a time when your own sense and rationality takes the place of every dogma that you might have lived by. What may have been a good ritual for centuries doesn't mean that it's still good.

19 – The Intact Penis

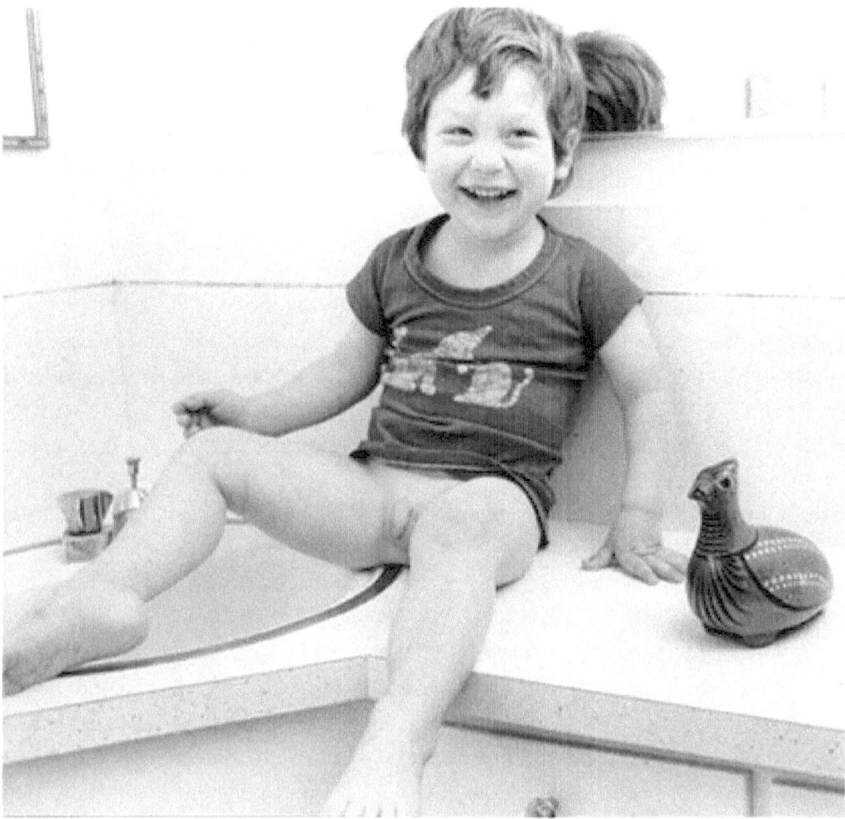

© *Suzanne Arms*

R: If a little boy is not circumcised, what is the nature of the infection that can develop? Is that a major concern? I've heard that they can get terrible infections under the foreskin.

F: No. It's a normal piece of tissue. My practice is not to do anything until they're a year old or more, and then push back and gently retract the foreskin and wash underneath when you bathe them[12]. When he gets older he can do this himself. When you're older, if you don't retract the foreskin it's possible to get bacteria or infection underneath it. Sometimes the foreskin can get swollen. An infection does not mean that the individual has to be circumcised to correct it.

R: If parents felt that they had to have their baby circumcised, what if they waited until the baby was older and had him anesthetized for the operation?

---

12 Dr. Fleiss later amended his advice and recommended that the foreskin be left entirely alone during infancy and early childhood.

F: Think of the cost! You're talking about several hundred dollars for an elective procedure!

R: How old or large would a baby have to be for that?

F: When I used to do circumcisions, we would do them in the office until 4 or 5 months of age. When they got too big to be strapped down, then we stopped.

R: Which doesn't mean it hurts any less when they're littler.

F: No.

R: In the Jewish ceremony they sometimes give the baby wine or alcohol of some kind to sedate him. Does that really make it easier for the baby?

F: I think it's mostly part of the ritual. Alcohol is a depressant and can't be used like an anesthetic. But why would you want to give a baby alcohol? Alcohol is a poison.

R: If circumcision is to be done, is there any one way that's better or less traumatic than the others?

F: No, I don't think there's any advantage to any of them. I feel very strongly that it simply should not be done.

R: Do you believe that the trauma of circumcision results in any long term psychological ill effects?

F: It seems to be a very brief moment in the baby's life. I don't think it's something to have guilt feelings about if a parent has already had a child circumcised. It was done to me. I did it to my boy. I've done thousands of them. We always thought that we were doing the right thing. But now we have a new awareness. Our whole opinion of what babies are has changed. All procedures like this are going to stop because babies begin to learn as soon as they're born. They need special treatment, *not* the treatment that we've been giving our children. That's a disaster!

Whether circumcision has any serious psychological consequences, I don't know. It wouldn't matter to me. Even if you found that there were absolutely no harmful psychological effects, it still would not justify doing an unnecessary procedure. You just should not be cruel to babies.

19.4.2 Interviews with Mothers

Tonya Brooks, Los Angeles, CA

Tonya: When my first son was born I was considering having him circumcised because my husband Bob was circumcised. I thought if our son wasn't circumcised he'd feel strange about it. I had also read Dr. Bradley's book *Husband-Coached Childbirth.* In it he recommends that *all* baby boys be circumcised. He also says *all* women should have episiotomies, so I wanted an episiotomy. Now I disagree and cannot recommend that book.

Bob was circumcised when he was five and remembers how it felt. He said "No, absolutely not!" So our boys have not been circumcised. Now I'm really glad.

There is so much wrong information about intact babies. With my first son Gabriel, the doctor convinced me that his foreskin was too tight. I watched my child be traumatized as she took tweezers and forced it open. He was just a newborn when that happened. I felt that some of the good effect of not having our child circumcised was negated by that. With my second son I resolved that nobody was going to mess with his foreskin! When he was four months old I took him to a pediatrician who said, "Look at all this smegma," and forced it open. Some smegma did come out, but he'd never had an infection. I didn't have time to stop the doctor.

From what I know now, the foreskin doesn't collect smegma as long as you leave it alone. I had been working with it to get the foreskin to retract. Now I know that it builds up because people bother it.

I've had no problems with my kids getting infections or getting it dirty. I find them sometimes in the bathtub pushing their foreskins back and there's no trauma. One time when Cyrus was four he woke up and the end of his penis under his foreskin was swollen and red. I thought "Oh dear, he's got an infection!" So I put him in the bathtub and had him soak in warm water and the foreskin retracted easily. By the end of the day the swelling was gone. He had slept in his underwear that night and it may have bound him. Maybe some mothers would have gone running to the doctor to have their kid circumcised over something like that.

Rosemary: Parents are often led to believe that circumcising the baby prevents "problems" when he gets older.

T: My oldest boy has never had the slightest problem. And Cyrus had only that one time. My kids are responsible for their own baths. I don't enforce baths. They have certainly been grimy sometimes and have gone a few days without baths, but there's never been a problem.

When you clean a baby girl you'll find smegma in the labia. You just wipe it out. It's very simple. I have never forced back my baby girls' clitorises to clean out smegma from under the hood. It never occurred to me to do so, nor on myself. It's so ridiculous because we never worry about it. I suppose they could offer similar arguments for female circumcision, that it would prevent vaginal infections or problems later.

R: Now that your sons are in school, have they had any problems with feeling different from their peers?

T: No. They also haven't worried about being different from their father. They simply have been told that they were not circumcised. My older son tells his friends, "I'm not circumcised," and then the other kids are fascinated.

Today increasing numbers of parents are choosing not to circumcise their sons anyway.

(Since this interview took place, Tonya has given birth to two more sons, Aaron and Ethan. They have both been left intact like their older brothers. Tonya also has two daughters, Shannon and Aleisha.)

Diane Cook

(Diane is the mother of five children, four of whom are boys. Her husband and oldest three boys have all been circumcised. Her youngest son, Joshua, is intact, Diane is also a La Leche League leader. She lived in Pt. Hueneme, CA at the time of this interview.)

Rosemary: You had your first three children in hospitals. What were the births like? Why did you choose circumcision?

Diane: We had the first two in the same hospital, but with different doctors. The births were natural, as best as I could do back then with no classes or doctors supporting natural childbirth at that time. I had Demerol with the first baby. The second time I had hypnosis. With the third, there were still no classes, but I got a lot of information from a friend who had all of her children naturally.

We didn't think we had a choice about circumcision. My husband had been circumcised. I guess we thought "We'll just carry on this family 'tradition'." I happened to be walking by the nursery window when they were circumcising my first son. I could see him screaming and throwing up and strapped down on his back. I was horrified, kind of paralyzed when I realized it was my own baby there. But then I walked back to my room and stopped thinking about it. Soon they brought the baby to me and he was fine. You would think that would have "cured" me. But no, we went ahead and had our second son circumcised, and then the third son. I thought they had to match. Now I think that's a ridiculous reason, but then I thought it was a valid reason.

After that we had Julie and then Joshua at home. I did more thinking about it and decided it was unnecessary. So we didn't have it done with Joshua.

R: Does it seem like he is "different" from the rest of the family?

D: No.

R: Are you concerned about problems later when he goes to school?

19 – The Intact Penis

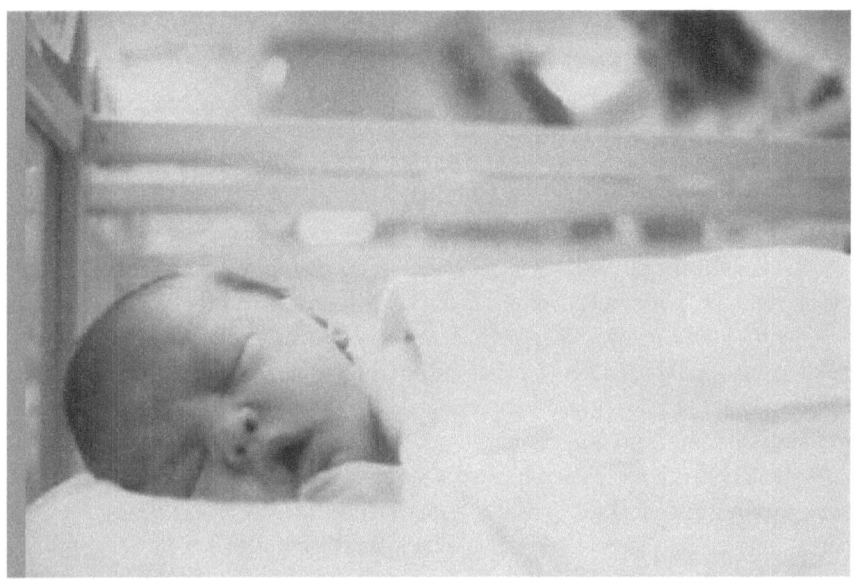

Reprinted with permission from the Saturday Evening Post Company © 1981

D: No. I think more parents are choosing non-circumcision. We also have not had any adhesion problems.

R: How did you care for his foreskin when he was a baby?

D: I didn't do anything for the first three months. Then a friend who had two boys who were not circumcised got me all worried. She said if you don't pull it back every day it will get problems with infections. I tried to pull it back and it was completely stuck. So I worked on it for a few minutes every day. After several months it started to get unstuck. It wasn't like those horrible moves that doctors sometimes do to forcefully yank it back. Now I don't do that anymore because he's very sensitive. He's not old enough yet to do it himself, so we just leave it alone.

Since then I've read that it normally takes about three years for the adhesions to naturally disappear. But in our case, what I did worked.

R: How did you make the decision not to have Joshua circumcised? Did your husband have strong feelings about it?

D: No. Anything that means saving money, he's for. We didn't even consider it. He doesn't really care one way or the other. I'm sorry now that I did all the rest of them, but what can you do?

R: Just make sure that they know that it's not necessary, so that when they have kids of their own they won't feel that their own sons have to be circumcised just because they are.

19.4.3 Letters from Parents of Intact Sons

Our son, Thomas Jonah, was born November 8, 1976. I had never considered having an uncircumcised child and when pregnant began talking to friends about circumcision and how it was done. We planned a home birth. Our doctor and nurse practitioner did not do circumcisions. After hearing descriptions of tying the child down or holding him forcibly and how most of them scream as no anesthetic is used, I began to question the practice. I read both pros and cons in several birthing books. Finally my husband Tom expressed his desire not to have it done. He is circumcised and does not feel that it has caused him any psychological damage. But he did feel that since we were searching for a positive birth experience with a loving atmosphere and caring attendants, a circumcision would be a less than positive event and certainly not peaceful. We decided against it.

The birthing was the most affirming and fulfilling moment of my life. My labor was peaceful and short. The support and assistance with relaxation that I got helped the birth to be peaceful. The child I held in my arms, touched, nursed, talked to, and massaged was also peaceful. He was alert, attentive, curious, and beautiful. I am so glad we decided against circumcision. Jonah means "peace" and that is what we call him.

Following our doctor's instructions I gently tried to retract the foreskin. Once it would retract easily I did it only once a week. After a few months we discontinued this and will resume it when he is old enough to continue it as part of his hygiene routine. We haven't experienced and don't anticipate any problems. If we have another son we will leave his foreskin alone until he is 4 or 5 years old and can care for his hygiene himself.

Jan, Tom, & Jonah Easterly, Petersburg, NY

(Jan & Tom have since had a second son, Teddy, born in 1980, He is also intact.)

♦

I am the mother of two sons, one circumcised and one not. Jeremiah, my 6 ½ year old was circumcised because no one ever offered me the choice. My obstetrician's fee had an extra $25 tacked on "if the baby is a boy" for circumcision. His circumcision is only a part of what I feel now was an early traumatic experience for him. Other than slight bleeding though, he suffered no noticeable ill effects. He did get a meatal ulcer at about one year of age concurrently with a fungal diaper rash.

The doctor who was to deliver Elisha, my second-born, at home, was very much against circumcision. By that time, I was too. I had read more about it, that it is painful and done without anesthesia to a newborn baby who is then left to scream in his plastic crib. Also I had become convinced that there is no medical justification for the operation. My husband, who is circumcised, decided he was also not in favor of it being done. Therefore Elisha was not circumcised.

He has never had any problems with his penis. When he was two months old we moved and took him to a new doctor for a check-up. This doctor, while professionally reassuring us "he didn't believe in circumcision either" and that "this wouldn't hurt," he'd "just break a few adhesions so we could clean beneath the foreskin to prevent infection" – forcibly yanked back Elisha's foreskin, causing it to bleed! It did seem to hurt a great deal and he screamed whenever he urinated for a day. We still can't retract his foreskin, are no longer concerned with doing so, and he has had no infections.[13]

I would advise any concerned parent of an intact son not to succumb to the "line" that this doctor handed us. The treatment is unnecessary and quite painful. If he gets an infection, it could hardly be worse than the "prevention." Cure it then, when (and if) it happens.

We know two adult men who are not circumcised and who have had no problems with their foreskins. Both say they took no special care of their foreskins till school age, when they learned to clean beneath the foreskin.

Vicki Meyer, Sandstone, West Virginia

♦

My son was born at home. My naturopathic chiropractor who attended our birth was against circumcision. I felt that if boys were born with coverings for their penises, there must be a good reason. It seemed a cruel, painful thing to do to a little one. I felt I would be able to teach my son cleanliness and to feel at ease with his body. When he got to be 1 ½ years old he was getting real squirmy about it. He'd get ornery and wrestle with me and giggle. So I gave him the cloth to clean it and he started getting involved in it and mellowed out. I pull his skin down, he squeezes warm water on his penis, then I wash it and quickly check it and then pull his skin

---

13 Repeated forcible retraction of an infant's foreskin is more likely to *cause* an infection. An intact baby is *less* likely to develop a penile infection if his foreskin is left alone. – R.R.

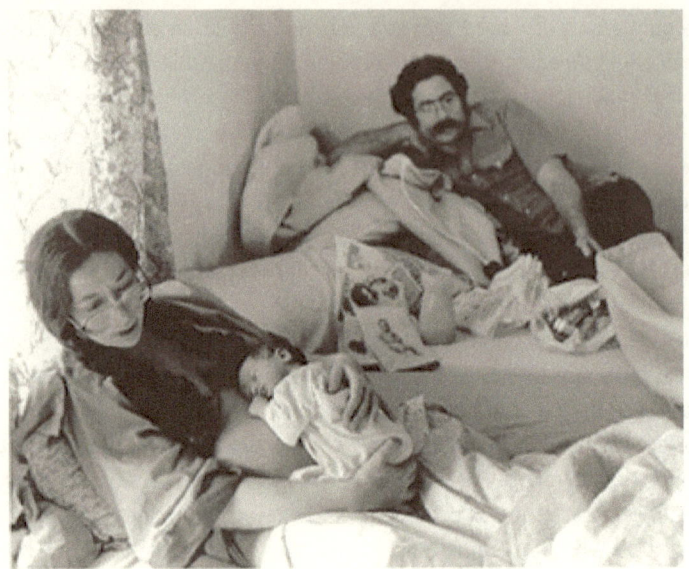

© Suzanne Arms

up. We do this after a bath along with cleaning toenails, fingernails, etc. It only takes a few minutes. Gradually he'll grow into caring for his cleanliness and his foreskin will be part of that.

We lived in the woods for a year and Ansel ran naked except in cold weather. I think the foreskin is handy when you're cruising through the bushes!

When Ansel was five months old he was in for a check-up and the doctor felt I should have circumcised Ansel. I explained my feelings. He said, "Well okay, if that's how you can do it." But he felt that I should let him separate the membranes that were keeping the foreskin attached to the penis. He said if I didn't do this now, I'd run into problems later with infections. Under pressure, misinformed, and wanting to do best, I agreed. My God, what an agonizing few minutes we spent!! Ansel was tense, red, and screaming with pain!! I felt helpless and "Oh no! What did I do?!" As soon as it was done, Ansel collapsed in my arms exhausted and frightened.

Now I know that that was an unnecessary, cruel thing to do. Now I know the membranes naturally separate by the time the boy is 3 or 4 and that he cannot get infected underneath the skin that has not separated yet.

I think that people have often been inhibited about natural occurrences. There is an idea of not touching one's body intimately. "This is bad, sick, might lead to who knows what! Mother has to touch her son's penis!!" if that boy has a foreskin. Well it's not a big deal. You brush your teeth, wash your ears ... so you clean the foreskin. Simple.

My husband is circumcised and he supported my decision. They don't feel concerned that they're "different." I think that's a heavy ego trip and no reason to do it.

Ansel's penis rarely has any white stuff on it. He is a clean, robust, healthy, strong boy. This is probably because of the way we eat and live. We are vegetarians, love our mother earth, fresh air, and good exercise. We work hard to help our planet earth and its creatures and peoples. We're low income so we don't have control over much, but we do what we can. You can always do more than you think.

Willow, James & Ansel Harvey, Missoula, MT

♦

My husband Stephen and I went through our first pregnancy and birth in 1970 in the midst of a great wave of "back to nature" enthusiasm. We were strong-willed and had great faith in the natural order of God's creation. Thus if God made penises with foreskins, who were we to say they shouldn't be there? So our firstborn son, Noah, remained intact without our being even slightly tempted to do otherwise. It seemed like common sense to us.

We have never had any physical problems resulting from Noah having his foreskin. I did not try to retract it for any reason such as cleaning, but did try very gently once or twice out of curiosity and found it very adherent. I wondered at this and looked for information but found none. It has only been in the past few years that I've read of the normalcy of this adherence and that I was right not to force it back.

Our second son, River, was born in 1972. Again we did not consider having him circumcised. He, like Noah, was born at home and both of them were untouched by medical hands until school physicals were required at around 5 years of age. Circumcision seems like a real nightmare of medical intervention! Unthinkable cruelty! River did have some occasional redness and swelling of his foreskin with general diaper rash, but leaving his diaper off always seemed to clear it up. His foreskin was also non-retractable. Now that they are older both of them can pull back their foreskins with no difficulty. I'm not sure when the change came – maybe at 4 years of age.

Socially we had no great pressure. My family wouldn't think of talking about something like circumcision. Stephen's family lived far away. Our peer group was generally in agreement with us. Occasionally we heard comments such as: 1.) "They won't 'look like' their dad. Won't that cause problems?" It hasn't so far. They've accepted easily the rational and loving reasons for not having something cut off. 2.) "The other boys will make fun of them." No problems so far.

A couple that we know with two intact sons who did foreskin retraction for cleaning – their sons had bad smegma buildup. The doctor had advised them to practice *daily* retraction and cleaning. I wonder … perhaps if you start doing it you have to do it continuously after that? But if the foreskin is left adherent, no smegma problem? Or is smegma buildup related to a general state of lowered resistance? I never saw smegma on our boys' penises.

I never paid any more attention to our sons' penises than I did to their ears, noses, or toes. They got baths once a week or so with hardly any soap used, just plain water, the best food we knew how to feed them and lots of exercise and fresh air. Their health has been very good.

I'm glad there's so much more information around today and that more babies are being spared that pain and insult.

Diane Brandon, W. Burke, VT

♦

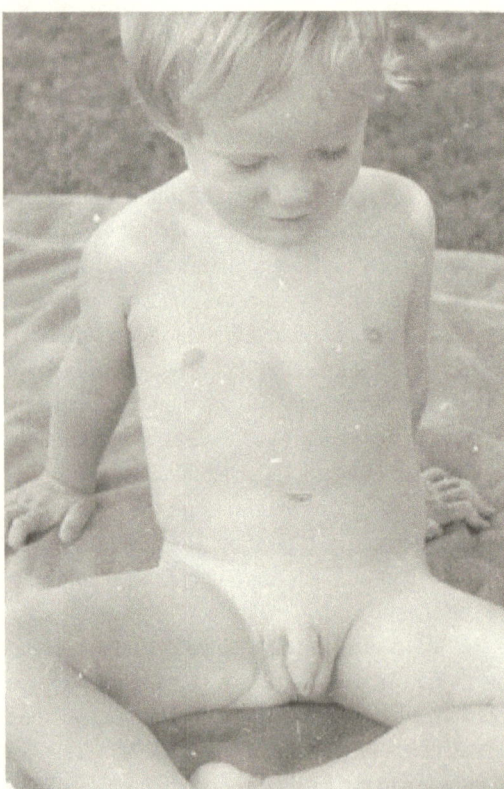

Steven Finch (contributed by Frances Finch.)

My husband and I decided while I was pregnant that if the baby was a boy he would not be circumcised. My husband is not circumcised and is perfectly healthy. He has never experienced any problems or criticism from schoolmates. His older two brothers were circumcised, but the doctor that delivered my husband said it wasn't necessary to circumcise him and my mother-in-law agreed.

The woman who taught our natural childbirth classes said she didn't have her six year-old son circumcised and he's just fine. Also our pediatrician said it is not necessary. The doctor who delivered our son was in favor of circumcision "for medical and social reasons." This amazed me since he is strictly a natural childbirth doctor. He uses the Leboyer method with dim lights, warm bath, etc.

He then has the babies come back one week later to be circumcised. There was no way I was going to take our son back for such a cruel procedure.

We have been criticized by my family for not having it done. My three brothers and nephews have all been circumcised. My mother and sisters-in-law never even questioned it.

At the local hospital, the standard admitting form for all patients says in the fine print that by signing to be admitted you are also authorizing circumcision if you have a baby boy. However, our son was born at the doctor's office. He has two rooms set up for births that are furnished with double beds, picture on the walls, printed sheets, etc.

I have been breastfeeding our son. I have been criticized by my mother for not putting him on the bottle and for waiting so long to start solids. She didn't nurse any of her children. I have had support from my mother-in-law and other friends who have nursed their babies.

One friend had a baby boy one week after ours was born and he wasn't circumcised either. Maybe one day it will no longer be "the thing to do."

Frances Finch, Fullerton, CA

◆

My husband is not circumcised. He's never had any kind of problem because of it. He's also a very good lover and does not have the premature ejaculation problem that so many circumcised men experience. I think there may be a connection.

As a nurse's aide at a hospital several years ago I witnessed a circumcision. It was the first and only time I have ever fainted. The poor infant screamed in pain. The whole procedure seemed incredibly sadistic. I decided right then that no son of mine would be subjected to that senseless torture and our son was not circumcised.

Some parents worry about junior looking different from papa if they don't circumcise their son. Fortunately we don't have that concern.

Debra Bottomly, Poughkeepsie, NY

◆

My wife and I are both doctors. She trained in Pediatrics and then Child Psychiatry. We were initially confused about circumcision when confronted with the task in

Circumcision – The Painful Dilemma

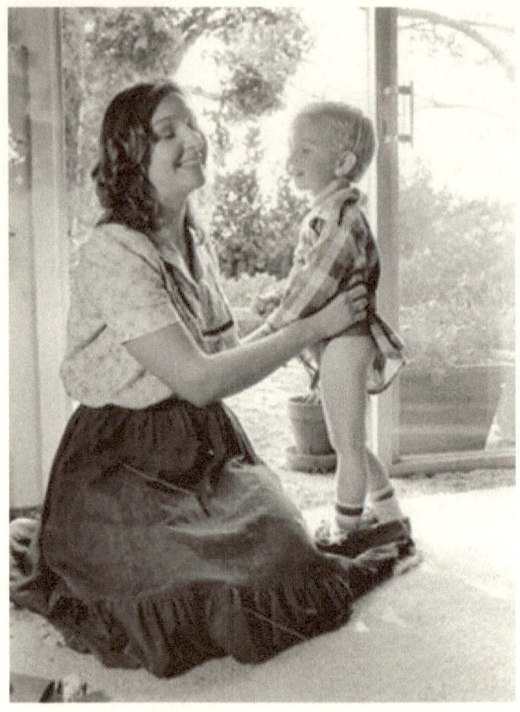

© Suzanne Arms

medical school. I chose to ignore the absurdity of the procedure and the baby's screaming and learn to do circumcisions. My wife absolutely refused to have anything to do with it.

When she went into Pediatrics, she was considered a bit odd, being unwilling to perform a simple procedure which is economically beneficial to the doctor. I went into Internal Medicine and had no further confrontation with the issue until my wife became pregnant. I was hoping to have a female baby so that I could avoid the issue. I had been circumcised. My major conflict was not whether I thought circumcision was beneficial, for I had long since decided that it was no more than a pagan ritual, but rather whether I wanted the baby to be like me or not.

In order to make a final decision I went to the newborn nursery at the hospital where I worked. I watched a circumcision being performed and immediately, without any question, knew that there was no way that I could have my newborn son tortured in such a manner. It seemed like the first time I had ever really watched the procedure *even though I had done several dozen in medical school.* The baby was absolutely panicked and exhibited the most shrill and desperate behavior one could imagine! The pediatrician performing the procedure continued his mutilation as if nothing were happening. I almost vomited.

We had a son and of course we did not circumcise him. We have had absolutely no problems and I am certain there will be none. I consider circumcision a vestige of savage ritualism. I am certain that it scars the psychological and sexual development of the human being.

Gregory E. Skipper, M.D., Newberg, OR

♦

My husband Philip and I decided not to have our son circumcised. Circumcision decreases sexual sensitivity and dries out the glans, whereas if he weren't circumcised there would be a natural lubricant which can aid in intercourse.

My midwife, (an elderly lady) told us that the baby had adhesions between the head of the penis and the foreskin and that some of these adhesions should be broken with a probe inserted into the opening. We were also told that this opening was too small for the head to be forced through and that we would probably need to have his penis circumcised.

Since then we've learned that the head should not be fully exposed by force. We got the opinions of three doctors, read two articles (which were hard to come by) and talked to some intact friends with intact babies before we decided that our son is a perfectly normal, healthy little boy with no reason to have this unnecessary operation performed on his sensitive little body.

We now know that the foreskin should be gently pulled back when bathing and that the head of the penis usually will not be completely exposed until approximately three years of age. The father can then teach his son how to clean it.

The only problem now will be what to say when Nicholas asks why he is "different" from Daddy.

Viki and Philip Morgan, Canyon Country, CA

♦

We decided not to have our son circumcised. Since he was born I've allowed myself to be unsure of my decision. Since the article about circumcision in *Mothering* ("Why Not to Circumcise Your Baby Boy" by Sylvia Topp, Jan. 1978, Vol. 6), I'm reassured now that we did the right thing.

I used to think that circumcision was right and normal. I never questioned it. But while I was pregnant I thought about it. We were having the baby at home, partly to protect him from insults and unkindnesses that would happen to him at the hospital.

It would be a paradox to put him through such a trauma after he had such a peaceful, calm birth.

The doctor I saw for prenatal care is Orthodox Jewish. When his son was born seven years before, he researched circumcision and found no evidence in favor of it, so he did not have his son circumcised. He will circumcise babies if the parents want it done, but the midwife that he works with told me that he doesn't perform the operation often. She told us that none of the younger pediatricians in town will do circumcisions. They consider it "cosmetic surgery." The obstetricians do them, though.

I am an R.N. and I should have known, but I honestly did not know the difference in appearance between circumcised and intact penises. All the men I've paid attention to looked the same and I didn't realize how very common circumcision was. I had thought they all must be uncircumcised. I realized what an intact penis looked like from our son Ethan. For a while I was sorry we hadn't had him circumcised because I thought that circumcised penises were more attractive.

But I really feel that God knew what He was doing when He designed people. He must have put foreskins there for a purpose. I think people should respect that. Also, I really believe babies shouldn't have to go through that!

I recently visited some old friends, including a doctor who is a very good friend. He made me feel really bad about not having Ethan circumcised. He said a lot about older men needing to be circumcised, peer acceptance, etc.

But now after reading the article in Mothering, I'm feeling a lot more confident in my decision. My husband left it up to me.

Even this article didn't describe how to clean under the foreskin. I've never read an article that did. You'd think I might have had the opportunity to learn in nursing school or working or just in life. It seems strange to me how uninformed I am and I consider myself a fairly bright, sophisticated person.

Susan Scott, Santa Fe, NM

◆

I am the mother of two children, a three-year-old girl and a five-month-old boy, both of whom were born at home.

When I was pregnant for the first time we discussed circumcision. I didn't want it, but my husband, who is circumcised, felt it was a good idea. I knew that he would be the one to make the final decision. Sighs of relief when Sarah arrived – no decision to make!

During my first pregnancy I read *The Hygienic Care of Children* by Herbert M. Shelton, which has a strongly anti-circumcision chapter entitled "Mutilation of Boy Babies." This, in conjunction with my European upbringing and sexual experiences with intact men convinced me that routine infant circumcision is unnecessary and undesirable.

In the interim between Sarah's birth and my second pregnancy my husband became more receptive to the idea of non-circumcision. This was a relief to me, since we both felt very strongly that I was carrying a boy. The chiropractor who assisted at Daniel's birth put no pressure on us one way or the other. We decided not to subject our beautiful, whole, newborn baby to mutilation and unnecessary pain.

I was unable to find any information on care of the intact baby. I was not sure if I should try to retract the foreskin forcibly or not. Asking other mothers produced the information that all their boys had been circumcised. I was beginning to feel like an "oddball!" Fortunately, Mothering magazine had an article that bolstered my instinct to "leave well enough alone" by telling me that the foreskin is not usually retractable until 1 ½ to 2 years.

This is an area of parenting that is still not considered deeply by many couples. I asked a close friend why their son had been circumcised. She said, "I thought you needed to! You mean you don't *have* to?" Too many parents say "yes" simply because they really don't know that they can say "no."

Lynne Knox, Cross City, FL

◆

My son has not been circumcised because I felt that a foreskin is a personal and private part of a man's body and I could not make the decision on having him circumcised. That decision is for him to make when he grows old enough to know whether or not he wants it done. It is a barbaric thing to do to a tiny baby. I have been in a clinic where it was done and have seen the trays that babies are strapped to. I shuddered when I saw them. Besides, what if the doctor should slip?

My son was born five weeks early and in breech position. I delivered at home as planned. The waters were clear so I anticipated no problems. However, my baby was born with Infant Respiratory Distress Syndrome. He was trying so hard to breathe that he couldn't take the breast. We took him to the hospital which had a Newborn Intensive Care Unit. I was glad I had him at home even with the problems we had because I couldn't have endured it in a hospital. This way, at least he was mine for a little while.

The doctors did not even bother to mention circumcision, since the babies in the NB-ICU were already traumatized enough.

One of my grandmothers told me that we should circumcise because uncircumcised boys would "play" with themselves. (So what!)

I have had no problems with my son's foreskin. I have left it alone as I have heard it is not a good idea to mess with it. I don't anticipate any trouble with his peers.

I saw the circumcision trays in the hospital after my son was born. It only reinforced my feelings. It seems quite barbaric to me. I could never do that to a little boy. It makes my mother's heart pain when I hear parents talking about having their sons circumcised.

(My correspondence with this mother continued for several months. I received the following, very sad letter):

Unfortunately my son has died as a result of the heart and lung problems he was born with. It is a very hard thing to lose a child when you have worked as hard as we did just to keep him alive. [Her son lived for about 5 months.]

(A couple of months later she wrote again:)

It wasn't too hard to let my son go because I knew that it was going to happen. Eric was born prematurely and had congenital heart disease. When he first looked into my eyes right after birth, I knew he would never grow up. It's better this way because he had a very painful life. It was amazing that he lived as long as he did. But we sure had love while it lasted.

We do plan to have more children. I may already be pregnant as it has been over a month and still no period. I hope I am. I'd like to have another chance as soon as possible.

Deborah & John Hollenbeck, Albuquerque, NM

(Deborah and John gave birth to their second son, Jacob, in November of 1978. He too has remained intact, and is thriving and healthy.)

◆

My son was born at home in Fairfax, California. The doctors that I saw for prenatal care were very open concerning the issue of circumcision. They saw no medical need for the operation. This concurred with my intuitive feeling on the subject. I feel that "nature" created us perfectly and it seemed bizarre to me that such a radical alteration was necessary. It made sense to me that the foreskin served in a protective capacity. That this should be removed because a small percentage of males had trouble with uncleanliness was analogous to dentists pushing tooth extraction and plates so that the maintenance problem be handled.

My main objection to circumcision, however, is that it is such a painful experience. I've come to recognize that much of the fabric out of which we operate consists of "forgotten" imprints. A trauma occurs and from this painful experience the child gets feedback from his/her environment ... "I am not safe here! Life is painful!" The child has no framework to modify the imprint such as "This procedure is for your future well-being." He receives a painful experience for which he has no means to assimilate except in the direct experience of hurt. People continually reconstruct reality as "unsafe," "detrimental" and with the feeling that other people can have power over their lives because of long forgotten (to the conscious mind) events.

My son is now 15 months old. I recently took him to a local doctor for an examination. The doctor was looking at him and explaining some things to me when he suddenly reached down and yanked my son's foreskin back! It was horrible! After months of dealing with conscientious doctors in California who developed a warm and respectful relationship with my son, I was filled with sorrow not only because of the pain he felt but because of the imprint that doctors and their environments aren't safe. He said my son definitely needed a circumcision and I set up a date which I later cancelled.

I still did not feel that circumcision was necessary even after another doctor examined him and said it was. This doctor's response to my questions and wanting to be with my son up to the time the anesthesia would be given and immediately afterwards while awakening, was "What's your hang-up?!" He figured that when the child cried out enough that signaled that he would be awake enough to be carried out to his parents ... I found the "professionals" to be totally insensitive to the human factors involved. They had no awareness of a child's needs or of the psychological implications of their actions.

I called my doctor in California. I related to him the whole situation and he told me that he recommends that nothing be done to the penis until the child reaches two years of age. At that time he said to begin gently retracting the foreskin. By the time the child is three the foreskin will be completely loosened and the child will be able to learn how to clean himself.

Around here it seems that most people consider not being circumcised "unheard of."

The Mothering issue with Sylvia Topp's article arrived three days after my experience with the doctor. I learned of acquired phimosis and was really crushed until I was reassured by the California doctor that one instance would not create scar tissue.

(The following is this mother's letter to the doctor who forcefully retracted her son's foreskin:)

"I am writing to express my concern over the recent experience my son Aleph and I had in your office.

You gave no indication to my child or to me that you were going to proceed so abruptly in your examination of his penis. With the knowledge that his foreskin was tight you yanked it back aggressively. You never acknowledged the child as a person, said anything to him, or touched him in a kindly way before doing something which you knew would be intensely painful for him.

A child is extremely impressionable. Until his experience with you, every visit he had ever made to a doctor's office was one in which he was treated with care and respect. He enjoyed going to the doctor's office and had no fear of examination.

You were appraising his condition and expressed the need for circumcision based on the fact that his skin tone had become leathery and tight, when you suddenly retracted it! I don't feel that you had to make your point by further illustration, especially when your action aggravated an existing condition, causing bleeding and severe pain which still persists. Last night he awakened repeatedly, crying, and now gives indication that he feels discomfort in this area.

I feel strongly that a requisite to the healing that a physician performs is an attitude of respect and compassion toward the people who are his patients. Human beings are more than their bodies and when this is overlooked the harm done to a person's psyche can be equal to or greater than the physical repair. This is even more important when dealing with children who have not yet evolved a framework in which to understand the "whys" of certain actions and interchanges.

Please cancel all the arrangements we made for circumcision. I will take my son to a physician whose qualifications include sensitivity and compassion as well as adeptness in surgical procedure."

Esther Frances Schrank, Bridgeton, NJ

◆

My first son was born when I was 18. I was naive about pregnancy and birth and had never read anything that was informative about circumcision. I had Solomon in a hospital and didn't have him circumcised because I felt it wasn't natural. When my dad noticed he wasn't, he expressed his disapproval saying it wasn't clean and that he should have it done right away.

I lived with my mother after the baby was born. (My boyfriend whom I had been living with shortly before Solomon's birth was out of the country and we planned on getting back together when he returned.) My mother and I had a talk about the baby's not being circumcised. She disapproved also, saying it wasn't clean. Not having *any* support, I gave in and had it done at a doctor's office. It was a very traumatic experience. We were separated and it took us a long time to get over it. I very much regret having had Solomon circumcised.

I knew I wasn't going to have my second son circumcised. At the time I had Silver, the first edition of *Spiritual Midwifery* was out. They recommended retraction of the foreskin for keeping it clean. I couldn't pull Silver's skin back so I took him to a woman doctor who did it. She wasn't nice and sent me out of the room while she did it. It was very painful also and I regret having let her send me out.

When I was pregnant for the third time I went to the Wisconsin Farm. (Sister Farm of the one in Tennessee where *Spiritual Midwifery* by Ina May Gaskin is published.) I read the revised edition of *Spiritual Midwifery* and it said retraction of the foreskin is not necessary. The Farm midwives neither encourage nor discourage circumcision. They circumcise boys if the parents wish and they do it in a religious manner, showing the baby and mother utmost respect and keeping the vibes holy.

The midwife who delivered my third son, Brook, circumcised her own baby and said she held him a lot afterwards. She, and also another woman there who had her son circumcised by Ina May, said if they had another boy they wouldn't have it done. Their reasons for circumcision were cleanliness but they felt the natural way was cool too. I didn't have Brook circumcised, but if I had wanted him to be I feel it would have been okay.

I don't think it matters about boys being embarrassed because they "look different." Lots of boys aren't being circumcised these days. I think children are growing up with a healthy attitude about their bodies and it probably does not matter to them. I had thought Solomon should look like his dad who was circumcised. My husband doesn't think it's an important factor for someone making this decision. The father can explain in an informative way why his penis is different. It's no big deal. I explained it to Solomon who is five now. He understood it and that was it. My other two are too young for explanations but I'm sure there won't be any problems just because they look different from daddy.

Most of the ladies I've met with boys have had their first boy circumcised and not their second son or any boys after that. This is because they weren't informed while pregnant with their first sons.

Linda Kehoe, Ball Club, MN

♦

We chose not to circumcise our son, but it was not an easy decision. I did not want it done because I believe it to be a trauma. We had our son at home to provide the most

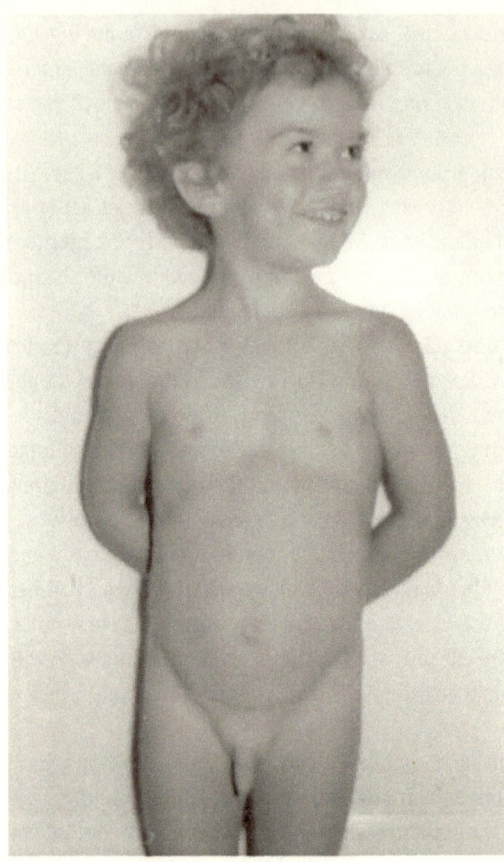

Aaron Altman (Photograph contributed by Maxine Altman)

pleasant birth experience for all of us.

My husband, who is of Jewish heritage, though not a practicing Jew, was more inclined toward having it done. He was less skeptical of the medical reasons. He also felt our son would wonder why he was different from the other boys and his father.

We anguished for months and he finally decided that I was correct or at least could have my way. He came to the conclusion that it was unnecessary surgery.

Aaron, our son, is 18 months old now and we are both glad we did not have him circumcised. We have never pushed his foreskin back. I'm sure it would not go back easily as it is very tight. He has had an infection once – after a doctor's visit during which the doctor pushed it back. It was red for a day and we put a cornstarch solution on it. Now we always state that we don't want his foreskin pushed back to any physician before we remove his diaper.

Maxine and Armand Altman, Kennebunkport, ME

◆

I split with Seagan's father when I was six months pregnant. We had never discussed circumcision. A few years before Seagan's conception I lived with a couple who had an intact child. Until recently we lived in Venice (Calif.). Many of the boys there are intact. Before Seagan was born I always thought intact penises were very "odd" looking until I would occasionally see a "naked" penis (one bare of foreskin). It always

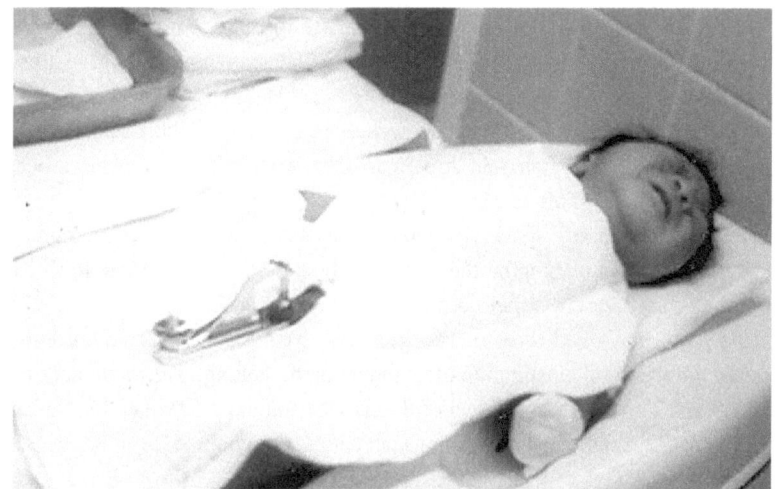

Photograph contributed by John C. Glaspey, MD.

had a raw, "uncovered" look to it. Adult penises always seemed like "adult penises" to me, but though looking a bit mutilated, don't seem as odd as a young child circumcised.

It also seemed, though we lived in a community where naked children are accepted as natural, that circumcised males chose to remain covered more often than intact ones. This could go in hand with parental hang-ups over "private" areas and cleanliness to these parts.

Seagan was born at a hospital with my mother at my side. I told my mother often (as I knew my belly was full of boy child) I would not have my son circumcised. After Seagan's birth I lay on this bed in the hallway with my still-nursing son an hour out of my womb. People were singing "Happy Birthday" and sipping orange juice. The pediatrician was asking if I wanted Seagan circumcised. I was saying "No," and my mom, seemingly shocked, was saying *"Yes."* Then she asks for the doctor's advice and that of his wife. They say they're biased to a mother's choice about her own child. My mother was frantically talking about cleanliness and what not ...

And Seagan, so young and sweet, nursing ... lying warm and naked next to my body ... trusting me to do the best I can for him ... with this argument/discussion about his penis ... such a small, tiny penis ... as new as he was.

In my mind I see picket lines of tormented males with signs saying "Save the Foreskin!" How odd, and what a fantasy!! [14]

---

[14] Not such an "odd" fantasy any more. Take a look at the "Bloodstained Men" protests going on! – R.R.

I am not often around relatives other than my immediate family, so I haven't had any pressure from my Jewish background other than my mother who to this day remarks how "funny" Seagan's penis looks.

For a short while I had an intact, very Italian, stepfather who couldn't relate to circumcision at all. He often said American men must have little penises because they were "half chopped off as a baby!"

Male friends with any sensitivity would react towards the idea of circumcision similarly to the way a nursing mother reacts to the thought of a cracked nipple. They reach for their penis or cross their legs and look very wounded.

In the past I have had three intact "intimate" friends. Two were more into "hiding" their penises and cleaning up after intercourse, making love in the dark or under the covers. The third was a wonderful man who felt most fortunate for having his foreskin intact. It is, amongst other things, an added attraction.

Laurie Levites, Los Angeles, CA

♦

I chose not to have my sons circumcised so they would remain whole and unmaimed. The foreskin acts as a shield that protects the end of the penis from desensitization from contact with underclothing and also functions as a flexible folding-unfolding sleeve during sexual intercourse for the increased pleasure of both partners.

Our first son was born in 1964. Prior to his birth we discussed circumcision with our family physician who recommended it for general hygiene. Other friends gave varying reasons – reduces masturbation, would be more painful later, or other boys in the locker room would tease. Since these ideas seemed vague at best, I made some cursory research and learned that circumcision was rarely necessary. The only substantial reason that I have found favoring it is for religious grounds.

When we were expecting our second child, my wife told our doctor that I did not want a male child circumcised and asked that I visit him to discuss it. His penile and cervical cancer scare did little good because I knew more about circumcision than he did.

In 1974 we found ourselves expecting another baby. By this time I was a virtual anti-circumcision fanatic. I suspect that circumcision can be related to homosexuality and high divorce rates. When my anti-circumcision stand was mentioned to the doctor he suggested that we make an appointment with him to discuss it. This physician said "Circumcision was so common that the hospital might as well do all male babies as routine." He did admit that many doctors did not find circumcision necessary. After I sent our doctor and the hospital a certified letter refusing permission for cir-

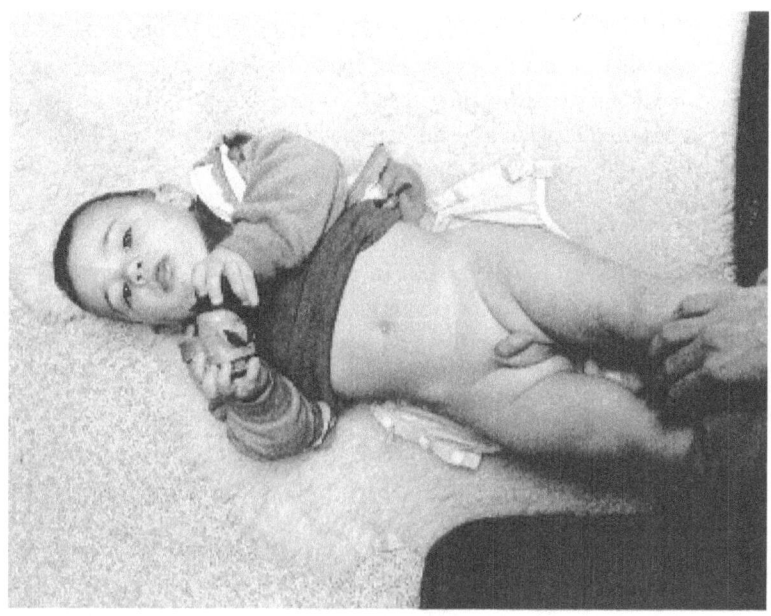

© *Suzanne Arms*

cumcision, our doctor threatened to drop my wife as a patient, but did not and never mentioned circumcision again. After our son was born his bassinet was marked with 4 inch letters "NO CIR."

(Name Withheld by Request)

♦

My husband, Larry, has a very good friend. This man had always been an analytical type – if you couldn't explain it mathematically, it couldn't be true. Several years ago he started to change and see things more "spiritually."

One afternoon he was working in his garden and suddenly felt very bad – so terrible that he didn't want to stay out there. He went inside to work out his problem. He had been practicing yoga, so he went into a meditative state. He began feeling extreme anger, humiliation, and frustration and realized that these feelings "reminded" him of his circumcision as an infant. A subconscious realization is very hard to describe to someone else, but Larry's impression was that his friend had *no doubt* that he had, indeed, recalled the operation and was feeling the same sensations and emotions he felt as a newborn.

Over the last few years I began to doubt the practice, but figured it must be very difficult to deal with an intact foreskin and perhaps it was best to remove it. However, I've come to realize how brainwashed I've been. If new mothers can be taught to clean their newborn daughters' genitals, then why not their sons'? If little girls can be taught to clean the myriad folds that we're blessed with, why not little boys?

My feelings toward circumcision are the same as my feelings about the entire birth experience. *Everything* that happens, from the onset of labor, if not before, is "remembered" by the subconscious. *Everything* changes us toward higher or lower potential as adults. *Any intervention* with the natural birth and mothering process, must be detrimental to the physical and emotional well-being of the newborn. Believing this, I must agree with my husband who says, "What kind of a way is that to start your life, getting the end of your penis cut off ?"

Debi Miller, Camarillo, CA

(Debi was pregnant when she wrote this. Their son, Bartholomew, was born at home, June 1978.)

♦

When I was pregnant with my first son, Terence, we found a wonderful doctor who would assist us with a home delivery. I asked him, "When do people have their babies circumcised?" thinking most people did this. I had never seen an intact penis. I am Jewish and my husband is Catholic. He had been circumcised and so had all the other males I had known.

The doctor said "Did you know circumcision is not necessary?" With all my knowledge about birth and pregnancy, I had to answer "No." No book that I had read was informative on the subject. We discussed the matter. He gave us some literature to read and said that if we chose to have it done he would do it three weeks after the birth. He felt that birth was traumatic enough and one should wait to circumcise.

We then researched the subject so we would make a responsible decision. We talked with male friends, some circumcised, others not. I wondered whether uncircumcised men had any difficulties. One friend had chosen to be circumcised when he found intercourse painful. It was an individual situation though. When he and the woman he lives with gave birth to their son, they chose not to circumcise even though the father had experienced a problem. What was most influential to my own decision not to have Terry circumcised was my husband's saying, "When I found out my foreskin had been cut off *without my permission,* I felt angry and cheated!" We decided we wanted it to be Terry's decision.

My mother was terribly upset and had one of my stepfather's colleagues write me a detailed letter about Terry's future as an uncircumcised male. My stepfather is a doctor. For a month my mother and I didn't speak. This was mostly my choice, for each conversation would come around to the horrors of non-circumcision. She would cut out clippings from medical journals that described phimosis and other such things. My dear grandfather said "We should have him circumcised because God wanted it that way." I couldn't get too angry at him because he's Orthodox Jewish. But I did reassure him that God really didn't make a mistake when he put the foreskin on.

When Terry was a little older I took him to a different doctor. The doctor saw that Terry's penis was not retractable (which I now know, was totally okay!). So he pulled it back, Terry cried, and he said to pull it back regularly so that the foreskin doesn't adhere to the head of the penis and the smegma is removed frequently. He was gentle about it. I did this. As Terry got older occasionally I did find a little smegma. Later he learned to clean himself. I explained to him how it is important to keep his penis clean along with all the other parts of his body. I talked to him about being uncircumcised and showed him pictures. We talked about his friends since occasionally it was noticed that he was "different." He has said he would like one like Peter (his Daddy). Peter and Terry talked together. Now Terry says, "Daddy wishes he had a cover on his penis like me."

Our second son, Kian, was born at home also. There was no question as to whether or not we'd circumcise him. When Kian was about four months old he became quite ill with a cold. My doctor was on vacation, so I saw the doctor who was on call. He examined him, removed his diaper, and exclaimed in a loud, disapproving voice, "You should have had this baby circumcised! His foreskin doesn't retract!" He then proceeded to pull it back and make it bleed ... Here was this very sick baby and the doctor was worrying about his foreskin not retracting!! My regular doctor had seen the same penis many times and nothing was said or done. On Sunday Kian was worse but I didn't want to see that doctor again. By Monday, Kian was in bad shape. I waited at my doctor's doorstep, was his first patient, and told him of my experience. He said "I'm sorry this happened, Julie. You're going to have to put Kian in the hospital. He's got pneumonia pretty bad. He's full of mucus and dehydrated." I asked, "What else can I do?" He knows I am an intelligent, responsible person and gave me an option to take Kian home, get four humidifiers, a breast pump, and push fluids. I was to call him every hour to let him know Kian's progress. Kian had become too weak to nurse so I was feeding him with an eyedropper, pumping my breasts, and suctioning out tons of mucus. If he hadn't looked better the following day the doctor would have admitted him to the hospital.

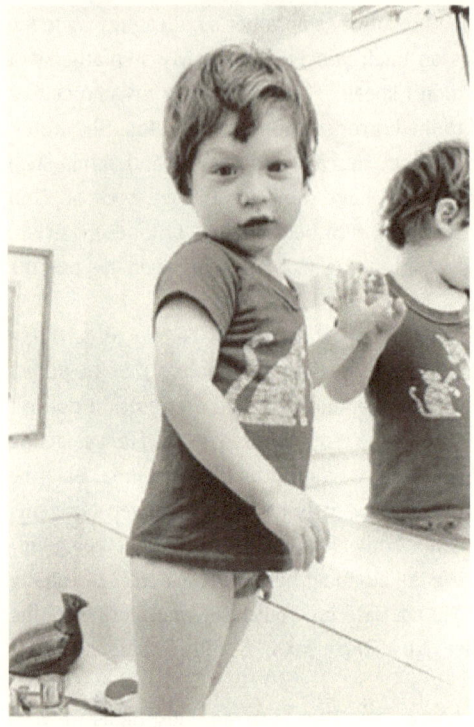
© *Suzanne Arms*

Thank God he progressed. I saw the doctor every day for two weeks. It was a horrible experience for our whole family. It took Kian three months to fully recover.

Then began my attempts to educate others, by giving articles to childbirth educators, doctors, ministers, etc., and by sharing my experience of having two healthy, happy boys who are intact and are having no problems.

I am not attempting to retract Kian's foreskin. I have friends in France and in Denmark. They have said that it is practically unheard of [in Europe] to mess about things like that. Everyone there seems to know that by age three or so the foreskin loosens naturally.

Julie Freitas, N. Hollywood, CA

♦

I have two boys, one born in 1966 and one in 1976. We also had three girls in between. My oldest son's birth was a typical uninformed first birth – induced labor, drugs, forceps. I didn't question any of that, and did not question the routine circumcision.

My birth experiences with each of the three girls got a little better. The oldest girl's birth was somewhat "prepared" with only a little medication, but my husband wasn't there. The next girl's birth was my husband's first time present at a birth. He got to stand in the delivery room doorway – a big concession for that hospital in 1970. The last girl's birth was a good hospital experience and we went home the next day.

With my fifth baby we planned a home birth. During this pregnancy we talked to other home birth couples about the unnecessary things done in hospitals. Nobody had any good reason why a boy child should be circumcised. I didn't want to subject my baby to it at all, but my husband felt strongly that if the baby was a boy he should be circumcised so that all the males in the family would "match!" Reluctantly I agreed.

When our second son was born in 1976, (a beautiful home birth!), my husband immediately started trying to arrange the circumcision. We are members of a group health plan, so he called the hospital and got started on the "merry-go-round!" Pediatrics wouldn't perform an outpatient circumcision because they didn't have the "equipment." Urology wouldn't perform a circumcision on a child under a year of age. The Health Plan office wouldn't pay for a circumcision performed by an "outside" doctor. He called a local synagogue (we are not Jewish) to see if they could recommend someone, but they couldn't. He called the Social Services Office at the hospital. The social worker called back the next day to report that Urology had told them that they didn't have to do it because the child wasn't born there! Finally my husband called the Chief of Staff obstetrician. The Chief of Staff said he'd do the circumcision himself.

I had to take Trent to the doctor myself as Paul couldn't get off work. I dreaded it and took a friend with me for support! When we arrived a nurse took the baby to get him ready while I signed a form stating that "I understood there is no medical reason for this procedure, but I wanted it done ..." My mothering instincts and common sense were fighting the whole thing, but I knew it meant a lot to my husband. So, against my better judgment, I went ahead.

I started into the examining room where they had taken Trent. I could hear him crying. It was the first time he had ever been away from me! The nurse tried to stop me, (my friend said it looked like she was going to slam the door in my face!) but I pushed on through. I found my poor little boy naked, strapped to a horrible contoured board with room for his legs, arms, head, etc. each in a compartment! He was painted with an orange antiseptic from the waist down. As soon as the nurse left I crawled up on the table next to Trent and by half-lying, half-standing I nursed him and tried to get across to him that I loved him and hated what I had to do to him. I think he got the message. He stopped crying and was peacefully nursing (as much as possible in that contraption!) when the doctor came in. He told me to leave. (I think he didn't want me to see such a personal "male" procedure!) I refused. He said that either I left or he would. Again, common sense was overcome by what I felt was "duty" to my husband, so I left and stood right outside the door.

A couple of minutes later the door opened. We had an "eleventh hour reprieve!!" Trent had a rash and he didn't feel he should do surgery without having someone look at it. The Chief of Pediatrics was called. I unstrapped Trent and held him. The pediatrician concurred that it was inadvisable to do a circumcision at that time because with the rash there was a good chance that the open wound would get infected.

Circumcision – The Painful Dilemma

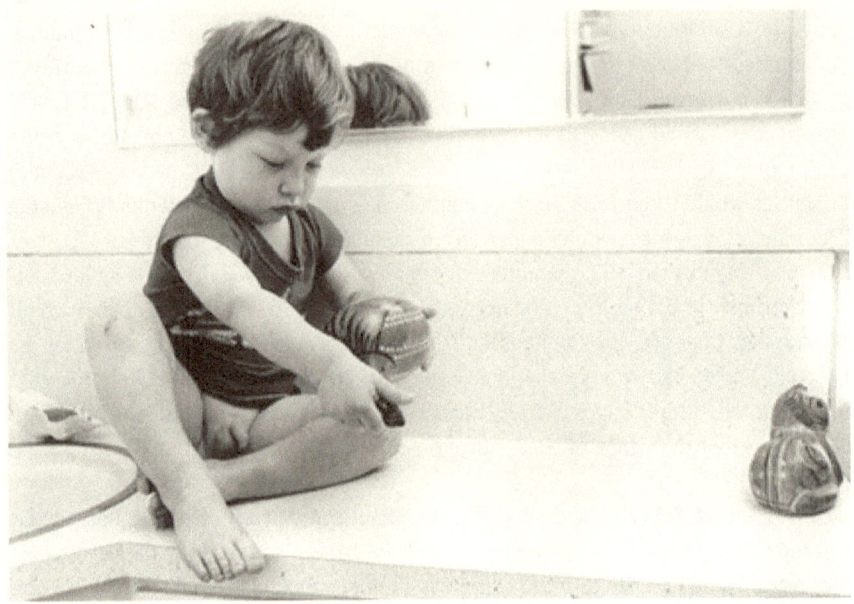

© *Suzanne Arms*

Thankfully I took my uncircumcised baby home, determined not to put him through THAT again! When I described the procedure to my husband and said, "If you want him circumcised, YOU get him circumcised!" he agreed that he didn't want his son to go through all that, even if it did mean they didn't "match!"

Paul isn't a cruel or unreasonable man. I'm sure if he had known what was involved he wouldn't have been so insistent on the procedure. Needless to say, if we ever have another son, we will also not have him circumcised.

My friend who accompanied me to the doctor's office had had a similar experience with her baby who was born six weeks before Trent, also at home. Her husband was in the military and she called four large military hospitals before she could find someone to do it. She also said, "Never again!" and tried to help me talk Paul out of it.

The pediatrician who examined Trent said that if we did decide to have it done after the rash had cleared, he would recommend using a general anesthetic!

Trent is seventeen months old now. We have never had any problems with the care of his penis. The foreskin retracts quite easily and although we aren't fanatical about cleaning it, he's never had any infections.

Dee Le Clair, Vallejo, CA

(Dee is also a La Leche League leader.)

19.5 MALE Circumcision REMOVES 16+ Functions. Do you know what they are?

19.5.1 Frenar Band, or Ridged Band

The frenar band is a group of soft ridges near the junction of the inner and outer foreskin. This region is the primary erogenous zone of the intact male body. Loss of this delicate belt of densely innervated, sexually responsive tissue reduces the fullness and intensity of sexual response.[15]

19.5.2 Mechanical Gliding Action

The foreskin's gliding action is a hallmark feature of the normal, natural, intact penis. This non-abrasive gliding of the penis in and out of its own shaft skin facilitates smooth, comfortable, pleasurable intercourse for both partners. Without this gliding action, the corona of the circumcised penis can function as a one-way valve, making artificial lubricants necessary for comfortable intercourse.[16]

19.5.3 Meissner's Corpuscles

Circumcision removes the most important sensory component of the foreskin – thousands of coiled fine-touch receptors called Meissner's corpuscles. Also lost are branches of the dorsal nerve, and between 10,000 and 20,000 specialized erotogenic nerve endings of several types. Together these detect subtle changes in motion and temperature, as well as fine gradations in texture.[17, 18]

19.5.4 Frenulum

The frenulum is a highly erogenous V-shaped structure on the underside of the glans that tethers the foreskin. During circumcision it is frequently either amputated with the foreskin or severed, which destroys or diminishes its sexual and physiological functions.[19, 20]

---

15 Taylor JR, et al. The Prepuce: Specialized Mucosa of the Penis and Its Loss to Circumcision. *Br J Urol.* 1996; 77: 291-5.
16 Fleiss PM. The Case Against Circumcision. *Mothering.* 1997/Winter: 36-45.
17 Winkelmann RK. The Erogenous Zones: Their Nerve Supply and Its Significance. *Proceedings of the Staff Meetings of the Mayo Clinic.* 1959; 34: 39-47.
18 Winkelmann RK. The Cutaneous Innervation of Human Newborn Prepuce. *JID.* 1956; 26: 53-67.
19 Cold C, Taylor J. The Prepuce. *BJU International.* 1999; 83(Suppl. 1): 34-44.
20 Kaplan GW. Complications of Circumcision. *Urol Clin N Am.* 1983; 10.

19.5.5 Dartos Fascia

Circumcision removes approximately half of this temperature-sensitive smooth muscle sheath which lies between the outer layer of skin and the corpus cavernosa.[21]

19.5.6 Immunological System

The soft mucosa (inner foreskin) contains its own immunological defense system which produces plasma cells. These cells secrete immunoglobulin antibodies as well as antibacterial and antiviral proteins, including the pathogen killing enzyme lysozyme.[22, 23]

19.5.7 Lymphatic Vessels

The loss of these vessels due to circumcision reduces the lymph flow within that part of the body's immune system.[24]

19.5.8 Estrogen Receptors

The presence of estrogen receptors within the foreskin has only recently been discovered. Their purpose is not yet understood and needs further study.[25]

19.5.9 Apocrine Glands

These glands of the inner foreskin produce pheromones – nature's powerful, silent, invisible behavioral signals to potential sexual partners. The effect of their absence on human sexuality has never been studied.[26]

---

21 Netter FH. Atlas of Human Anatomy. *Novartis.* 1997, 2nd edition, plates 234, 329, 338, 354, 355.
22 Ahmed A, Jones AW. Apocrine Cystadenoma: A Report of Two Cases Occurring on the Prepuce. *Br J Dermatol.* 1969; 81: 899-901.
23 Flower PJ, et al. An Immunopathologic Study of the Bovine Prepuce. *Veterinary Pathology.* 1983; 20: 189-202.
24 Netter FH. Atlas of Human Anatomy. *Novartis.* 1997, 2nd edition, plate 379.
25 Hausmann R, et al. The Forensic Value of the Immunohistochemical Detection of Oestrogen Receptors in Vaginal Epithelium. *International Journal of Legal Medicine.* 1996; 109: 10-30.
26 Ahmed A, Jones AW. Apocrine Cystadenoma: A Report of Two Cases Occurring on the Prepuce. *Br J Dermatol.* 1969; 81: 899-901.

19.5.10 Sebaceous Glands

The sebaceous glands may lubricate and moisturize the foreskin and glans, which is normally a protected internal organ. Not all men have sebaceous glands on their inner foreskin.[27]

19.5.11 Natural Glans Coloration

The natural coloration of the glans and inner foreskin (usually hidden and only visible to others when sexually aroused) is considerably more intense than the permanently exposed and keratinized coloration of a circumcised penis. The socio-biological function of this visual stimulus has never been studied.

The glans ranges from pink to red to dark purple among intact men of Northern European ancestry, and from pinkish to mahogany to dark brown among intact men of Color. If circumcision is performed on an infant or young boy, the connective tissue which protectively fuses the foreskin and glans together is ripped apart. This leaves the glans raw and subject to infection, scarring, pitting, shrinkage, and eventual discoloration. Over a period of years the glans becomes keratinized, adding additional layers of tissue in order to adequately protect itself, which further contributes to discoloration. Many restoring men report dramatic changes in glans color and appearance, and that these changes closely mirror the natural coloration and smooth, glossy appearance of the glans seen in intact men.[16]

19.5.12 Length and Circumference

Circumcision removes some of the length and girth of the penis – its double-layered wrapping of loose and usually overhanging foreskin is removed. A circumcised penis is truncated and thinner than it would have been if left intact.[28]

19.5.13 Blood Vessels

Several feet of blood vessels, including the frenular artery and branches of the dorsal artery, are removed in circumcision. The loss of this rich vascularization interrupts

---

27 Hyman AB, Brownstein MH. Tyson's Glands: Ectopic Sebaceous Glands and Papillomatosis Penis. *Arch Dermatol.* 1969; 99: 31-7.
28 Talarico RD, Jasaitis JE. Concealed Penis: A Complication of Neonatal Circumcision. *J Urol.* 1973; 110: 732-3.

normal blood flow to the shaft and glans of the penis, damaging the natural function of the penis and altering its development.[29, 30]

19.5.14 Sensation of the Prepuce
19.5.15 Sensation of the Corpora Cavernosa
19.5.16 Sensation of the Glans

The terminal branch of the pudendal nerve connects to the skin of the penis, the prepuce, the corpora cavernosa, and the glans. Destruction of these nerves is a rare but devastating complication of circumcision. If cut during circumcision, the top two-thirds of the penis will be almost completely without sensation.[31, 32]

19.6 Other Losses

- Circumcision performed during infancy disrupts the bonding process between child and mother. There are indications that the innate sense of trust in intimate human contact is inhibited or lost. It can also have significant adverse effects on neurological development.
  Additionally, an infant's self-confidence and hardiness is diminished by forcing the newborn victim into a defensive psychological state of "learned helplessness" or "acquired passivity" to cope with the excruciating pain which he can neither fight nor flee.
- The trauma of this early pain lowers a circumcised boy's pain threshold below that of intact boys and girls. This has been proven in a study during vaccination time.[33, 34]
- Every year some boys lose their entire penises from circumcision accidents and infections. They are then "sexually reassigned" by castration and transgender surgery, and are expected to live their lives as females.[35, 36]

---

29 Bazett HC, et al. Depth, Distribution and Probable Identification in the Prepuce of Sensory End-Organs Concerned in Sensations of Temperature and Touch; Thermometric Conductivity. *AMA Arch NeurPsych.* 1932; 27: 489-517.
30 Netter FH. Atlas of Human Anatomy. *Novartis.* 1997, 2nd edition, plates 238, 239.
31 Agur AMR (ed.). Grant's Atlas of Anatomy. Williams and Wilkins, 1991. 9th edition: 188-90.
32 Netter FH. Atlas of Human Anatomy. *Novartis.* 1997, 2nd edition, plates 380, 387.
33 Goldman G. *Circumcision: The Hidden Trauma.* Boston: Vanguard; 1997: 139-175.
34 Taddio A, et al. Effect of Neonatal Circumcision on Pain Responses during Vaccination in Boys. *Lancet.* 1995; 345: 291-2.
35 Gearhart JP, Rock JA. Total Ablation of the Penis after Circumcision with Electrocautery: A Method of Management and Long-Term Followup. *J Urol.* 1989; 142: 799-801.
36 Diamond M, Sigmundson HK. Sex Reassignment at Birth: Long-Term Review and Clinical Implications. *Arch Pediatr Adolesc Med.* 1997; 151: 298-304.

- Every year many boys in the United States and elsewhere lose their lives as a result of circumcision – a fact that is routinely ignored or obscured.[37, 38]

19.7 Informational Resources

- 16+ Functions Lost to Male Circumcision: dropbox.com/s/xoq9y67hhunkyrx/foreskinfunctions.jpg
- A Booklet for Boys: peacefulbeginningsrosemary.wordpress.com/infant-care/booklet-for-boys
- A Chronology of the Foreskin and Circumcision: Medical claims begin:
    circumstitions.com/Chronology.html#Sayre
- A Historical and Medical Critique of Circumcision (Brilliant Video):
    hooded2016.wordpress.com/2016/04/16/brilliant-video-a-historical-and-medical-critique-of-circumcision
- AAP waves white flag as Vikings storm fortress circumcision: circinfo.org/AAP_in_retreat.html
- American Academy of Pediatrics Releases – Neutral Statement on Infant Circumcision *(response to AAP)*:
    peacefulbeginningsrosemary.wordpress.com/circ-information/letter-to-aap-response
- Answers for Boys: peacefulbeginningsrosemary.wordpress.com/infant-care/answers-for-boys
- Answers to Your Questions about Avoiding Circumcision After the Neonatal Period:
    nocirc.org/publish/7pam.pdf
- Answers to Your Questions about Care of the Intact Penis in theGeriatric/ Disabled Population:
    nocirc.org/publish/8pam.pdf
- Answers to Your Questions about Premature (Forcible) Retraction of Your Young Son's Foreskin:
    nocirc.org/publish/6pam.pdf
- Answers to Your Questions About Your Young Son's Intact Penis: cirp.org/pages/parents/care
- Answers to Your Questions about Your Young Son's Intact Penis: nocirc.org/publish/4pam.pdf
- Ask the Doctor: Is it safe to keep taking steroids for two years?: dailymail.co.uk/health/article-3569818
- Ask the Experts: Forced Foreskin Retraction:
    www.drmomma.org/2009/09/ask-experts-forced-foreskin-retraction.html
- Attorneys for the Rights of the Child, Newsletter 10/4: arclaw.org/wp-content/uploads/Newsletter-10-3.pdf
- Ballooning in the Intact Child: www.drmomma.org/2011/06/ballooning-in-intact-child.html
- Basic Care of the Intact Child: www.drmomma.org/2010/01/basic-care-of-intact-child.html
- Brickhouse Projects profound film on the Bloodstained Men:
    facebook.com/groups/IntactivistsStopCircumcision/permalink/883181045198074
- Care of the Intact (Not Circumcised) Penis in the Young Child:
    doctorsopposingcircumcision.org/for-professionals/care-of-the-intact-penis
- Caring for Intact Boy: peacefulbeginningsrosemary.wordpress.com/infant-care/caring-for
- Catheters & Intact Boys: What's the Proper Procedure?:
    thewholenetwork.org/twn-news/catheters-intact-boys-whats-the-proper-procedure
- Celebrities Against Circumcision: organiclifestylemagazine.com/celebrities-against-circumcision

---

37 Kaplan GW. Complications of Circumcision. *Urol Clin N Am.* 1983; 10: 543-9.
38 Thompson RS. Routine Circumcision in the Newborn: An Opposing View. *J Fam Pract.* 1990; 31: 189-96.

- Circumcision and the American Academy of Pediatrics: Should Scientific Misconduct Result in Trade Association Liability?: facebook.com/notes/bloodstained-kansas-city/circumcision-and-the-american-academy-of-pediatrics-should-scientific-misconduct/1036828516482728/
- Circumcision Is Male Genital Mutilation: returntonow.net/2016/05/10/circumcision-male-genital-mutilation
- Circumcision: don't do it for baby's health #genitalintegrity:
  web.archive.org/web/20160504080753/http://gloriabrame.com/circumcision-dont-do-it-for-babys-health-genitalintegrity
- Court's circumcision ruling welcomed by secular medic:
  hooded2016.wordpress.com/2016/04/23/courts-circumcision-ruling-welcomed-by-secular-medic
- Development of Retractile Foreskin:
  doctorsopposingcircumcision.org/wp-content/uploads/2016/07/development-of-retractile-foreskin.pdf
- Doctor Ignorance of Male Anatomy Harms Boys:
  psychologytoday.com/intl/blog/moral-landscapes/201110/doctor-ignorance-male-anatomy-harms-boys
- Doctors Doing Harm: peacefulbeginningsrosemary.wordpress.com/circ-information/doctors-doing-harm
- Dr Martin Scurr: 'Why I think the circumcision of boys is wrong':
  j4mb.org.uk/2016/05/03/dr-martin-scurr-why-i-think-the-circumcision-of-boys-is-wrong
- Dying to Cut – Unnecessary Surgeries You May Want to Avoid, and Why:
  organiclifestylemagazine.com/dying-to-cut-unnecessary-surgeries-you-may-want-to-avoid-and-why
- Forced Retraction: i2researchhub.org/articles/doctors-opposing-circumcision-forced-retraction
- Forced Retraction: Don't Let it Happen to Your Son:
  www.drmomma.org/2010/11/forced-retraction-dont-let-it-happen-to.html
- Forced Retraction: What to do Now & How to Clean: thewholenetwork.org/twn-news/forced-retraction
- Forced Retraction: What to Do Now?: www.drmomma.org/2009/12/forced-retraction-what-now.html
- Foreskin care for boys: ccdimager.net/familypracticesource/Urology/Patient%20information%20Handouts/Pediatric%20Urology/Foreskin%20Care%20in%20Boys.pdf
- Foreskin Care Information:
  web.archive.org/web/20201019104307/http://www.icgi.org/information/penile-care-information
- Foreskin Care: A Guide for Parents: web.archive.org/web/20171014100419/http://intactamerica.org/sites/default/files/Foreskin_Care_Guide_for_Parents.pdf
- Foreskin Care: A Parent's Guide:
  web.archive.org/web/20191229023817/http://circumcisiondecisionmaker.com/downloads/foreskin-guide-pamphlet.pdf
- Foreskin Facts: facebook.com/photo.php?fbid=10152925459483693&set=p.10152925459483693
- Foreskin Morbidity in Uncircumcised Males:
  pediatrics.aappublications.org/content/early/2016/04/04/peds.2015-4340
- Foreskin Wars: Why is the United States so Addicted to Circumcision?:
  goodmenproject.com/ethics-values/foreskin-wars-why-is-the-united-states-so-addicted-to-circumcision-gmp
- Foreskin: It's Not 'Icky': www.drmomma.org/2010/12/foreskin-its-not-icky.html

- Foreskin: The Most Under Appreciated Body Part of Them All?:
    hooded2016.wordpress.com/2016/04/12/foreskin-the-most-under-appreciated-body-part-of-them-all
- Functions of the Foreskin: Purposes of the Prepuce:
    www.drmomma.org/2009/09/functions-of-foreskin-purposes-of.html
- Genital Care: peacefulbeginningsrosemary.wordpress.com/infant-care/genital-care
- German court rules circumcision goes against "fundamental right of the child to bodily integrity":
    cbsnews.com/news/german-court-rules-circumcision-goes-against-fundamental-right-of-the-child-to-bodily-integrity
- Graphic Circumcision Post Sparks Heated Debate on What Baby Boys Actually Experience:
    cafemom.com/parenting/211186-what-babies-feel-during-circumcision
- Guidelines and Suggestions for presenting information questioning and opposing infant circumcision to the public and in classes for expectant parents: peacefulbeginningsrosemary.wordpress.com/circ-information/guidelines
- Having a Foreskin: The Unspoken Aspects of having a Foreskin:
    peacefulbeginningsrosemary.wordpress.com/circ-information/having-a-foreskin
- Heart of the Issue: peacefulbeginningsrosemary.wordpress.com/circ-information/heart-of-the-issue
- Historic Highlights: nocirc.org/milestones
- How Circumcision Broke the Internet: slate.com/technology/2013/09/intactivists-online-a-fringe-group-turned-the-internet-against-circumcision.html
- How the Foreskin Protects Against UTI (urinary tract infection):
    www.drmomma.org/2009/12/how-foreskin-protects-against-uti.html
- How To Care For Your Child's Foreskin: kidshealth.org.nz/how-care-your-childs-foreskin
- How to Care for Your Intact Son: www.drmomma.org/2009/06/how-to-care-for-intact-penis-protect.html
- Humanistic Judaism and anti-circumcision Intactivism:
    jewishbusinessnews.com/2016/04/06/humanistic-judaism-and-anti-circumcision-intactivism
- Infant Rights: peacefulbeginningsrosemary.wordpress.com/infant-care/infant-rights
- Informal Survey of Prisoners Reflects Variety of Attitudes about Infant Circumcision:
    peacefulbeginningsrosemary.wordpress.com/circ-information/informal-survey
- Intact-Friendly Doctors: thewholenetwork.org/intact-friendly-doctors
- Intactivism Burn Out: peacefulbeginningsrosemary.wordpress.com/circ-information/intactivism-burn-out
- Intactivist: Definition and Resources: peacefulbeginningsrosemary.wordpress.com/circ-information/intactivist
- Is His Uncircumcised Penis Dangerous?:
    womenshealthmag.com/relationships/a19925433/is-his-uncircumcised-penis-dangerous
- Jessicah's Story: "I'm not saying your son is dirty, but his foreskin is":
    littleimages.org/blog/jessicahs-story-im-not-saying-your-son-is-dirty-but-his-foreskin-is
- Jonathon Conte: Motivations of an Intactivist:
    web.archive.org/web/20180617092132/http://intactnews.org/node/134/1318099689/jonathon-conte-motivations-intactivist
- Land of Yu-Phonia: peacefulbeginningsrosemary.wordpress.com/circ-information/land-of-yu-phonia

- Leave de Boy Penis ALONE!!! (Aka: He is Intact, Do Not Retract):
    web.archive.org/web/20130515141632/http://onelovelivity.com/childofnatureblog/leave-de-boy-penis-alone-aka-he-is-intact-do-not-retract
- Leave It Alone: peacefulbeginningsrosemary.wordpress.com/circ-information/leave-it-alone
- Letter to AAP 1988-1989: peacefulbeginningsrosemary.wordpress.com/circ-information/letter-to-aap
- Letters To AAP 2011 -: peacefulbeginningsrosemary.wordpress.com/circ-information/letters-to-aap
- Look Like Daddy: peacefulbeginningsrosemary.wordpress.com/circ-information/look-like-daddy
- 'Love ALL of him': Billboard asks parents to rethink circumcision:
    post-gazette.com/news/health/2018/07/07/Billboard-asks-parents-to-rethink-circumcision-parents-infant-male/stories/201807060178
- 'Make home circumcision illegal':
    hooded2016.wordpress.com/2016/04/19/uk-2012-make-home-circumcision-illegal
- Male Circumcision as a Feminist Issue:
    peacefulbeginningsrosemary.wordpress.com/circ-information/feminist-issue
- Minority Rules: Scientists Discover Tipping Point for the Spread of Ideas: news.rpi.edu/luwakkey/2902
- More Circumcision Myths You May Believe: Hygiene and STDs: psychologytoday.com/intl/blog/moral-landscapes/201109/more-circumcision-myths-you-may-believe-hygiene-and-stds
- NOCIRC Pamphlets: nocirc.org/publish
- Non-surgical treatment of foreskin problems (foreskin care): circinfo.org/alternatives.html
- Non-therapeutic circumcision of male minors:
    knmg.nl/zoekresultaten.htm?keyword=Non-therapeutic+circumcision+of+male+minors
- Normal Feet: peacefulbeginningsrosemary.wordpress.com/circ-information/normal-feet
- Notes on Care: peacefulbeginningsrosemary.wordpress.com/infant-care/notes-on-care
- Nurse's View on Circumcision: peacefulbeginningsrosemary.wordpress.com/circ-information/nurses-view
- One Baby's Experience: peacefulbeginningsrosemary.wordpress.com/home/babys-experience
- Only Clean What Is Seen: Reversing the Epidemic of Forcible Retraction:
    www.drmomma.org/2009/09/only-clean-what-is-seen-reversing.html
- Painful Urination During Prepuce Separation:
    www.drmomma.org/2010/01/painful-urination-during-prepuce.html
- Parents Cancel Son's Circumcision Just in Time... "I Want him Back!":
    yourwholebaby.org/blog/lucky-mom-cancels-circumcision
- Penile hygiene for intact (non-circumcised) males: cirp.org/library/hygiene
- Penis and foreskin care: rch.org.au/kidsinfo/fact_sheets/Penis_and_foreskin_care
- Penis care (uncircumcised): medlineplus.gov/ency/article/001917.htm
- Pro Circ Profile: peacefulbeginningsrosemary.wordpress.com/circ-information/pro-circ-profile
- Pro-Parental Choice Versus Pro-Circumcision: A Distinction Without a Difference:
    dbalablog.blogspot.com/2018/05/pro-parental-choice-versus-pro.html
- Proper Care of the Intact Penis (From Baby to Teenager):
    thewholenetwork.org/twn-news/proper-care-of-the-intact-penis-from-baby-to-teenager

- Protect Your Intact Son: Medical Advice for Parents When Your Doctor Says to Circumcise: www.drmomma.org/2009/08/protect-your-uncircumcised-son-expert.html
- Public Comments on Proposed CDC Circumcision Guidelines: web.archive.org/web/20190407233525/http://cdc.intactivist.net
- Questions Regarding Normal Separation of the Prepuce: www.drmomma.org/2010/01/common-questions-regarding-normal.html
- Raising Intact Boys *(private Facebook group)*: facebook.com/groups/RaisingIntactBoys
- Raising Intact Sons: www.drmomma.org/2009/11/raising-intact-sons.html
- Real Stories: I changed my mind about circumcision and left my second son intact: web.archive.org/web/20150317043202/http://www.moralogous.com/2013/07/22/real-stories-i-changed-my-mind-about-circumcision
- Red Foreskins in Children: What Does it Mean?: thewholenetwork.org/twn-news/red-foreskins-in-children-what-does-it-mean
- Remembering Elizabeth Noble and Her Contributions to Maternal Infant Health: lamaze.org/Connecting-the-Dots/Post/remembering-elizabeth-noble-and-her-contributions-to-maternal-infant-health
- Ridged Band: facebook.com/SavingOurSons/photos/a.1085533248132462.1073741850.166998263319303/1085533261465794
- Should Your Baby Boy Be Circumcised?: peacefulbeginningsrosemary.wordpress.com/circ-information/should-your-baby
- Societal Justification for Neonatal Circumcision in America (Symposium Speech): peacefulbeginningsrosemary.wordpress.com/circ-information/symposium-speech
- Some Statements About Circumcision By Circumcised Men: peacefulbeginningsrosemary.wordpress.com/circ-information/comments-from-men
- Ten Things You Should Know About the Foreskin: web.archive.org/web/20140809225627/http://www.intactamerica.org/sites/default/files/ForeskinFactsMay2011.pdf
- The Big Circumpendium: abgeblogged.rz-etelsen.net/wp-content/uploads/2014/12/The_big_Circumpendium.pdf
- The case that could end ritual male circumcision in the UK: theconversation.com/the-case-that-could-end-ritual-male-circumcision-in-the-uk-94873
- The Circ Room: peacefulbeginningsrosemary.wordpress.com/circ-information/the-circ-room
- The Circumcision Debate: circumcisiondebate.org
- The Collateral Damage of Circumcision: peacefulbeginningsrosemary.wordpress.com/circ-information/hurt-egos
- The Development of Foreskin Retraction in the Child & Adolescent: thewholenetwork.org/twn-news/the-development-of-foreskin-retraction
- The Forced Retraction of My Son: www.drmomma.org/2011/07/forced-retraction-of-my-son.html
- The Hundredth Monkey: peacefulbeginningsrosemary.wordpress.com/circ-information/hundredth-monkey

- The law will not end infant circumcisions, but education just might:
  hooded2016.wordpress.com/2016/04/21/uk-april-2016guardian-the-law-will-not-end-infant-circumcisions-but-education-just-might
- The Phony Phimosis Diagnosis: www.drmomma.org/2010/01/phony-phimosis-diagnosis.html
- The Vulnerability of Men *(Vincent Bach)*:
  web.archive.org/web/20170723175630/http://www.coloradonocirc.org/files/handouts/Vulnerability_of_Men.doc
- UTI Testing on Boys: DO NOT RETRACT!:
  www.drmomma.org/2009/09/uti-testing-on-boys-do-not-retract.html
- What exactly is circumcision and what is it not? *(Not a study, but an essay at CIRP. It's actually a great paper, but I don't think it has ever been published. The "triple whammy" really says it all):*
  cirp.org/library/anatomy/garcia
- What Is the Greatest Danger for an Uncircumcised Boy?:
  psychologytoday.com/intl/blog/moral-landscapes/201110/what-is-the-greatest-danger-uncircumcised-boy
- Why Is Circumcision So Popular in America?:
  matthewtontonoz.com/2015/01/05/why-is-circumcision-so-popular-in-america

Videos:
- Brother K and the Uncut Truth: vimeo.com/256436369
- Circumcision: The Whole Story: youtu.be/SeAXantm4tE
- Frontline and Online: Intactivist Strategies of Resistance – Brother K: youtu.be/9LI9-lNIJXY
- How Do We Talk About Circumcision?: youtu.be/f9S86vgkeCI
- Is Infant Circumcision Ethical? A Discussion with Brian D. Earp: youtu.be/mDr5ahWWV4E
- Mischief: Circumcise Me?: vimeo.com/9031078
- "Rabbi, in the kitchen ... now!": facebook.com/brotherk.bloodstainedman/videos/977345859089235
- Rosemary's Story: The Painful Dilemma: youtu.be/8LjEI9Z8N6k
- Say No to Circumcision: Leave those Babies Alone: youtu.be/SNN3Xv-q0CQ
- Sex & Circumcision: An American Love Story by Eric Clopper: youtu.be/FCuy163srRc
- Snip-Snip: vimeo.com/39719765

20 Timeline

12th Century
A very early contribution to intactivism comes from the 12th century Jewish scholar Moses Maimonides who wrote *The Guide for the Perplexed* (NY: Dover Publications). His words about the weakening, sexually diminishing effect of circumcision prove to be an essential observation and foundation for our present day work. This was one of the first books I purchased. It's copyright date is 1954. The first translation into English was in 1904.

1947
Felix Bryk authored the book *Sex and Circumcision: A Study of Phallic Worship and Mutilation in Men and Women* (Brandon House).

1949
- Joseph Lewis authored an angry tirade against genital cutting: *In The Name of Humanity* (NY: Eugenics Publishing).
- Douglas Gairdner's article "The Fate of the Foreskin – A Study of Circumcision" was published in the *British Medical Journal*, leading to a rapid decline of infant circumcision rate in Great Britain.

1971
- The American Academy of Pediatrics made the official statement: "There are no valid medical indications for circumcision in the neonatal period."
- During the early 70's Van Lewis and his brother protested circumcision on the streets in Florida and were arrested.[1]

1975
- The American Academy of Pediatrics re-stated "There is no absolute medical indication for routine circumcision of the newborn." (With much explanation of details.)
- Kenneth Hopkins and Carole Anne Babyak began lobbying people about circumcision with informal discussions in Southern California. They first went "Public" at the university of California, Santa Barbara, in the summer of 1979 when they handed out an information sheet at an anthropological speech on female circumcision by a professor.

---

1 intactamerica.org/iotm-van-lewis/

- Suzanne Arms' book *Immaculate Deception* (Boston, MA: Houghton Mifflin), highly questioned the hospital/medical system in its treatment of parents and babies during birth, thus implementing many changes in how we view childbirth.

1976
- Dr. Frederick Leboyer's book *Birth Without Violence* (NY, Alfred A. Knopf), awakened the world's awareness to the feelings and needs of infants.
- Roger Saquet wrote "Circumcision in Social Perspective", published in *Country Lady's Daybook*.

1977
- Joseph Chilton Pearce's book *Magical Child* (NY: E.P. Dutton), another inspiring book educating the public on infant awareness including strong denunciation of infant genital cutting
- Jeannine Parvati Baker's books, including *Prenatal Yoga, Conscious Conception, Hygieia* (Freestone Publishing), and many other writings during the 70's and 80's all contributed to our awareness of infants' needs and possibilities of alternative lifestyles.[2, 3, 4]
- Elizabeth Noble's books and writings, including *The Joy of Being a Boy, Primal Connections* (Simon & Schuster, 1993) and many others (*Childbirth With Insight* (1983) were invaluable to intactivism.
- Bud Berkeley – a San Francisco gay rights activist – published several articles during the 70's and 80's.
- The American Academy of Pediatrics again stated:
  "There are no medical indications for routine circumcisions, and the procedure cannot be considered an essential components of health care."
- Constance Bean's book *Labor and Delivery: An Observer's Diary* (NY: Doubleday) included a chapter "The Circ Room" (now available on the Peaceful Beginnings website). Her observations are immensely disturbing and eye opening.
- Paul Zimmer's article "Modern Ritualistic Surgery – A Layman's View of Non-ritual Neonatal Circumcision" was published in *Clinical Pediatrics*.
- Rosemary Romberg's 3rd son was born at home in Thousand Oaks, CA. The baby's circumcision caused Ms. Romberg intense emotional distress and regret. Her research began during the months that followed.

---

2 https://en.wikipedia.org/wiki/Jeannine_Parvati_Baker
3 http://marcyaxness.com/parenting-for-peace/jeannine-parvati-baker-65/
4 http://wisewomanwayofbirth.com/remembering-jeanine-parvati-baker/

1978

- Jeffrey R. Wood founded INTACT Educational Foundation, worked together via correspondence with Rosemary Romberg and wrote several articles including "The Circumcision Controversy" during the late 70's and 80's.
- Sylvia Topp's article "Why Not to Circumcise Your Baby Boy" was published in *Mothering Magazine*.

1979

- The American Academy of Pediatrics slightly backpedaled their stance by issuing the statement:
  "Newborn circumcision has potential medical benefits and advantages as well as disadvantages and risks. When circumcision is being considered, the benefits and risks should be explained to the parents and informed consent obtained."
- Kenneth Hopkins and Carole Anne Babyak first went "public" with their opposition to circumcision at the University of California, Santa Barbara, by handing out an information sheet at an anthropological speech on female circumcision by a professor
- Publication of Nicholas Carter's book *Routine Circumcision: The Tragic Myth*, (London, England: Londinium Press).
- Marilyn Milos, as a nursing student, witnessed an infant undergoing circumcision. What she observed of the infant's reaction was so upsetting that it changed her life forever. Her organization, NOCIRC, was founded in 1985, shortly after she was forced to resign from the hospital where she worked because she was giving new parents accurate information about circumcision before they signed a consent form, and she has been one of the leading voices in intactivism ever since.

1980

Publication of Edward Wallerstein's book *Circumcision: An American Health Fallacy* (Springer Publishing).

1980 – 1981

- Kenneth Hopkins and Carole Babyak did protests in the summer of 1980 & winter 1981 in the Northern California cities of Arcata, Eureka, San Francisco and Sacramento. The Associated Press and UPI carried the story and photos.[5]
- Summer of 1981 – *NBC Magazine* interviewed and then televised "The Casual Cut" feature on their show. Intactivists interviewed included Marilyn Milos, RN, Rosemary Romberg, Dr. Paul Fleiss, and Edward Wallerstein.

---

5 https://www.facebook.com/photo.php?fbid=1054798296091808&set=pb.100004414898074.-2207520000.1470254979.&type=3&theater

- December of 1981 – *The Saturday Evening Post* featured an article by Cory Servaas, M.D. "Groups Conclude: 'Routine Circumcision Not Recommended' ". This featured a graphic picture series of a baby undergoing circumcision. The slides were later sold to Rosemary Romberg who duplicated them in bulk and sold them at cost to childbirth educators and other interested people. They are now shown on line on the Peaceful Beginnings website as "One Baby's Experience." [6]

1983

- Rosemary Romberg resigned from Wood's INTACT Educational Foundation and began *Peaceful Beginnings*. At the time it consisted of instructional slides and written material concerning circumcision and other pregnancy, birth and infancy related issues. Today it continues as an online website.[7]
- Production of the film "The Circumcision Question" by Perennial Education, Highland Park, IL.
- Production of the film "A Matter of Choice" by Orion Express, Sausalito, CA.

1984

- Publication of Anne Brigg's book *Circumcision: What Every Parent Should Know* (Earlysville, VA: Birth and Parenting Publications).
- The AAP's pamphlet on intact care stated:

"The function of the foreskin and the glans at birth is delicate and easily irritated by urine and feces. The foreskin shields the glans. With circumcision this protection is lost. In such cases, the glans and especially the urinary opening (meatus) may become irritated or infected, causing ulcers, meatitis (inflammation of the meatus) and meatal stenosis (a narrowing of the urinary opening.) Such problems virtually never occur in uncircumcised penises. The foreskin protects the glans throughout life."

In 1990, the AAP removed the above with no explanation.

1985

Publication of Rosemary Romberg's book *Circumcision: The Painful Dilemma* (S. Hadley, MA: Bergin and Garvey).

1986

Kenneth Hopkins legally changed his name to Brother K as an expression of rejecting his birth name which he associated with his hospital circumcision.

---

6   https://peacefulbeginningsrosemary.wordpress.com/home/babys-experience/
7   http://peacefulbeginningsrosemary.wordpress.com

1989
- First NOCIRC Symposium was held in Anaheim, CA.
- N.O.R.M. (National Organization for Restoring Men") was founded by R. Wayne Griffiths and Tim Hammond.[8]

1990
Publication of Billy Ray Boyd's book *Circumcision: What it Does* (San Francisco, CA: Taterhill Press).

1992
- Second NOCIRC Symposium was held in San Francisco, CA.
- Publication of Jim Bigelow's book *The Joy of Uncircumcising* (Pacific Grove, CA: Hourglass Publishing).
- Publication of Thomas J. Ritter, M.D.'s book *Say No to Circumcision!* (Pacific Grove, CA: Hourglass Publishing).
- Publication of Thomas J. Ritter, M.D. and George C. Denniston, M.D.'s book *Doctors Re-Examine Circumcision* (Seattle, WA: Third Millennium Publishing).
- Publication of Tim Hammond's book *Male Circumcision in America, Violating Human Rights*.

1993
- Publication of Bud Berkeley's book *Foreskin, A Closer Look*.
- Publication of "Circumcision: The Rest of the Story", Peggy O'Mara, ed. 1993. *Mothering Magazine*, Santa Fe, NM.

1994
- Publication of "To Mutilate in the Name of Jehovah or Allah: Legitimization of Male and Female Circumcision", Sami A. Aldeeb. NOHARMM, San Francisco, CA.
- Third International Symposium on Circumcision was held in College Park, Maryland.

1996
- American Cancer Society stated in a letter that circumcision is not a factor in penile, prostate or cervical cancer.[9]
- Fourth International Symposium on Sexual Mutilation was held in Lausanne, Switzerland.

---

8 http://norm.org/
9 http://www.cirp.org/library/statements/letters /1996-02_ACS/

1997

- The American Academy of Pediatrics issued the following statement:
  "It is emphasized that newborn circumcision is an elective procedure to be performed at the request of the parents when the infant is physiologically and clinically stable. Because of the lack of hard scientific data, a firm recommendation for appropriate method of pain control was not provided. The AAP has recently convened a task force to review new information available since the writing of the Guidelines with the goal of making specific recommendations on this issue."
- Female genital mutilation (even a tiny, "ceremonial" nick) was made illegal in the United States. (Males were left unprotected by legislation.)
- Publication of Ronald Goldman's book *Circumcision: The Hidden Trauma* (Boston, MA: Vanguard Publications).
- Publication of "Sexual Mutilations: A Human Tragedy", George C. Denniston and Marilyn Fayre Milos, eds. Proceedings of the Fourth International Symposium on Sexual Mutilations, Lausanne, Switzerland, 1996. Plenum Publishers.

1998

- Fifth International Symposium on Circumcision and Genital Integrity was held in Oxford, England.
- Hugh Young published the first of The Intactivism Pages[10], a comprehensive compilation of the case for leaving babies of all sexes intact, featuring lists of foreskin functions, bad reasons to cut, intact celebrities, etc.
- Publication of Billy Ray Boyd's books Circumcision Exposed, The Crossing Press, Freedom, CA and "Circumcision: What it Does", Tatterhill Press, San Francisco, CA.
- Publication of Ronald Goldman's book *Questioning Circumcision: A Jewish Perspective* (Boston, MA: Circumcision Resource Center).

1999

- Publication of "Male and Female Circumcision: Medical, Legal, and Ethical Considerations in Pediatric Practice", George C. Denniston, Frederick Mansfield Hodges, Marilyn Fayre Milos, eds. Proceedings of the Fifth International Symposium on Sexual Mutilations, Oxford, UK, August 5-7, 1998. Kluwer Academic/Plenum Publishers.

2000

- Sixth International Symposium on Circumcision and Genital Integrity was held in Sydney, Australia.

---

10 http://www.circumstitions.com

- Publication of David L. Gollaher's book *Circumcision: A History of the World's Most Controversial Surgery* (Boston, MA: Vanguard Publications).
- Publication of "Sweet Dreams: A Pediatricians Secrets for Your Child's Good Night's Sleep" by Paul M. Fleiss, MD, MPH, FAAP with Frederick M. Hodges, DPhil (Oxon), Lowell House.
- Publication of John Colapinto's book *As Nature Made Him: The Boy Who Was Raised As a Girl* (NY: HarperCollins Publishers).

2001

- Publication of *Doctors Re-examine Circumcision*, 3rd edition, Thomas J. Ritter, M.D. and George C. Denniston, M.D., Third Millennium Publishing Co., Mountville, PA.
- Publication of "Understanding Circumcision: A Multi-Disciplinary Approach to a Multi-Dimensional Problem", George C. Denniston, Frederick Mansfield Hodges, Marilyn Fayre Milos, eds. Proceedings of the Sixth International Symposium on Genital Integrity, Sydney, Australia, December 7-9, 2000. Kluwer Academic/ Plenum Publishers.

2002

- Seventh International Symposium on Circumcision, Human Rights and Modern Society was held in Washington, D.C.
- Publication of Paul M. Fleiss, M.D. and Frederick M. Hodges, D.Phil's book *What Your Doctor May Not Tell You About Circumcision* (NY: Warner Books).

2004

- Eighth International symposium on Circumcision and Human Rights was held in Padua, Italy.
- Publication of "Flesh and Blood: Perspectives on the Problem of Circumcision in Contemporary Society", George C. Denniston, Frederick Mansfield Hodges, Marilyn Fayre Milos, eds. Proceedings of the Seventh International Symposium on Human Rights and Modern Society, Washington, DC, USA, April 4-7, 2002. Kluwer Academic/Plenum Publishers.

2005

- The magicians Penn & Teller produced their film: *Circumcision is BULLSH*T!* [11]
- Publication of Leonard Glick's book *Marked in Your Flesh: Circumcision from Ancient Judea to Modern America* (Oxford University Press).

---

11 www.liveleak.com/view?i=416_1218124584

- The Peaceful Parenting Network was first established by Danelle Frisbie and a few fellow professors to increase awareness and educate on baby/child-friendly ways of parenting and living (which of course includes genital autonomy); The DrMomma.org site came not long after merely as a way to share information that we'd previously always been emailing to interested persons and students (we taught workshops at the time).

2006

- Ninth International Symposium on Circumcision, Genital Integrity and Human Rights was held in Seattle, Washington.
- Publication of "Bodily Integrity and the Politics of Circumcision: Culture, Controversy, and Change", George C. Denniston, Frederick Mansfield Hodges, Marilyn Fayre Milos, eds. Proceedings of the Eighth International Symposium on Circumcision and Human Rights: An Anthropological, Medical, Legal, and Ethical Analysis, Padua Italy, September 2-4, 2004. Springer
- Publication of Robert Darby's book *A Surgical Temptation: The Demonization of the Foreskin & the Rise of Circumcision in Britain* (University of Chicago Press).

2007

Production of *CUT: Slicing Through the Myths*, by Eliyahu Ungar-Sargon.[12]

2008

- Tenth International Symposium on Circumcision, Genital Integrity and Human Rights was held in Staffordshire, U.K.
- Saving Our Sons was founded by Danelle Frisbie as an intact-specific educational effort.
- Intact America was founded.

2009

Peter Keay started Little Images[13] to research and work towards ending the genital cutting of minors, specifically within Christian communities.

2010

- Eleventh International Symposium on Circumcision, Genital Integrity and Human Rights was held in Berkeley, CA.
- Glen Callender founds the Canadian Foreskin Awareness Project (CAN-FAP).

---

12 https://www.youtube.com/watch?v=VkBsrBHpbDs
13 littleimages.org

- "Bloodstained Man in London" Richard Duncker introduced the idea of male protesters wearing white painters' overalls, marked with red crotches, hence making his wound visible to the world. Brother K conceived the name "Bloodstained Men" and wore the suit for the first time in March 2010.
- The INTACT Network was established as a grassroots effort to duplicate and disseminate efforts at the local level by advocates across the board.
- Publication of Lisa Braver Moss' book *The Measure of His Grief*.
- The WHOLE Network was founded by Lauren Jenks soon after having her son. She dreamed of an organization dedicated to providing accurate information about circumcision and proper intact care. TWN is now fueled by a team of directors who supply information to both medical professionals and the general public, both in the United States and abroad.

2011

Production of the film *An Elephant in the Hospital* by Ryan McAllister.[14]

2012

- Twelfth International Symposium on Law, Genital Integrity and Human Rights was held in Helsinki, Finland.
- American Academy of Pediatrics back-pedaled on its pronouncement on the non-necessity of circumcision, insisting that it has "some benefits:"
  "Evaluation of current evidence indicates that the health benefits of newborn male circumcision outweigh the risks and that the procedure's benefits justify access to this procedure for families who choose it. Parents ultimately should decide whether circumcision is in the best interests of their male child. They will need to weigh medical information in the context of their own religious, ethical, and cultural beliefs and practices. The medical benefits alone may not outweigh these other considerations for individual families."
- The 2012 statement has received an extraordinary level of critical comment. The AAP's position on male circumcision is markedly different from the positions of other medical societies.
  - The Circumcision Reference Library believes that the critical comment should be published along with the statements and that the public should read the critical comment before drawing any conclusions about the contents of the Circumcision Policy Statement and its supporting Male Circumcision statement.
  - Staff. (2012) Commentary on American Academy of Pediatrics 2012 Circumcision Policy Statement. Doctors Opposing Circumcision. Seattle.
  - Young H. (2012) Comment. The Intactivism Pages. New Zealand.

14 https://www.youtube.com/watch?v=Ceht-3xu84I

- Svoboda JS. Van Howe RS. Out of step: fatal flaws in the latest AAP policy report on neonatal circumcision. *J Med Ethics*. 2013;00:1-8.
- Frisch M, Aigrain Y, Barauskas V, et al. Cultural bias in the AAP's 2012 technical report and policy statement on male circumcision. *Pediatrics* 2013; 131(4): 1-5.
- Jonathon Conte brought the concept of men wearing "blood-stained" white pants to the United States at the protest of the AAP conference[15] in New Orleans. Brother K morphed this concept into his current "Bloodstained men and their Friends" [16] as it exists now in the U.S.
- The first Blood Stained Men protest was held in the United States. James Loewen photographed & videoed the spectacle, and the shock of attendees at the AAP convention.[17]

2014
- Thirteenth International Symposium Genital Autonomy and Human Rights was held in Boulder, Colorado.
- Your Whole Baby[18] was founded by Jennifer Williams to provide gentle education on the lifelong harms of circumcision as well as information on the functions and proper care of the foreskin in an effort to end infant genital cutting.
- Tim Hammond directed and produced *Circumcision: Whose Body, Whose Rights?*[19]
- Publication of Lindsay R. Watson's book *Unspeakable Mutilations – Men Do Complain* (KDP).

2015
- Publication of Lisa Braver Moss and Rebecca Wald's book *Celebrating Brit Shalom*.
- Publication of Samuel M. Carnes' book The Foreskin and Why You Should Keep It.

2016
The 14th Genital Integrity symposium was held at Keele University in England.

---

15 mendocomplain.com/2012/10/28/no-prosecutions
16 bloodstainedmen.com
17 facebook.com/photo.php?fbid=131826253641204&set=oa.446304585417033&type=3&theater
18 YourWholeBaby.org
19 youtu.be/8GmIQH-Dujs

2018
- The 15th Genital Integrity symposium was held at the Kabuki Hotel in San Francisco, U.S.
- Brendon Marotta produced the film "American Circumcision".
- Eric Clopper produced the film "Sex and Circumcision: An American Love Story."
- The state of California (U.S.), condemned surgery for intersex children.
- USA Federal Judge ruled Congress lacked authority to adopt 1996 Anti-FGM law based on states' rights.

2020
"Is Circumcision a Fraud?" paper by Peter W. Adler published at Cornell Journal of Law and Public Policy.

2021
Lawsuit filed against American Academy of Pediatrics based on Peter W. Adler's "Is Circumcision a Fraud?" paper.

21 Use of Infant Foreskins in Cosmetics, Skin Grafts and Other Industries

"Imagine some weird sci-fi story about a land where they extract cells containing the vibrancy and purity from the body tissue of their newborns. These cells are then mixed with other strange concoctions and applied to their wealthier elderly citizens supposedly to restore their youth and energy. Like soylent green, almost everyone is oblivious to this macabre practice.

Oh ... wait a minute!! Where would this possibly happen??"– R.R.

In 1971 the American Academy of Pediatrics pronounced infant circumcision not medically necessary, i.e. "Not an essential element of total health care." In 1975 The American Academy of Pediatrics re-stated "There is no absolute medical indication for routine circumcision of the newborn." (With much explanation of details.) In 1977 The American Academy of Pediatrics again stated "There are no medical indications for routine circumcisions, and the procedure cannot be considered an essential components of health care." 1984 – The AAP's pamphlet on intact care stated: "The function of the foreskin and the glans at birth is delicate and easily irritated by urine and feces. The foreskin shields the glans. With circumcision this protection is lost. In such cases, the glans and especially the urinary opening (meatus) may become irritated or infected, causing ulcers, meatitis (inflammation of the meatus) and meatal stenosis (a narrowing of the urinary opening.) Such problems virtually never occur in uncircumcised penises. The foreskin protects the glans throughout life."

In the 1980's I personally sent each member of the AAP task force a xeroxed copy of the complications chapter in this book and a complimentary copy of my book to the AAP. This information was never acknowledged. They still claim that the complications of circumcision are "unknown." In 1990 the AAP removed the above foreskin information with no valid explanation. They then issued their new statement that infant circumcision "may have health benefits as well as disadvantages and risks." In 1997 The American Academy of Pediatrics issued the following statement: "It is emphasized that newborn circumcision is an elective procedure to be performed at the request of the parents when the infant is physiologically and clinically stable. Because of the lack of hard scientific data, a firm recommendation for appropriate method of pain control was not provided. The AAP has recently convened a task force to review new information available since the writing of the guidelines with the goal of making specific recommendations on this issue." Their response was identical in 2012. More recent but less official statements acknowledge that other non-medical issues are the more recognized explanations surrounding circumcision, i.e. family expectations, social pressures, etc., which should not be an expected part of the medical realm, especially with non-consenting minors.

Meanwhile, one can only wonder what egotism and sense of elitism must take place within the medical establishment. Certainly anyone's valid, scholarly efforts deserve respect, both in and outside of official academic establishments. Should a plaque on someone's wall (which may represent only a sentence or two of knowledge about infant circumcision) outweigh the countless hours and mountains of research done by another?

Is any challenge to their status quo world that threatening because it has come from a collective group, many of whom are doctors, nurses and other medical professionals themselves standing alongside remorseful parents, angry grown men, and countless other concerned citizens that are questioning their protected bubble of "authority." Do they perceive us as some sub-human species, expected to bow and scrape to their every whim, no matter how much knowledge and wisdom we may have to offer?

While doing research for this chapter I have labeled this investigation "The Smoking Gun" because there is strong evidence of yet another motivation to preserve infant circumcision as a monetary source within the U.S. medical establishment.

As early as 1977 Dr. Fleiss offered us the following warning:

> "Parents should be wary of anyone who tries to retract their child's foreskin, and especially wary of anyone who wants to cut it off. Human foreskins are in great demand for any number of commercial enterprises and the marketing of purloined baby foreskins is a multi million dollar a year industry." [1]

A flurry of magazine articles in recent years have brought much more of this to the attention of the public:

According to a "Mail on Line" article: "Dubbed a HydraFacial, the treatment's key ingredient is stem cells from an infant's foreskin. Described as a 'multi-step treatment that promises to erase wrinkles, reverse sun damage, lighten dark spots and prevent acne." [2]

Dr. Gail Naughton, speaking to NY Magazine has said: "As we age our cells divide at a slower rate which contribute to the telltale signs of aging such as wrinkles. ... Growth factors captured from the donated foreskin of a baby, ... when applied topically, spur adult skin cells to regenerate." [3]

---

1   Fleiss PM. Foreskins For Sale – Where is My Foreskin? The Case Against Circumcision. *Mothering.* 1977/Winter: 39.
2   Is This the Most Disgusting Beauty Trend Yet? – Salons in New York are Using FORESKIN in their Facials ... and Fans Say Treatment Gives Them 'Beyonce Level Confidence'. *Daily Mail.* 2015-04-23.
3   ibid.

The 30 minute treatment involves a cleansing process using salicylic and glycolic acid peel and an extraction to remove blackheads and dead skin. This process is followed by a mask packed with hydrating hyaluronic acid and a serum with foreskin extracts and then some light therapy.[4]

Another online publication has made a similar statement:

"A key ingredient in ('Miracle Wrinkle Cream') is the foreskin of a circumcised baby. It's in the antiwrinkle gel called TNS Recovery Complex. Betsy Rubenstone is the aesthetician in the plastic surgery department at the University of Pennsylvania. She knows why the foreskin is used. 'It's filled with everything we begin to lose as we age (including) growth factors, amino acids, proteins, collage, elastin and hyaluronic acid.' ... Thomas Jefferson University Hospital dermatologist Paul Bujanauskas says while TNS might have merit, he would not prescribe it for his patients because no scientific research proving its value has been published in medical journals. The cost of one bottle of TNS is about $130 and will last about a month and a half. According to people who have used it (the smell is) ... 'disgusting. It has a sour smell to it that makes you want to gag.' "[5]

Huffington Post has also announced the following:

"Anti-aging products and services is a multi-billion dollar industry. Many women and men are willing to try just about anything in order to achieve a more youthful appearance. ... HydraFacial, a facial treatment that uses (cells derived from) baby foreskin to fight acne, treat hyper-pigmentation and reduce wrinkles. The growth factors obtained from the foreskin is at a microscopic level."[6]

Scientific American provides the following explanation of the process:

"Each vial of Vavelta (enough for treating about four square centimeters of skin) ... consists of about 20 million live fibroblasts – cells that produce a skin-firming protein collagen. ... Fibroblasts also make elastin, a protein that allows the skin to snap back to its original shape, ... as well as hyaluronic acid which locks moisture in the skin. The fibroblasts are isolated from the foreskins taken from baby boys, given several months to grow and multiply in the lab and then pack-

---

4 ibid.
5 The Skinny On 'Miracle' Wrinkle Cream. *SkinMedia.com*. 2002-11.
6 Oliver D. Is Baby Foreskin The Key to Youthful Skin? *Huff Post*. 2015-04-10.

aged into treatment vials that are shipped to a select group of U.K. physicians. Each vial costs approximately 750 pounds or $1,000." [7]

Skin cells extracted from baby foreskins have also been used to create artificial skin for various medical applications: "One educated nurse from San Antonio told me they have to save infants' amputated foreskins because the hospital's Department of Oral Surgery uses them for reconstructive surgery of the inner lining of the mouth!" [8] A brief post by Reuters has stated the following:

"Apligraf (FDA approved in 1998) is made from human skin cells mixed with collagen from cattle. Made by Organogenesis, Canton, MA. Used to treat venous skin ulcers, Novarti Pharmaceuticals Corp. has global marketing rights to Apligraf, ... made with live cells from the foreskin of a newborn's penis, mixed with tissue from a cow." [9]

The U.S. Food and Drug Administration (FDA) has signed in with their approval:

"The U.S. FDA committee recommended approval of Dermagraft, artificial skin made from circumcised baby foreskins to treat diabetic foot ulcers on condition that the manufacturer, Advanced Tissue Sciences, Inc., do a post-marketing study. NOCIRC's attorney was given just five minutes to speak to the committee in defense of the babies whose foreskins are cut off and marketed without their consent. [10]

From Business Week:

"Into these tubs the workers add skin cells harvested from the foreskins of circumcised newborns (is the beginning of the process done by) Organogenesis, Inc. of Canton, MA & Advanced Tissue Sciences Inc. of La Jolla, CA. One piece of foreskin can produce four acres of engineered skin with a 5 day shelf life. [11]

The Latest From the Labs: Human Skin: "The FDA is about to approve commercial use of living tissue grown by (these two) biotech outfits." [12]

---

7   Ballantyne C. A Cut above the Rest?: Wrinkle Treatment Uses Babies' Foreskins. *Scientific American.* 2009-02-12.
8   DeSeabra R. Report on the 1995 American Academy of Pediatrics, San Francisco Convention. *Intact Network Newsletter.* 1995-11-01.
9   Reuters, 29 May 1998 [no online source available any longer].
10 NOCIRC Annual Report. La Jolla, CA. 1998/Spring.
11 Science and Technology. *Business Week.* 1988-05: 118-122.
12 Ibid.

Adding to this scandal is the usage of baby foreskins being used to create vaccines (which has undergone much misunderstanding.) Variations of one recently published article have shown up repeatedly on the internet and elsewhere.

> "Every year some infants are circumcised. During this surgical procedure part of the child's protective penile tissue is removed. This tissue removed from his penis may be sold to companies and institutions seeking the rich human fibroblast cells and other cells it contains. ... Certain microorganisms used by vaccine companies need living human cells to replicate. The cells within foreskin are being used for this purpose. Foreskin cells can be used to turn a wild-type microorganism found in nature into a genetically modified microorganism for use in vaccines." [13] (This was published by an organization which is strongly opposed to vaccines of all types.)

Other articles have stressed that the foreskin cells are only used to create cell lines which are used in testing and developing the vaccines. Foreskin cells are not used directly in the vaccines themselves.[14] In any event this does illustrate yet another example of commercial use of body tissue being taken from our babies.

The following article which appeared in The New York Daily News is one which I find curious since infant circumcision is rare in most parts of Europe:

> "German scientists have created a machine that manufactures human skin using cells from a baby's foreskin. The scientists at the Fraunhofer Institute hope the skin they've been able to produce will provide a humane [?!] alternative to using animals in testing of cosmetics and other products, a German news service, the Deutsche Presse Agentur reported:
>
> Invented by Teads, the machine has been dubbed the 'skin factory.' It is about 22 feet long, 10 feet tall and 10 feet wide. It fosters the growth of skin samples from cells extracted from foreskins of boys 4 years old or younger who are circumcised. ... After the cells from the foreskins have multiplied inside the machine, they're injected into a gel that forces them to grow into a sheet that simulates the epidermis – the outermost layer of human skin. To create a model that simulates human skin, three of these layers are fused together. The process of growing new skin takes about six weeks. At present, the Fraunhofer Institutes is producing about 5,000 new samples per month." [15]

---

13 Ursino A. Baby Foreskin is Being Used to Make Vaccines. *Vactruth.com.* 2917-09-28.
14 Human foreskin in vaccines – another anti-vaccine zombie myth. *The Original Skeptical Raptor.* 2017-10-09.
15 German Scientists Grow Artificial Skin Using Cells From Babies' Foreskins. *NY Daily News.*

Yet another resource has reported the following:

"ICCPR's (International Covenant on Civil and Political Rights) UN GA Resolution 2200 A (XXI) slavery, forced labor and traffic in persons includes the industry of a growing number of American medical hospitals and medical professionals colluding with scientific agencies harvesting neonatal foreskins for skin grafts, i.e. as compulsory organ donation." [16]

According to Forbes:

"Advanced Tissue Sciences (La Jolla, CA) retrieves foreskins from hospitals. One foreskin can create 250,000 square feet of dermis. The annual market could be 1-2 Billion $. Advanced Tissue Sciences has sold about $1 million worth of cultured dermis to Procter & Gamble, Helene Curtis and other businesses. Advanced Tissue Science's foreskin-derived merchandise held a $32 million stock offering in 1992. (The 32 page Advanced Tissue Sciences, Inc. 1997 Annual Report refers to 'fibroblasts' but does not contain the word "foreskin.")" [17]

In the business section of the Boston Globe business section, BioSurface Technology of Cambridge, MA is mentioned. These companies face no shortage of hoarding and retailing foreskins. Dr. Tania Phillips, professor of dermatology at Boston University of Medicine has stated: "Foreskin gathering and cultivating is scientifically and technologically very promising." [18]

Some of the justifications for harvesting baby foreskins have been quite strange. One example of this has come from the animal rights groups who have been deeply concerned about the use of animal testing in laboratories, including those of various cosmetic companies:

The Coriell Institute for Medical Research has stated: "Animal testing is an incredibly outdated method that should be replaced by more modern Institute for in Vitro Sciences' in vitro process." [19]

This group's website includes an Outreach section with a page dedicated to the Animal Protection Community saying: "The activities of the animal protection community have had a significant role in driving the search for valid non-animal

---

16 Brewer S. New Skin Twin Life – and Look Saver. *Longevity.* 1992-09.
17 Pitta J. Biosynthetics. *Forbes.* 1992-05-10: 170-1.
18 Rosenberg R. Companies See $1.5b Market in Replacement Skin Products. *The Boston Globe.* 1992-10-19: 22-3.
19 Animal testing versus... human animal testing. The profits of circumcision! *CircWatch.* 2016-03-06.

methods", but is it really a non-animal method if it depends on the amputation of genital tissue from human babies?[20]

> "Are PETA, the Humane Society of the U.S., and the other listed 'animal protection outreach partners' aware of the use of genital tissue removed from American babies in this 'non-animal method?' or are they so culturally ingrained in the rite of circumcision that they no longer see it as a cruel action? ... Protecting animals from testing by using harvested genital tissue forcefully amputated from non-consenting individuals is hypocritical. How does it feel to feed the machine and treat our children as little more than guinea pigs? Why have we allowed the biomedical industry to turn our children's genitals into a commodity for the cosmetic industry?" [21]

First place in hypocrisy goes to the world famous Talk Show Maven, Oprah Winfrey, who has been an outspoken opponent of female genital mutilation, animal rights and protection of the earth's resources. According to David Balashinsky:

> "Oprah Winfrey has endorsed Meatless Mondays, and organization founded for protection of animals, promotion of health and protection of the earth's resources. ... (Yet) Winfrey has also gone on national television for Skin Medica, a company that manufactures anti-wrinkle face cream that is made from a line of fibroblasts harvested from the prepuce of infants who were subjected to non-therapeutic circumcision – a totally unnecessary genital modification surgery that causes infants excruciating pain, violates their right of bodily integrity, permanently removes a normal, sensitive and functional body part, kills over 100 of them [per year] and leaves over one million more scarred for life in the United States every year." [22]

> "Winfrey's hypocrisy has been noted by human rights advocates who have rhetorically questioned whether she would similarly endorse beauty products manufacturers with the excised genital tissue of girls, given Winfrey's opposition to the practice of female genital mutilation. Winfrey's double standard regarding the right to bodily integrity of boys is thrown into relief more generally by her robust advocacy on behalf of protecting children." [23]

---

20 ibid.
21 ibid.
22 Balashinsky D. Meatless Mondays, Oprah Winfrey and the Humane Society of the United States. *Balablog*. 2016-08-29.
23 ibid.

The late John Erickson posted the following:

"I wrote to the American Cancer Society May 1, 1987, and asked if it was true that one of the sources of the interferon used in cancer research in this country was the foreskins of circumcised human babies. A few days later, John Stevens at the American Cancer Society called and told me that the answer to my question was 'yes'."

"How much does one infant foreskin sell for? (I received an email January 1997 from someone who prefers to remain anonymous who said that the going rate for infant foreskins at a large hospital in the greater San Diego area was $35 each *[certainly much higher than that today – R.R.]* – and that 'ethical' doctors deducted that amount from their circumcision fees.)

[Whether or not he received any other answers to the following questions is not stated. – R.R.]

How many foreskins have been sold?

Who sells them? Doctors? Midwives? Mohels? Hospitals?

Who buys them?

Are there any 'middle men,' and if so, who are they?

Are the foreskins sold 'per foreskin' or by weight? (Do circumcisers have a financial incentive to cut off as much skin as possible?)

Is a foreskin still marketable if it has been covered with or injected with anesthetic? (Do circumcisers have a financial incentive not to use an anesthetic?)

Are some types of foreskin more in demand than others (w*hite*, Black, Latino, Asian)?

Are parents told that their baby's foreskin will be sold? Are they asked if their baby's foreskin may be sold?

Who is the legal owner of a baby's foreskin after it's been cut off?

Is it ethical to cut off a baby's foreskin, charge his parents for the operation, sell his foreskin without telling his parents, and keep the money? Is it legal?

Are the foreskins of children and adults being sold too?

Are other parts of people's bodies being cut off – or out – and sold without their knowledge or consent?

If someone cuts part of another person's body off – or out – and sells it without obtaining signed legal consent from the person cut, and the person who buys it makes money from it, who does that money rightfully belong to?

Does Diane Sawyer know about this?" – JAE[24]

---

24 Erickson JA. Foreskins For Sale. *Foreskin.org.*

Understandably, virtually everyone who has questioned any aspect of infant circumcision has become up in arms about this scandal.

> "Putting a baby's foreskin on your face might sound more suited to a Satanic ritual. ... A fibroblast is a piece of skin used as a culture to grow other skin cells. Baby foreskins are young and unadulterated, untouched by free radicals and environmental toxins. Their identifying proteins haven't fully developed. They are also used for growing skin for burn victims and diabetics with ulcers, eyelid replacement and skin graft surgeries. Foreskin fibroblasts are thought to secrete large amounts of human growth factor proteins which stimulate cell regeneration and collagen production, making the skin appear younger." [25]

Money has been rightfully dubbed "the root of all evil." Reports of the going prices paid for freshly amputated baby foreskins, and the costs of ensuing facial treatments bear this out.

Cate Blanchett told Vogue magazine about a treatment she received at Georgia Louise, an upmarket New York salon. ... She gives what we call the 'penis facial.' Business insider reports that the treatment costs $650 U.S. dollars and has a two year wait list.[25]

Australia based InVitro Technologies sells neonatal foreskin fibroblasts online via ATCC. One milliliter costs $427 US. dollars.[25]

Babble.com, a parenting magazine and blog network, reports that some hospitals sell foreskins to third parties and that "companies will pay thousands of dollars for a single foreskin".[25]

There is a current worldwide downward trend in the rates of circumcision, but an increasing bio-technological interest in foreskins. According to Dr. Chris Coughran (an anti-circumcision advocate):

> "The use of newborn baby foreskin cells in biotechnology for various purposes has been a driver of male circumcision since the early 1990's (interview with VICE). ... The commercialization of male circumcision is a much larger story than 'skincare product X.' It involves billions of dollars of public and private investment on a transnational, intergovernmental scale." [25]

Some readers may have visions of chopped up bits of baby foreskin being mixed in with skin cream ingredients and other substances. The actual process is intricately more complicated than this. The internet is replete with detailed, scientific descriptions of exactly how cells are extracted from infant foreskins and grown into artificial

---

25   Kesa I. Beauty Industry Part of Foreskin Flesh Trade, Anti-Circumcision Activists Warn. *Vice.com.* 2018-03-27.

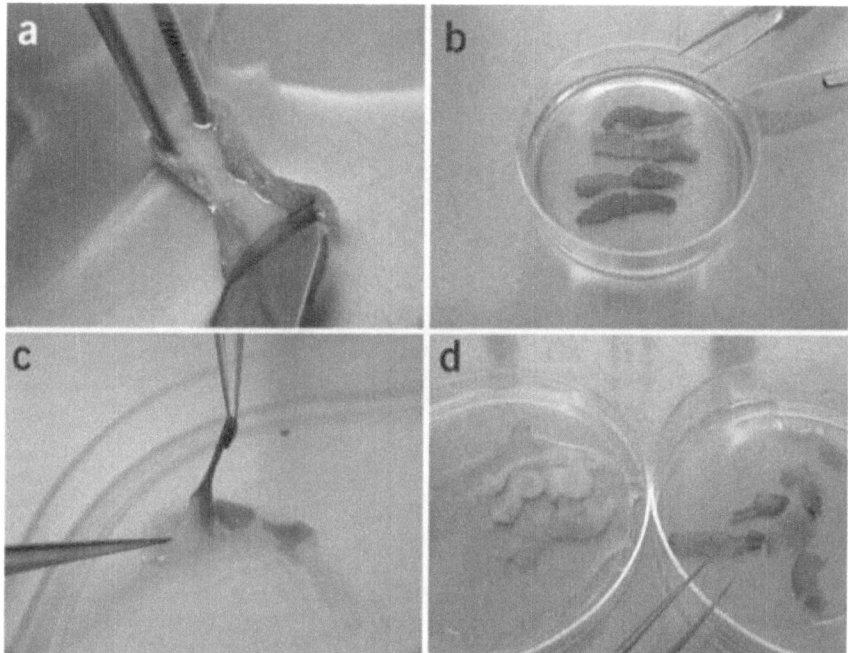

Cutting Foreskins

skin or substances to add to skin treatments. Most of this is probably beyond the interest or understanding of most of us outside of the scientific/medical realm. The following is just one example of the descriptions available:

> "Foreskins were obtained from newborn babies after circumcision and donated by parents. Foreskins were washed, minced by scissors and dissociated to single cells by trypsinization. The resulting cells were grown in a culture medium of 80% Dulbecco modified Eagle medium, no pyruvate, high glucose formulation, supplemented with either 20% fetal bovine serum or 20% human serum. Foreskin cells were split using trypsin. Feeder layers were later transferred to the human ES cell medium supplemented with 20% SR. Cells were frozen in liquid nitrogen. Human ES cell lines were initially cultured with MEF and then transferred to the foreskin lines.
>
> All foreskin lines tested gave rise to fibroblast-like lines which were grown and split for more than 25 consecutive passages. ... No reduction in the rate of growth or the ability to support human ES growth was noted after using high-passage foreskin cells or after freeze and thaw cycles. When in culture, foreskin fibroblasts are known to grow at least 42 passages before senescence. Human ES

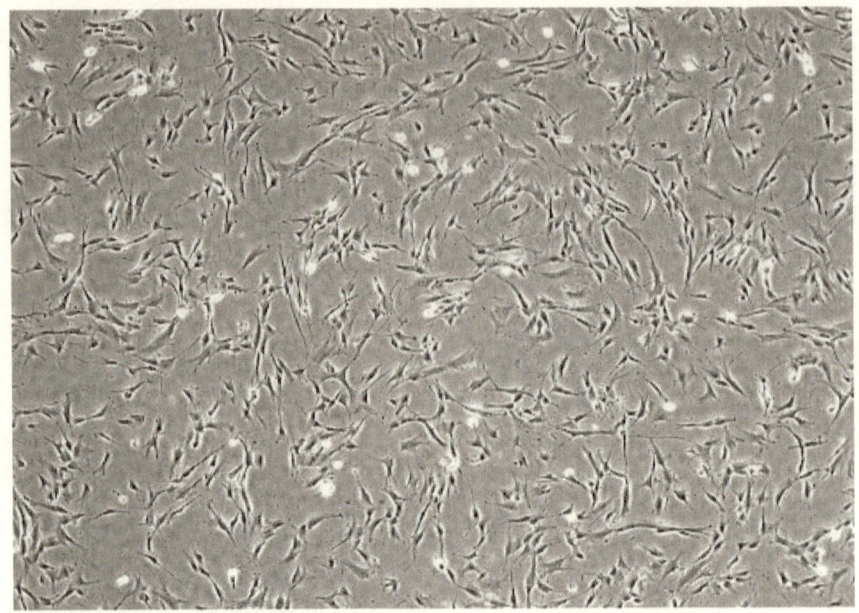

Microscopic view of foreskin cells

cell lines were easily transferred to the foreskin feeders. Each transferred line continued to proliferate and maintained normal ES features." [26]

With the huge profit potential in harvested baby foreskins is it any wonder that the AAP continues to drag its feet about the "benefits versus risks" of infant circumcision? Doctors get paid for doing the procedure (usually through reimbursements from insurance companies.) More profit is made by selling foreskins to the various pharmaceutical and cosmetic companies who benefit widely from the sale of their product. Further money is earned for treating the many complications of circumcision, not to mention the plethora of sexual lubricants and erectile dysfunction medications purchased later in life as a result of lack of the natural gliding function that a foreskin affords.

More recent statements from the AAP appear to be increasingly waffling about any true medical benefits of cutting a baby's genitals.

"The AAPs' task force published in 2012: 'The health benefits of newborn male circumcision outweigh the risks.' ... This formulation of the debate, 'benefits

---

26 Amit M, Margulets V, Segev H, Shariki K, Laevsky I, Coleman R, Itskovitz-Eldor J. Human Feeder Layers for Human Embryonic Stem Cells. *Biol Reprod.* 2003-06-01; 68(6): 2150-6.

versus risks' rather than 'medical necessity' resulted in wide-ranging ramifications. ... This was vigorously criticized by anti-circumcision activists as well as many primarily European physicians and medical societies. Difficulties with this approach included the lack of a universally accepted metric to accurately measure or balance the risks and benefits. ... (There has been) insufficient information about the actual incidence and burden of non acute complications. ... 'The procedure's benefits justify access to this procedure for families who choose it,' and later 'health benefits are not great enough to recommend routine circumcision,' ... What was the task force really saying?

The health issues are only one small piece of the puzzle. In much of the world, newborn circumcision is not primarily a medical decision. Most circumcisions are done due to religious and cultural tradition. ... Parents choose what they want for a wide variety of non-medical reasons. (It is usually a) non-therapeutic, only partially medical decision. ... As physicians, although we claim authority in the medical realm, we have no standing to judge on these other elements. The ethical standard used was 'the best interest of the child.'

In this setting the well-informed parent was felt to be the best proxy to pass this judgment. Protecting this option was not an idle concern at a time when there are serious efforts in both the U.S. and Europe to ban the procedure outright.

In circumcision, what we have is a messy immeasurable choice that we leave to the parents to process and decide.

To the anti-circumcision activists ... educate and promote the prepuce positively, to win in the court of public opinion, and to change the culture, so as to make having a foreskin be the 'popular thing to do.' " [27]

In my opinion, although the challenge to change public attitudes is an excellent idea, and much of our actions as intactivists include this, Freedman is passing the buck. (Or as the late Edward Wallerstein firmly announced on NBC Magazine's television article in 1981 "The Casual Cut" – a "cop out.")

As a seasoned childbirth educator during the 70's and 80's decades I have witnessed how parents and activists have struggled to make changes within the birthing scene, especially in hospitals. Parents have pleaded to have immediate access to their babies following birth, only to be forced to accept a waiting period. Mothers have begged not to be given routine episiotomies to no avail. Parents have fought to have their breastfed babies be given no supplementary water or formula. I could continue here with a long list of urgently wanted changes in how birth and infant care is handled. Change has been steady but sometimes much too slow, while hospital per-

---

[27] Freedman A. The Circumcision Debate: Beyond Benefits and Risks. *Pediatrics.* 2016-05; 137(5): e20160594.

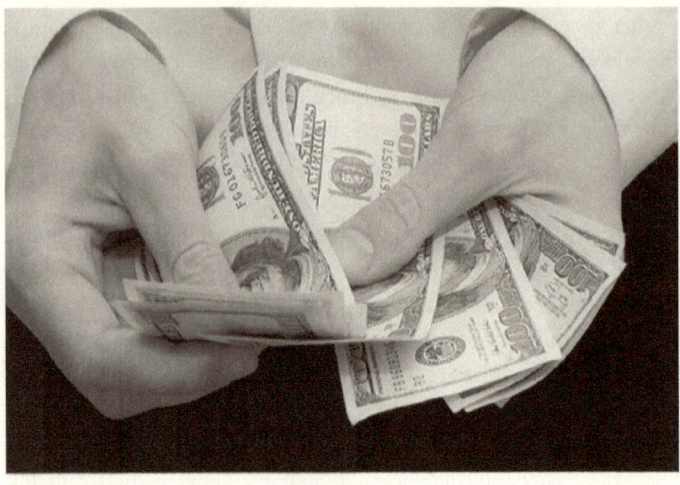

sonnel have stubbornly fought against suggested challenges to their long established system, as if non-medical people were some sort of ignorant subspecies.

Now, as to circumcision, suddenly we're asked to make our own choice? This may be a good idea on paper, yet we hear countless stories of parents wishing to leave their sons intact being harassed and bullied by hospital personnel during their stay. Parents have had to say no repeatedly as one nurse after another asks them about circumcision. As intactivists we have had to provide parents with infant t-shirts, wrist or leg bands and signs to attach to the baby isolettes or incubators which say "Do Not Circumcise" and "Do Not Retract Foreskin." Sadly, some parents who have wished to leave their sons intact have been heavily pressured by doctors or other personnel until they finally agreed to it.

The medical system is challenged to take a positive, ethical stand against circumcision. Freedman has clearly stated, most of the considerations surrounding circumcision are not medical concerns, hence outside of the medical arena. No other body part is treated this way, as if slated for destruction over the slightest problem or at the whims of the adults involved. If a parent were to ask for the amputation of any other normal body part of their infant, such as chopping off his feet or hands, no sane doctor would agree and the parents would at least be slated for mental health evaluation if not imprisonment. A sane and ethical society would quickly recognize amputation of normal genital tissue from a non-consenting infant as preposterous. But endless craving for money and cultural/religious conformity blinds our sensibilities while positions of authority bloats our egos. Sadly this has serious hampered American doctors and other medical personnel – people whose role is supposed to be one of caring and service to all of humanity.

21 – Use of Infant Foreskins in Cosmetics, Skin Grafts and Other Industries

21.1   As Concerned Consumers What Can We Do?

We are often asked if there are certain products we should boycott. The facial substances and treatments derived from infant foreskins are quite expensive and appear to be primarily available at high priced salons catering to celebrities and other wealthy people. To the best of my knowledge foreskin based concoctions are not available on the shelves at ordinary drug stores or other outlets. (Hopefully this will not become an omen for products of the future.) As of now it appears that we are not harming boys by purchasing reasonably priced products or making our own recipes for facial care. At one time someone advised me that "pentapeptides" was the code word to look for in the fine print details of product ingredients. This left me dismayed as I found this word listed on various low priced skin care substances. Later, another person told me that pentapeptides can come from a variety of protein sources, so apparently these easily purchased items under suspect were now off the hook.

If we become medical patients in need of any type of skin graft, it is hoped that we or our caretakers can know of our wishes and insist that no product derived from infant foreskin be used. (Dedicated vegans make similar stipulations to avoid use of any animal sourced product when medical intervention is needed.)

The overall rates of newborn circumcision are continually dropping while commercial demand for infant foreskins continues to increase. Therefore our hope is that alternative substances can be found for their "miracle cream" and other products. Hospital maternity wards are replete with placentas and umbilical cords which are not normally needed after birth. (Use of animal based products is a separate "can of worms." Other groups are avidly voicing their objection to this. Some have suggested use of body tissue from miscarriages, still births or neonatal deaths could be used. Undoubtedly many parents would find this objectionable. Use of fetal cells and body parts from deliberate abortions is yet another scandal, regardless of what personal circumstance or tragedy may have led any woman to the abortionist.)

As I am writing this, I am now in my 70's. I'm a proud grandma of four beautiful grandchildren and have many memories of my sparkling days of youth. I'm now going for a "not too bad for my age" appearance. Us "70 somethings" cannot expect to look like 20 year olds. Some would say "we've earned our age lines."

There are many ways to keep our skin vibrant and healthy well into our later years without spending a fortune or extracting cells from non-consenting infants. I've obtained many ideas from my own use and from suggestions given by friends:

1. Abstain from smoking, especially tobacco cigarettes which are well known to contribute to aging, health hazards and skin damage.

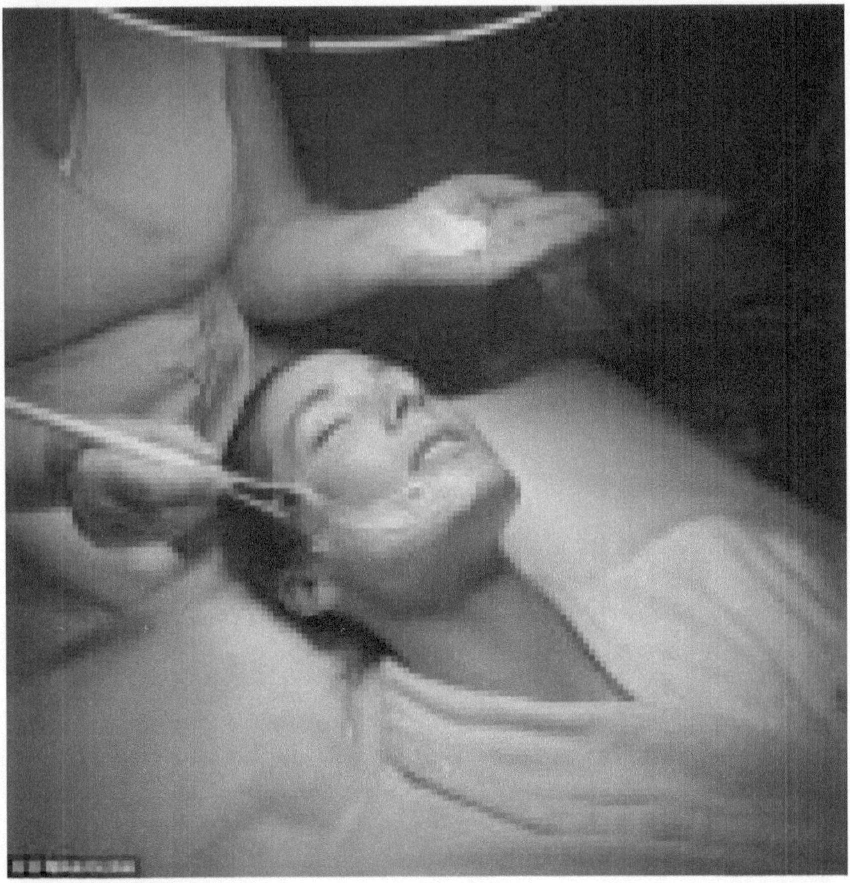

Circumcision – The Painful Dilemma

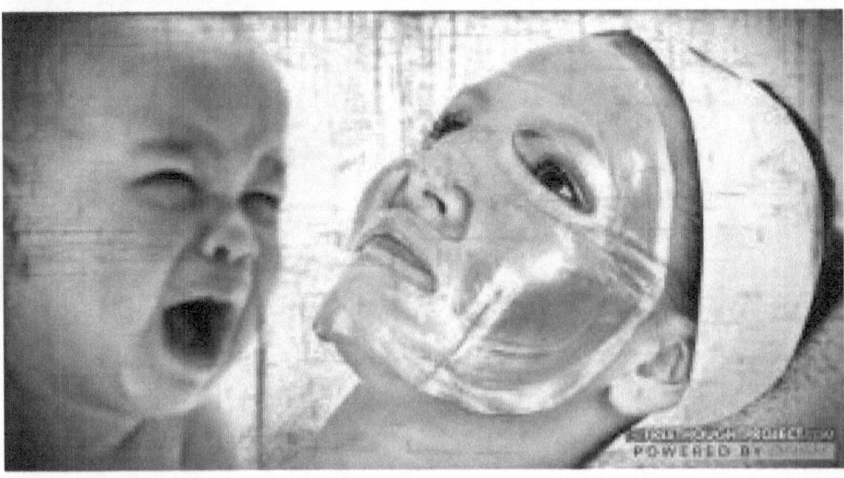

21 – Use of Infant Foreskins in Cosmetics, Skin Grafts and Other Industries

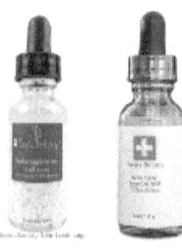 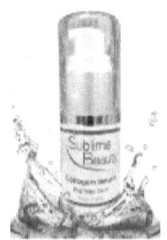 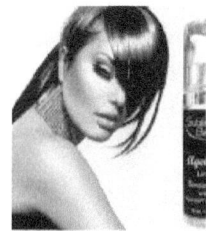

2. Limit sun exposure, especially in tropical environments. There are healthy and environmentally safe sunscreens available. Sun hats and loose but body covering clothing can be helpful. There are also "rash guard" types of long sleeved or long legged clothing which are specially made for swimming while protecting the body from sun damage.
3. Follow a healthy and moderate diet. Fresh fruits and vegetables, nuts and seeds, and healthy grains like brown or black rice and whole wheat breads are almost always advisable (barring personal allergies.) I've heard from carnivore advocates who recommend copious amounts of meats, eggs and other animal based products. I've also heard from vegans and vegetarians who have expounded on the cruelty of animal slaughtering and the dangers of meat eating. I am not making any stand on either extreme. One can be extremely healthy and long lived without the use of animal products, but for those who choose not to be a total vegan or vegetarian, I would recommend keeping such products down to a minimum. Also we all know that sugar and other junk foods offer no nutritional value. Either abstain from them, or at least keep such things down to a minimum (which is what I do.)
4. Over use of alcohol can exacerbate aging. Some of this may be related to the overall lifestyle and diet of a heavy drinker. Abstaining from alcohol or limiting it to occasional social events is the better choice. Most alcoholic drinks can be classified along with empty calories and junk food, although some people laud the health benefits of wine with meals.
5. Do use ample moisturizer. There are many, inexpensive and beneficial oils and healthfully based skin products on the market that contain no human cell based products (some also have no animal products or animal cruelty used in testing.) There are also recipes available for making ones own skin moisturizers from household products or substances available from health food stores.
6. Stay hydrated. The best substance for this is water. Drink plenty of water or other healthy liquids, especially in hot weather or when physically active.

7. Vitamins and other nutritional supplements are purported to be of help to retaining our youth. If possible, supplements should be pure and organic. (The many that have been suggested by others have included multivitamins, vitamins C, B, D & E, calcium, collagen, turmeric, cranberry oil, fish oil and flax seed oil.)
8. Get adequate sleep. No one looks or feels their best when overly fatigued or sleep deprived.

Skin care suggestions from others have included lemon essential oil and coconut oil (applied directly or in the bath water), essential oils such as frankincense and lavender, carrot seed oil, olive oil, tea tree oil, hemp oil, argan oil, jojoba oil, almond oil, vitamin E oil, aloe vera, red light therapy, urine therapy [!], avocados (as face cream), water cleansing, oil cleansing, barley water, banana peels, and even semen as a facial emollient. Fasting, bone broth, saunas and avoiding petrochemical products have also been suggested.

As a final consideration: **Why the fixation on youth?** The progression of age only goes forward. Should age be considered shameful? Age-ism has never made sense. There is a season to every phase of life. Should wrinkled skin or graying hair be considered ugly or something to be disguised? As a child I never understood why adults acted ashamed of telling their age. (After all, the number of years we have been on this planet is beyond our control.) I vowed to myself in early childhood that when I grew up I would never hide my age. (As of this writing I am now 71 years old.) What we may have lost in energy and physical strength we gain in wisdom and the long term perspective of a life that continually changes. There are other measure of beauty besides the taut skin of youth. Those of us who have reached our senior years are experiencing a privilege that not everyone attains.

(Skin care suggestions have been provided by Mary Minshall, Douglas Pythagoria, Sandy Gerstner, Madeline Gill, Christoph Dollis, Kim Helm, Kevin Hoffman, Eliza Bryan Tropez, Karl Remmen, Neely Murphy, Marla May, Daniel Rold & R. Van Den Kerkhof.)

21.2   Informational Resources

- 3 Ways Corporations Profit Off Harvesting Baby Foreskin:
  thinkaboutnow.com/2016/03/3-wayscorporationsprofitoffbaby-foreskin14
- A Cost-Utility Analysis of Neonatal Circumcision: journals.sagepub.com/doi/abs/10.1177/0272989x04271039
- A culture system using human foreskin fibroblasts as feeder cells allows production of human embryonic stem cells: pubmed.ncbi.nlm.nih.gov/12832363

21 – Use of Infant Foreskins in Cosmetics, Skin Grafts and Other Industries

- A Cut above the Rest?: Wrinkle Treatment Uses Babies' Foreskins:
  scientificamerican.com/article/a-cut-above-the-rest-wrin
- AAP Pamphlet "Care of the Uncircumcised Penis" Included Foreskin Functions *(foreskin info once published, now deleted by AAP)*:
  circumcision.org/aap-pamphlet-care-of-the-uncircumcised-penis-included-foreskin-functions
- Allergan and SkinMedica Face Class Action over Potential NouriCel Cancer Risk:
  bigclassaction.com/lawsuit/allergan-skinmedica-face-class-action-over-potential.php
- Animal testing versus… human animal testing. The profits of circumcision!:
  circwatch.org/animal-testing-versus-human-animal-testing-the-profits-of-circumcision
- Can Cells From a Baby's Foreskin Give You Youthful Skin?:
  web.archive.org/web/20181114083917/http://nymag.com/next/2015/03/can-a-babys-foreskin-give-you-youthful-skin.html
- Canadian Anti-Circumcision Protesters Target Oprah Over Foreskin Face Cream:
  huffingtonpost.ca/2013/04/10/oprah-skin-cream-foreskin-protest_n_3053871.html
- CCD-1112Sk (ATCC® CRL-2429™) *(foreskin product)*: lgcstandards-atcc.org/products/all/CRL-2429.aspx
- CD13 Antibody (BR2): sc-53970 *(foreskin product)*: scbt.com/p/cd13-antibody-br2
- Circumcision: Who Profits?: thewellspring.com/flex/myth-circumcision-is-neither-harmful-nor-painful/2617/circumcision-who-profits.cfm.html
- Co-culturing mammalian embryonic stem cells with human foreskin fibroblasts:
  patents.google.com/patent/US8318486
- Companies that sell foreskin cells *(IntactiWiki)*: en.intactiwiki.org/wiki/Companies_that_sell_foreskin_cells
- Each Year, over 1 million baby boys lose part of their body:
  facebook.com/photo.php?fbid=10203171066632303&set=p.10203171066632303
- Effects of N-terminal extension peptides on the structure and stability of bovine pancreatic trypsin inhibitor studied by 1H n.m.r: pubmed.ncbi.nlm.nih.gov/1282363
- Fibroblast foreskin sale *(Google results)*: google.com/search?q=fibroblast+foreskin+sale
- Fibroblast Skin Care Products at Amazon: amazon.com/s?k=fibroblast+skin
- Foreskin Products *(Coriell Institute)*: catalog.coriell.org/Search?q=foreskin
- Foreskin products by ATCC: lgcstandards-atcc.org/search#q=skin%20foreskin&sort=relevancy
- Foreskins For Sale: foreskin.org/f4sale.htm
- German scientists grow artificial skin using cells from babies' foreskins:
  web.archive.org/web/20130422154317/http://www.nydailynews.com/life-style/health/german-scientists-grow-artificial-skin-cells-baby-foreskins-article-1.994464
- Hagens Berman: Pharmaceutical Company SkinMedica Selling Misbranded Drug Products as Cosmeceuticals: businesswire.com/news/home/20140319006554/en
- HGM of Boys: Baby Genitalia Parts Sold:
  hooded2016.wordpress.com/2016/04/07/hgm-of-boys-baby-genitalia-parts-sold
- HUFO – The Missing Piece: kickstarter.com/projects/1337054006/hufo-the-missing-piece
- Human adipose-derived stem cell transplantation as a potential therapy for collagen VI-related congenital

- muscular dystrophy: stemcellres.biomedcentral.com/articles/10.1186/scrt411
- Human Body: 18 Amazing Facts:
    web.archive.org/web/20150328144609/http://tribesports.com/infographics/human-body-18-amazing-facts
- Human Dermal Fibroblasts: thermofisher.com/search/results?query=Human%20Fibroblasts
- Human Dermal Fibroblasts, neonatal (HDFn): thermofisher.com/order/catalog/product/C0045C#
- Human feeder layers for human embryonic stem cells: pubmed.ncbi.nlm.nih.gov/12606388
- Human Foreskin Fibroblast Whole Cell Lysate: rockland-inc.com/Product.aspx?id=40484
- Human Primary Neonatal Fibroblasts:
    web.archive.org/web/20170727032806/https://www.abmgood.com/Neonatal-Fibroblasts-T4104.html
- Is Baby Foreskin The Key To Youthful Skin?: huffpost.com/entry/7040808
- Is this the most disgusting beauty trend yet? Salons in New York are using FORESKIN in their facials... and fans say treatment gives them 'Beyonce level confidence': dailymail.co.uk/femail/article-3051982
- Man Accused of Stealing Human Skin From Hospital:
    nbcphiladelphia.com/news/national-international/man-accused-of-stealing-human-skin-from-hospital/70612
- Merchants of Doubt: How a Handful of Scientists Obscured the Truth on Issues from Tobacco Smoke to Global Warming: headbutler.com/reviews/merchants-doubt-how-handful-scientists-obscured-truth-issues-tobacco-smoke-global
- New controversy about circumcision raising eyebrows:
    askdrmanny.com/new-controversy-about-circumcision-raising-eyebrows
- NHFK: Epidermal keratinocytes – pooled, cultures established on collagen IV, Derivation: Neonatal foreskins:
    catalog.coriell.org/0/Sections/Search/NHFK.aspx?Ref=NHFK&PgId=202
- Normal Human Dermal Fibroblasts (NHDF): promocell.com/product/normal-human-dermal-fibroblasts-nhdf
- Oprah Draws Criticism for Endorsing Face Cream Made From Foreskins:
    web.archive.org/web/20140716002110/http://www.ecouterre.com/oprah-draws-criticism-for-endorsing-face-cream-made-from-foreskins
- "Parents love genital cutting more than they love their own children": Two "intactivists" tell Salon about foreskin restoration:
    salon.com/2015/01/31/%E2%80%9Cparents_love_genital_cutting_more_than_they_love_their_own_children%E2%80%9D_two_intactivists_tell_salon_about_foreskin_restoration
- Primary Epidermal Keratinocytes; Normal, Human, Neonatal Foreskin (HEKn) (ATCC® PCS-200-010™):
    lgcstandards-atcc.org/products/all/PCS-200-010.aspx
- Researchers transplant human hair onto mice using infant foreskins:
    web.archive.org/web/20160617075723/http://www.nydailynews.com/life-style/health/researchers-transplant-human-hair-mice-article-1.1492475
- Skin rejuvenation using cosmetic products containing growth factors, cytokines, and matrikines: a review of the literature: ncbi.nlm.nih.gov/pmc/articles/PMC5108505
- Stimulation of Collagen Production in Human Fibroblasts: dr-baumann-international.co.uk/science/Stimulation%20of%20Collagen%20Production%20in%20Human%20Fibroblasts%20with%20Vitamin%20C.pdf

- Structure and Functions of the Foreskin *(AAP)*:
  facebook.com/photo.php?fbid=10203362271092295&set=p.10203362271092295
- Sustained ability for fibroblast outgrowth from stored neonatal foreskin: a model for studying mechanisms of fibroblast outgrowth: pubmed.ncbi.nlm.nih.gov/11858954
- The Bizarrely Profitable Business Of Baby Foreskins:
  knowledgenuts.com/2013/09/23/the-bizarrely-profitable-business-of-baby-foreskins
- The Foreskin in Oprah's Facecream: www.drmomma.org/2009/10/foreskins-in-oprahs-facecream.html
- The Skin Factory: Scientists at secret German lab grow human tissue from baby foreskins in bid to end animal testing: dailymail.co.uk/news/article-2076666
- The Skinny On 'Miracle' Wrinkle Cream:
  web.archive.org/web/20080204011552/http://www.nbc10.com/health/1808693/detail.html
- TNS Essential Serum: skinmedica.com/products/correct/tnsessentialserum
- TNS Recovery Complex: skinmedica.com/products/correct/tnsrecoverycomplex
- US Doctors Are Increasingly "Self-Referring" Patients For Profit:
  exposingtruth.com/us-doctors-increasingly-self-referring-patients-profit
- When they say it's not the money... it's the money: circumstitions.com/$$$.html
- Yes, Facial Cream Is Made From Foreskins... Why, Does That Bother You?:
  familyfriendlydaddyblog.com/2014/07/06/yes-facial-cream-is-made-from-foreskins-why-does-that-bother-you
- Your son's foreskin is valuable:
  facebook.com/photo.php?fbid=1014083708614083&set=p.1014083708614083

22   Humane Alternatives in Infant Circumcision?

This book was originally intended to be an investigation, rather than a *denunciation* of infant circumcision. I began my research with a *neutral* stance on the subject. My only concern was the pain experienced by the infant. I imagined that the operation conferred many benefits. This is what the American middle class has been led to believe. I had originally planned that this book would simply guide parents to *either* decision, rather than specifically influence them against circumcision. And in my original plans it was very important that I discuss humane alternatives for those who did choose circumcision, so as to help alleviate the infant's pain.

Today I have found myself on a soapbox crusading against infant circumcision. But in the early stages of my research I was uncertain over whether I had made the right decision for my sons and undecided over whether or not I would ever have another son circumcised. I often became angry and bewildered to find so many people adamantly opposed to the operation! Even though this book has turned out to be a polemic, strongly opposing infant circumcision, I was actually several months into my research before the overwhelming facts and heartrending personal experiences convinced me that babies should not have their foreskins cut off.

It is ironic that today some people label *me* as "dogmatic" or "biased" about this issue, and are unaware of my neutral beginnings. When I hear other people's uncertain or noncommittal viewpoints about circumcision, all I am hearing are my own views before I became deeply involved in this research.

Shortly after my son Ryan was born, when my concerns about circumcision were first dawning, I had a friend who gave birth to a baby boy who was born with a naturally short foreskin which made it appear as if he had been circumcised. At the time, this event seemed to me the "ideal solution" – to have a baby boy whose penis looked like our culturally accepted norm without having to undergo the pain of circumcision. I believed that if there was some way that the pain of the operation could be eliminated or greatly minimized for the infant, then the "problem" would be solved. I had no comprehension that foreskins were of any value to the individual. I had absolutely no concern over which "style" of penis males happened to have. I had never imagined that any man had ever been dissatisfied over his lack of foreskin. Nor did I have any awareness that the presence or absence of the foreskin could make any difference sexually. *Women rarely have had any knowledge of such things.* However, these issues are of crucial, central importance to most of the men who are concerned about circumcision.

When I was originally collecting information and working on this book my three circumcised sons were my only children. Eric was 5, Jason 3, and Ryan just a few months old when I first decided to write my book. They were still little guys, in a constant state of small child immodesty and continual need of mother's attention in dressing, bathing, etc. Therefore, I was continually reminded of my own little sons' circumcised states while researching a continued stream of literature and communications repeatedly informing me (sadly), too late, of the operation's cruelty and non-necessity. (I conducted some of the interviews in this book while holding my youngest baby in my arms!) I believe that I have been a caring, sensitive mother in almost every other respect. If any mother in the world has ever wanted to believe that what was done to her own children was something beneficial and positive, it would have been me! I am certain that I battled internally with what I was learning far more intensely than most people who have researched this subject. But the overwhelming facts have won out over my initial determination to be "impartial." Some of my childbirth education peers have tried to insist upon "neutrality" on this (and other emotional issues surrounding birth.) My answer: It is easy to be "neutral" about something if one does not know very much about it. I simply have heard and learned too much. "Neutrality" for me would mean shutting down my brain and closing my heart. I am incapable of reverting back to my previous state of ignorance.

Although the issue of pain experienced by infants has been of primary importance to *me* as a mother, it is of *secondary* importance to the overall anti-circumcision concern. The *central* issue is that the infant's penis should be left in its natural state *regardless of the pain*. One cannot improve on the body by cutting any part off. The other chapters in this book have uncovered some disastrous consequences of circumcision. But even *if* cutting off the foreskin conferred minor benefits, or made absolutely no difference to the well-being of the individual, the operation, when performed on an infant is a violation of essential human rights because the infant does not have a *choice* over whether or not he should have his foreskin. Circumcision of an infant is taking away something that belongs to that individual – painful or not!

Nonetheless, fair coverage should be given to the use of anesthetics and efforts to minimize the pain felt by infants undergoing circumcision.

Ever since people first began cutting off the foreskins of infants, many have insisted that the baby feels little or no pain. Usually this is simply a means of placating one's own conscience about the matter! Others, while not thinking to question the loss of a useful piece of body tissue, *have* been conscious and aware enough to have heartfelt concern for the baby's distress, and have sought measures to alleviate the infant's pain.

Dr. Weiss, a Jewish physician who has written many articles expressing concern over the pain experienced by infants undergoing circumcision comments:

"The suffering of circumcised infants is referred to in the classical literature. Recent investigations indicate that they go through a period of stress, since they are irritable and show oozing and edema of their wounds for several days.

Throughout the ages attempts were made to decrease the pain of this operation. Some offered up special prayers in their behalf; others drowned out their cries by loud songs. During the nineteenth century the French physician du Havre pleaded for the use of an anesthetic – a plea subsequently repeated by medical men in the United States, New Zealand, and Germany." [1]

Frequently during the Jewish ritual the infant is given a small amount of wine from a spoon or to suck from a small piece of cloth. It is doubtful that the infant ingests enough wine for the alcohol to have an anesthetic effect. If an infant were actually given enough alcohol to make him drunk this would be dangerous to his system. But the sucking action may have some value in helping the infant cope with the stress of the operation.

Older children and adults are usually given general anesthesia if they are to undergo circumcision. Could this method be employed for newborns? Newborn infants *are* usually given general anesthesia if they have to have serious, necessary surgery.

General anesthesia requires the use of an operating room and an anesthesiologist on duty. If all male neonates undergoing routine circumcision were being given general anesthesia, this would tie up the use of valuable hospital facilities and personnel, making them unavailable for more necessary, life-saving procedures. General anesthesia would add greatly to the expense of the operation, as well as lengthen the baby's hospital stay after birth. *If* general anesthesia were deemed necessary for infant circumcision, this would force most parents and medical practitioners to *think* about the necessity of the operation. People would have to realize that circumcision *is* surgery. More parents would decide against infant circumcision. Insurance companies would be reluctant to cover the operation. Doctors would usually advise parents against it.

General anesthesia can result in complications. Its use *is* riskier when administered to a tiny baby. There is no question that if the millions of newborn male infants who undergo circumcision each year were all given general anesthesia, a number of these would experience dangerous complications and a few would die. For this reason alone, few people would wish to adopt its use.

For many, the most common "solution" has been to disregard the infant's distress from circumcision by insisting that the baby feels little or nothing. For many others, the preferred "solution" is to leave the baby as nature made him.

---

1   Weiss C. Does Circumcision of the Newborn Require an Anaesthetic? *CLP.* 1968-03; 7(3): 128-9.

22 – Humane Alternatives in Infant Circumcision?

There is one other alternative that some doctors have tried. In June 1978 *The Journal of Pediatrics* published an article describing the use of a penile dorsal nerve block for infant circumcision.

The penis has two main nerves called dorsal nerves because they are situated along the upper surface of the penile shaft. In the procedure described, two injections of lidocaine are administered into the infant's penis at the site of these two nerves, prior to circumcision.

> "Stabilizing the organ with gentle traction of the skin of the penis at an angle of about 20 to 25 degrees, the skin is pierced at one of the dorsolateral positions and the needle advanced posteromedially into the subcutaneous tissue. The depth of the needle need not be more than 0.25 to 0.5 cm. There should be no further resistance felt after the skin is penetrated, the top of the needle remaining freely movable. At this point infiltration of 0.2 to 0.4 ml. of 1% lidocaine is made, taking great care to avoid accidental vascular injection. Under no circumstance should the infiltration be made as the needle is being advanced or withdrawn. The same procedure is repeated at the other dorsolateral position." [2]

The authors conclude that this technique renders the operation painless and non-traumatic for the infant.

Had I come across this article early in my research, before I was aware of the many other issues surrounding circumcision, I may have pronounced this the "ideal solution." However, this technique demands many considerations. The authors do exhibit a certain amount of humanitarianism for their concern about the feelings of the infant. But it is questionable that this method renders circumcision totally painfree and non-traumatic for the baby. And, as previously stated, pain is certainly not the only consideration surrounding circumcision. It appears that in response to the concern that has been expressed over the infant's pain from circumcision, some medical professionals have simply sought less painful methods of operating, rather than taken the time to question the wisdom of cutting off part of someone's body.

When the dorsal nerve block is used, the infant is still strapped down to a Circumstraint board. Being forcibly restrained, strapped to a plastic board, and worked over by a giant adult, may be a more significant element in circumcision trauma than the actual pain. In Leslie Pam's primal therapy experience (see interview in Chapter 18.5) the feelings of fear, total helplessness, and being "numb" with terror at the time of the actual cutting, were more crucial than the pain itself.

---

2   Kirya C, Werthmann MW Jr. Neonatal Circumcision and Penile Dorsal Nerve Block – A Painless Procedure. *J Pediatr.* 1978-06; 92(6): 998-1000.

Additionally, two injections into the penis are certainly not without pain. Would an adult or child be nonchalant about needles being stuck into his penis? (I can bear personal witness to this. A recent fall on the ice caused me to need stitches on the inner part of my upper lip. An injection of local anesthesia was needed. I learned that the ultra sensitive tissue inside the mouth is NOT a comfortable place to receive an injection! I am an adult yet was screaming "bloody murder" as the needle went in! Of course genital tissue is the same kind of extremely sensitive tissue. One only needs to consider this.) This brings us back to the "babies don't feel pain" hoax.

Certainly complications can result from this method, either from adverse reaction to the lidocaine or from mistakes in administering the injection. A newborn infant's penis is quite tiny and the procedure does require great care and skill. Dr. Call mentions that a local injection presents a problem with swelling of tissues and resultant difficulty in making an even cut. (See interview in Chapter 18.7.)

Finally, the effects of lidocaine wear off completely in a short time. However, it is well known that the soreness, swelling, pain upon urination, and general discomfort in healing of the infant's penis last for several days. The surface of the freshly circumcised infant's glans is raw, newly-exposed tissue from which the foreskin has literally been torn away. This cannot be disregarded.

Perhaps the most significant function of the dorsal nerve block is that it alleviates the consciences of the *adults* involved.

A more recent article has suggested introduction of a sweetened substance as a means of alleviating pain of circumcision for a baby. Babies are naturally attuned to sweet tastes and mothers' milk is highly sweet in flavor. The author derived his idea from having observed the wine soaked cloths given to a babies during Jewish bris ceremonies. For hospital circumcisions he tested the use of sugar based solutions. (Elsewhere candied "ring pops" have been used.) As expected the use of a sugared substance decreased the infant crying time, and as adult we presume crying to indicate a measure of pain experienced. Obviously a baby cannot suckle and cry out at the same time. It may be that the action of suckling itself distracts the baby from the pain.[3]

However, now that we have the documented study that has verified the obvious, that infants experience pain equal to if not more than adults, we must question the "sugar as pain relief" finding.[4] How many adults would accept a lollipop or a bottle of sweetened soft drink as effective anesthesia for surgery on an exquisitely sensitive body part?

I find it difficult to believe that anyone after reading this book in its entirety would still wish to have their infant son circumcised. Even *if* a method could be

---

3   Gaff T. Sweet Solutions Can Help Manage Pain. *Kpcnnews*. 2017-01-07.
4   McIntosh J. World-first MRI Study Shows Babies Experience Pain 'Like Adults'. *MNT.* 2015-04.

devised that would render neonatal circumcision totally painless and non-traumatic, a consideration of the horrendous complications that have resulted, the sexual advantages of possessing one's foreskin, the ethics of altering another person's body without his permission, and the simple, common-sense value of leaving the body in its natural state should certainly convince most people that the operation should not be done.

However, there are some parents who still decide, after reading all the literature and arguments opposing the operation, that their sons must be circumcised. Parents who already have one or more circumcised sons sometimes find it extremely difficult to make the decision not to have it done to a subsequent son. I have also seen parents in strong disagreement over the decision. Usually it has been the mother who wants with all her heart to protect her baby from any harm while the father callously insists that his son must "match" him. (This is why I am especially angered when some people insist on blaming *mothers* for perpetuating the practice!) Parents who cannot make the decision to leave their sons as nature made them should consider alerting their doctor to the dorsal nerve block procedure, in the hopes that this will at least partly alleviate some of the baby's pain.

Jewish parents who believe that circumcision of their newborn sons is an expression of their "covenant with God" may wish to consider incorporating the dorsal nerve block procedure into the Jewish ritual. Different mohelim will undoubtedly have varying feelings about using this technique. However, I know of no stipulation in Jewish law that would prohibit this. The procedure definitely involves administering medication. Therefore a mohel would probably not be qualified to perform this part of the operation. If the parents believe that a mohel must perform the circumcision, they may have to employ a doctor to administer the anesthetic beforehand. This method may involve some additional expense, but some parents will consider it worth it if it will alleviate some of the baby's pain.

Jeffrey R. Wood has suggested yet another alternative to "conventional" routine circumcision. Some parents have chosen to have only the tip of their baby's foreskin severed without separating the remaining foreskin from the glans. If this is done with an extremely sharp blade this should be no more painful than an injection and would not involve any accompanying risks of anesthesia. The operator would have to employ unusual skill and caution, however, not to damage the glans, since no protective "bell" device would be used.[5]

This option, or other variations of the "mini" circumcision, *would* afford the individual the opportunity to stretch his remaining foreskin over his glans should he later decide that he prefers the intact appearance.

---

5   Wood JR, (personal correspondence).

It must be emphasized, however, that cutting off even a tiny amount of foreskin *still* involves strapping the baby down in the conventional manner. It *still* involves hurting his penis and exposing him to trauma and risk of complications.

There have been parents who have read our literature and have agonized over the circumcision decision, and have finally opted for a "partial" circumcision such as this as a "compromise." Most anti-circumcision activists have difficulty understanding such people. *Why* can't they be motivated to simply leave the baby's penis alone?!

Yet just as in other countries where female circumcision is common, many people today are opting for less radical variations of the operation because the custom is too culturally ingrained to be totally abandoned, there are some American parents who can not be persuaded to leave their sons totally intact, but can be persuaded to accept *partial* circumcision for their sons. It will probably take many years for American parents and doctors to totally do away with routine infant circumcision. However, perhaps many of the "partially" circumcised baby boys of today, born to parents who cannot let go of the circumcision concept, will some day, as fathers, be more willing to leave their own sons intact.

22.1 Informational Resources

- Anesthesia May Harm Children's Brains:
    webmd.com/parenting/baby/news/20120820/anesthesia-may-harm-childrens-brains
- Babies feel pain 'like adults': Most babies not given pain meds for surgery:
    sciencedaily.com/releases/2015/04/150421084812.htm
- Cathejell Lidocaine, Dynexan, EMLA, Jelliproct, Orofar, Strepsil Plus, Xylestesin-A, Xylonor *(Lidocaine)*:
    hma.eu/fileadmin/dateien/Human_Medicines/CMD_h_/Paediatric_Regulation/Assessment_Reports/Article_45_work-sharing/Lidocaine_2013_07_45_PdAR.pdf
- Circumcision and Pain: circumstitions.com/Pain.html
- Circumcision: Techniques, Results, Complications *(shows use of dorsal nerve block)*:
    coloradonocirc.org/files/handouts/Circumcision_Techniques_and_Complications.pdf
- Lidocaine toxicity secondary to local anesthesia administered in the community for elective circumcision:
    pubmed.ncbi.nlm.nih.gov/22059457
- Neonatal Cortisol Response to Circumcision with Anesthesia:
    journals.sagepub.com/doi/abs/10.1177/000992288602500807
- Oral sucrose as an analgesic drug for procedural pain in newborn infants: a randomised trial:
    thelancet.com/journals/lancet/article/PIIS0140-6736%2810%2961303-7/fulltext
- Pain in babies *(Wikipedia)*: en.wikipedia.org/wiki/Pain_in_babies
- Pain of circumcision and pain control: cirp.org/library/pain
- Pain relief for neonatal circumcision: cochrane.org/CD004217
- Sucrose as an Analgesic for Newborn Infants: pediatrics.aappublications.org/content/87/2/215

- Sugar Does Not Relieve Newborn Pain:
    www.drmomma.org/2010/09/sugar-does-not-relieve-newborn-pain.html
- Sugar-Coating a Pacifier Helps Ease Infants' Pain:
    webmd.com/parenting/baby/news/19991202/sugar-coating-pacifier-ease-infants-pain
- Sweet Ease 15ml cup: usa.philips.com/healthcare/product/HC99044/sweet-ease-15ml-cup-infant-soothing
- The Effectiveness of Anesthesia for Circumcision Pain:
    www.drmomma.org/2008/11/the-effectiveness-of-anesthesia-for.html
- The GoMo study: a randomized clinical trial assessing neonatal pain with Gomco vs Mogen clamp circumcision: ajog.org/article/S0002-9378%2815%2900249-5/abstract
- "What About Local Anesthesia?":
    peacefulbeginningsrosemary.wordpress.com/circ-information/local-anesthesia

Video:
- Infant Circumcision Operation: youtu.be/W2PKdDOjooA

Appendix A: Glossary

Some of these definitions were found with the help of:
a) Taber. *Cyclopedic Medical Dictionary.* 13th ed. 1977;
b) Webster. *7th New Collegiate Dictionary.* Springfield, MA: C & C Merriam; 1967.

amputation
The permanent loss of a normal body structure, resulting from accident, surgical intervention due to irreparable injury or disease, or as religious ritual or medical routine. Circumcision involves the surgical *amputation* of the foreskin of the penis.

balanitis
Inflammation and infection of the glans penis and mucous membrane immediately behind it.

balanoposthitis
Inflammation and infection of the glans penis and prepuce, caused by ammonia irritation during the diaper-wearing period, or by very poor hygiene in the older individual. Usually this can be resolved by simple measures and need not be treated by amputation of the foreskin (circumcision).

brith
A Hebrew word meaning "covenant" or promise (with God). Alternate spellings: "bris," "brit," "berith," or "briss." Pertains to the Jewish ritual circumcision ceremony which is normally performed on the eighth day of the male baby's life.

carcinoma
Cancer. A growth of malignant cells which may affect almost any part of the body.

carcinogen
A substance which is known to cause or stimulate the growth of cancer.

chordee
Downward curvature of the penis on erection, which is sometimes painful. This can occur as a result of a congenital anomaly, a urethral infection such as gonorrhea, or as a complication of circumcision due to excessive removal of foreskin.

circumcision
(Latin derivatives – "circum" – "around" or "in a circle"; "cisio" – "cutting")

> **enforced circumcision:** The cutting off of an individual's foreskin against his or her will. Examples: Forcible circumcision of war captives by conquering armies as an act of subjugation and humiliation; forcible circumcision of slaves as a means of identification; forcible circumcision of mental incompetents, infants, and small children. Forcible circumcision is usually performed without anesthesia.

female circumcision: The surgical amputation of the prepuce ("hood") of the clitoris, so that the glans of the clitoris is exposed. Variations include amputation of the outer part of the clitoris and labia minora (clitorectomy). Female circumcision is rarely performed in the United States or done to infants.

male circumcision: The surgical amputation of the prepuce (foreskin), which normally covers the glans penis.

voluntary circumcision: The personal decision of an adult to have his or her foreskin cut off. Usually performed under anesthesia by a doctor.

Almost all cases of amputation of the foreskin, throughout history and today, have not been the personal choice of the individual.

Circumstraint

A plastic tray molded to fit the shape of an infant's body, in which he is placed on his back with his arms and legs secured with straps for the circumcision operation. Manufactured by the Olympic Medical Company, Seattle, WA (ed. note: now bought out by Natus Medical Inc.). (See photo on page 195.)

corona

(The Greek word "korone" means "crown.") A structure resembling a crown.

corona glandis

The circular border of the glans penis.

coronal sulcus

The circular indented area or groove beneath the corona of the glans penis.

covenant

A promise or pledge. A sacred religious agreement to perform a certain act. In the case of Jewish ritual circumcision, an agreement for the Jews to mark the body in a certain way to show that they are God's "chosen people."

dorsal nerve block

A technique of injecting a local anesthetic (lidocaine) into the dorsal nerve of the penis prior to circumcision.

dorsal slit

A procedure in which a hemostat is applied to the foreskin, effectively crushing the blood vessels, after which a slit is made at that site to enlarge the opening of the foreskin.

The dorsal slit can be an effective alternative to circumcision for the purpose of enlarging and loosening a tight, non-retractable prepuce.

The dorsal slit is the first step in some methods of infant circumcision. When the Plastibell and Gomco Clamp devices are used, the normally tiny opening of the infant's foreskin must first be enlarged before the "bell" can be inserted under the foreskin and over the glans.

The dorsal slit should not be performed on intact infants or small boys for the purpose of loosening the foreskin, as it is painful and unnecessary. The foreskin normally loosens and enlarges spontaneously during the first few years of the child's life.

episiotomy
An incision made in the female perineum at the time of giving birth, for the purpose of enlarging the vaginal opening and enabling the baby to be born more quickly. After delivery this incision is repaired with stitches. Episiotomy is not necessary for the majority of vaginal births, although many doctors perform it routinely.

fistula
An abnormal, tube like passage between two parts of the body, or between one part of the body to an outside surface. A fistula may be a congenital defect due to incomplete closure of parts during development, or may result from an injury, abscess, or inflammatory process. A fistula occurring between the urethra and the outside of the shaft of the penis is a rare complication of circumcision.

foreskin
The skin which normally covers the glans penis or the clitoris. Technical term – *prepuce*. (Originally "foreskin" referred only to the portion of penile skin extending beyond the tip of the glans in the infant which usually later "disappears" as the penis grows to fill it.)

frenulum
A fold of membrane which connects two parts of the body, one part being moveable, and serves to control the movement of that part.

>**frenulum preputii:** The membrane which unites the prepuce to the glans along the underside of the penis. A frenulum develops along the line where two halves of an organ began separately and later joined during prenatal development.

glans
(Derived from the Latin word for "acorn" due to physical resemblance.) In the male: the "head" of the penis. In the female: the outer part of the clitoris. Normally the glans is covered by the prepuce and is essentially an internal organ.

Gomco clamp
A 20th century circumcision device, invented in 1934 by Aaron Goldstein, and manufactured by the Gomco Surgical Manufacturing Corp., Buffalo, N.Y. ("Gomco" is derived from "**GO**ldstein **M**edical **CO**mpany"). Also known as the *Yellen* clamp, after Hiram S. Yellen, M.D., who developed a precursor to this device during the 1800's. The device consists of a metal "bell" which is inserted under the foreskin and over the glans, and a large metal clamp which is then screwed over the foreskin and bell to crush the foreskin. The Gomco clamp is left in place for five minutes, the foreskin is then cut off and the clamp removed. (See picture display on page 184.)

hemorrhage

Excessive bleeding from an injury, surgical incision, tooth extraction, childbirth, abortion, menstruation – any event which causes rupture of blood vessels. Excessive blood loss can result in anemia (insufficient red blood cells). Severe hemorrhage may be treated by blood transfusion. Death can result from hemorrhage. Hemorrhage is an occasional complication of circumcision.

hemostat

A scissors-like clamp frequently used during surgical procedures to pinch off blood vessels or pieces of skin or to hold body tissue out of the way. One method of infant circumcision involves pulling the foreskin up beyond the glans, crushing it straight across with a hemostat, and cutting off the foreskin at that site. The dorsal slit procedure involves inserting a hemostat into the opening of the foreskin to crush the skin and blood vessels, so that it then may be enlarged without undue bleeding.

hypospadias

An abnormal opening of the male urethra onto the undersurface of the penile shaft, caused by incomplete closure during prenatal development. An infant born with hypospadias should not be routinely circumcised as the prepuce provides an effective skin graft to correct the defect. In some cases hypospadias can be corrected easily or lived with without surgery or sacrificing the foreskin.

iatrogenic

Induced by a doctor or medical practitioner, medical procedure, medication, or condition within a medical establishment. Particularly used to describe an injury, disease, or ailment (usually inadvertently) caused by the above.

infibulation

female infibulation

A form of genital mutilation, usually accompanied by primitive forms of female circumcision (clitorectomy) in which the vaginal opening is stitched closed as a method of preserving virginity. A second operation to open the vagina is required at the time of marriage.

male infibulation

The stitching or otherwise fastening of the foreskin together in front of the glans as a means of preventing masturbation.

intact

Untouched, especially by anything that harms or diminishes. Having no relevant component removed or destroyed. The adjective "intact" is currently being used to describe the individual who has his foreskin.

meatal stenosis

A condition in which the urinary opening of the glans penis becomes constricted due to repeated irritation from ammonia in urine-soaked diapers. This condition does not occur in the child with a foreskin which covers the glans, as this protects the glans from irritation. This condition only occurs in the circumcised male child whose glans is exposed.

meatal ulceration
"Burns" consisting of sores and blisters on the sensitive glans penis, especially around the urethral opening, of the circumcised child. Caused by ammonia irritation from urine as it collects in the diaper. Both male and female children may develop similar "burns" in other parts of the diaper area. The male child with a foreskin may develop similar ulcerations on the less sensitive outside of the foreskin. Urine burns are treated by frequent diaper changing, warm baths, ointments, and use of diaper liners or disposal diapers (which help draw urine away from the skin), but can be a persistent and troublesome problem. Meatal ulceration does not occur in the female child, or the intact male child, as the outer skin protects the more sensitive glans.

meatotomy
An operation to enlarge the urinary opening, done to correct severe cases of meatal stenosis, in which the irritated meatus has become so small that it is difficult to pass urine.

meatus
> **female meatus:** the passage for urine, located between the clitoris and the vaginal opening.
>
> **male meatus:** The opening in the glans of the penis, from which urine and semen are discharged.

mezizah
Hebrew term for the third step of the Jewish circumcision ritual, in which the mohel applies his mouth to the freshly circumcised infant's penis and sucks up the first drops of blood. In more recent times this procedure has been carried out via a tube, as infections, venereal disease, and tuberculosis, sometimes resulting in the death of the infant, have occurred due to contamination of the wound. Most Jewish circumcisors today have eliminated this step from the circumcision ritual. Critics have attributed sadistic and homosexual implications to this practice, while defenders claim that this was simply all that was known during ancient times to stop the bleeding.

micturition
The voiding of urine.

milah
Hebrew term for the amputation of the prepuce which is the first step of the circumcision ceremony. In ancient times this was done with a sharp stone or knife. In modern times, most mohelim use the same clamps and devices that are used by the

medical profession. (Orthodox Jews, however, prohibit the use of clamps, as they believe that not enough blood is shed with these devices.)

mitzvah

A Hebrew term meaning "religious duty." Also interpreted as "good deed" or "blessed occasion." The term "mitzvah" is used to describe the circumcision ritual.

mohel (pl. "mohelim')

A Jewish ritual circumcisor, usually a rabbi, who has special training and certification to do this operation. In former times mohelim learned from each other. In modern times, mohelim usually train in hospitals and learn from doctors who do routine (non-religious) circumcisions on newborn babies. Mohelim are licensed by their state to perform ritual circumcision on Jewish babies.

mutilate

To cut off or permanently destroy a limb or part of, to cut up or alter radically so as to make imperfect.

nachas

A Hebrew term for "parental bliss," which Jewish parents are expected to feel when their newborn infant son undergoes the circumcision ritual.

neonate

A newborn baby during the first four weeks of life.

neonatal

Of or pertaining to babies during the first four weeks of life.

non-REM sleep

A state of deep sleep without rapid eye movements, described as a "low point on an arousal continuum." Prolonged sleep beginning with a lengthy, behaviorally inactive sleep period without rapid eye movements is not normally characteristic in the sleeping patterns of newborn infants but is observed as a response following circumcision. This behavior is consistent with a theory of conservation-withdrawal in response to stressful stimulation.

paraphimosis

A condition in which the infant's normally tight foreskin is forcefully retracted beyond the glans, constricts and becomes stuck. The glans then swells and the foreskin cannot be easily replaced. The condition is extremely painful for the baby. Some doctors will immediately amputate the foreskin of a baby with this condition, although in most cases it can be corrected with warm water to ease the swelling and gentle easing back of the foreskin. If the parents or caretaker know to leave the foreskin alone during infancy this problem will not occur.

periah

A Hebrew term for the second step of the Jewish circumcision ritual, in which after the foreskin is amputated, the inner membrane is then torn away from the glans and pushed back with the mohel's thumbnail. (This step was devised to prevent the individual from later undergoing an operation to become "uncircumcised" – drawing his remaining foreskin forward to make it appear that he had never been circumcised, thereby concealing his identity as a Jew.) Modern clamp devices for circumcision eliminate the need for this step as the membranes are first separated before the insertion of the clamp and "bell."

perineum
The external region between the vulva and the anus in the female or between the scrotum and the anus in the male. This is the area that is cut when a woman has an episiotomy.

phimosis
A condition in which the foreskin is either adhered to the glans penis or tightly constricted over the glans and cannot be retracted.

> **acquired phimosis**
> A complication caused by forceful retraction of the infant's foreskin before it has separated naturally. Forcefully retracting the naturally tight foreskin of the infant will break adhesions and cause it to bleed. The foreskin and glans may heal together when the foreskin is replaced (much as two fingers, with the skin injured, would join together if bandaged together). With acquired phimosis, scar tissue develops between the foreskin and glans and the foreskin cannot be retracted. This condition can usually be corrected by gradual easing back of the foreskin over time, applying petroleum jelly or similar ointments to prevent the two surfaces from rejoining, or warm baths. However, some doctors prescribe amputation of the foreskin to correct this condition.

> **congenital or "true" phimosis**
> A rare condition in which the naturally tight foreskin, left alone from infancy, still cannot be retracted during late childhood or teenage years. Like acquired phimosis, this can usually be corrected by gradual easing back of the foreskin and warm baths, although some doctors will prescribe circumcision.

> **neonatal tightness of the foreskin**
> In the newborn infant the foreskin is *normally* adhered to the glans and has a very tiny opening. "Phimosis" is an incorrect term for this condition. The opening does not enlarge and the prepuce and glans usually do not separate until months or years later in life. The parent or medical practitioner should not attempt to loosen or retract the foreskin during infancy.

Plastibell
A circumcision device manufactured by Hollister Corporation, Chicago, IL. The device consists of a plastic "bell" which is placed over the glans and under the foreskin. A string is then tied over the foreskin and the bell, part of the foreskin is cut off, the

handle of the bell removed, and the ring of plastic stays in place. Within ten days the remaining foreskin dries up and the plastic ring normally falls off. (See picture display on page 186.)

posthitis
Inflamed condition of the foreskin.

prepuce
> **female:** The skin that covers the clitoris, sometimes called the "hood" of the clitoris. This piece of skin is cut off during female circumcision.
> **male:** The skin which normally covers the glans of the penis, commonly known as the "foreskin." This skin is what is cut off during circumcision.

priapism
Abnormal, painful and continued erection of the penis due to disease and usually without sexual desire.

pseudo
False. Used in this book to describe the modern medical establishment as a "pseudo-religion."

raphe
A seam or ridge originating in embryonic development in which two halves of an organ that begin separately are later joined. The raphe of the penis and scrotum is a ridge which extends along the posterior surface of the penis and extends through the midline of the scrotum.

retraction (of foreskin)
The pulling back of the foreskin to expose the glans. Usually this is only necessary when washing. Normally in the young boy or adult this procedure is simple. This should not be done to an infant until the foreskin has naturally loosened from the glans and can be retracted easily.

routine
A procedure that is done automatically, without question, especially by a system or organization. Pertaining to hospitals – a procedure that is done automatically to all patients in a given situation. For example: all patients admitted to a hospital will probably have a *routine* blood sample taken. Routine procedures are usually not essential life-saving procedures, but are often done as precautionary measures, or simply because that hospital staff always does things in that particular way. Therefore a mother giving birth in a hospital may have a *routine* enema, *routine* pubic shave, *routine* medication, or a *routine* separation from her baby for several hours after birth.

routine neonatal circumcision
All or nearly all newborn male infants born in a hospital have their foreskins amputated, for non-religious reasons, shortly after birth. While at least one parent is

usually asked to sign a consent form, parents are usually inclined to cooperate with hospital procedures and therefore sign it "routinely."

sandek
A Hebrew term meaning "Godfather." A man who holds the infant during the Jewish circumcision ritual. This is considered to be a position of high honor.

Sheldon clamp
A circumcision device manufactured by the Olympic Medical Supplies Company, Seattle, WA. With this method, the infant's foreskin is stretched up over the glans, smashed by this clamp, and cut off. No protective "bell" is used to cover the glans. *(This device was taken off the market during the 1980's, probably due to the greater risk of damage to the glans. – R.R.)*

smegma
The naturally occurring substance that collects beneath the foreskin of the penis and around the clitoris and labia. It is mainly composed of dead skin cells. Smegma is easily washed away while bathing. If the individual does not bathe for several days, smegma will develop an unpleasant odor (as will feet, mouths, underarms, and all parts of the body). Smegma has not been proven to be carcinogenic despite repeated tests with laboratory animals.

trauma
An event which causes great physical pain and/or psychological upset to the individual, which may have lasting repercussions affecting that person's future and/or nature. Intense fear, anger, shame, or remorse may be emotional reactions to trauma. Amputation of the foreskin (circumcision) is a *trauma* to a newborn baby. The procedure is also frequently an emotional *trauma* to new parents.

Appendix B: Bibliography

1. Abeshouse BS, Abeshouse GA. Metastatic Tumors of the Penis: A Review of the Literature and a Report of Two Cases. *J Urol.* 1961-07; 86(1): 99-112.
2. Airola P. The Circumcision Decision (ch. 19). In: *Every Woman's Book.* Phoenix, AZ: Health Plus. 1979: 263-7.
3. Aitken-Swan J, Baird D. Circumcision and Cancer of the Cervix. *Br J Cancer.* 1965-06; 19(2): 217-227.
4. Alexander IE, Blackman S. Castration, Circumcision, and Anti-Semitism. *J Abnorm Psychol.* 1957-07; 55(1): 143-4.
5. Allen JS, Summers JL, Wilkerson JE. Meatal Calibration of Newborn Boys. *J Urol.* 1972; 107: 498.
6. Anders TF, Chalemian RJ. The Effects of Circumcision on Sleep-Wake States in Human Neonates. *Psychosom Med.* 1974/Mar-Apr; 36(2): 174-9.
7. Anderson SH. A Plea for Gentleness to the Newborn. *NYT.* 1978-01-15: 48.
8. Anna-Munthrodo H. Carcinoma of the Penis in Jamaica. *J Int Coll Surg.* 1961; 35:21-31.
9. Annunziato D, Goldblum L. Staphylococcal Scalded Skin Syndrome – A Complication of Circumcision. *Am J Dis Child.* 1978-12; 132: 1187-8.
10. Apt A. Circumcision and Prostatic Cancer. *Acta Med Scand.* 1965; 178: 493-504.
11. Arms S. *Immaculate Deception.* Boston: Houghton Mifflin. 1975: 22.
12. Arnold SJ. Stenotic Meatus in Children: An Analysis of 160 Cases. *J Urol.* 1964-04; 91(4): 357-360.
13. Atkinson EM. *Behind the Mask of Medicine.* NY: Charles Scribners House. 1941: 174-183.
14. Auerbach MR, Scanlon JW. Recurrence of Pneumothorax as a Possible Complication of Elective Circumcision. *AJOG.* 1978-11-01; 132(5): 583.
15. Baker RL. Newborn Male Circumcision Needless and Dangerous. *Sex Med Today.* 1979-11; 3(11).
16. Baker TJ, Gonzalez MA. A Complication of Circumcision. *SMJ.* 1961-07; 54: 815.
17. Ball JRB, Grounds AD. Head Injury, Hypopituitarism and Paranoid Psychosis – Circumcision for the 'Singapore Virus'. *Med J Aust.* 1974-09-14: 403-5.
18. Banister PG. Circumcision. *Lancet.* 1953; 265: 401.
19. Barker-Benfield G. *The Horrors of the Half-Known Life.* New York: Harper Colophon Books. 1976.
20. Barney JD. Epithelioma of the Penis. An Analysis of One Hundred Cases. *Ann Surg.* 1907; 46: 890-914.
21. Baron SW. The Modern Age. In: Schwarz LW, ed. *Great Ages and Ideas of the Jewish People.* 1956: 366.
22. Barrie H, Huntingford PJ, Gough MH. The Plastibell Technique for Circumcision. *BMJ.* 1965-07-31: 273-4.
23. Bassett JW. Carcinoma of the Penis. *Cancer.* 1952-05; 3(3): 530-8.
24. Bean C. The Circ Room (ch. 12). In: *Labor and Delivery; An Observer's Diary.* NY: Doubleday & Co. 1977: 154-8.
25. Bergman RT, Howard AH, Barnes RW. Plastic Reconstruction of the Penis. *J Urol. 1943;* 59: 1171-1182.
26. Berkeley B. A History of Foreskin. *Drummer.* 1982-07; 54: 24-8.
27. Berkeley B. A History of Foreskin Part II. *Drummer.* 1982-08; 55: 26-28, 80-1.
28. Berkeley B. Excerpts from an Underground Newsletter. San Francisco, CA.
29. Berman W. Urinary Retention Due to Ritual Circumcision. *Pediatrics.* 1975-10; 56(4): 621.
30. Berry CD Jr, Cross RR Jr. Urethral Meatal Caliber in Circumcised and Uncircumcised Males. *AMA J Dis Child. 1956;* 92: 152-5.
31. Bettelheim B. Symbolic Wounds. In: Lessa WA, Vogt EZ, eds. *Reader in Comparative Religion.* 2nd ed. NY: Harper & Row. 1965: 230-240.
32. Bird B. A Study of the Bisexual Meaning of the Foreskin. *J Am Psychoanal Assoc.* 1958-04; 6(2): 287-304.
33. Birnbaum P. Circumcision, Brith. In: *A Book of Jewish Concepts.* NY: Hebrew Publishing. 1964: 102-3.
34. Birrell RG. A Case Against Circumcision. *Med J Aust.* 1965; 2: 393.
35. Birrell RG. Circumcision. *Aust Pediatr J.* 1970-06; 6(1): 66-7.
36. Bleich AR. Prophylaxis of Penile Carcinoma. *JAMA.* 1950-07-22; 143(12): 1054-7.
37. Bloch I. *Odoratus Sexualis.* NY: Ams Press. 1976 (reprint, original ed. 1934).

38. Bolande RP. Ritualistic Surgery – Circumcision and Tonsillectomy. *N Engl J Med.* 1969-03-13; 280(11): 591-5.
39. Boston Women's Health Book Collective, The. (information on sexually transmitted disease) *Our Bodies, Ourselves.* 2nd ed. NY: Simon and Schuster. 1971, 1973, & 1976: 168-170, 191.
40. Brackbill Y, Schroeder K. Circumcision, Gender Differences, and Neonatal Behavior: An Update. *Dev. Psychobiol.* 1980-11; 13(6): 607-614.
41. Bradley RA. Does My Wife Have to be Cut? / If We Have a Boy, Should He be Circumcised? In: *Husband-Coached Childbirth.* NY: Harper & Row. 1965: 136-143 / 159-160.
42. Brennemann J. The Ulcerated Meatus in the Circumcised Child. *Am J Dis Child.* 1920; 21: 38-47.
43. Brewer GS, Greene JP. Circumcision – Ritual Care (ch. 7). In: *Right From the Start.* Emmaus, PA: Rodale Press. 1981: 120-8.
44. Brodny ML, Robins SA. Urethrocystography in the Male Child. *JAMA.* 1948-04-21; 137(17): 1511-7.
45. Bromely RI. Circumcision. *Medical Journal and Records.* 1929-08-21; 130: 212-3.
46. Brooke BN, Walker FC. Circumcision Without Catgut. *Br J Urol.* 1964-03; 36: 106-9.
47. Brown JB. Restoration of the Entire Skin of the Penis. *Surg Gynecol Obstet.* 1937-09; 65: 362-5.
48. Browne D, Parker G, Doll R, Hadley AL, Royde CA. Fate of the Foreskin. (separate letters to the editor) *BMJ.* 1950-01-21: 181-2.
49. Bruhl P. Problems of Therapeutic Surgery in Penis Carcinoma. In: *Recent Results Cancer Res.* Bonn, Germany: Dept. of Urology, University of Bonn. 1977; (60): 120-6.
50. Bryk F. *Sex & Circumcision: A Study of Phallic Worship and Mutilation in Men and Women.* North Hollywood, CA: Brandon House. 1967.
51. Bryk F. *Circumcision in Man and Woman.* NY: American Ethnological Press. 1934.
52. Burger R. Dr. Burger Replies. *Pediatrics.* 1975-08; 56(2): 340-1.
53. Burger R, Guthrie TH. Why Circumcision? *Pediatrics.* 1974-09; 54: 362-4.
54. Burns NR. Alternative Circumcision? *Mothering.* 1979/Fall; 12: 85.
55. Butler J. Is It Wise to Circumcise? In: *Childbirth Education Newsletter.* Lewis, KS: Partal Post. 1978-06.
56. Byars LT, Trier WC. Some Complications of Circumcision and Their Surgical Repair. *AMA Arch Surg.* 1958-03; 76: 477-481.
57. Calnan J, Copenhagen H. Circumcision for the Newborn. *Br J Surg.* 1966-05; 53(5): 427-9.
58. Campbell ME. Stenosis of the External Urethral Meatus. *J Urol.* 1943; 50: 740-6.
59. Campbell ME. Stricture of the Urethra in Children. *J Pediatr.* 1949; 35: 169.
60. Canice M. Circumcision of the Newborn. *Am J Nurs.* 1960-10; 60(10): 1431-2.
61. Cansever G. Psychological Effects of Circumcision. *Br J Med Psychol.* 1965; 38: 321-331.
62. Caper P. Value of Common Medical Procedures. *N Engl J Med.* 1975-03-06; 292(10): 538.
63. Carne S. Incidence of Tonsillectomy, Circumcision, and Appendicectomy Among R.A.F. Recruits. *BMJ.* 1956-07-07; 2: 19-23.
64. Carpenter GG, Hervada AR. More Criticism of Circumcision. *Pediatrics.* 1956; 56(2): 338-9.
65. Carter N. Brutal Operation. *The Enterprise,* Riverside, CA. 1977-04-09.
66. Carter N. Brutalizing Infants. *The Enterprise,* Riverside, CA. 1975-04-09.
67. Carter N. Medical Myths. *The Enterprise,* Riverside, CA. 1975-10-04.
68. Carter N. *Routine Circumcision: The Tragic Myth.* London, England: Londinium Press. 1979.
69. Ciaglia P. The 'David' of Michelangelo or (Why the Foreskin?). *JAMA.* 1971-11-22; 218(8): 1304.
70. Cohen R. A New Circumcision Instrument. *Calif Med.* 1960-09; 93(3).
71. Colon JE. Carcinoma of the Penis. *J Urol.* 1952-05; 67(5): 702-8.
72. Comfort A. Foreskin. In: *The Joy of Sex.* Simon & Schuster. 1972: 65.
73. Conard R. Side Lights on the History of Circumcision. *Ohio State Med J.* 1954-08; 50(8): 770-3.
74. Conaway T. The First Rip-Off. *Hustler.* 1979-06: 38, 95-7.
75. Conrad A. What's Behind the Sports Myths About Sex? *Sex Med Today,* p. 26-31.
76. Conn R. Circumcision Value Questioned: Many M.D's Say Not To. *Charlotte Observer.* 1977-09-19.
77. Cooke RA, Rodrigue RB. Amoebic Balanitis. *Med J Aust.* 1964-01-25: 114-6.

78. Cozzarelli JJ, Little JA, Kariher D, Speert H. Questions and Answers – Circumcision. *JAMA*. 1965-10-18; 194(3): 205.
79. Cullen J. Circumcision: A Medical and Cultural Dilemma? *Cleo Magazine* (Australia). 1981-11: 99-105.
80. Curtis JEA. Circumcision Complicated by Pulmonary Embolism. *Nursing Mirror*. 1971; 132(25): 28-30.
81. Dagher R, Selzer ML, Lapides J. Carcinoma of the Penis and the Anti-Circumcision Crusade. *J Urol*. 1973-07; 110: 79-80.
82. Daly M. Chinese Footbinding: On Footnoting the Three-Inch 'Lotus Hooks' (ch. 4) / African Genital Mutilation:The Unspeakable Atrocities (ch. 5). In: *Gyn/Ecology – The Metaethics of Radical Feminism*. Boston: Beacon Press. 1978: 134-152 / 153-177.
83. Damjanovski L, Marcekic V, Miletic M. Circumcision and Carcinoma Colli Uteri in Macedonia, Yugoslavia. *Br J Cancer*. 1963-05-15; 17: 406-9.
84. Dańczak-Ginalska Z. Treatment of Penis Carcinoma with Interstitially Administered Iridium; Comparison with Radium Therapy. In: Grundmann E, Vahlensieck W (eds). *Tumors of the Male Genital System. Recent Results in Cancer Research*. Berlin/Heidelberg: Springer. 1977; 60: 127:134.
85. Datta NS. Simple Circumcision Dressing. *Urology*. 1976-11; 8(5): 495.
86. Datta NS, Zinner NR. Complication from Plastibell Circumcision Ring. *Urology*. 1977-01; 9(1): 57-8.
87. Davidson F. Yeasts and Circumcision in the Male. *Br J Ven Dis*. 1977; 53: 121-2.
88. Day DH. Men on the Island of Wogeo Attempt to Simulate Menstruation (letter to editor). *Ms*. 1979-02: 7.
89. DeLee JB. *Obstetrics for Nurses*. 7th ed. Philadelphia, PA: W.B. Saunders. 1924: 436-440.
90. Demetrakopoulos GE. A Different View of the Facts. Pediatrics. 1975-08; 56(2): 339-340.
91. Denton J, Schreiner RL, Pearson J. Circumcision Complication. *CLP*. 1978-03; 17: 285-6.
92. Derbes VJ. The Keepers of the Bed – Castration and Religion. *JAMA*. 1970-04-06; 212(1): 97-100.
93. Devereux G. The Significance of the External Female Genitalia and of Female Orgasm for the Male. *J Am Psychoanal Assoc*. 1958-04; 6(2): 278-286.
94. Dewhurst CJ, Michelson A. Infibulation Complicating Pregnancy. *BMJ*. 1964-12-05; 2: 1442.
95. Diaz A, Kantor HI. Dorsal Slit: A Circumcision Alternative. *Obstet Gynecol*. 1971; 37(4): 619-622.
96. Dinari G, Haimov H, Geiffman M. Umbilical Arteritis and Phlebitis with Scrotal Abscess and Peritonitis. *J Pediatr Surg*. 1971-04; 6: 176.
97. Dodge OG, Linsell CA. Carcinoma of the Penis in Uganda and Kenya Africans. *Cancer*. 1963-10; 16(10): 1255-1263.
98. Dolf RH. Answer to a Letter on Fate of the Foreskin (Gairdner). *BMJ*. 1950; 1: 181.
99. Donin HH. Kindness: A Means and an End / Briss: The Covenant of Circumcision. In: *To Be A Jew*. NY: Basic Books. 1972: 41-5, 54, 56-7 / 273-4.
100. Dranov P. Tonsillectomies May Be Dangerous to Your Health. *Family Weekly* (Newspaper Supplement). 1979-03-11: 25.
101. Drew JH. Bloodless Circumcision. *Med J Aust*. 1968-02-10; 1: 220-1.
102. Dunn JE Jr, Buell P. Association of Cervical Cancer with Circumcision of Sexual Partner. *JNCI. 1959-04*; 22(4): 749-764.
103. Dunn J. The Newborn Baby – Sex Differences. In: Bruner J, Cole M, Lloyd B, series eds. *Distress and Comfort. The Developing Child – series*. Cambridge, MA: Harvard University Press. 1977: 13-4.
104. Eastman R. Circumcision (letter to ed.) *Playgirl*. 1974-03; 1(10).
105. Edwards ML Sr. Pleased With Similar Views. *MedTrib*. 1965-07-05; 80: 11.
106. Emde RN, Harmon RJ, Metcalf D, Koenig KL, Wagonfeld S. Stress and Neonatal Sleep. *Psychosom Med*. 1971/Nov-Dec; 33(6): 491-7.
107. Eser SR. Circumcision and Cervical Cancer. *BMJ. 1964-10-24;* 2: 1073-4.
108. Faber MM. Circumcision Revisited. *Birth and the Family Journal*. 1974/Spring; 1(2): 19-21.
109. Falliers CJ, Freedman LD, Nadel RS, Daley MC, Preston EN. Circumcision (letters to editor). *JAMA*. 1970-12-21; 214(12): 2194-5.
110. Feehan EB. A Way of Handling Circumcisions and Consent Forms. *Pediatrics*. 1977-10; 60(4): 566.
111. Feehan EB. Information Sheet (for use in private practice).
112. Filton R. A Note on Circumcision in Infants. *N Z Med J:* 176-7.

113. Fisher TL. Complicated Circumcision. *CMAJ.* 1967-11-25; 97: 1345.
114. Fisher TL. Office Surgery. *CMAJ.* 1954-10; 71: 395.
115. Fishman M, Shear MJ, Friedman HF, Stewart HL. Studies in Carcinogenesis. Local Effect of Repeated Application of 3,4 Benzpyrene and of Human Smegma to the Vagina and Cervix of Mice. *JNCI:* 361-6.
116. Fitzgerald WD. Circumcision is Barbarous. *Northwest Med.* 1971-10; 70: 681-2.
117. Fleiss PM, Douglass J. The Case Against Neonatal Circumcision. *BMJ.* 1979-09: 554.
118. Foley JM. The Unkindest Cut of All. *Fact.* 1966/Jul-Aug; 3(4): 309.
119. Frand M, Berant N, Brand N, Rotem Y. Complication of Ritual Circumcision in Israel. *Pediatrics.* 1974-10; 54(4).
120. Fredman RM. Neonatal Circumcision: A General Practitioner Survey. *Med J Aust.* 1969-01-18; 1: 117-9.
121. Freud P. The Ulcerated Meatus in Male Children. *J Pediatr.* 1947-08; 31(2): 131-141.
122. Friederich L. Zachary's Circumcision. *Mothering.* 1979/Summer; 12: 79-80.
123. Furlong JH Jr, Uhle CAW. Cancer of Penis: A Report of Eighty-Eight Cases. *J Urol.* 1953-04; 69(4): 550-5.
124. Gairdner D. The Fate of the Foreskin – A Study of Circumcision. *BMJ.* 1949-12-24: 1433-7.
125. Gallagher AGP. Complications of Circumcision. *Br J Urol.* 1972-12; 44(6): 720-1.
126. Garvin CH, Persky L. Circumcision: Is It Justified in Infancy? *J Natl Med Assoc.* 1966-07; 58(4): 233-8.
127. Gee WF, Ansell JS. Neonatal Circumcision: A Ten-Year Overview: With Comparison of the Gomco Clamp and the Plastibell Device. *Pediatrics.* 1976; 58: 824-7.
128. Gellis SS. Circumcision. *Am J Dis Child.* 1978-12; 132: 1168.
129. Gibbens J. Circumcision. In: *The Care of Young Babies.* London: J & A Churchill. 1959: 194-5.
130. Girgis B. Infibulation. *Lancet.* 1936-01-18: 170.
131. Glaspey J. Circumcision Imposes Needless Pain, Expense. *ICEA News.* 1980-02; 19(1).
132. Glenn J. Circumcision and Anti-Semitism. *Psychoanal Q.* 1960; 29: 395-8.
133. Gottschalk EC Jr. Living With Hemophilia. *Fam Circle.* 1979-04-24: 14.
134. Graber B, Kline-Graber G. *Woman's Orgasm.* NY: Popular Library. 1975: 96-8.
135. Greenblatt J. Circumcision on the Newborn. *Am J Dis Child.* 1966-04; 3: 448.
136. Greenhill JP. Circumcision (ch. 84). In: *Obstetrics.* Philadelphia, PA: W.B. Saunders. 1965: 1190-3.
137. Grimes DA. Routine Circumcision of the Newborn Infant; A Reappraisal. *AJOG.* 1978-01-15; 130(2): 125-9.
138. Grimes DA. Routine Circumcision Reconsidered. *Am J Nurs.* 1980-01: 108-9.
139. Grossberg P, Hardy KJ. Carcinoma of the Penis. *Med J Aust.* 1973-12-08; 2: 1050.
140. Grossman EA. *Circumcision; A Pictorial Atlas of its History, Instrument Development and Operative Techniques.* Great Neck, NY: Todd & Honeywell. 1982.
141. Haar H, Shanbrom E, Miller S. The Treatment of Leukemic Priapism with A-139. *J Urol.* 1960-04; 83(4): 429-432.
142. Hall G. Circumcision. *Med J Aust.* 1971-07-24: 223.
143. Halpin J. Circumcision in the Military. *QQ Magazine.* 1978/Jan-Feb: 13, 15, 44.
144. Hamm WG, Kanthak FF. Gangrene of the Penis Following Circumcision with High Frequency Current. *SMJ.* 1949-08; 42(8): 657-9.
145. Hathout HM. Some Aspects of Female Circumcision – With Case Report of a Rare Complication. *Obstet Gynecol.* 1963-06; 70: 505-7.
146. Hazell LD. *Commonsense Childbirth.* NY: G.P. Putnam's Sons. 1976: 16.
147. Heins HC Jr, Dennis EJ, Pratt-Thomas HR. The Possible Role of Smegma in Carcinoma of the Cervix. *AJOG.* 1958-10; 76(4): 726-735.
148. Hellman LM, Pritchard JA. *Williams Obstetrics.* 14th ed. NY: Appleton-Century Crofts. 1971: 490.
149. Herrera A, Cochran B, Herrera A, Wallace B. Parental Information and Circumcision in Highly Motivated Couples with Higher Education. *Pediatrics.* 1983-02; 71(2): 233-4.
150. Herskowitz MS. The Mechanistic Distortion in Treatment of Infants and Children. *J Amer Coll Neuropsych.* 1964-06; 3: 13-8.
151. Hertzberg A. Circumcision. In: *Judaism.* Washington Square Press. 1961: 74-5.
152. Homan WE. How Necessary is Circumcision? *Mother's Manual.* 1978/May-June: 43-4.
153. Horn J. Are Male Infants More Active Than Females at Birth? *Psychol Today.* 1978-09: 26-8.

154. Horwitz J, Schusseim A, Scalettar HE. Abdominal Distension Following Ritual Circumcision *Pediatrics.* 1976-04; 57(4): 579.
155. Hous R. *Thus Spake St. Paul* (on circumcision) (unpublished).
156. Howard M. *Only Human.* NY: Seabury Press. 1975: 143.
157. Huddleston CE. Female Circumcision in the Sudan. *Lancet.* 1949-04-09; 1: 626.
158. Hutchings G. Should He Be Circumcised? – First published in the *New Zealand Family Doctor*, and with permission reprinted in the *Bulletin of the Federation of New Zealand Parents Centre.* 1964-11.
159. Hutchins P, Dunlop EMC, Rodin P. Benign Transient Lymphangiectasis (Sclerosing Lymphangitis) of the Penis. *Br J Ven Dis.* 1977; 53: 379-387.
160. Hyman AB, Brownstein M II. Tyson's 'Glands'. *Arch Dermatol.* 1969-01; 99: 31-6.
161. Isaac E. The Enigma of Circumcision. *Commentary.* 1967-01: 51-5.
162. Isenberg S, Elting LM. *The Consumer's Guide to Successful Surgery.* NY: St. Martin's. 1976: 269-275.
163. James T. A Causerie on Circumcision, Congenital and Acquired. *SAMJ.* 1971-02-06; 45: 151-4.
164. James T. Philo on Circumcision. *SAMJ.* 1976-08-21: 1409-1412.
165. Janov A. *The Feeling Child.* Touchstone Books, Simon & Schuster. 1973.
166. Janov A. *The Primal Revolution.* Touchstone Books, Simon & Schuster. 1972.
167. Janov A. *The Primal Scream.* NY: Dell Publishing. 1970.
168. Janus, RB. Abnormalities of the Prepuce. In: *Essentials of Pediatrics.* 4th ed. Lippencott Press; p. 275.
169. Jefferson G. The Peripenic Muscle: Some Observations on the Anatomy of Phimosis. *Surg Gynecol Obstet.* 1916; 23: 177-181.
170. Johannesen GT Jr. A Question for Prospective Parents. 1977 (unpublished).
171. Johnson S. Persistent Urethral Fistula Following Circumcision. *U S Nav Med Bull.* 1949/Jan-Feb; 49(1): 120-2.
172. Johnson WR, Belzer EG. *Human Sexual Behavior and Sex Education.* Philadelphia, PA: Lea & Febiger. 1973: 38.
173. Johnsonbaugh RE, Meyer BP, Catalano JD. Complication of a Circumcision Performed with a Plastic Bell Clamp. *Am J Dis Child.* 1969-11; 118(5): 781.
174. Jolly H. Circumcision. *The Practitioner.* 1964-02; 192: 257.
175. Jonas G. Retention of a Plastibell Circumcision Ring. *Obstet Gynecol.* 1964-12; 24(6): 835.
176. Jones FW. The Development and Malformations of the Glans and Prepuce. *BMJ.* 1910-01-15: 137-8.
177. Jones FW. The Morphology of the External Genitalia of the Mammals. *Lancet.* 1914-04-18: 1099-1103.
178. Kantor HI. Circumcision – A Simple and Rapid Technic. *Obstet Gynecol.* 1960-01; 15(1): 89-92.
179. Kantor HI. History of Circumcision – Introduction of a New Instrument. *Tex State J Med.* 1953-02; 49(2): 75-7.
180. Kaplan GW. *Circumcision – An Overview. Current Problems in Pediatrics* (Year Book). Chicago, IL: Medical Publishers. 1977-03; 7(5).
181. Kaplan GW. The Incidence of Carcinoma of the Prostate in Jews and Gentiles. *JAMA.* 1966-05-30; 196(9): 123.
182. Kariher DH, Smith TW. Immediate Circumcision of the Newborn. *Obstet Gynecol.* 1956-01; 7(1: 50-2.
183. Kass LR. Ethical Dilemmas in the Care of the Ill. I. What is the Physician's Service?. *JAMA.* 1980-10-17; 244(16): 1811-6.
184. Katz J. The Question of Circumcision. *Int J Surg.* 1977-09; 62: 490-2.
185. Kennaway EL. Cancer of the Penis and Circumcision in Relation to the Incubation Period of Cancer. *Br J Cancer.* 1947-12; 1(4): 335-344.
186. Kennaway EL, Kennaway NM. The Social Distribution of Cancer of the Scrotum and Cancer of the Penis. *Cancer Res.* 1946-02; 6(2): 49-53.
187. Kiester E Jr. To Circumcise or Not to Circumcise? *Today's Health.* 1975-12: 6.
188. King LR. The Pros and Cons of Neonatal Circumcision (unpublished personal study).
189. Kirkpatrick BV, Eitzman DV. Neonatal Septicemia After Circumcision. *CLP.* 1974-09; 13(9): 767-8.
190. Kirya C, Werthmann MW Jr. Neonatal Circumcision and Penile Dorsal Nerve Block-A Painless Procedure. *J Pediatr.* 1978-06; 92(6): 998-1000.

191. Kiser EF. Ceremonial Circumcision. *N Engl J Med.* 1930-10-23; 203(17): 835-6.
192. Kitahara M. A Cross-cultural Test of the Freudian Theory of Circumcision. *Int J Psychoanal Psychother.* 1976-01-01; 5: 535-546.
193. Klauber GT. Circumcision and Phallic Fallacies or The Case Against Routine Circumcision. *Connecticut Mag.* 1973-09; 37(9): 445-7.
194. Klauber GT, Boyle J. Preputial Skin-Bridging; Complication of Circumcision. *Urology.* 1974-06; 3(6): 722-3.
195. Klaus MH, Kennell JH. *Maternal-Infant Bonding.* Saint Louis: C.V. Mosby. 1976.
196. Kmet J, Damjanovski L, Stucin M, Bonta S, Cakmakov A. Circumcision and Carcinoma Colli Uteri in Macedonia, Yugoslavia. Results from a Field Study. *Br J Cancer.* 1965-05-15; 17: 391-9.
197. Korones SB. Vitamin K. In: *High-Risk Newborn Infants.* St. Louis: C.V. Mosby. 1976: 188-9.
198. Kravitz H, Murphy JB, Edadi K, Rosetti A, Ashraf H. Effect of Hexachlorophene-Detergent Baths in a Newborn Nursery, With Emphasis on the Care of Circumcisions. *Ill Med J.* 1962-08; 122(2): 133-9.
199. Kunz J. Special Problems of Infants and Children-Should I Have My Son Circumcised? In: *American Medical Association Family Medical Guide.* NY: Random House. 1982: 644.
200. Lackey JT, Mannion RA, Kerr JE. Urethral Fistula Following Circumcision. *JAMA.* 1968-12-02; 206(10): 2318.
201. Lamb L. Doctor's Mailbag. *The Scranton Times-Tribune.* 1978-03-27: 22.
202. La Roc C. Circumcision Not for Everyone (letter to ed.). *Playgirl.* 1975-02; 2(9).
203. Lawrie R. Minor Surgical Prodecures – X11: Circumcision. *Practitioner.* 1958-11; 181(1085): 650-7.
204. Leboyer F. *Birth Without Violence.* NY: Alfred A. Knopf. 1976.
205. Le Doc E. The Value of Common Medical Procedures. *N Engl J Med.* 1975-03-06; 202(10): 538.
206. Leiter E, Lefkovits A. Circumcision and Penile Carcinoma. *NY State J Med.* 1975: 75(9): 1520-2.
207. Lenowitz H, Graham AP. Carcinoma of the Penis. *J Urol.* 1946; 56: 458-484.
208. Levin HA. Lateral-Slit Circumcision. *Med Times.* 1952-08; 80(8): 493-5.
209. Levin ML, Kress LC, Goldstein H. Syphilis and Cancer. *NY State J Med.* 1942-09-15: 1737-1745.
210. Levin S. Brit Milah: Ritual Circumcision. *SAMJ.* 1965-12-11; 39(44): 1125-7.
211. Levin S. Circumcision and Uncircumcision. *SAMJ.* 1976-06-05: 913.
212. Levitt SB, Smith RB, Ship AG. Iatrogenic Microphallus Secondary to Circumcision. *Urology.* 1976-11; 6(5): 472-4.
213. Lewin P. Ritual Circumcision Sequel. *CLP.* 1971-10: 583.
214. Lewis J. *In The Name of Humanity.* NY: Eugenics Publishing. 1956.
215. Lichtenauer P, Scheer H, Louton T. On the Classification of Penis Carcinoma and Its 10-year Survival. *Recent Results Cancer Res.* Bonn, Germany: Dept. of Urology, University of Bonn. 1977; (60): 110-9.
216. Licklider S. Jewish Penile Carcinoma. *J Urol.* 1961-07; 86(1): 98.
217. Lilienfeld AM, Graham S. Validity of Determining Circumcision Status by Questionnaire as Related to Epidemiological Studies of Cancer of the Cervix. *JNCI.* 1958-10; 21(4): 713-720.
218. Limaye RD, Hancock RA. Penile Urethral Fistula as a Complication of Circumcision. *J Pediatr.* 1968-01; 72(1): 105-6.
219. Loeb EM. The Blood Sacrifice Complex. *AAA Memoirs.* Periodicals Service. 1924; 30: 3-40.
220. Long WW Jr, Derrick FC Jr. Use of Polyglycolic Acid Suture in Circumcision. *SMJ.* 1972-06; 65(6): 761.
221. Lyster WR. Uterine Cancer in the Circumcised and Uncircumcised Populations of Fiji. *Med J Aust.* 1967-11-25: 998.
222. MacCarthy D, Douglas JWB, Mogford C. Circumcision in a National Sample of 4-Year-Old Children. *BMJ.* 1952-10-04: 755-6.
223. Macfarlane A. Feeling Pain. In: Bruner J, Cole M, Lloyd B, series eds. *The Psychology of Childbirth – The Developing Child series.* Cambridge, MA: Harvard University Press. 1977: 86-7.
224. Mackenzie AR. Meatal Ulceration Following Neonatal Circumcision. *Obstet Gynecol.* 1966-08; 28(2): 221-3.
225. Maimonides M. *The Guide for the Perplexed.* NY: Dover Publications. 1954: 378-379 (orig. transl. 1904) (orig.: 12th century).
226. Malev M. The Jewish Orthodox Circumcision Ceremony. *J Am Psychoanal Assoc.* 1966; 14(3): 510-5.

227. Malherbe WDF. Injuries to the Skin of the Male External Genitalia in Southern Africa. *SAMJ*. 1975-02-01; 49(5): 147-152.
228. Malo T, Bontorte RJ. Hazards of Plastic Bell Circumcisions. *Obstet Gynecol*. 1969-06; 33(6): 869.
229. Masters WH, Johnson VE. Circumcision. In: *Human Sexual Response*. London: J & A Churchill. 1966: 189-191.
230. Mass L, Stambolian G. The Unkindest Cut of All. *Christopher Street Magazine*. 1981-11-23; 64: 21-5.
231. McConckie BR. Circumcision. In: *Mormon Doctrine;* p. 142-4.
232. McDonald CF. Circumcision of the Female. *GP.* 1958-09; 18(3): 98.
233. McGowan AJ Jr. A Complication of Circumcision. *JAMA*. 1969-03-17; 207(11): 2104-5.
234. McWilliams PC. Secrets of the Foreskin. *Forum*. 1982-12: 54-61.
235. Melges FJ. Newborn Circumcision With a New Disposable Instrument. *Obstet Gynecol*. 1972-03; 39(3): 470-3.
236. Mendelsohn RA. People's Doctor – Circumcision Views Solicited. *Hayward*, CA (newspaper). 1978.
237. Menninger KA. *Man Against Himself*. Harcourt, Brace & World. 1966: 223-225 (paperback ed.).
238. Miller RL, Snyder DC. Immediate Circumcision of the Newborn Male. *AJOG*. 1953-01; 65(1): 1-11.
239. Miner H. Body Ritual Among the Nacirema. In: Lessa WA, Vogt EZ, eds. *Reader in Comparative Religion.* 2nd ed. NY: Harper & Row. 1965: 414-8.
240. Mohl PC, Adams R, Greer DM, Sheley KA. Prepuce Restoration Seekers: Psychiatric Aspects. *Arch Sex Behav*. 1984; 10(4): 383-393.
241. Money J. Ablatio Penis: Normal Male Infant Sex-Reassigned as a Girl. *Arch Sex Behav*. 1975; 4(1): 65-71.
242. More E, Venkade G, et al. Cutting Remarks (letters to editor). *Hustler*. 1979-08: 12.
243. Morgan R, Steinem G. The International Crime of Genital Mutilation. *Ms*. 1980-03: 65-7, 98, 100.
244. Morgan WKC. Penile Plunder. *Med J Aust*. 1967-03-27; 1: 1102.
245. Morgan WKC. Reply to Dr. Greenblatt. *Am J Dis Child*. 1966-04; 3: 448-9.
246. Morgan WKC. The Rape of the Phallus. *JAMA*. 1965-07-19; 193(3): 223-4.
247. Morrison J. The Origins of the Practices of Circumcision and Subincision Among the Australian Aborigines. *Med J Aust*. 1967-01-21: 125-217.
248. Mouzas GL, Pompa P. The Use of Dexon and Plain Catgut in Circumcision. *Br J Surg*. 1974; 61: 313-7.
249. Mueser AM, Verrilli GE. Circumcision: Yes or No? / Circumcision Care. In: *Welcome Baby: A Guide to the First Six Weeks*. NY: St. Martin's Press. 1981: 8-9 / 50.
250. Muschat Maurice. Occlusion of Urethral Meatus. *Am J Dis Child*. 1944; 67: 275-7.
251. Mustafa AZ. Female Circumcision and Infibulation in the Sudan. *J Obstet Gynaecol Br Commonw*. 1966-40; 73: 302-6.
252. Newhill R, Woodmansey AC, Pearsons DE, Lawton NM. Circumcision (separate letters to editor). *BMJ*. 1965-08-14; 2: 419-420.
253. Nicholas P. The Lasting Impact, In: Ward C, Ward F. *The Home Birth Book*. Washington: Inscape. 1976: 77-84.
254. Nunberg H. *Problems of Bisexuality as Reflected in Circumcision*. London: Imago Publishing. 1949.
255. Onuigbo W. Vulval Epidermoid Cysts in the Igbos of Nigeria (complication of female circumcision). *Arch Dermatol*. 1976-10; 112: 1405-1416.
256. Otten C. The Case Against Newborn Circumcision. *Saturday Evening Post*. 1981-12; 253(9): 30-1, 116.
257. Øster J. Further Fate of the Foreskin – Incidence of Preputial Adhesions, Phimosis, and Smegma among Danish Schoolboys. *Arch Dis Childh*. 1968-04; 43: 200-3.
258. Ozturk OM. Ritual Circumcision and Castration Anxiety. *Psychiatry*. 1973-02; 36: 49-60.
259. Packard JH. On Congenital Phimosis. *Am J Med Sci*. 1970-10; 60: 384-9.
260. Paige KE. The Ritual of Circumcision. *Hum Nat*. 1978-05: 40-8.
261. Panter GG. Circumcision: Making the Choice. *Parents*. 1981-07; 56(7): 82, 84.
262. Parker JH, Haber HF. Circumcision (separate letters to editor). *Med J Aust*. 1971-06-19: 1352.
263. Patel DA, Flaherty EG, Dunn J. Factors Affecting the Practice of Circumcision. *Am J Dis Child*. 1982-07; 136: 634-6.
264. Patel H. The Problem of Routine Circumcision. *CMAJ*. 1966-09-10; 95: 576-581.

265. Paymaster JC, Gangadharan P. *Cancer of the Penis in India.* Parel, Bombay, India: Tata Memorial Hospital; p. 110-2.
266. Pearce JC. *Magical Child.* NY: E.P. Dutton. 1977.
267. Pearlman CK. Circumcision. *Med Trib.* 1965-07-26; 89: 15.
268. Pearlman CK. Reconstruction Following Iatrogenic Burn of the Penis. *J Pediatr Surg.* 1976-02;11(1):121-2.
269. Penn J. Penile Reform. *British Journal of Plastic Surgery.* 1963; 16: 287-8.
270. Persky L. Commentary on Adult Circumcision by Valentine. *Med Aspect Hum Sex.* 1974-01: 50, 55.
271. Persky L. Epidemiology of Cancer of the Penis. *Recent Results of Cancer Res.* (Berlin). 1977: 97-109.
272. Pfeiffer CF. Men and Tribes (ch. 4) / "The Patriarchal Institutions" (Circumcision) / Law in Patriarchal Times. In: *Old Testament History.* Grand Rapids, MI: Baker Book House. 1973: 32-3 / 98-9 / 114-5.
273. Philip AGS. Urologist's Views Challenged. *Pediatrics.* 1975-08; 56(2): 238.
274. Philipson D. *The Reform Movement in Judaism.* Nabu Press. 2014: p. 280.
275. Pickard-Ginsberg M. Jesse's Circumcision. *Mothering.* 1979/Spring; 11: 80.
276. Pietzsch TT. Fifty Consecutive cases of Circumcision with the 'Plastibell' Circumcision Device. *Med J Aust.* 1971-06-26: 1380-2.
277. Pirie GR. The Story of Circumcision. *CMAJ.* 1927-12; 17(12): 1540-2.
278. Plaut A, Kohn-Speyer AC. The Carcinogenic Action of Smegma. *Science.* 1947; 105: 391-2.
279. Policzer M. Jewish Parents Sue Hospital Over Circumcision. *Los Angeles Herald Examiner.* 1979-03-18.
280. Pomeroy WB. *Boys and Sex.* NY: Delacourt Press. 1968: 138.
281. Pratt-Thomas HR, Heins HC, Latham E, Dennis EJ, McIver FA. The Carcinogenic Effect of Human Smegma: An Experimental Study. *Cancer.* 1956/Jul-Aug; 9(4): 671-680.
282. Preston EN. Whither the Foreskin? *JAMA.* 1970-09-14; 213(11): 1853-8.
283. Pugh WS. *Circumcision.* NY: Surgical Clinics of North America. 1935-04: 461.
284. Rathmann WG. Female Circumcision, Indications and a New Technique. *GP.* 1959-09; 20(3): 115-120.
285. Ravich A. Circumcision: Arguments Pro. *Med Trib.* 1965-07-10/11; 82: 4.
286. Ravich A. *Preventing V.D. and Cancer by Circumcision.* NY: Philosophical Library. 1973.
287. Ravich A. The Relationship of Circumcision to Cancer of the Prostate. *J Urol.* 1942; 48: 298-9.
288. Rawlings DJ, Miller PA, Engel RR. The Effect of Circumcision on Transcutaneous P02 in Term Infants. *Am J Dis Child.* 1980-07; 134: 676-8.
289. Raynal M, Chassagne D, Decroix Y, Peirquin B. [Endocurietherapy for carcinoma of the penis (author's transl.) [Article in French]. *J Radiol Electrol Med Nucl.* 1977-05; 58(5): 399-403.
290. Reddy CRRM, et al. A Study of 80 Patients with Penile Carcinoma Combined with Cervical Biopsy of Their Wives. *Int J Surg.* 1977-10; 62(10): 549-553.
291. Reddy DG, Baruah IKSM. Carcinogenic Action of Human Smegma. *Arch Pathol.* 1963-04; 75: 414-420.
292. Redman JF, Scriber L, Bissada NK. Postcircumcision Phimosis and Its Management. *CLP.* 1975-04; 14(4): 407-9.
293. Reichelderfer TE, Fraga JR. In: Shepard KS (ed.): *Care of the Well Baby* (reprint). J.B. Lippencott. 1968: 10.
294. Reid BL, French PW, Singer A, Hagan BE, Coppleson M. Sperm Basic Proteins in Cervical Carcinogenesis: Correlation with socioeconomic class. *Lancet.* 1978-07-08; 2(8080): 60-2.
295. Remondino PC. *History of Circumcision from Earliest Times to the Present.* NY: Ams Press. 1974.
296. Richards MPM, Bernal JF, Brackbill Y. Early Behavioral Differences: Gender or Circumcision? *Dev. Psychobiol.* 1976; 9(1): 89-95.
297. Rieser C. Circumcision and Cancer. *SMJ.* 1961-10: 1133-4.
298. Rieser C, Robertson W0, Stankewick WR, Vermooten V, Glenn JF, Diddle AW, Fielding IM. Should Circumcision be Done Routinely? *Med Aspect Hum Sex.* 1967-12: 26-33.
299. Riley HD Jr, Schwartz T. Your Newborn's Appearance and How it Will Change. *American Baby.* 1979-09: 59, 63.
300. Ritter TJ. Circumcision Criticized. *American Medical News.* 1980-01-25: 5.
301. Ritter TJ. Correspondence. 1978-02-01.

302. Ritter TJ. Correspondence to *Cosmopolitan Magazine* re an article about circumcision pros and cons. 1980-02-15.
303. Ritter TJ. Iatrogenic Urethral Meatal Stenosis in the Male. Letter sent to *JAMA*. 1978-01-24.
304. Ritter TJ. Personal Notes on Circumcision (unpublished). 1977.
305. Ritter TW. Personal Studies on Cancer of the Penis (unpublished).
306. Robertson W0 Jr. Commentary on Adult Circumcision by Valentine. *Med Aspect Hum Sex*. 1974-01: 48-9.
307. Rodgers W. Circumcision: Pro and Con (letter to ed.). *Playgirl*. 1974-06; 2(1).
308. Rodin P, Kolater B. Carriage of Yeasts on the Penis. *BMJ*. 1976-05-08: 1123-4.
309. Rodrique RB. Amebic Balanitis. *JAMA*. 1978-01-09; 239(2): 109.
310. Rosefsky JB. Glans Necrosis as a Complication of Circumcision. *Pediatrics*. 1967; 39: 744-5.
311. Rosenstein JL. Wound Diphtheria in the Newborn Infant Following Circumcision. *J Pediatr*. 1941-05; 18: 657-8.
312. Rosenzweig EM. Circumcision. In: *We Jews – Invitation to Dialogue*. NY: Hawthorn Books. 1977: 82-3.
    Rosner F. Circumcision – Attempt at Clearer Understanding. *NY State J Med*. 1966-11-15: 2919-2922.
313. Rothenberg R. The Male Genitals. In: *Understanding Surgery*. Pocket Books. 1955: 424-5, 436.
314. Rotkin ID. Relation of Adolescent Coitus to Cervical Cancer Risk. *JAMA*. 1962-02-17; 179(7): 486-491.
315. Rubenstein MM, Bason WM. Complication of Circumcision Done With a Plastic Bell Clamp. *Am J Dis Child*. 1968-10; 116: 381-2.
316. Saadawi N el. The Question No One Would Answer (female circumcision). *Ms*. 1980-03: 68-9.
317. Safren C. How Children Feel About Their Bodies. *Redbook*. 1979-06: 21, 140, 142, 144, & 148.
318. St. John-Hunt D. Circumcision and Tonsillectomy. *N Engl J Med*. 1969-09-11; 281(11): 621.
319. St. John-Hunt D. Circumcision as a Hygienic Procedure. *Med J Aust*. 1972-03-18; 1: 607.
320. St. John-Hunt D, Newill RGD, Gibson OB. Three Englishmen Favor Circumcision and Why They Do. *Pediatrics*. 1977-10; 60(4): 563-4.
321. Samuels N, Samuels M. Circumcision, Medical Facts Today are Challenging Popular Beliefs. *Fam J*. 1982/Sep-Oct; 11(5): 27-32.
322. Saquet R. Circumcision in Social Perspective. *Country Lady's Daybook*. 1976-03.
323. Sanjurjo LA, Flores BG. Carcinoma of the Penis. *J Urol*. 1960-04; 83(4): 133-7.
324. Sauer LW. Fatal Staphylococcus Bronchopneumonia Following Ritual Circumcision. *AJOG*. 1943; 1(46): 583.
325. Saxton L. *The Individual, Marriage, and the Family*. Belmont, CA: Wadsworth Publishing. 1968: 81, 426.
326. Scarzella GI. Circumcision: modified circular cuff technique. *Med Ann Dist Columbia*. 1970-08;39(8): 420-1.
327. Schaefer G. Female Circumcision. *Obstet Gynecol*. 1955; 6(2): 235-7.
328. Schaff P, Herzog JJ. Circumcision: In: *Schaff-Herzog Encyclopedia of Religious Knowledge;* 1: 486-7.
329. Schechet J. *The Layman's Guide to the Covenant of Circumcision*. Los Angeles, CA. 1973.
330. Schinella RA, Miranda D. Posthitis Xerotica Obliterans in Circumcision Specimens. *Urology*. 1974-03; 3(3): 348-351.
331. Schlosberg C. Thirty Years of Ritual Circumcisions. *CLP*. 1971-04; 10(4).
332. Schlossman HH. Circumcision as Defense – A Study in Psychoanalysis and Religion. *Psychoanal Q*. 1966-07; 35: 340-356.
333. Schneider T. Circumcision and 'Uncircumcision'. *SAMJ*. 1976-03-27: 556-8.
334. Schrek R. The Racial Distribution of Cancer; 11 – Tumors of the Kidney, Bladder and Male Genital Organs. *Ann. Surg*. 1944-11; 120(5): 809-812.
335. Schrek R, Lenowitz H. Etiologic Factors in Carcinoma of the Penis. *Cancer Res*. (From the Tumor Research Unit and the Dept. of Urology, Veterans Administration, Hines, Ill.) 1946-11-12: 180-7.
336. Schultz T. Female Circumcision: Operation Orgasm. *Viva*. 1975; 2(6): 53-4, 104-5.
337. Schultz T. A Nurse's View on Circumcision. *Mothering*. 1979/Summer; 12: 83.
338. Schwark TE. Do Edicts Have Any Effect on Circumcision Rate? *Pediatrics*. 1977-10; 60(4): 563.
339. Scurlock JM, Pemberton PJ. Neonatal Meningitis and Circumcision. *Med J Aust*. 1977-03-05: 332-4.
340. Seaman B. Circumcision: The Pros and Cons. *Woman's Day*. 1976-08: 40, 152.
341. Seligmann J. To Circumcise or Not? *Newsweek*. 1979-10-01: 40.

342. Sequeira JH. Female Circumcision and Infibulation. *Lancet.* 1931-11-07: 1054-5.
343. SerVaas C. Health Groups Conclude: 'Routine Circumcision Not Recommended'. *Saturday Evening Post.* 1981-12; 253(9): 26-9, 110.
344. Sexty L. Jared's Ordeal. *Mothering.* 1979/Summer; 12: 84-5.
345. Shabad AL. Some Aspects of Etiology and Prevention of Penile Cancer. *J Urol.* 1964-12; 92(6): 696-702.
346. Sharma SK, Bapna BC. Preputial Calculi. *Int J Surg.* 1977-10; 62(10): 553-4.
347. Shelton H. Circumcision. *Dr Shelton's Hygienic Review.* 1943-05: 201-2.
348. Shelton H. Do Boys Require Mutilation? *Dr. Shelton's Hygienic Review.* 1943-10: 38-9, 45.
349. Shelton HM. Mutilation of Male Babies (ch. 8). In: *The Hygienic Care of Children.* Bridgeport, CT: Natural Hygiene Press. 1981: 87-105.
350. Shelton H. To Circumcise or Not to Circumcise? *Dr. Shelton's Hygienic Review.* 1944-02: 136, 140, 142.
351. Shepard M. *Ecstasy: The Moneysworth Marriage Manual.* NY: Moneysworth. 1977: 12, 13, 16-7, 35-6.
352. Sherline DM. Circumcision at Birth In: Landers A. (ed.) *The Ann Landers Encyclopedia;* p. 257-8.
353. Sherwood J. The Leboyer Method offers 'Gentle' Childbirth. *Bellingham (WA) Herald.* 1979.
354. Shiraki IW. Congenital Megalourethra With Urethrocutaneous Fistula Following Circumcision: A Case Report. *J Urol.* 1973-04; 109: 723-5.
355. Shulman J, Ben-Hur N, Newman Z (Israel). Surgical Complications of Circumcision. *Am J Dis Child.* 1961-02; 107: 149-154.
356. Singh B, Kim H, Wax SH. Strangulation of Glans Penis by Hair. *Urology.* 1978-02; 11(2): 170-2.
357. Smith ED. Another View of Circumcision. *Austr Paediatr J.* 1970-06; 6: 67-9.
358. Snell JA. A Method of Bloodless Circumcision. *Med J Aust.* 1975-09-20: 474-5.
359. Snell JA. Bloodless Circumcision is Practical for All Ages. *Mod Med.* 1976-08-01: 146.
360. Spence GR. Chilling of Newborn Infants: Its Relation to Circumcision Immediately Following Birth. *SMJ.* 1970-03; 63: 309-311.
361. Spitz RA. Authority and Masturbation (ch. 16). In: Marcus IM, Francis JJ, eds. *Masturbation: From Infancy to Senescence.* NY: National Universities Press. 1975: 381-409.
362. Sorrells ML. Still More Criticism. *Pediatrics.* 1975-08; 56(2): 339.
363. Soule G. Circumcision Speech. *Partal Post, Childbirth Education Newsletter*, Lewis, KS. 1980/Winter.
364. Speert H. Circumcision of the Newborn. *Obstet Gynecol.* 1953-08; 2(2): 164-172.
365. Spock B. *Baby and Child Care.* Pocket Books, Simon & Schuster, 1976: 191-2.
366. Stagg D. A Basis for Decision on Circumcision. In: *Compulsory Hospitalization or Freedom of Choice in Childbirth*, Vol. III. Stewart & Stewart, transcript of 1978 NAPSAC Convention, p. 831-843.
367. Stein L. Ambivalence (letter to editor). *JAMA.* 1971-03-08; 215(10).
368. Stern E, Dixon WJ. Cancer of the Cervix-A Biometric Approach to Etiology. *Cancer.* 1961/Jan-Feb; 14(1): 153-160.
369. Stern E, Lachenbruch PA. Circumcision Information in a Cancer Detection Center Population. *Int J Chronic Dis.* 1968; 21: 117-124.
370. Stern E, Neely PM. Cancer of the Cervix in Reference to Circumcision and Marital History. *J Am Med Womens Assoc.* 1962-09; 17(9): 739-740.
371. Stinson JM. Impotence and Adult Circumcision. *J Nat Med Assoc.* 1973-03; 65(2): 161.
372. Strage M. Improving on Nature, How and Why (ch. 4). In: *The Durable Fig Leaf; A Historical, Cultural, Medical, Social, Literary and Iconographic Account of Man's Relations with His Penis.* NY: William Morrow. 1980: 141-159.
373. Street R. The Case Against Circumcision. In: *Modern Sex Techniques.* NY: Archer House. 1959: 203-210.
374. Sussman SJ, Schiller RP, Shashikumar VL. Fournier's Syndrome. *Am J Dis Child.* 1978-12; 132: 1189-1191.
375. Swafford TD. More About Circumcision. *CMAJ.* 1967-01-28; 96: 228.
376. Swyer GIM. Contraceptives and Cervical Carcinoma. *BMJ.* 1969-08-23: 3(5668): 71.
377. Talarico RD, Jasaitis JE. Concealed Penis, A Complication of Neonatal Circumcision. *J Urol.* 1973-12; 110: 732-3.

378. Talbert LM, Kraybill EN, Potter HD. Adrenal Cortical Response to Circumcision in the Neonate. *Obstet Gynecol.* 1976-08; 48(2): 208-210.
379. Tan RE. Observations on Frequency of Carcinoma of the Penis at Macassar and its Environs (South Celebes). *J Urol.* 1963-05; 80(5): 704-5.
380. Taylor JN. Circumcision of Adults. In: Landers A. (ed.) *The Ann Landers Encyclopedia;* p. 258-9.
381. Taylor PK, Rodin P. Herpes Genitalis and Circumcision. *Br J Ven Dis.* 1975; 51: 274-7.
382. Tedeschi CG, Eckert WG, Tedeschi LG. Mechanical Trauma / Circumcision Injuries. In: *Forensic Medicine – A Study in Trauma and Environmental Hazards,* Vol. I. Philadelphia: W.B. Saunders. 1977: 240-1.
383. Terris M. Epidemiology of Cervical Cancer. *Ann N Y Acad Sci.* 1962; 97: 808-813.
384. Terris M, Fitzpatrick W, Nelson JH Jr. Relation of Circumcision to Cancer of the Cervix. *AJOG.* 1973-12-15; 117(8): 1056-1066.
385. Terris M, Oalmann MC. Carcinoma of the Cervix – An Epidemiologic Study. *JAMA.* 1960-12-03; 174(14): 1847-1851.
386. Thomas CL (ed.). Circumcision / Foreskin. In: *Taber's Cyclopedic Medical Dictionary.* Philadelphia, PA: F.A. Davis, p. C-75 / F-37.
387. Thompson HC. The Task Force Replies. *Pediatrics.* 1977-10; 60(4): 564.
388. Thompson HC, King LR, Knox E, Korones SB. Ad Hoc Task Force on Circumcision – Report. *Pediatrics.* 1975-10; 56(4).
389. Thompson RK, Askovitz SI, Marshall VF. More on Circumcision (separate letters to editor). *Med Trib.* 1965-07-05; 80: 11.
390. Toguri AG, Light RA, Warren MM. Penile Tourniquet Syndrome Caused by Hair. *SMJ.* 1979-05; 72(5).
391. Topp S. The Argument Over Circumcision – The Case Against. & Misurella F. The Case For. *Village Voice.* 1975-06-16: 8-10.
392. Topp S. Why Not to Circumcise Your Baby Boy. *Mothering.* 1978-01; 6: 69-77.
393. Towne JE. Carcinoma of the Cervix in Nulliparous and Celibate Women. *AJOG.* 1965-03; 69(3): 606-613.
394. Trainin N. Cervical Carcinoma and Circumcision. *Isr J Med Sci.* 1965; 1: 303-4.
395. Trier WC, Drach GW. Concealed Penis – Another Complication of Circumcision. *Am J Dis Child.* 1973-02; 125: 276.
396. Tushnet L. Uncircumcision. *Med Times.* 1965-06; 93(6): 588-593.
397. Valdés-Dapena MA. *Sudden Unexplained Infant Death.* Rockville, MD: U.S. Dept. H.E.W. 1978.
398. Valentine FC. Surgical Circumcision. *JAMA.* 1901-03-16: 712-3.
399. Valentine RJ (pseudonym). Adult Circumcision: A Personal Report. *Med Aspect Hum Sex.* 1974-01: 31-48.
400. Van Duyn J, Warr WS. Excessive Penile Skin Loss from Circumcision. *JMA Georgia.* 1962-08; 51: 394-6.
401. Vanns JL. Circumcision: Pro and Con (letter to ed.). *Playgirl.* 1974-06; 2(1).
402. Van Zante P, Butterfield RM, Van Duyn J (interviewees). Circumcision is Still Given Loud Yeas and Nays. *Med Trib.* 1965-06-12/13; 70(Weekend Edition).
403. Verzin JA. Circumcision and Cervical Cancer. *BMJ. 1964-12-12;* 2(5432): 1531-2.
404. Vidal G. *Myra Breckenridge.* Boston, MA: Little, Brown. 1968-02: 93, 127.
405. Viola M. In Response to Jesse's Circumcision. *Mothering.* 1979/Summer; 12: 79.
406. Vitale E, Abdel-Haqq Muhammad K. More on the Controversy over Circumcision (letters to ed.). *American Baby.* 1982-02: 58.
407. Waddell WW Jr, Guerry D III. Effect of Vitamin K on the Clotting Time of the Prothrombin and the Blood. *JAMA.* 1925-06-03; 112(22).
408. Wade TR, Kopf AW, Ackerman AB. Bowenoid Papulosis of the Penis. *Cancer.* 1978-10; 42: 1890-1903.
409. Walker K. Special Procedures in General Practice – Circumcision. *BMJ.* 1938: 1377-8.
410. Wall RL Jr. Routine Circumcision? Recent Trends and Concepts. *N C Med J.* 1968-03; 29: 103-7.
411. Wallerstein E. *Circumcision: An American Health Fallacy.* NY: Springer Publishing. 1980.
412. Wallerstein E. *The Circumcision Decision* (information pamphlet). Seattle, WA: Pennypress. 1980.
413. Wallerstein E. *When Your Baby Boy is Not Circumcised* (information pamphlet). Seattle, WA: Pennypress. 1982.
414. Walton V. *Have It Your Way.* Seattle, WA: Henry Philips Publishing. 1976: 191-2.

415. Waszak SJ. The Historic Significance of Circumcision. *Obstet Gynecol.* 1978-04; 51(4): 499-501.
416. Weiss C. Circumcision in Infancy, A New Look At An Old Operation. *CLP.* 1964-09; 3(9) 560-3.
417. Weiss C. Does Circumcision of the Newborn Require an Anaesthetic? *CLP.* 1968-03; 7(3): 128-9.
418. Weiss C. Ritual Circumcision – Comments on Current Practices in American Hospitals. *CLP.* 1962-10: 65-72.
419. Wertz RW, Wertz DC. *Lying-In, A History of Childbirth in America.* NY: Schocken Books. 1979.
420. Wessel H. *The Joy of Natural Childbirth.* NY: Harper & Row. 1973: 242-3.
421. Wheat W. Cancer-Free Society Called not 'Realistic'. *Bellingham Herald* (WA). 1979-09-30: 3D.
422. Whelan P. Male Dyspareunia Due to Short Frenulum: An Indication for Adult Circumcision. *BMJ.* 1977-12: 1633-4.
423. Whiddon D. Should Baby be Circumcised? *Lancet.* 1953-08-15: 337-8.
424. Whiteford CH. A Case of Epithelioma of the Penis Following Incomplete Circumcision. *Lancet.* 1920-12-25: 1304.
425. Williams H. The Foreskin File. *CoEvolution Quarterly.* 1980/Winter: 68-77.
426. Williams LP. Common Operations and Circumcision (ch. 12). In: *How to Avoid Unnecessary Surgery.* Los Angeles, CA: Nash Publishing. 1971: 105-113.
427. Williamson PS, Williamson ML. Physiologic Stress Reduction by a Local Anesthetic During Newborn Circumcision. *Pediatrics.* 1983-01; 71(1): 36-40.
428. Williamson TV. Phimosed Preputial Sac Serving as an Adventitious Urinary Reservoir. *JAMA.* 1932; 99(10): 831.
429. Wilson CL, Wilson MC. Plastic Repair of the Denuded Penis. *SMJ.* 1959-05; 52: 288-290.
430. Wilson DC. Female Circumcision and the Age of the Menarche. *BMJ.* 1955-06-04: 1375.
431. Wilson RA. Circumcision. *CMA Journal.* 1977-04-09; 116: 715.
432. Winkelmann RK. The Erogenous Zones: Their Nerve Supply and its Significance. *Proc Staff Meet Mayo Clin.* 1959-01-21; 34(2): 39.
433. Winsey V. Parents Choose Sides Over Circumcision. *The Sun.* 1978-01-26: B5.
434. Winterbotham LP. Ceremonial Circumcision. *Med J Aust.* 1959-03-21; 46(12): 412-3.
435. Wirth JL. Health Insurance Statistics on Circumcision in Australia. *Med J Aust.* 1977-05-14: 760.
436. Wirth JL. Statistics on Circumcision in Canada and Australia. *AJOG.* 1978-01-15; 130(2): 236-9.
437. Wolbarst AL. Circumcision and Penile Cancer. *Lancet.* 1932-01-16: 150-3.
438. Wood JR. Alternatives to Circumcision in the Treatment of Phimosis (reprint). *INTACT Educational Foundation,* Wilbraham (MA).
439. Wood JR. The Circumcision Controversy (reprint). *INTACT Educational Foundation.* INTACT Educational Foundation, Wilbraham (MA). 1979-05-10.
440. Wood JR. What They Say (reprint). *INTACT Educational Foundation,* Wilbraham (MA). 1976, rev. 1981-11.
441. Worsely A. Infibulation and Female Circumcision – A Study of a Little-Known Custom. *J Obstet Gynecol Br Emp.* 1938; 45: 686-691.
442. Wrana P. Historical Review – Circumcision. *Arch Pediatr.* 1939; 56: 385-392.
443. Wright JE. Non-Therapeutic Circumcision. *Med J Aust.* 1967-05-27: 1033-4.
444. Wright RA, Judson FN. Penile Venereal Edema. *JAMA.* 1979-01-12; 241(2): 157-8.
445. Wynder EL, Cornfield J, Schroff PD, Doraiswami KR. A Study of Environmental Factors in Carcinoma of the Cervix. *AJOG. 1954-10;* 68(4): 1016-1952.
446. Wynder EL, Licklider SD. The Question of Circumcision. *Cancer.* 1960/May-Jun; 13(3): 442-5.
447. Wynder EL, Mantel N, Licklider SD. Statistical Considerations on Circumcision and Cervical Cancer. *AJOG.* 1960-05; 79(5): 1026-1030.
448. Yannaccone K. The Controversy Over Circumcision. *American Baby.* 1981-11; 43(20): 35, 37.
449. Yazmajian RV. A Circumcision Fantasy. *Psychoanal Q.* 1965; 34: 108-9.
450. Yellen HS, Brodie EL. Discussions of Bloodless Circumcision. *Gomco Surgical Manufacturing Corp. brochure,* information taken from *AJOG.* 1935-07; *Medical Record.* 1935-06-05; *Surgery.* 1939-02.
451. Yellen HS. Bloodless Circumcision of the Newborn. *AJOG. 1935;* 30: 146-7.
452. Young HH. A Radical Operation for the Cure of Cancer of the Penis. *J Urol.* 1931-08; 26(2): 285-316.

453. Zborowski M, Herzog E. *Life is With People; The Culture of The Shtetl.* NY: Schocken Books. 1952: 318-321.
454. Zimmer PJ. Modern Ritualistic Surgery-A Layman's View of Nonritual Neonatal Circumcision. *CLP.* 1977-06; 16(6): 503-6.
455. Zimmer PJ. Notes on Circumcision (unpublished).

No authors listed:

456. Before 20 Sex Linked by Doctor to Cervical Cancer. *CDN.* 1972-11-04: 27.
457. Case Against Circumcision, The. *Time.* 1970-10-19: 58.
458. Circumcision. *The Interpretor's Dictionary of the Bible* Vol. I, p. 629-631.
459. Circumcision. *Group Health Cooperative of Puget Sound* information hand-out. 1972-03.
460. Circumcision. *JAMA.* 1970-12-21; 214(12): 2194-2195.
461. Circumcision and Cervical Cancer. *BMJ.* 1964-08-15: 397-8.
462. Circumcision and Cervical Cancer. *Lancet.* 1966-01-15; 1(7429): 137.
463. Circumcision as a Hygiene Measure. *Med J Aust.* 1971-05-29; 1: 175-6.
464. Circumcision as a Hygiene Measure. *Med J Aust.* 1971-07-24; 1: 175.
465. Circumcision – Barbaric or Healthy? *New Age.* 1980-05: 13-4.
466. Circumcision 'Nonessential' Pediatrics Academy is Told. *NHF Bull.* 1970-01: 24.
467. Circumcision Not Health Requirement. *Kalamazoo Gazette* (MI). 1976-01-02.
468. Circumcision – Right or Wrong? *Playgirl.*
469. Circumcision vs. Circumspection. *Sci Am.* 1970-11: 45.
470. Circumcisional Hazards. *Emerg Med.* 1979-04-15: 145-7.
471. Cleanliness, Continence, Constancy, and Cervical Carcinoma. *CMAJ.* 1964-05-09; 90: 1132.
472. Death by Fright. *Time.* 1980-03-24.
473. Dog Fanciers Urged to be Less Fancy (cutting ears & tails of dogs). *Prevention.* 1974-03: 131, 134.
474. First Week of Life, The. *American Baby Magazine.* 1979: 19-21.
475. Foreskin Reconstruction (anonymous personal report). *Texas Medical Center.* 1972-08-24.
476. Foreskin Saga, The. *Time.* 1971-09-20: 59.
477. Genital Mutilation of Females Protested. *The Times-Picayune.* 1979-11-01.
478. Malpractice Leads to Sex Change. *Philadelphia Inquirer.* 1975-10-31.
479. One Circumcision Experience or Never Trust an Adult. (unpublished account by "Bill".)
480. Our Recent Article on Circumcision Hit a Sore Spot With Many Readers (letters to ed.). *Moneysworth.* 1976-03-29.
481. Playgirl Answers. *Playgirl.* 1974-03.
482. *Pregnancy, Birth, & the Newborn Baby.* Boston Medical Center Delacourt Press. 1971-1972: 284-5.
483. Rape of the Phallus, The – A Sequel (letters in response to Morgan WKC. The Rape of the Phallus). *JAMA.* 1965-10-18; 194(3): 195-7.
484. Spence on Circumcision. *Parents Centres New Zealand.* 1953-08-22: 401.
485. Responses to Foley JM. The Unkindest Cut of All. *Fact.* 1967/Jan-Feb: 29.
486. Responses to Foley JM. The Unkindest Cut of All. *Fact.* 1967/May-Jun: 29.
487. Responses to Foley JM. The Unkindest Cut of All. *Fact.* 1967/Jul-Aug: 37.
488. Unkindest Cut of All, The (anonymous). *Playgirl.* 1979-07: 108, 111.
489. Uncircumcised How To (letter to ed., name withheld). *Playgirl.* 1974-12; 2(7).
490. Who Wrote My Baby's Story? (name withheld). *Mothering.* 1979/Summer; 12: 79.

Appendix C: Books About

Appendix C.1: Male Genital Mutilation / Intactivism

- Aldeeb SA. *To Mutilate in the Name of Jehovah or Allah: Legitimization of Male and Female Circumcision.* San Francisco, CA: NOHARMM. 1994.
- Auslander S. *Foreskin's Lament: A Memoir.* Riverhead Books. 2008.
- Benatar D. *The Second Sexism.* Wiley-Blackwell. 2012.
- Berkeley B. *Foreskin, A Closer Look.* Boston, MA: Alyson Publications. 1993.
- Bigelow J. *The Joy of Uncircumcising.* Pacific Grove, CA: Hourglass Publishing. 1992.
- Bisque L. *You Call This Love? The Real Reason Women Don't Like Sex.* iUniverse. 2000.
- Boyd BR. *Circumcision Exposed.* Freedom, CA: The Crossing Press. 1988.
- Boyd BR. *Circumcision: What it Does.* San Francisco, CA: Taterhill Press. 1990.
- Briggs A. *Circumcision: What Every Parent Should Know.* Earlysville, VA: Birth and Parenting. 1984.
- Bryk F. *Sex & Circumcision: A Study of Phallic Worship and Mutilation in Men and Women.* North Hollywood, CA: Brandon House; 1967.
- Carlquist S. *UNCUT.* Santa Barbara, CA: Pinecone Press. 2000.
- Carmack A. *The Good Mommy's Guide to Her Little Boy's Penis.* KDP (CreateSpace). 2015.
- Carnes SM. *The Foreskin and Why You Should Keep It.* KDP (CreateSpace). 2015.
- Carter N. *Routine Circumcision: The Tragic Myth.* London, England: Londinium Press. 1979.
- Colapinto J. *As Nature Made Him: The Boy Who Was Raised As a Girl.* NY: HarperCollins. 2000.
- Countryman WL. *Dirt, Greed and Sex: Sexual Ethics in the New Testament and Their Implications for Today.* Fortress Press. 2007.
- Darby R. *A Surgical Temptation.* Chicago, IL: University of Chicago Press. 2005.
- Darby R. *The Sorcerer's Apprentice.* SJF Publishing. 2013.
- Denniston GC, Milos MF. *Sexual Mutilations: A Human Tragedy, Proceedings of the Fourth International Symposium on Sexual Mutilations, Lausanne, Switzerland.* Plenum Publishers. 1996.
- Denniston GC, Hodges FM, Milos MF. *Male and Female Circumcision: Medical, Legal, and Ethical Considerations in Pediatric Practice, Proceedings of the Fifth International Symposium on Sexual Mutilations, Oxford, UK, August 5-7, 1998.* NY: Kluwer Academic/Plenum Publishers. 1999.
- Denniston GC, Hodges FM, Milos MF (eds.) *Understanding Circumcision: A Multi-Disciplinary Approach to a Multi-Dimensional Problem, Proceedings of the Sixth International Symposium on Genital Integrity, Sydney, Australia, December 7-9, 2000.* NY: Kluwer Academic/Plenum Publishers. 2001.
- Denniston GC, Hodges FM, Milos MF (eds.) *Flesh and Blood: Perspectives on the Problem of Circumcision in Contemporary Society, Proceedings of the Seventh International Symposium on Human Rights and Modern Society: Advancing Human Dignity and the Legal Right to Bodily Integrity in the 21st Century, Washington, DC, April 4-7, 2002.* NY: Kluwer Academic/Plenum Publishers. 2004.
- Denniston GC, Hodges FM, Milos MF (eds.) *Bodily Integrity and the Politics of Circumcision: Culture, Controversy, and Change, Proceedings of the Eighth International Symposium on Circumcision and Human Rights: An Anthropological, Medical, Legal, and Ethical Analysis, Padua Italy, September 2-4, 2004.* NY: Springer. 2006.
- Denniston GC, Hodges FM, Milos MF. *Genital Autonomy: Protecting Personal Choice.* NY: Springer. 2010.
- Elium D & J. *Raising a Son: Parents and the Making of a Healthy Man.* Celestial Arts. 2004.
- Fleiss PM, Hodges FM. *Sweet Dreams: A Pediatricians Secrets for Your Child's Good Night's Sleep.* Lowell House. 2000.
- Fleiss PM, Hodges D. *What Your Doctor May Not Tell You About Circumcision.* NY: Warner Books. 2002.
- Friedman DM. *A Mind of Its Own: A Cultural History of the Penis.* Penguin. 2003.
- Glick LB. *Marked in Your Flesh: Circumcision from Ancient Judea to Modern America.* Oxford: Oxford University Press. 2005.

- Goldman R. *Circumcision: The Hidden Trauma.* Boston, MA: Vanguard. 1997.
- Goldman R. *Circumcision: A Jewish Perspective.* Boston, MA: Vanguard. 1998.
- Gollaher DL. *Circumcision: A History of the World's Most Controversial Surgery.* NY: Perseus Books. 2000.
- Griffin GM. *Decircumcision.* Los Angeles, CA: Added Dimensions. 1991.
- Hammond T. *Male Circumcision in America, Violating Human Rights.* San Francisco, CA: NOHARMM. 1992.
- Heimlich J. *Breaking Their Will: Shedding Light on Religious Child Maltreatment.* Prometheus. 2011.
- Hoffman L. *Covenant of Blood: Circumcision and Gender in Rabbinic Judaism* (Chicago Studies in the History of Judaism). Chicago: University of Chicago Press. 2001.
- Hulms R. *Please Don't Circumcise Your Baby Boy: The Inarguable Case Against Infant Male Circumcision.* Kindle. 2015.
- Legler K. *What happened? A guide to help children understand the intact and circumcised penis.* KDP (Createspace). 2010.
- Lewis J. *In The Name of Humanity.* NY: Eugenics Publishing. 1949.
- Lightfood-Klein H. *Children's Genitals Under the Knife: Social Imperatives, Secrecy and Shame.* Nunzio Press. 2008.
- Matteoli RL. *The Munchhausen Complex.* Monterey, CA: Nemean Press. 2010.
- Moss LB. *The Measure of His Grief.* First Notim Press. 2010.
- Moss LB, Wald R. *Celebrating Brit Shalom.* 2015.
- Noble E. *The Joy of Being a Boy.* New Life Images. 1994.
- O'Hara Kr. *Sex as Nature Intended It.* MA: Turning Point Publications. 2002.
- O'Mara P. *Circumcision: The Rest of the Story.* Santa Fe, NM: Mothering Magazine. 1993.
- Ritter TJ. *Say No to Circumcision!* Aptos, CA: Hourglass Book Publishing. 1992.
- Ritter TJ, Denniston GC. *Doctors Re-examine Circumcision.* Seattle, WA: Third Millennium Publishing. 2001.
- Watson LR. *Unspeakable Mutilations – Men Do Complain.* KDP (CreateSpace). 2015.
- Wallerstein E. *Circumcision: An American Health Fallacy.* NY: Springer. 1980.

Appendix C.2: Female Genital Mutilation

- Abdelmagied A, Salah W, ElTahir N, NurEldin T, Shareef S. Perception and Attitudes of Religious Groups Towards Female Genital Mutilation. *Ahfad Journal.* 2005-12; 22(2).
- Abusharaf RM. *Female Circumcision, Multicultural Perspectives.* University of Pennsylvania Press. 2006.
- Barker-Benfield GJ. *The Horrors of the Half-Known Life.* NY: Harper & Row. 1976.
- Bekers E. *Rising Anthills: African and African American Writing on Female Genital Excision, 1960-2000.* University of Wisconsin Press. 2010.
- Burrage Hilary. *Eradicating Female Genital Mutilation: A UK Perspective.* Ashgate Publishing. 2015.
- Caney S. *Justice Beyond Borders: A Global Political Theory.* Oxford University Press. 2005.
- Chavkin W, Chesler E. *Where Human Rights Begin: Health, Sexuality and Women in the New Millennium.* Rutgers University Press. 2005.
- Corea G. *The Hidden Malpractice: How American Medicine Treats Women as Patients and Professionals.* William Morrow. 1977.
- Dally A. *Women Under the Knife: A History of Surgery.* NY: Castle Books. 2006.
- Daly M. *Gyn/Ecology, The Meta Ethics of Radical Feminism.* Boston, MA: Beacon Press. 1978.
- Dirie W, Miller C. *Desert Flower: The Extraordinary Journey of a Desert Nomad.* Harper Collins. 2009.
- Ezzat D. A Savage Surgery. *The Middle East* (journal). 1994-01.
- Foster C. On the Trail of a Taboo: Female Circumcision in the Islamic World. *Contemporary Review.* 1994-05; 264(1540).
- Gruenbaum E. *The Female Circumcision Controversy: An Anthropological Perspective.* University of Pennsylvania Press. 2001.

- Herndlund Y, Shell-Duncan B. *Female Circumcision in Africa: Culture, Controversy and Change.* Lynne Reiner. 2000.
- Herndlund Y, Shell-Duncan B. *Transcultural Bodies: Female Genital Cutting in Global Context.* Rutgers University Press. 2007.
- Ian P. Responding to Female Genital Mutilation: The Australian Experience in Context. *Aust J Soc Iss.* 2001-02; 36(1).
- Koso-Thomas O. *The Circumcision of Women: A Strategy for Eradication.* NY: Zed Books. 1987.
- Lightfoot-Klein H. *Prisoners of Ritual: An Odyssey into Female Genital Circumcision in Africa.* NY: Hayworth Press. 1989.
- Lightfoot-Klein H. *Secret Wounds.* Authorhouse. 2003.
- Lightfoot-Klein H. *Children's Genitals Under the Knife: Social Imperatives, Secrecy and Shame.* Nunzio Press. 2008.
- Mire S. *The Girl With Three Legs: A Memoir.* Chicago Review Press. 2011.
- Mohammed HN. *Can FGM be Eradicated Through an Alternate Means?* GRIN. 2009.
- Nnaemeka O. *Female Circumcision and the Politics of Knowledge.* Westport, CT: Praeger. 2005.
- Raya PD. Female Genital Mutilation and the Perpetuation of Multigenerational Trauma. *J Psychohist.* 2010/Spring; 37(4).
- Robinett P. *The Rape of Innocence: Female Genital Mutilation & Circumcision in the USA; Connecting the Dots ... Where Personal, Social, Medical & Economic Interests Intersect.* Eugene, OR: Nunzio Press. 2010.
- Rodriguez SB. *Female Circumcision and Clitoridectomy in the United States.* Rochester, NY: University of Rochester Press. 2014.
- Ross SD. *Women's Human Rights: The International and Comparative Law Case Book.* University of California Press. 2003.
- Sands KM. *God Forbid: Religion and Sex in American Public Life.* Oxford University Press. 2000.
- Thomas LM. *Politics of the Womb: Women, Reproduction and the State in Kenya.* University of California Press. 2003.
- Thomas J. Female Genital Mutilations Lead to Lost Lives and High Costs. *Int Perspect Sex Reprod Health.* 2010-09; 36(3).
- Tong R, Anderson G, Santos A. *Globalizing Feminist Bioethics: Crosscultural Perspectives.* Westview Press. 2001.
- Wangila MN. *Female Circumcision: The Interplay of Religion, Culture and Gender in Kenya.* Maryknoll, NY: Orbis Books. 2007.
- White AE. Female Genital Mutilation in America: The Federal Dilemma. *Texas J Women Gender Law.* 2001-04; 10(2).

Appendix C.3: Pregnancy, Birth, Infancy & Child Raising

- Arms S. *Immaculate Deception.* Boston: Houghton Mifflin. 1975.
- Baker JP. *Hygieia: A Woman's Herbal.* Freestone Publishing. 1979.
- Baker JP. *Prenatal Yoga & Natural Birth.* North Atlantic Books. 1986.
- Baker JP. *Conscious Conception: Elemental Journey Through the Labyrinth of Sexuality.* North Atlantic Books. 1986.
- Bean C. *Labor and Delivery: An Observer's Diary.* NY: Doubleday. 1977.
- Brewer GS, Greene JP. *Right From the Start.* Emmaus, PA: Rodale Press. 1981.
- Buckley S. *Gentle Birth, Gentle Mothering.* Celestial Arts. 2012.
- Chamberlain D. *The Mind of your Newborn Baby.* North Atlantic Books. 1998.
- Chamberlain D. *Windows to the Womb: Revealing the Conscious Baby from Conception to Birth.* North Atlantic Books. 2013.
- Eanes R. *Positive Parenting: An Essential Guide.* Tarcher Perigree. 2016.
- Garbarino J. *Children and the Dark Side of Human Experience.* NY: Springer. 2008.

Appendix C – Books About

- Gerhardt S. *Why Love Matters: How Affection Shapes a Baby's Brain.* Routledge. 2004.
- Granju KA, Kennedy B, Sears W. *Attachment Parenting: Instinctive Care For Your Baby and Young Child.* Atria Books. 1999.
- Grille R. *Parenting for a Peaceful World.* Vox Cordis Press. 2013.
- Gurmuker KK. *Bountiful, Beautiful, Blissful: Experience the Natural Power of Pregnancy and Birth With Kundalini Yoga & Meditation.* St. Martin's Griffin. 2004.
- Halfmoon H. *Primal Mothering in a Modern World.* Sunfood Nutrition. 1988.
- Heath A, Bainbridge N. *Baby Massage: The Calming Power.* DK Publishing. 2004.
- Heimlich J. *Breaking Their Will: Shedding Light on Religious Child Maltreatment.* Prometheus Books. 2011.
- Heller S. *The Vital Touch; How Intimate Contact With Your Baby Leads to Happier, Healthier Development.* Hold Paperbacks. 1997.
- Hunt J. *The Natural Child, Parenting From the Heart.* New Society Publishers. 2001.
- Janov A. *The Primal Scream.* NY: Dell. 1970.
- Janov A. *The Primal Revolution.* NY: Touchstone Books, Simon & Schuster. 1972.
- Janov A. *The Feeling Child.* NY: Touchstone Books, Simon & Schuster. 1973.
- Janov A. *The Biology of Love.* Prometheus Books. 2000.
- Johnson E. *The Children's Bill of Emotional Rights: A Guide to the Needs of Children.* Jason Aronson. 2011.
- Knost LR. *The Gentle Parent: Positive, Practical, Effective Discipline.* Little Hearts Books. 2013.
- Lang R. *The Birth Book.* Ben Lomond, CA: Genesis Press. 1972.
- Leboyer F. *Birth Without Violence.* NY: Alfred A. Knopf. 1976.
- Liedloff J. *The Continuum Concept: In Search of Happiness Lost.* Perseus Books. 1986.
- Makichen W. *Spirit Babies: How to Communicate With the Child You're Meant to Have.* Delta. 2005.
- Margulis J. *The Business of Baby.* NY: Scribner (Simon & Schuster). 2013.
- Margulis J. *Your Baby, Your Way: Taking Charge of Your Pregnancy, Childbirth and Parenting Decisions.* NY: Simon & Schuster. 2015.
- McClure V. *The Tao of Motherhood.* New World Library. 1997.
- McClure V. *Infant Massage. Revised Edition: A Handbook for Loving Parents.* Bantam Books. 2000.
- McGrory Massaro M, Katz MJ. *The Other Baby Book, A Natural Approach to Baby's First Year.* Full Cup Press. 2013.
- Miller A. *For Your Own Good: Hidden Cruelty in Child-Rearing and the Roots of Violence.* Farrar Straus Girau. 1990.
- Morell SF, Cowan RS. *The Nourishing Traditions Book of Baby & Child Care.* New trends Publishing. 2013.
- Nagel R. *Healing Our Children.* Golden Child Publishing. 2015.
- Newton R. *The Attachment Connection.* New Harbinger Publications. 2008.
- Nicholson B. *Attached at the Heart.* iUniverse. 2009.
- Noble E. *Essential Exercises for the Childbearing Year.* New Life Images. 2003.
- Noble E. *The Joy of Being a Boy.* New Life Images. 2004.
- Odent M. *The Scientification of Love.* Free Association Books. 1999.
- Odent M. *Primal Health: Understanding the Critical Period Between Conception and Birth.* Clairview Books. 2002.
- O'Mara P. *Natural Family Living: The Mothering Magazine Guide to Parenting.* Atria Books. 2000.
- Palmer LF. *The Baby Bond: The New Science Behind What's Really Important for Your Baby.* Source Books. 2009.
- Palmer LF. *Baby Matters.* 3rd. ed. Baby Reference. 2015-05.
- Pantley E. *The No Cry Sleep Solution.* McGraw Hill. 2002.
- Payne KJ, Roos LM. *Simplicity Parenting: Using the Extraordinary Power of Less to Raise Calmer, Happier & More Secure Kids.* Ballantine Books. 2010.
- Pearce JC. *Magical Child.* NY: E.P. Dutton. 1977.
- Perry BD, Szalavitz M. *Born for Love: Why Empathy is Essential and Endangered.* William Morrow Paperbacks. 2011.
- Petrillo M, Sanger S. *Emotional Care of Hospitalized Children.* Philadelphia, PA: J.B. Lippincott. 1980.

- Placksin S. *Mothering the New Mother: Women's Feelings & Needs After Childbirth: A Support and Resource Guide.* Newmarket Press. 2000.
- Pollack W. *Real Boys: Rescuing Our Sons from the Myths of Boyhood.* Owl Books. 1999.
- Sears M & W. *The Complete Book of Christian Parenting and Child Care.* B & H Books. 1997.
- Sears W & M. *The Attachment Parenting Book.* Boston, MA: Little, Brown. 2001.
- Sears W & M & R & J. *The Baby Book: Everything You Need to Know About Your Baby From Birth to Age Two.* Boston, MA: Little, Brown. 2013.
- Silverstone A. *The Kind Mama.* NY: Rodale. 2014.
- Small MF. *Our Babies, Ourselves: How Biology and Culture Shape the Way We Parent.* Anchor Books. 1999.
- Stadlen N. *What Mothers Do, Especially When It Lookis Like Nothing.* Tarcher, Perigree. 2007.
- Stadlen N. *How Mothers Love: And How Relationships are Born.* Piatkus Books. 2012.
- Sunderland M. *The Science of Parenting.* DK Adult. 2008.
- Verrilli GE, Mueser AM. *While Waiting.* NY: St. Martin's Press. 1981.
- Ward C & F. *The Home Birth Book.* Washington: Inscape. 1976.
- Wells HM. *The Sensuous Child.* NY: Stein & Day. 1978.
- Wertz RW & DC. *Lying-In: A History of Childbirth in America.* NY: Schocken Books. 1979.,
- Wiessinger D, West D, Pitman T. *The Womanly Art of Breastfeeding: Completely Revised and Updated.* 8th ed. Hachette Book Group. 2013.
- Wootan G, Verney S. *Take Charge of Your Child's Health.* Marlowe. 2015.

Appendix D: Resources Online

Appendix D.1: Facebook Sites & Groups

- Africans against circumcision (NO FGM or MGM): facebook.com/groups/447691211931944
- Beyond the Bris: facebook.com/beyondthebris
- Children Are Circumcised Because They Can't Say NO!: facebook.com/groups/405795696164453
- Circumcision is Mutilation: facebook.com/groups/411675378894954
- #Circumcision Kills: facebook.com/groups/circumcionkills
- Circumcision Re-Education Network (Intact Support): facebook.com/groups/1725068757740900
- Future Doctors and Nurses who oppose circumcision: facebook.com/groups/495705067197409
- Genital Cutting is NOT a Parental Right: facebook.com/groups/230772543600809
- Gentle Intactivism Support Group: facebook.com/groups/892162834178807
- #IfiHadKnownThen – Circ Regret Parents: facebook.com/groups/317393261755258
- Intact Jewish Network: facebook.com/JewishNetwork
- Intact: Healthy, Happy, Whole: facebook.com/groups/IntactHealthy
- Intactivist Library: facebook.com/groups/379115088775825
- Intactivist Memes: facebook.com/IntactivistMemes
- INTACTIVISTS: facebook.com/groups/INTACTIVISTS
- Intactivists in the Middle East: facebook.com/groups/intactivist.me
- INTACTIVISTS Stop Circumcision: facebook.com/groups/1744214872475763
- Jews Against Circumcision: facebook.com/Jews-Against-Circumcision-165424110207450
- Keeping Future Sons Intact: facebook.com/FutureSons
- Medical Professionals for Genital Autonomy: facebook.com/IntactCare
- Opposing circumcision מתנגדים לברית מילה: facebook.com/groups/opposingcircumcision
- Pagans Against Circumcision: facebook.com/groups/82262004273
- Parents of Intact Boys: facebook.com/groups/529750937046430
- Parents Regretting Circumcision: facebook.com/groups/175347165878088
- peaceful parenting: facebook.com/peacefulparenting
- Saving Our Sons Community: facebook.com/groups/SavingOurSons
- Stop Routine Infant Circumcision!: facebook.com/groups/2209115729
- The Intact Generation: facebook.com/groups/919601681451136
- The Intact Network: facebook.com/TheIntactNetwork/
- We Learned Better And Did Better – Parents With Cut AND Intact Sons: facebook.com/groups/411953809001548
- Whole Christian Community: facebook.com/groups/WholeChristian
- Your Whole Baby: A Community for Learning: facebook.com/groups/YWBCommunity

Appendix D.2: Websites

- A Bill to End Male Genital Mutilation in the U.S.: mgmbill.org
- AIDS Circumcision Fallacy: studentsforgenitalintegrity.org
- Attorneys for the Rights of the Child: arclaw.org
- Beyond the Bris: beyondthebris.com
- Catholics Against Circumcision: catholicsagainstcircumcision.org
- Circumcision – Does the Qur'an Approve it?: quranicpath.com/misconceptions/circumcision.html
- Circumcision Resource Center: circumcision.org
- CircWatch: circwatch.org
- CIRP: Circumcision Information and Resource Pages: cirp.org
- Doctors Opposing Circumcision (D.O.C.): doctorsopposingcircumcision.org
- Dr. Momma – peaceful parenting: www.drmomma.org
- foregen: Regenerating the foreskin with its natural benefits and functions: foregen.org
- Foreskin Restoration Intactivist Network: foreskinrestoration.vbulletin.net
- Genital Autonomy America: gaamerica.org
- Genital Autonomy Society: genitalautonomysociety.org
- Historical Medical Quotes on Circumcision: circumcisionquotes.com
- In Memory of the Sexually Mutilated Child: sexuallymutilatedchild.org
- Infant Circumcision Information for Parents: circinfosite.info
- Intact America: intactamerica.org
- IntactiWiki: en.intactiwiki.org
- International Coalition for Genital Integrity *(ICGI, archived)*:
    archive.crin.org/en/library/organisations/international-coalition-genital-integrity.html
- Jewish Circumcision Resource Center: jewishcircumcision.org
- Joseph4GI: The Angry Intactivist: joseph4gi.com
- *Link list at Circumstitions*: circumstitions.com/links.html#general
- Little Images: Help us save babies from unnecessary cutting: littleimages.org
- Mothering Magazine: mothering.com
- Mothers Against Circumcision: mothersagainstcirc.org
- NOCIRC: National Organization of Circumcision Information Resource Centers: nocirc.org
- NOHARMM: National Organization to Halt the Abuse and Routine Mutilation of Males: noharmm.org
- NORM: The National Organization of Restoring Men: norm.org
- Not Just Skin: notjustskin.org
- Nurses for the Rights of the Child: childrightsnurses.org
- Peaceful Beginnings *(the author's website)*: peacefulbeginningsrosemary.wordpress.com
- Restoring Tally: restoringtally.com
- Saving Our Sons: www.savingsons.org
- Sex As Nature Intended It: sexasnatureintendedit.com

Appendix D – Resources Online

- Stop Infant Circumcision Society (SIC Society): stopinfantcircumcision.org
- The Circumcision Debate: circumcisiondebate.org
- The Intact Network: intactnetwork.org
- The Intactivism Pages: circumstitions.com
- Whole Christian: wholechristian.com